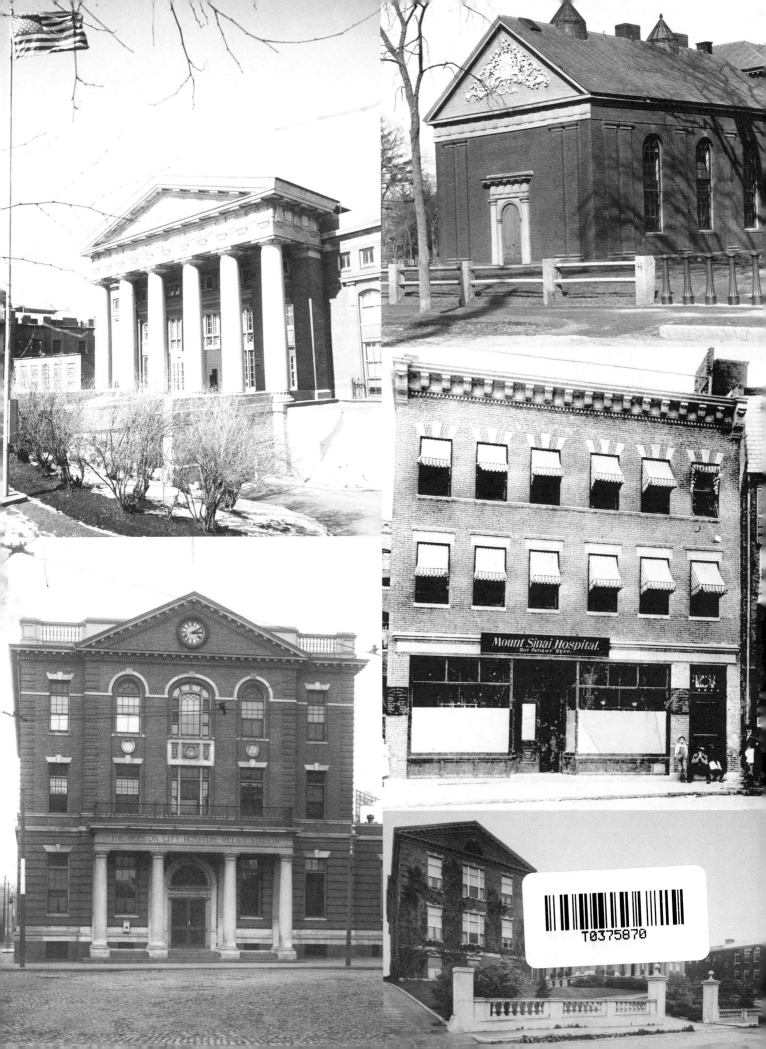

BIRTH *of a* SPECIALTY

BIRTH of a SPECIALTY

A History of Orthopaedics at Harvard and Its Teaching Hospitals

VOLUME 3

by

James H. Herndon, MD, MBA

Peter E. Randall Publisher
Portsmouth, New Hampshire
2021

© 2021 James H. Herndon
All rights reserved.

ISBN: 978-1-942155-36-2
Library of Congress Control Number: 2021916147

Published by
Peter E. Randall Publisher LLC
Portsmouth, NH 03801
www.perpublisher.com

Printed volumes;
Volume 1: Harvard Medical School
Volume 2: Boston Children's Hospital
Volume 3: Massachusetts General Hospital
Volume 4: Brigham and Women's Hospital, Beth Israel Deaconess Medical Center, Boston City Hospital, World War I, and World War II
Volume 5: Bibliography (available only in PDF form, visit www.birthofaspecialty.com)

Cover images:
Front:
Volume 1: Boston Medical Library collection, Center for the History of Medicine in the Francis A. Countway Library.
Volume 2: *Images of America. Children's Hospital Boston.* Charleston, SC: Arcadia Publishing, 2005. Boston Children's Hospital Archives, Boston, Massachusetts.
Volume 3: Massachusetts General Hospital, Archives and Special Collections.
Volume 4: Brigham and Women's Hospital Archives.

Back:
Volumes 1–4: Warren Anatomical Museum collection, Center for the History of Medicine in the Francis A. Countway Library.

Endpaper images:
Front: **Top:** (l) Exterior view of the Old Harvard Medical School, Boston, Mass, ca. 1880. Photograph by Baldwin Coolidge. Courtesy of Historic New England; (cl) Boston Children's Hospital Archives, Boston, Massachusetts; (cr) Brigham and Women's Hospital Archives; (r) Theodore Roosevelt Collection in the Houghton Library, Harvard University.
Center: (l) The Ruth and David Freiman Archives at Beth Israel Deaconess Medical Center; (c) Boston Children's Hospital Archives, Boston, Massachusetts; (r) The Ruth and David Freiman Archives at Beth Israel Deaconess Medical Center.
Bottom: (l) Massachusetts General Hospital, Archives and Special Collections; (c) Boston City Archives; (r) Brigham and Women's Hospital Archives.
Back: All: Kael E. Randall/Kael Randall Images

All reasonable efforts have been made to obtain necessary copyright permissions. Grateful acknowledgment for these permissions is made at point of use (for images) and in Volume 5 (for text). Any omissions or errors are unintentional and will, if brought to the attention of the author, be resolved.

Book design by Tim Holtz

Printed in the United States of America

Contents

Section 5 Massachusetts General Hospital

Chapter 29	Massachusetts General Hospital: The Beginning	3
Chapter 30	Henry J. Bigelow: The First Orthopaedic Surgeon at MGH	23
Chapter 31	Charles L. Scudder: Strong Advocate for Accurate Open Reduction and Internal Fixation of Fractures	53
Chapter 32	Orthopaedics Becomes a Department at MGH: Ward I	67
Chapter 33	Joel E. Goldthwait: First Chief of the Department of Orthopaedic Surgery at MGH	77
Chapter 34	Ernest A. Codman: Father of the "End-Result Idea" Movement	93
Chapter 35	Elliott G. Brackett: His Character Was a Jewel with Many Facets	147
Chapter 36	Nathaniel Allison: A Focus on Research and Education	163
Chapter 37	Marius N. Smith-Petersen: Prolific Inventor in Orthopaedics	179
Chapter 38	Joseph S. Barr: A "Gentle Scholar" and a Great Teacher	201
Chapter 39	William H. Harris: Innovator in Hip Replacement Surgery	215
Chapter 40	MGH: Other Surgeon Scholars (1900–1970)	227
Chapter 41	Henry J. Mankin: Prolific Researcher and Dedicated Educator	381
Chapter 42	MGH: Other Surgeon Scholars (1970–2000)	395
Chapter 43	MGH: Modernization and Preparation for the Twenty-First Century	453
	Index	465

Volume 1 Contents

	Acknowledgements	xiii
	Foreword	xv
	Preface	xvii
	Introduction	xix
	About the Author	xxv

Section 1   The First Family of Surgery in the United States

Chapter 1	Joseph Warren: Physician Before the Revolution	3
Chapter 2	John Warren: Father of Harvard Medical School	21
Chapter 3	John Collins Warren: Co-Founder of the Massachusetts General Hospital	31
Chapter 4	Warren Family: Tradition of Medical Leaders Continues into the Twentieth Century	71

Section 2   Orthopaedics Emerges as a Focus of Clinical Care

Chapter 5	John Ball Brown: The First American Orthopaedic Surgeon	95
Chapter 6	Buckminster Brown: Founder of the John Ball & Buckminster Brown Chair	105
Chapter 7	The Boston Orthopedic Institution: America's First Orthopaedic Hospital	113
Chapter 8	House of the Good Samaritan: America's First Orthopaedic Ward	123

Section 3   Harvard Medical School

Chapter 9	Orthopaedic Curriculum	133
Chapter 10	The Evolution of the Organization and Department of Orthopaedic Surgery	171
Chapter 11	The Harvard Combined Orthopaedic Residency Program	183
Chapter 12	Harvard Sports Medicine	245
Chapter 13	Murder at Harvard	291

Volume 2 Contents

Section 4 Boston Children's Hospital

Chapter 14 Boston Children's Hospital: The Beginning — 3

Chapter 15 Edward H. Bradford: Boston's Foremost Pioneer Orthopaedic Surgeon — 19

Chapter 16 Robert W. Lovett: The First John Ball and Buckminster Brown Professor of Orthopaedic Surgery — 45

Chapter 17 James W. Sever: Medical Director of the Industrial School for Crippled and Deformed Children — 83

Chapter 18 Arthur T. Legg: Dedicated to Disabled Children — 101

Chapter 19 Robert B. Osgood: Advocate for Orthopaedics as a Profession of Physicians and Surgeons Who Restore Function — 113

Chapter 20 Frank R. Ober: Caring Clinician and Skilled Educator — 143

Chapter 21 William T. Green: Master in Pediatric Orthopaedics — 167

Chapter 22 David S. Grice: Advocate for Polio Treatment — 207

Chapter 23 BCH: Other Surgeon-Scholars (1900–1970) — 217

Chapter 24 Melvin J. Glimcher: Father of the Bone Field — 319

Chapter 25 John E. Hall: Mentor to Many and Master Surgeon — 333

Chapter 26 Paul P. Griffin: Southern Gentleman and Disciple of Dr. William T. Green — 349

Chapter 27 BCH Other Surgeon Scholars (1970–2000) — 357

Chapter 28 Boston Children's Hospital: Modernization and Preparation for the Twenty-First Century — 427

Volume 4 Contents

Section 6   Brigham and Women's Hospital

Chapter 44   Peter Bent Brigham Hospital and Robert Breck Brigham Hospital: The Beginning   1

Chapter 45   Robert Breck Brigham Hospital and Peter Bent Brigham Hospital: Orthopaedic Service Chiefs   43
    Robert Breck Brigham Hospital   44
    Peter Bent Brigham Hospital   72

Chapter 46   RBBH and PBBH: Other Surgeon Scholars, 1900–1970   79
    Robert Breck Brigham Hospital   80
    Peter Bent Brigham Hospital   104

Chapter 47   Origins of BWH and Organizing Orthopaedics as a Department   113

Chapter 48   Clement B. Sledge: Clinician Scientist   125

Chapter 49   BWH: Other Surgeon Scholars: 1970–2000   143

Chapter 50   BWH's Modernization and Preparation for the Twenty-First Century   191

Section 7   Beth Israel Deaconess Medical Center

Chapter 51   Beth Israel Hospital: The Beginning   199

Chapter 52   Albert Ehrenfried: Surgeon Leader at Mount Sinai and Beth Israel Hospital   215

Chapter 53   Beth Israel Hospital: Orthopaedic Division Chiefs   223

Chapter 54   Augustus A. White III: First Orthopaedic Surgeon-in-Chief at Beth Israel Hospital   257

Chapter 55   Stephen J. Lipson: Chief of Orthopaedics at Beth Israel Hospital and Beth Israel Deaconess Medical Center   267

Chapter 56   Beth Israel Deaconess Medical Center: A History of New England Deaconess Hospital and Its Merger with Beth Israel Hospital   273

Chapter 57   BIDMC: Modernization and Preparation for the Twenty-First Century   283

Section 8 Boston City Hospital

Chapter 58 Boston City Hospital (Harvard Service): The Beginning — 293

Chapter 59 Frederic J. Cotton: Orthopaedic Renaissance Man — 309

Chapter 60 The Bone and Joint Service at Boston City Hospital: Other Surgeons-in-Chief — 333

Chapter 61 Boston City Hospital: Other Surgeon Scholars — 357

Chapter 62 Pedagogical Changes: Harvard Leaves Boston City Hospital — 377

Section 9 Harvard Orthopaedists in the World Wars

Chapter 63 World War I: Trench Warfare — 385

Chapter 64 World War II: Mobile Warfare — 463

Volume 5 Contents

Bibliography

Copyright Acknowledgments

"Military Orthopedic Surgery," World War I by R. W. Lovett

Harvard Faculty Who Served as Presidents of Major Professional Organizations

James H. Herndon, MD, MBA Curriculum Vitae

Volume 5 is available as an electronic version only and is included with purchase. It is available for download at www.birthofaspecialty.com.

To access link directly, go to https://pathway-book-service-cart.mypinnaclecart.com//peter-e-randall/birth-of-a-specialty-bibliography-only/

SECTION 5

MASSACHUSETTS GENERAL HOSPITAL

"It is a hospital for the care of the sick…a fellowship of research…a company of trained physicians and surgeons…a school for…the training of doctors and nurses. But in addition, the Hospital has an intangible quality impossible to describe, an atmosphere created through the devotion of literally thousands of men and women over a period of more than one hundred years. Generations of benefactors, trustees, officers, physicians, surgeons, nurses and employees have contributed to this continuing life and spirit. In the corridors and wards, we feel the great and noble tradition of high purpose in great accomplishment."

—**Henry Knox Sherrill**, foreword to *The Massachusetts General Hospital, Its Development, 1900–1935*, by Frederick Washburn (Houghton Mifflin, 1939).

"We stand on the shoulders of our predecessors…the common character trait among them that led to success was their unwillingness to accept any defeat as final and a burning steadfastness of purpose in pursuing what were to become major contributions to their selected field of interest. I salute their courage and tenacious quest for truth on unchartered seas, which enable them to make their contributions and bring their patients to safe harbor."

—**Edward D. Churchill**, MD, MGH, Chief of Surgery.
Quoted by Dr. Tom Dodson, *MGH Surgical Society Newsletter* 9, no. 11 (Fall 2008).

"Hospitals…those larger laboratories, private and public, which nature fills with her mistakes and experiments."

—**Sir William Osler**, 1930

"It is essential, if we are to shape our course rightly, that the foundations of our work be known and studied. Knowledge of this sort not only helps us in matters of direction of our efforts, but also saves what would otherwise be much duplication of effort."

—**Joel E. Goldthwait, MD**. Robert Jones Lecture. Published in the *Journal of Bone and Joint Surgery* 15 (1933): 279.

CHAPTER 29

Massachusetts General Hospital
The Beginning

Communities in New York and Pennsylvania had hospitals already operating as the nineteenth century began. Massachusetts, however, had none—though "there were various indications... that the want of such establishments was beginning to be felt in [the] community" (Bowditch 1851). At that time, people received medical care in their homes; the homeless and very poor received their care in a poorhouse, also referred to as an almshouse. Although the first almshouse in Boston was built in the 1660s, a century later other cities in the Northeast, such as Philadelphia and New York, had larger almshouses that cared for more people. In the mid-1700s, the almshouse in Boston was located at Beacon and Park Streets, just near Boston Common. It was closed in 1801, and a larger house (with eight beds) was opened on Leverett Street in the West End. At the turn of the nineteenth century, the almshouse was caring each year for 300 people among Boston's population of 6,000. Sick people who could not afford medical care could seek medical attention not only at the almshouse but also at the Boston Dispensary; "those who applied to the Dispensary for aid were visited at their homes. It was not until 1856, sixty years after its founding, that 'clinics' were begun, although they had been suggested by Dr. Oliver Wendell Holmes in 1837 when he was serving as a district physician" (Myers 1929).

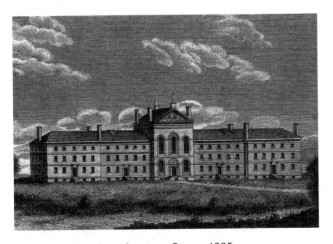

Boston Almshouse on Leverett Street, 1825.

Engraver: Abel Bowen. Originally published in *A History of Boston* by Caleb Snow, 2nd edition, 1828. Print Department, Boston Public Library.

A HOSPITAL IS NECESSARY

Reverend John Bartlett had been the chaplain at the Boston Almshouse from 1807 to 1810, when he resigned to take a position as pastor of the Second Congregational Church in Marblehead, Massachusetts. In an 1839 letter to his son, he explained his influence on the establishment of the Massachusetts General Hospital. He noted that much of his time at the almshouse was spent caring for the sick, but he was most interested in those who were "insane." "There were generally from 10 to 20 in the house...yet there was no proper place for their confinement and rest...several cells [with] a board[, a] birth, with loose straw, a pail for necessary purposes, was their only accommodation." (Bartlett, quoted in Myers 1929). He referred to the physicians working at the almshouse as "good men" but said they did not understand the condition of insanity, and he insisted that no appropriate facilities existed to care for patients who were considered insane:

> At that time there were no places of refuge for the insane in Massachusetts except in a few private houses in the country, owned and managed by Doctors...The mode of managing the insane then was most cruel, and unfavorable to recovery. Whipping, etc., was often resorted to...in these country places...No facilities were afforded them for the employment of those moral remedies which Pinel and others had so successfully applied in France...I went to Philadelphia, New York, examined the hospitals there, read Pinel and all the accounts I could procure of the Asylum's in France and England. I became deeply convinced of the importance of a similar Asylum in Massachusetts. (Bartlett, quoted in Myers 1929)

Bartlett took action, setting out to garner support for establishing a hospital that could provide appropriate care and treatment to such patients:

> I sat down to my desk and wrote from 15 to 25 billets addressed to some of the wealthiest and most respectable gentlemen of Boston, requesting them to meet at Conant Hall [to discuss] measures for the establishment of the Hospital for the Insane. Among these...were Drs. J. C. Warren, James Jackson, Jno. [John] Gorham, several others...They listened and agreed that something should be done...and formed themselves into a society for the purpose...When they met, Drs. Warren and Jackson, and Gorham suggested the Expediency of uniting with this object, the establishment of a Hospital for the sick. Some fears were expressed that by proposing too much, neither object could be obtained. Consequently, subscriptions were first solicited for the Insane Hospital. Lt. Gov. Phillips subscribed $20,000. (Bartlett, quoted in Myers 1929)

A general hospital and a hospital for mentally ill patients would have obvious needs, but students and professors at the medical school at Harvard also needed access to patients. "In 1784 a petition had been presented to the Overseers of the Poor of the Town of Boston, to allow professors and lecturers from the medical department of Harvard College, with a limited number of their pupils, to attend the sick poor at the Almshouse for the purpose of clinical teaching. For various reasons–expense probably playing a large part–this petition was denied" (Myers 1929).

In May 1810, the Harvard Corporation sent another petition asking the Overseers of the Poor to reconsider their position. The Overseers met to vote on the subject in July of that year. They agreed that "the said Professors...be permitted to visit the sick in the Almshouse for the purpose expressed... with such number of pupils as the professors may think proper...provided that the sick...who fall under the care of the professors, should receive from them all necessary medical attention and medicine, free from expense to the Town" (Myers 1929). After this victory, in October, professors from Harvard who cared for patients at the almshouse met to determine how to incorporate students and teaching into their process. They made various relevant decisions: "1st. That the patients in the Almshouse be divided into two classes, medical and surgical. 2nd. That Dr. J. C. Warren take charge of the surgical patients through the year. 3rd. That Dr. [James] Jackson take charge of the medical patients for three months from November 1, 1810, and for one month longer, if circumstances require...8th. That House Pupils shall be permitted to attend the Almshouse for the sum of $50 for the year" (Myers 1929). Thus, until

Massachusetts General Hospital opened in 1821, for 11 years, "the Almshouse served as a place for clinical instruction" (Myers 1929). For years, other individuals had also supported the establishment of a hospital in Boston. In 1798, Thomas Boylston, head of the prominent Boylston family of Boston, named in his will the town of Boston as a residuary devisee, to receive all property remaining after other obligations such as debts and bequests have been fulfilled. The town was to build on the property a "small-pox hospital and a lunatic hospital" (Bowditch 1851). Boylston lost money, however, when a firm in which he had invested became insolvent. Nonetheless, a judge allowed a codicil of William Phillips—on April 18, 1797, and proved in 1804—bequeathing to Boston $5,000 to be used to build a hospital. In August, 1810 Drs. James Jackson and John C. Warren—two of those whom, upon Bartlett's urging, had created a society to establish a hospital in Boston—wrote a circular letter to prominent Bostonites imploring them to help fund such a venture. A portion of their letter is reprinted in **Box 29.1**.

THE HOSPITAL BECOMES A REALITY

The hard work by Bartlett, Jackson, Warren, and others paid off quickly. On February 25, 1811, the state legislature granted a charter to 26 "of the most distinguished inhabitants of the various towns of the Commonwealth" (Bowditch 1851). The charter incorporated those individuals under the name "Massachusetts General Hospital." "The report of the legislative committee which recommended approval of the charter…reveals the purposes for which the Massachusetts General Hospital was established" (Garland 2008). It mentions two elements that "define the purpose of our modern voluntary hospital system" (Garland 2008): the provision of skillful care to all patients and the teaching of students and new physicians:

> The Hospital…is intended to be a receptacle for patients from all parts of the Commonwealth afflicted with diseases [and] requiring the most skillful treatment, and presenting cases for instruction in the study and practice of surgery and physic…Persons of every age and sex whether permanent residents…or occasional residents…citizens of every part of the Commonwealth, as well as strangers, from other states and countries, those in indigent circumstances…Persons requiring the best surgical and medical aid and having the means of defraying the moderate expenses…will [also] resort to a hospital, as permitting the most convenient accommodations, and the surest means of restoration to health…It cannot be doubted that the plan of a general hospital is the offspring of [an] expansive benevolence [that is] seeking…

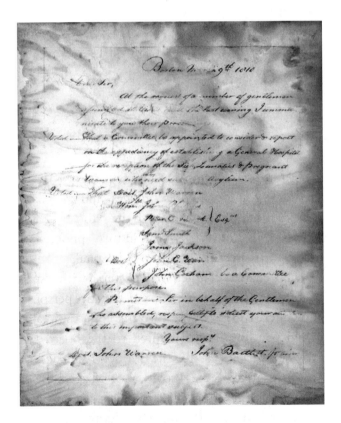

Letter from John Warren and John Bartlett stating that a committee had been formed to establish a general hospital in Boston. March 1810. Massachusetts General Hospital, Archives and Special Collections.

Box 29.1. *Circular Letter from Jackson and Warren Regarding Establishing a Hospital in Boston*

> Sir, —It has appeared very desirable to a number of respectable gentlemen, that a hospital for the reception of lunatics and other sick persons should be established in this town...We therefore beg leave to submit for your consideration proposals for the institution of a hospital, and to state to you some of the reasons in favor of such an establishment.
>
> It is unnecessary to urge the propriety and even obligation of succoring the poor in sickness...and in Christian countries...it must always be considered the first duties to visit and to heal the sick...
>
> The relief to be afforded to the poor, in a country so rich as ours, should perhaps be measured only by their necessities. We have, then, to inquire into the situation of the poor in sickness, and to learn what are their wants...
>
> In cases of long-protracted disease, instances...do occur amongst those of the most industrious class...[and are] less rare among...women who are...widowed...[and] the children of such families...are not rare of real suffering in sickness. To all...a hospital would supply every thing which is needful...In a well-regulated hospital, they would find a comfortable lodging...would receive food...and would be attended by kind and discrete nurses, under the directions of a physician...
>
> There is one class of sufferers who particularly claim all that benevolence can bestow, and for when a hospital is most especially required...[those] with diseases of the mind...The expense which is attached to the care of the insane in private families is extremely great...as to ruin a whole family...when called upon to support one of its members in this situation...
>
> Of another class, whose necessities would be removed by the establishment of the hospital, are women who are unable to provide for their own welfare...Houses for lying-in women have been found extremely useful in the large cities of Europe...
>
> There are many others who would find great relief in a hospital, and many times have life preserved when otherwise it would be lost. Such especially are the subjects of accidental wounds and fractures among the poorer classes of our citizens; and the subjects of extraordinary diseases, in any part of the Commonwealth, who may require the long and careful attention of either the physician or surgeon...
>
> In addition to what has already been stated, there are number of collateral advantages that would attend the establishment of a hospital in this place. These are facilities for acquiring knowledge, which it would give to the solace and comfort among the whole family of man!...The location of the proposed hospital is intended...to accommodate students in the metropolis and at the University in Cambridge, and the skill thus required, by the increased means of instruction, will be gradually and constantly diffused through every section of the Commonwealth. (quoted in Garland 2008)

Funding

The charter from the commonwealth of Massachusetts allowed the hospital to maintain yearly an estate valued at $30,000. Leaders in the commonwealth government—governor, lieutenant governor, president of the state Senate, speaker of the state House of Representatives, and the chaplains of both the Senate and the House—comprised a board of visitors, who in turn appointed 4 of the 12 trustees to manage the hospital.

The charter charged the hospital with "supporting thirty of the sick and lunatic persons" (Bowditch 1851), whose care the commonwealth would pay for. It also granted to the board the Province House estate, the former residence of the governors of the Province of Massachusetts Bay, one of the original 13 colonies; at that time, it was valued at $20,000. The charter provision requiring the commonwealth to pay for patients' care was then modified by an act that made "the number of patients...supported depend on the

> students in the medical school established in this town. The means of medical education in New England are at present very limited and totally inadequate to so important a purpose. Students of medicine cannot qualify themselves properly for their profession, without incurring heavy expenses, such as a very few of them are able to defray. The only medical school of eminence in this country is that at Philadelphia, nearly four hundred miles distant from Boston; and the expense of attending that is so great, that students from this quarter remain at it longer than one year. Even this advantage is enjoyed by very few…Those who are educated in New England have so few opportunities to the practice of physic, that they find it impossible to learn some of the most important elements of the science of medicine, until after they have undertaken for themselves the care of the health and lives of their fellow–citizens. This care they undertake with very little knowledge, except that acquired from books…With such deficiencies in medical education, it is needless to show to what evils the community is exposed.
>
> To remedy evils so important and so extensive, it is necessary to have a medical school in New England. All the materials necessary to form this school exist among us… Every one is liable to suffer from the want of such a school; every one may derive, directly or indirectly, the greatest benefits from its establishment.
>
> A hospital is an institution absolutely essential to a medical school, and one which would afford relief and comfort to thousands of the sick and miserable. On what other objects can the superfluities of the rich be so well bestowed?
>
> The amount required for the institution proposed may, at first site, appear large. But it will cease to appear so, when one considers that it is to afford relief… to erect a most honorable monument of the munificence of the present times, which will ensure to its founders the blessings of thousands in ages to come… that this amount may be raised at once, if a few opulent men will contribute only their superfluous income for one year…
>
> Hospitals and infirmaries are found in all the Christian cities of the Old World; and our large cities in the Middle States have institutions of this sort, which do grant honor to the liberality and benevolence of their founders… Boston may ere long assert her claim to equal praise.
>
> We are, sir, very respectfully, your obedient servants,
> James Jackson
> John C. Warren
> August 20, 1810
>
> (Reprinted from Bowditch 1851)

actual income derived from the Province House" (Bowditch 1851). Alternatively, the hospital could sell the house and use the profit as capital, with the stipulation that it obtain an additional $100,000 in private funding within 5 years.

The War of 1812 had extensive effects on the economy of Boston, and thus the board had to suspend its "plans for raising funds to meet the Legislature's Province House condition" (Garland 2008). The government enacted a law in June 1813 giving the hospital trustees another five years to raise funds, and they began doing so in April 1816. Those donating could select whether their contribution supported "the general hospital or the asylum" (Garland 2008); some donated to both. "Overall 1,047 individuals became subscribers; 245 gave over $100 and were made members of the Corporation" (Bowditch 1851).

> [Upon being] granted four acres of land… known as Prince's Pasture, west of the Leverett Street almshouse, the board officially launched its fund-raising drive on December 26, 1816[;] subscriptions exceeded $107,000. The largest gift was that of William Philips, Jr., who quadrupled his father's bequest in 1797, donating $20,000. The smallest alternation was 25 cents, given by a poor black man…The hospital met the requirement for a grant of the old Province House [and] the Trustees…abandoned the idea of using it as a temporary hospital. (Garland 2008)

State charter authorizing 56 prominent Bostonians to start a hospital. February 25, 1811.

Massachusetts General Hospital, Archives and Special Collections.

The hospital leased Province House in 1817 and made only a small income from it; thus the "additional Act" forcing the hospital to rely on only that income was repealed. The lease expired in 1916, at which time the property was valued at ~$1.5 million.

The hospital found another source of funding as well—life insurance. In February 1814, the commonwealth passed a law that allowed the Massachusetts Hospital Life Insurance Company to begin providing life insurance. At first, "one-third of [the company's] whole net profits from insurance on lives [was] made payable to the Hospital" (Bowditch 1851). Ten years later, a second act allocated to the Hospital "one-third of all the earnings of [the] Insurance Company, over and above six per cent...The regular annual dividends for several years have been nine per cent..." (Bowditch 1851).

With the dividends from the life insurance company; the small regular income from Providence House; and donations, which continued to flow in, the hospital could begin developing in earnest. Bowditch (1851) exclaimed that "the Corporation will live forever [, initially supported by that] first donation made to the institution... the Massachusetts General Hospital!"

Building

Now that funds were available, the trustees had to begin the task of creating the physical hospital itself. Because the board and those supporting the hospital "were at least as concerned with the mentally ill as they were with the physically sick [they] assigned priority to the opening of an insane asylum" (Garland 2008). To this end, they purchased a portion of Joseph Barrell's estate in Charlestown,

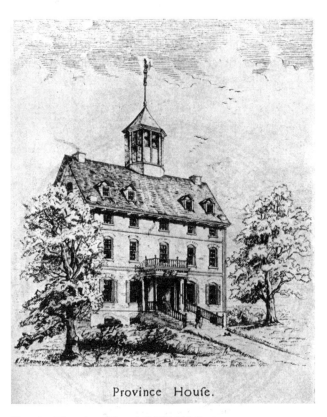

Sketch of Province House (1679–1864).
The Massachusetts General Hospital: Its Development, 1900–1935 by Frederic A. Washburn. Houghton Mifflin, 1939. Massachusetts General Hospital, Archives and Special Collections.

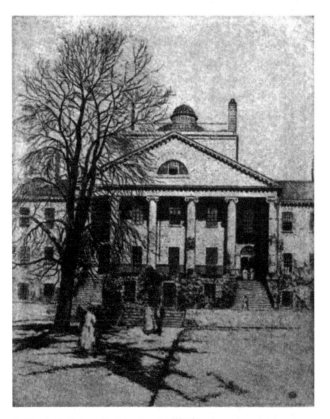

Bulfinch Building. Etching by R. S. Gallagher.
R. S. Gallagher's Etchings of Boston by Louis A. Holman. Boston: Charles E. Goodspeed & Co., 1920.

comprising 18 acres of land and the house, in 1816. "Meanwhile plans for the Massachusetts General Hospital moved forward. Four acres of a field [Prince's Pasture] on the bank of the Charles River in the West end of Boston…were acquired" (Garland 2008). The location of the hospital along the river "allows it to be approached by water by all the New England States which border on the ocean" (Myers 1929).

The board selected "Charles Bulfinch, the leading architect of the period and designer of the State House and [University Hall at Harvard]" (Garland 2008), to design the project. Bulfinch "took a personal interest in institutional architecture and new amenities like interior heating and sanitation" (Bull and Bull 2011). "He specified gray Chelmsford granite as building stone" (Bull and Bull 2011), and an 1817 law specified that "the stone for the erection of the Hospital should be hammered and fitted for use by the convicts in the State Prison [at Charlestown]" (Bowditch 1851).

Bulfinch designed a three-story building: "the first floor included wards for moribund cases, as well as a morgue, laundry, small sickroom, and kitchen-scullery. The two upper stories of the three-story building were dedicated to the care of the sick" (Bull and Bull 2011), with 60 beds in total. It also included living space for those staff who lived on site. John C. Warren and James Jackson—two of those who, along with Bartlett, drove the initial plan for creating and funding the hospital—were heavily involved in "perfect[ing] plans for the building's interior" (Bull and Bull 2011). In her 1929 history of MGH, Grace Whiting Myers described the layout of the hospital:

> In the centre, are the rooms for the Superintendent, the Apothecary, attendants, and the kitchen. In the upper part of the centre is also the operating theater [the Ether Dome]. The wings are divided into apartments for patients; those of the males being distinct from

First published plot plan of the MGH, 1823.
The Massachusetts General Hospital, 1935–1955 by Nathaniel W. Faxon. Cambridge: Harvard University Press, 1959. Massachusetts General Hospital, Archives and Special Collections.

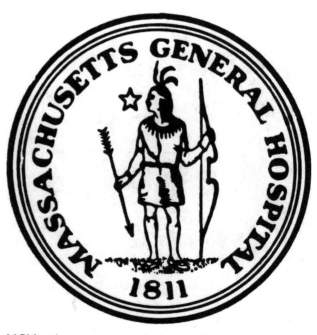

MGH seal. Massachusetts General Hospital, Archives and Special Collections.

the females. The stair cases and entries are of stone. The apartments are supplied with heat by pipes from a furnace in the cellar—They are also supplied with water…

The surgical environment was considered carefully in the planning:

There is a room expressly prepared for this purpose [performing surgery], with a light adapted to [it], and in case of accident or emergency, there are instruments, dressings, medicines and skillful attendants, all within call and reach of the operator. And also, in case of pain or accident following an operation there is always a Physician in the place ready to administer relief both day and night. (Myers 1929)

On November 24, 1817, the board requested that a common seal be made for the hospital. A week later, it was presented, "the device being an Indian with his bow in one hand, and an arrow in the other; and on his right a star, being encircled with the inscription, 'Massachusetts General Hospital, 1811'" (Bowditch 1851). The builders laid the cornerstone on the United States' 43rd Independence Day—July 4, 1818. "[It] contained several coins and an engraved [silver] tablet describing the benefactors of the hospital and citing the generosity of the people of Massachusetts" (Bull and Bull 2011).

The Grand Opening

On August 21, 1821—about six years after the building process had begun—Jackson and Warren were notified that "the Hospital will be ready for patients on Sept[ember] 1" (Bowditch 1851). Over the first 20 days only one patient, who had syphilis, was admitted; "not a single other application was made for admission" (Bowditch 1851). Visits did, however, begin to pick up, and the hospital provided care to 18 patients between October 1821 and February 1822. (See the first orthopaedic case discussed in chapter 3; see also a list of the illustrious surgeons who served as department chair in **Box 29.2**.) Throughout the rest of 1822, 122 patients were seen. In 1823 the building was finally completed, now holding 73 beds. Of this total, "the Trustees have appropriated six

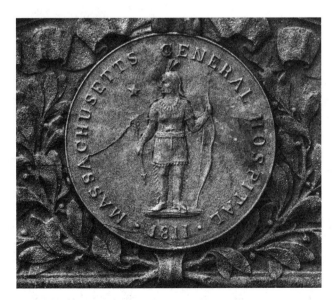

Original seal of MGH. Currently preserved at the entrance to the Resident Physician's House. Kael E. Randall/Kael Randall Images.

Box 29.2. *Orthopaedic Chairpersons*

Joel E. Goldthwait 1904–1908
Elliott G. Brackett 1911–1918
Interim: Mark Rogers 1918
Robert B. Osgood 1919–1922
Interim: Mark Rogers 1922
Nathaniel Allison 1923–1929
Marius N. Smith-Petersen 1929–1946
Interim: George W. Van Gorder 1946
Joseph S. Barr 1947–1964
Interim: Thornton Brown 1964–1965
Melvin J. Glimcher 1965–1970
Interim: Thornton Brown 1970–1972
Henry J. Mankin 1972–1996
Interim: William Tomford 1996–1998
Harry E. Rubash 1998–2018

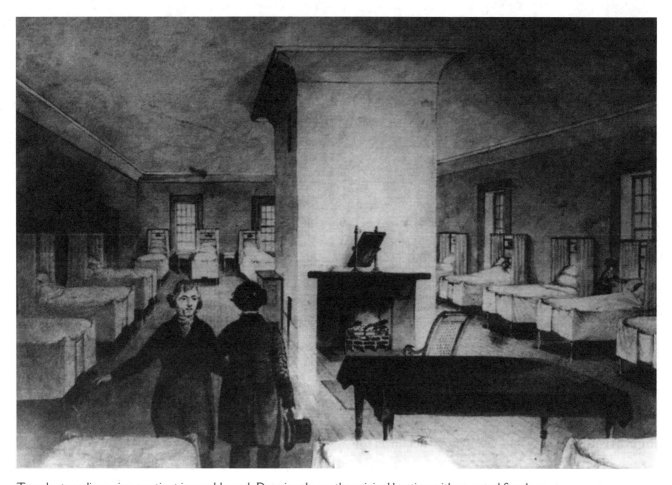

Two doctors discussing a patient in an old ward. Drawing shows the original heating with a central fireplace.
Every Man Our Neighbor: A Brief History of the Massachusetts General Hospital, 1811–1961 by Joseph E. Garland. Boston: Little, Brown and Company, 1961. 2nd edition, 2008. Massachusetts General Hospital, Archives and Special Collections.

beds [3 medical and 3 surgical] to poor patients" (Myers 1929); they hoped that the care of those patients would be offset by donations from the public.

According to Garland (2008), "The personalities of Drs. Jackson and Warren forcefully molded the developing character of the hospital until their retirements in 1837 and 1852 [respectively]." (Actually, Warren retired shortly after the first public demonstration of ether in 1846 but remained a consultant until 1852.) They had influenced every aspect of the hospital so far—from garnering support for the initial idea, to obtaining funding, to overseeing the construction. They both began caring for patients at the hospital, as well. In addition, Jackson held one weekly clinic and Warren, two. Warren remained the only surgeon at MGH for five years (except for John Ball Brown, who was appointed as a junior surgeon in November 1823, a position in which he remained until February 1826; see chapter 5) until 1826, when he was joined by George Hayward, who remained at MGH until he retired in 1851.

Jackson, the hospital physician, "initiated no radical departures from the therapeutic modes of this time, [but] his methods of treatment were relatively mild and conservative" (Garland 2008). At this time, however, there was considerably less emphasis on bleeding, purging, and puking than in the country-side generally. This and other rather terrible medical holdovers from the Middle Ages were finally knocked into limbo in 1835 when Dr. Jacob Bigelow published his classic "A Discourse on Self-Limited Diseases." Dr. O. W.

Massachusetts General Hospital

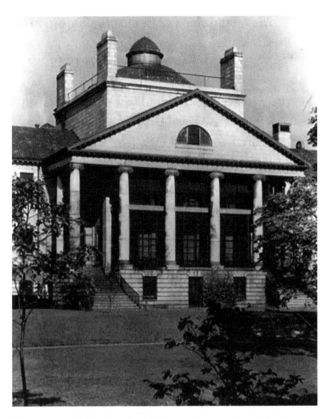

Entrance to the Bulfinch Building. Massachusetts General Hospital, Archives and Special Collections.

Box 29.3. *The Case of Charles Lowell*

"Dr. Warren described his treatment in December 1821 of a dislocated hip in one of his early patients, Charles Lowell:

"'A person came to the hospital for the purpose of having some effort made to restore a dislocation of the hip joint. He had met with this accident three months before; and there being, in such cases, no probability, nor scarcely possibility, of reducing the bone, he was told that his case was past the reach of surgical aid; but that if he desired, he might have efforts made with a view to give him a fair trial for the restoration of his limb. The most powerful means were employed for this purpose; the success was no better than what had been expected and promised. He left the hospital in the same state in which he entered it'."

(Myers 1929).

Holmes later wrote that this "did more than any other work or essay in our own language to rescue the practice of medicine from the slavery of the drugging system which was part of the inheritance of the profession" (Garland 2008). Both Jackson and Warren "vigorously advocated using the Hospital for clinical research, and Dr. Jackson carried on a number of investigations at the bedside, especially [of] typhoid fever" (Garland 2008). Performing research in a hospital was a new idea in the first quarter of the nineteenth century, and "the MGH was one of the few in the world where it was implemented in a planned way" (Garland 2008). The hospital quickly became a "training ground" for students at Harvard Medical School—much like the almshouse had been over the preceding decade—and "established Boston as an independent center of medical education on a par with New York and Philadelphia" (Garland 2008).

A superintendent handled the day-to-day running of the hospital. Some of the trustees would inspect the hospital each week, and the full board met there every two weeks. Again, Jackson and Warren—despite their more senior positions as hospital physician and hospital surgeon—acted as attending physicians throughout the week, providing care to outpatients.

Six months after the hospital opened, they began reporting on the patients they had cared for, "in the form of brief abstracts of the cases" (Myers 1929); at the time they created such reports for seven patients. Dr. Warren's first report described the case of Charles Lowell (**Box 29.3**; see also chapter 3). Although "[the] hospital has treated 'out patients' ever since it opened" (Myers 1929), such patients weren't described in the hospital's annual report until 1844, and the hospital didn't start maintaining records for such patients until 1846. And despite an ophthalmology service at the hospital since its early days, such care wasn't provided to outpatients until 1873.

FACILITIES AND STAFF EXPAND

For almost the first decade of the hospital's existence, reports of its financial standing were published only every three years, the first in 1824 and the second in 1827. Only in 1830 did the hospital begin disseminating annual reports. The surgical staff had continued to grow as the midcentury approached. In 1839, Warren and Hayward were joined by a third surgeon, Dr. Solomon D. Townsend. Oliver Wendell Holmes was a consulting surgeon from 1840 to 1845.

On December 31, 1843, the trustees sent out a notice of the next annual meeting. That notice included a request "that the present and past Physicians and Surgeons of the Institution…suggest to this board any changes in the management or arrangements of the Hospital, which in their view would increase its usefulness, and to express their opinion of the necessity of enlarging the buildings" (Bowditch 1851). The trustees received four requests:

1. A larger ward for male patients
2. More rooms for patients who were able to pay for their care ($20–40 a week)
3. An "additional isolation room for offensive patients"
4. A "new autopsy room" (Myers 1929)

The trustees considered these requests and decided to add two wings (each 50-square feet). The estimated cost: $50,000. To raise this money, "the Trustees organized the largest fund-raising drive since 1816" (Bull and Bull 2011). In their appeal to the public, they "recalled the participation of many Bostonians [in] the last drive" (Bull and Bull 2011). The trustees emphasized:

> the insufficient accommodations of the Hospital, by reason of the great increase of the population of Boston, only provides one bed for every 1,666 individuals, while Paris provides one for every 250 persons, and London for every 500; –that the wealth of Boston has kept pace with its population…
>
> To found and maintain institutions for the relief of the sick and afflicted is not only the mark but the privilege of civilization; and he who gives evidence…will leave a memento of himself, that shall outlive his generation, and be dear to the hearts of his children and of every true man (Bowditch 1851).

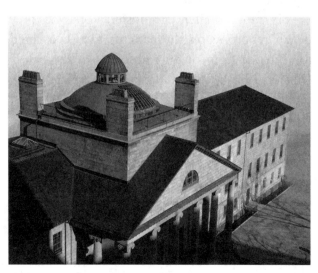

Aerial view of the Ether Dome. Massachusetts General Hospital, Archives and Special Collections.

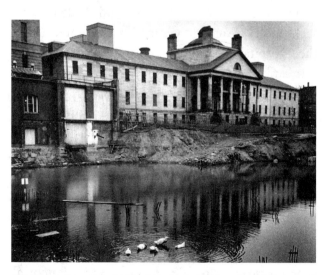

Addition of the East Wing (surgical), 1847 and the West Wing (medical), 1846, to the original Bulfinch Building. Massachusetts General Hospital, Archives and Special Collections.

During this period—just before both the wide use of ether and Warren's retirement—two more surgeons came aboard as staff in 1846: Dr. Henry J. Bigelow, who remained until 1885 (see chapter 30), and Dr. Samuel Parkman, who remained until 1854. During the years 1846 to 1867, J. Mason Warren was also a staff surgeon at MGH. The two new wings were then added to the Bulfinch building: the west wing, for medical patients, that same year in 1846, and the east wing, for surgical patients, in 1847. In addition, an "octagonal building in [the] rear for kitchen, laundry and apothecary were added to the Bulfinch building– the first enlargement of the hospital. Its capacity was thus increased from 60 to 141 beds" (Washburn 1939). Until 1867, when the Bigelow building was built, the Bulfinch building was the main location where care was provided. Outpatients received care in the north wing. The wards were located on the second and third floors of the east and west wings, and each had a medical and surgical suite; "hence came the terms East and West Medical and East and West Surgical. The East... Surgical [suites were] 16 and 31[;] the West Surgical [suites were] 28 and 29" (Myers 1929). Also, on the second floor, between the wings, were the trustees' suites and the resident physician's office. Just above those rooms, on the third floor, were two rooms referred to as "Ward 10," which was probably used exclusively to house private patients.

During this exciting period of expansion, a review of the surgical records from January 1, 1848, through May 12, 1851, revealed that among 350 procedures, sulfuric ether had been used in 186 cases, chloric ether in 138 cases, chloroform in 25 cases, and nitrous oxide in 1 case. Despite the hospital's blossoming growth and leading role in medical advances, however, it had its problematic history too. In the mid-nineteenth century, institutional racism was widespread—even at MGH. In his *History of the Massachusetts General Hospital*, published in 1851, Nathaniel Bowditch expressed what a "violation of the intent of [the hospital's] original founders" the large number of foreign patients presented:

> The Admitting Physician has been requested to use the utmost vigilance on this point, that none may be received who should properly be sent to the city institutions at South Boston. The admission of such patients creates in the minds of our own citizens a prejudice against the Hospital, making them unwilling to enter it, –and thus tends directly to lower the general standing and character of its inmates. Some such admissions must unavoidably take place.

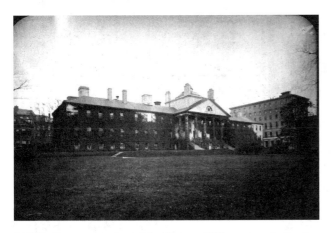

MGH after completion of the East and West wings before the addition of pavilions. Massachusetts General Hospital, Archives and Special Collections.

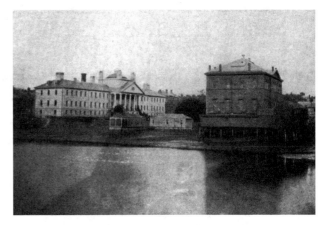

MGH (left) with the new medical school (right) on North Grove Street and the banks of the Charles River, 1853.
Massachusetts General Hospital: Memorial and Historical Volume. Boston: Griffith-Stillings Press, 1921. Massachusetts General Hospital, Archives and Special Collections.

There has always existed a most excellent rule, that every case of sudden accident may at once be brought to the Hospital. A broken arm or leg is a plenary certificate, entitling the bearer to all its benefits.

However, the hospital did provide equal treatment for patients regardless of ability to pay and included advanced planning to accommodate a larger number of patients who were unable to pay the fees. In 1851, the hospital had 80 beds for patients who could not pay; the other 40 beds for patients who *could* pay the $3.00 fee, which was only ~50% of the actual cost. Admitting physicians were paid a salary of $200; house pupils were paid $50.

By 1864, "the hospital had 'seven private rooms of different sizes and grades situated in different parts of the institution, not in a separate building...Some of these rooms were fitted up quite luxuriantly, and very little about them suggested a sick room'" (Myers 1929). On the fourth floor were the Ether Dome and the attic. Surgeries were performed in the Ether Dome: patients would be anesthetized with ether in the hallway, operated on in the dome itself, and then taken down to the wards to recuperate. In 1868, when all surgical procedures moved to the new Bigelow building, the Ether Dome was converted from an operating room into seven rooms that "gave much needed additional sleeping room for female employees, and also six beds which might be occupied at night by convalescing female patients. A bathroom was [also put there] for employees" (Myers 1929). The Ether Dome was renovated twice more before 1900: it "was converted to a dining room for the nurses" in 1889 (Myers 1929), and then to a lecture hall in 1892. That lecture hall is still used today. When the new operating space was unveiled in the Bigelow building in 1867, "all the surgical patients [were] moved to the west side of the hospital in order to

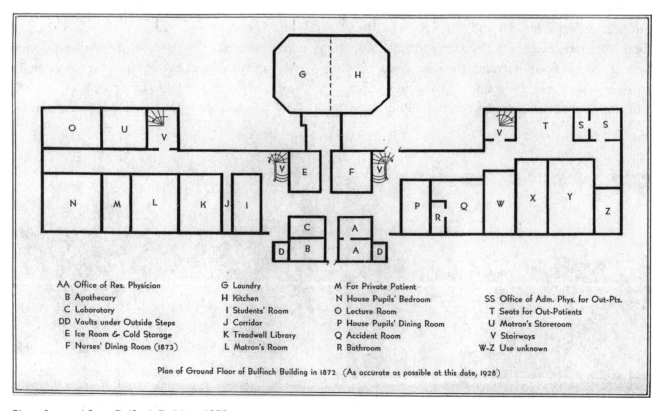

Plan of ground floor, Bulfinch Building, 1872. *History of the Massachusetts General Hospital: June, 1872, to December, 1900* by Grace W. Myers. Boston: Griffith-Stillings Press, 1929. Massachusetts General Hospital, Archives and Special Collections.

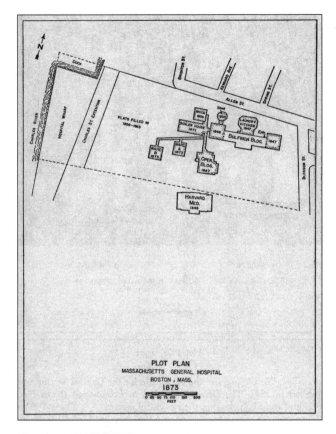

Plot plan of MGH, 1873.
The Massachusetts General Hospital, 1935–1955 by Nathaniel W. Faxon. Cambridge: Harvard University Press, 1959. Massachusetts General Hospital, Archives and Special Collections.

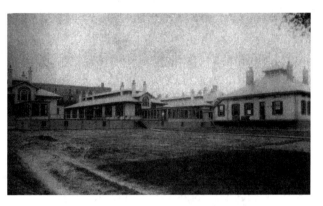

Pavilion Wards. Erected southwest of the Bulfinch Building, 1873.
Something in the Ether: A Bicentennial History of Massachusetts General Hospital, 1811 to 2011 by Webster Bull and Martha Bull. Memoirs Unlimited, 2010. Massachusetts General Hospital, Archives and Special Collections.

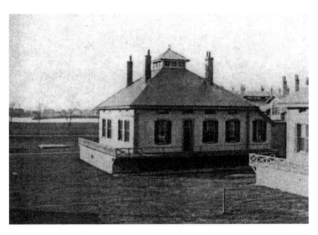

Wards A (Warren) and B (Jackson). 1873. Charles River in the background.
History of the Massachusetts General Hospital: June, 1872, to December, 1900 by Grace W. Myers. Boston: Griffith-Stillings Press, 1929. Massachusetts General Hospital, Archives and Special Collections.

bring them in close proximity to the operating room" (Myers 1929).

The hospital expansion in the mid-nineteenth century exposed some of the problematic issues with organization. After some back-and-forth with the house officers—and against the wishes of the hospital's board of physicians and surgeons—the trustees named a resident physician as the hospital superintendent. (Since 1921 this has been the role of director.) The superintendent supervised the admitting physician. No longer did the trustees visit the hospital regularly; now, they liaised with the superintendent regarding administrative issues.

In 1867, the Bigelow Surgical Building (and the Bigelow Operating Theatre within it) was completed. The building was also home to a new outpatient department. A corridor connected the Bigelow building to the west wing of the Bulfinch building. The expansion of new buildings continued westward on the hospital's property, toward the Charles River, with the additions of Ward A, the Warren building, and Ward B, the Jackson building—named "in memory of the valuable services of the late Drs. James Jackson and J. Mason Warren" (Washburn 1939). Both were completed around 1873 and were connected by covered corridors. Ward C, named after Henry Bigelow, was also completed in 1873; here, patients who needed to be isolated were housed and treated. The Allen

Street House, constructed beginning in 1874, was the autopsy building and morgue. Ward D, named after Solomon D. Townsend and used as another isolation ward, was built in 1875.

This expansion didn't slow in the last quarter of the nineteenth century. **Box 29.4** lists further hospital development projects in the 1880s and 1890s.

Box 29.4. MGH Expands in the Late 1800s

1880	A convalescent home was built in Waverly, MA
1881	A lodge was built at the hospital's Blossom Street entrance
1883	The Thayer Building for Nurses and the Gay Ward for outpatients were constructed
1885–1886	Sanitary towers were added to the Bulfinch building
1888	Ward E and its operating room opened; the building was named after J. Putnam Bradlee
1894	Ward F was built, named after George A. Gardner, a wealthy businessman and director of the Merchant's National Bank
1896	Both the clinical-pathological laboratory and a house for the resident physician (at the intersection of Blossom and Allen Streets) were constructed

Washburn 1939.

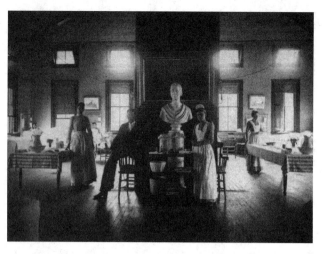

Ward A or Warren Ward in honor of John Collins Warren. The first pavilion ward, 1885. The central chimney had fireplaces on all four sides.

Something in the Ether: A Bicentennial History of Massachusetts General Hospital, 1811 to 2011 by Webster Bull and Martha Bull. Memoirs Unlimited, 2010. Massachusetts General Hospital, Archives and Special Collections.

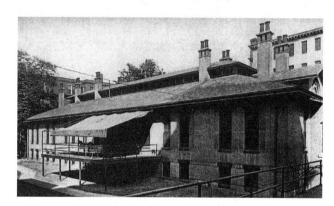

Ward D (Townsend Ward), 1875. Named for surgeon Solomon D. Townsend.

History of the Massachusetts General Hospital: June, 1872, to December, 1900 by Grace W. Myers. Boston: Griffith-Stillings Press, 1929. Massachusetts General Hospital, Archives and Special Collections.

In 1888 the hospital received a $50,000 donation from Helen C. Bradlee. This generous gift was allocated to build what would be Ward E, which was named after her brother, J. Putnam Bradlee and referred to as the Bradlee Building, where patients undergoing abdominal and head surgeries would be treated. Surgeons had long been pushing for such a dedicated space, particularly one that would focus on aseptic procedures and techniques. Upon the construction of Ward E, Dr. Maurice H. Richardson wrote:

> Abdominal surgery is now a field where the most brilliant successes are to be attained. No branch of surgery can compare with it for a moment…It is from the work we are now doing and hope to do in abdominal surgery (and I would include cerebral surgery as well) that the Hospital must gain its position among the Hospitals of the World at the end of the next ten years. We have the chance now to take the lead. (Quoted in Washburn 1939)

In the hospital's 1890 annual report, the trustees asked, "Who will imitate the liberal giver of

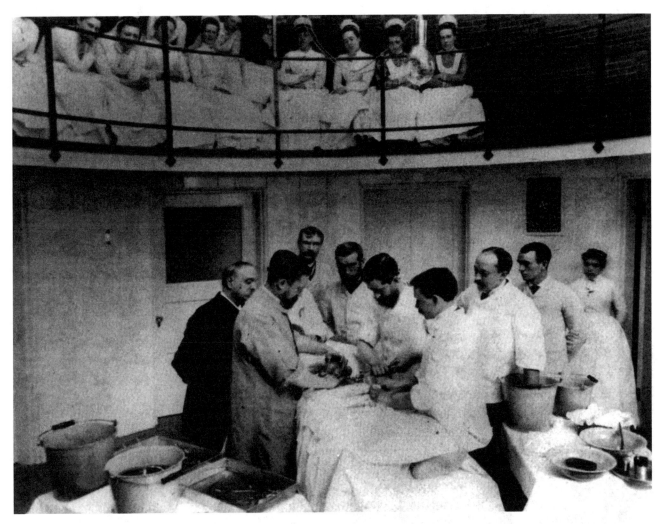

First aseptic operation in 1899 in the Bradley (Ward E) Ward operating room. J. Collins ("Coll") Warren assisted by Samuel J. Mixter.
Every Man Our Neighbor: A Brief History of the Massachusetts General Hospital, 1811-1961 by Joseph E. Garland. Boston: Little, Brown and Company, 1961. 2nd edition, 2008. Massachusetts General Hospital, Archives and Special Collections.

the Bradlee Ward, and provide the Hospital with a ward for contagious diseases?" (Washburn 1939). Donors stepped up, and with the funds they provided the hospital built the George A. Gardner building (Ward F) in 1894: "It was located beyond Ward B and opposite Ward E[; it] had two wings containing six single rooms each, and there was a 'nursery' accommodating three or four cribs…It supplied a long felt want in the hospital, affording a suitable place for the care of accidental and unavoidable cases of contagious disease; also affording a place where patients might be secluded [who] might be disturbing to patients in the general wards" (Washburn 1939).

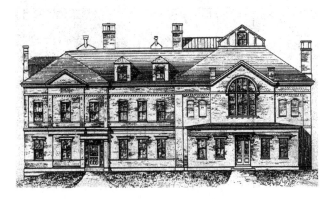

The Gay Ward (Outpatient Building), 1883.
History of the Massachusetts General Hospital: June, 1872, to December, 1900 by Grace W. Myers. Boston: Griffith-Stillings Press, 1929. Massachusetts General Hospital, Archives and Special Collections.

EXPANSION OF TREATMENTS AND TECHNIQUES

Not only did MGH expand its facilities and infrastructure toward the end of the 1800s, the physicians and staff working at the hospital also pushed ahead with the use of new techniques and treatments.

In 1895, Walter J. Dodd was promoted to the position of the apothecary. He had been working at MGH for three years as the head pharmacist and the hospital's photographer. After the announcement of the discovery of x-rays in December 1895, Dodd began building his own x-ray equipment.

"Early in 1896 [using his apparatus he] took the first successful radiograph in the Nerve Room of the Out-Patient Department. It required much labor and much time to take a picture of even the small parts of the body, but the work which Mr. Dodd accomplished with this amateur apparatus was so much appreciated by the surgeons... that the taking of the x-rays of the extremities... came into general use" (Washburn 1939). Dodd worked with x-rays, unprotected, since that first use in early 1896. "In April 1897 he developed a severe radio-dermatitis of the hands and was admitted to the surgical ward for treatment. This was the first of many operations that he was obliged to undergo as a result of the injuries [from his] early experimental work" (Holmes 1921). (Lead screens weren't used to protect the radiographer until 1900.) The hospital's 1897 annual report shows "the first record of expenditure for x-ray apparatus" (Holmes 1921).

"In 1900, the x-ray room was moved from the old West Room [in the old outpatient building] to the domestic building [just north of the old outpatient building at the west end of the west wing of the Bulfinch building]" (Holmes 1921). In 1907,

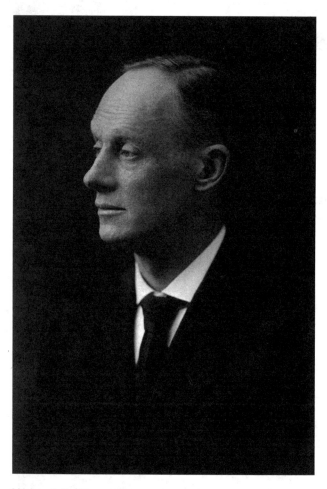

Walter J. Dodd.

Something in the Ether: A Bicentennial History of Massachusetts General Hospital, 1811 to 2011 by Webster Bull and Martha Bull. Memoirs Unlimited, 2010. Massachusetts General Hospital, Archives and Special Collections.

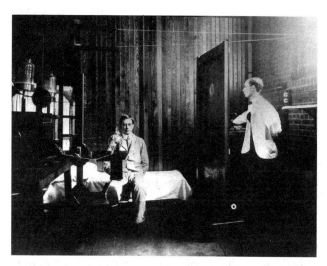

Walter Dodd (right) taking an x-ray of a patient's knee using an early x-ray machine.

Every Man Our Neighbor: A Brief History of the Massachusetts General Hospital, 1811–1961 by Joseph E. Garland. Boston: Little, Brown and Company, 1961. 2nd edition, 2008. Massachusetts General Hospital, Archives and Special Collections.

the hospital set up a roentgenology department, appointing Dodd—who by that time had obtained an MD degree from the University of Vermont—as a roentgenologist. The administration soon recognized the need for a teaching program in roentgenology, and in 1915 the hospital "appoint[ed] of a house pupil, [a] resident in the hospital, who would devote his entire time to work in the X-ray Department" (Holmes 1921). Dodd spent almost another decade at MGH; unfortunately, after returning from a visit to France in October 1915, "the injuries from which he had suffered so long became rapidly worse, and he died on December 18, 1916" (Homes 1921).

The hospital also made strides in pathology. Visiting physicians and surgeons at MGH took it upon themselves to develop "plans for a pathological and bacteriological laboratory" (Myers 1929). In June 1895, they sent the hospital trustees their plans for such a lab and shared their fundraising efforts for the purpose; their goal was $100,000. The trustees didn't hesitate to approve the physicians' project. "The pathological laboratory... was officially opened on October 16 [1896]" (Myers 1929).

In the last few years of the decade, MGH continued its burgeoning tradition of treating all patients and unusual diseases. In 1898, during the Spanish-American War, the hospital took in soldiers who were injured or ill, mainly with typhoid and malaria. On the lawn behind the outpatient building, "Tents had been put up to accommodate a large number of [men]" (Myers 1929). Over just three months in 1898 the hospital physicians treated 221 soldiers. To put this in perspective, throughout the five years of the Civil War (1861–1865), they had treated a total of 483 soldiers.

As the century came to a close, MGH trustees were pushed to consider the development of separate departments that focused on particular specialties. In 1897, a physician who treated patients with nervous diseases described to the trustees a donor who wanted to give "$100,000 to endow a department for the sole treatment of such affections" (Myers 1929). The trustees hesitated to do so, laying out some conditions:

> The acceptance of the proposed bequest would seem to involve a change in the policy hitherto pursued by the Hospital, in that it would set apart a special department for a special class of cases, and would thus afford a precedent for the establishment of perhaps a number of other special departments. The board can see no serious objection...provided that—1st, the establishment of a special ward should not result in a monopoly of the class of cases for which it was designed...cases being excluded from the general medical and surgical wards. A special ward should be complimentary to the general wards. Otherwise, the general wards would gradually become specialized, and the Hospital would be converted into a collection of special departments...inconsistent with the best interests of the Hospital and the community. (quoted in Myers 1929)

During the last quarter of the nineteenth century (1875–1899), MGH took in "gifts and bequests [totaling] $3,487,109.99" (Myers 1929). In 2020 dollars, this would amount to just shy of $100 million. All departments combined provided care to almost 40,000 patients in 1899; this fast-growing patient volume would require continual expansion of buildings and treatment space, and it forced physicians to expedite patient care: "'In 1855, the average length of time of stay for free patients was 81 days. The corresponding time for paying and free patients during 1899'...was 20 days. In other words, 292 beds were now doing the work which would have been done by 1,182 beds forty-five years before" (Myers 1929).

Fee structures kept changing. The hospital began charging surgical outpatients in 1894 "as a means towards abolishing the abuse of hospital charity" (Myers 1929). In 1894, all 25,113 of such patients "were charged ten cents for each visit, and

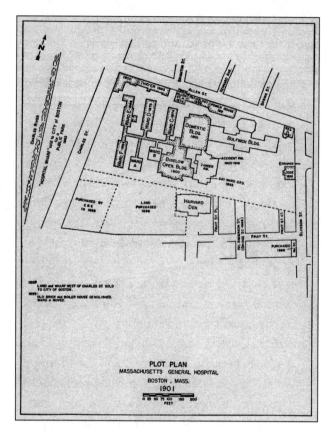

Plot plan of MGH, 1901.

The Massachusetts General Hospital, 1935-1955 by Nathaniel W. Faxon. Cambridge: Harvard University Press, 1959. Massachusetts General Hospital, Archives and Special Collections.

the cost price for splints, crutches and other apparatus, to be repaid on return of the articles in good condition" (Myers 1929). In 1895 patients undergoing a surgical procedure under ether anesthesia in the outpatient department were charged $5.00, and lock-boxes were placed in rooms so patients could make voluntary donations. By 1908, however, "the hospital cared for the poor only, and no physician was allowed to charge a fee to one of its patients. There were, for bed patients, only the wards of the General Hospital–those in the Bulfinch Building and the one-story so-called 'lower' wards. There was an Out–Patient Department and an Accident Service. In 1934 the Hospital was caring for all groups in the community" (Washburn 1939).

Additional changes at MGH (facilities and services) are found in the following chapters in section 5, notably in the chapter when orthopaedics becomes a department (chapter 32) and the last chapter on the transition to the twenty-first century (chapter 43).

CHAPTER 30

Henry J. Bigelow
The First Orthopaedic Surgeon at MGH

Henry Jacob Bigelow, the third to carry the family name in succession, was born on March 11, 1818, on Summer Street in Boston. He was the first child of Jacob Bigelow and Mary Scollay Bigelow, and four other children followed, two boys and two girls—though both boys died during childhood. His father, Jacob, had graduated from Harvard and the University of Pennsylvania School of Medicine. He was the first professor of materia medica at Harvard Medical School and was dean there for one year (1820–1821). He was also a well-known medical botanist and was most known "for his discourse on self-limited diseases, delivered to this society [the Massachusetts Medical Society] in 1835 which was a major and effective attack on Benjamin Rush's theory of 'one cause for all disease'... [and] which 'had more influence on medical practice in America than any other...treatise'" (Byrne 1981). Jacob also was largely responsible for the development of the Mount Auburn Cemetery in Cambridge.

Henry began his education at a Miss Ayer's school, then spent a year in Thayer's private school. For the next five years, he attended the Public Latin School under the tutelage of Master Leverett. When Leverett left Public Latin to establish a new private school, Henry followed him. Henry's son, W. S. Bigelow, later described his father as a young man in the 1894 memoir:

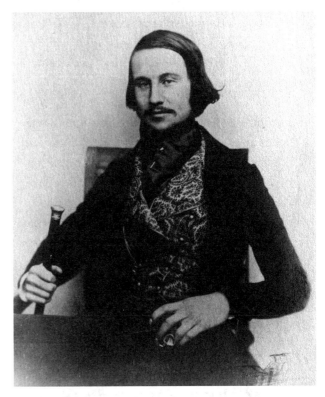

Henry Jacob Bigelow, age 23. Daguerreotype by Léon Foucault in Paris, 1841. Harvard Medical Library in the Francis A. Countway Library of Medicine.

Physician Snapshot

Henry J. Bigelow
BORN: 1818
DIED: 1890

SIGNIFICANT CONTRIBUTIONS: Described the Y-ligament; introduced the flexion method to reduce dislocated hips; performed the first excision of the hip joint (1852); developed the rapid litholapaxy procedure

23

"a very handsome boy"..."with red cheeks, blue eyes, and light hair, and a goodly figure." Possessed of a pleasant and companionable disposition, brimming over with spirits, and always on the alert, he was "the light and delight of his home, the most charming, affectionate, gay, and cheery son and brother." He was adept at dancing...as well as "an expert in swimming and in the gymnasium," and indeed whatever agility was a requisite. Endowed with remarkable ingenuity in mechanics, he was fertile in contrivances of all sorts. His traits, tastes, and parentage early earned for him, among his comrades, the nickname of "doctor."

Henry's closest friend, Henry Lee, remembered him as:

> a most entertaining companion, not only because of his keen observation of men and things, but also, as well, because of his eccentricities, –his intermittent activity and repose; his relentless, exhaustive unraveling of some tangled skein, or eager pursuit and abrupt abandonment of one hobby after another; his absorption in all he was doing, and consequent absent-mindedness; his intense curiosity about matters (some intrinsically interesting, some uninteresting); his secretiveness, or (to say the least) his excessive wariness. (W. S. Bigelow 1894)

EARLY LIFE AND TRAINING

In 1833, Henry, then 15 years old, began courses at Harvard College. At that time, the college had both a small faculty (fewer than 10 professors and tutors) and a small student body (~230 students). While there, he was a member of the Pierian Sodality, "a musical organization, in which he played the French horn" (W. S. Bigelow 1894), as well as the Rumford Chemical Society, "in connection with [which] he first became familiar with nitrous oxide, or laughing gas...In those days its administration to students, under the supervision of the Professor of Chemistry, was an annual frolic, held on a small common near the college; and Henry Bigelow manufactured the gas, in large gasometers, for use on some of these occasions" (W. S. Bigelow 1894). Despite his exuberance for life, the young Bigelow was serious in his pursuit of becoming a surgeon:

> Indeed, he declared that he never thought of choosing any other [profession]. He had definitely determined to be a surgeon, and, as a matter of course, a surgeon of eminence... Bigelow [was not] to be diverted from his purpose. Dr. James Jackson, whom Dr. Jacob Bigelow [Henry's father] regarded with profound esteem and respect...told the young man that his determination to be a surgeon was an immense mistake, as the surgery of Boston was already monopolized by a few individuals..."Your father is a medical, not a surgical practitioner. You want to forsake your best chance, and to try to practice in that corner of the room, when all your interests and opportunities are with him, over in the other corner!" To this advice the youth replied, "I'll be damned if I won't be a surgeon!" (W. S. Bigelow 1894)

Bigelow's medical education began with his father, whom he shadowed for three years. He attended lectures at a medical school over eight months and received an even broader experience than most students through:

> constant companionship with his father and his father's friends, particularly with two who were then in private practice, –Dr. James Jackson [cofounder of and chief physician at MGH], in whose family he spent a long summer at Waltham, and Dr. Oliver Wendell Holmes [who was just nine years older than Bigelow], with whom he went to Hanover, New Hampshire, to attend a course of lectures delivered by that distinguished teacher [Holmes] as Professor of

Anatomy and Physiology at the Medical School of Dartmouth College. (W. S. Bigelow 1894)

However, Bigelow experienced "threatening pulmonary symptoms" during his time in New Hampshire, which were "attributed to inhalation of nitrous oxide gas" (W. S. Bigelow 1894). Others speculated that he had pulmonary tuberculosis. According to Holmes, Bigelow "was 'perfectly cool about the matter [and]...his natural cheerfulness remained unabated,' although the condition of his health boded ill for the anticipations of an active and laborious life" (W. S. Bigelow 1894).

Bigelow returned to Boston and took a position as house surgeon at Massachusetts General Hospital, where he spent two years (1838–1839). But because of continuing health problems, he spent that winter in Cuba and then went to Europe with Dr. Samuel Cabot. He returned in 1841 solely to receive his degree from Harvard Medical School, after which he returned to Europe to continue his study of medicine. By that time, his health had rebounded, and "he devoted himself with great zeal to his professional pursuits, studying chiefly in Paris, then the acknowledged centre of all that was best and most advanced in medical science" (W. S. Bigelow 1894). In Paris, Bigelow lived on Rue de Tournon, in a house he shared with Dr. Jeffries Wyman; this was "the beginning of a long and intimate relations between them. No other contemporary did he hold in such high esteem" (W. S. Bigelow 1894). During his time in Paris, Bigelow was interested in the use of improved microscopes, especially their value in surgery, as demonstrated by lectures on the pathology of surgical diseases by Sir James Paget of London. Bigelow traveled to London from Paris each week to listen to Paget's lectures. Despite his improved health, "while in Paris, Bigelow had typhoid fever...On his recovery he went to Italy, spending several months in Rome, where he devoted himself to the art of drawing...From Italy [he] went to Egypt [to visit] the city of Thebes" (W. S. Bigelow 1894).

After almost five years away, "Bigelow returned to Boston in 1844, and immediately began practice in a familiar locality on Summer Street...Dr. Jeffries Wyman live[d] in the same house" (W. S. Bigelow 1894). At that time, Boston's population was approximately 150,000, and the Boston Medical Association had only 162 members. Then, at age 26, Bigelow still retained that headstrong confidence he had exhibited when he first declared his intention to become a preeminent surgeon:

[He] had little respect for tradition. He intended to be the founder of his own fortune, and to be dependent upon no one but himself for promotion. He made no concealment of his aspirations...mapping out his own path by sheer force and independence of character, undeterred by the fear of seniors or rivals and undisturbed by criticism. "If he does not become a distinguished man," Dr. James Jackson is declared to have said of Dr. Bigelow, "it will be because Boston is not a large enough field for his ability." From the moment of...[his] permanent establishment in Boston he became what he always remained, –a [handsome] prominent figure in social life as well as in medical and scientific circles...his fashionable and faultless dress were unfamiliar spectacles to the staid medical community. (W. S. Bigelow 1894)

During his first few years in practice, Bigelow worked with the artist Oscar Wallis to produce a series of illustrations of surgical specimens, especially tumors, and their histology. He eventually presented these to Harvard Medical School much later, in 1890. They remain unpublished.

The year 1844 was a busy one for Bigelow. He not only started his medical practice but also wrote and presented his dissertation, titled "Manual of Orthopedic Surgery," to the Boylston Medical Society at Harvard Medical School. In it he answered the question: "In what cases and to what extent is the division of muscles, tendons, or other parts proper for the relief of deformity or

MANUAL
OF
ORTHOPEDIC SURGERY,
BEING
A DISSERTATION
WHICH OBTAINED
THE BOYLSTON PRIZE FOR 1844,
ON THE FOLLOWING QUESTION:
"IN WHAT CASES AND TO WHAT EXTENT IS THE DIVISION OF MUSCLES, TENDONS, OR OTHER PARTS PROPER FOR THE RELIEF OF DEFORMITY OR LAMENESS?"
BY
HENRY JACOB BIGELOW, M. D.

"Eripiunt omnes ***** sine vulnere nervos."
OVID. REMED. AMORIS, V. 147.

BOSTON:
WILLIAM D. TICKNOR & CO.
CORNER OF WASHINGTON AND SCHOOL STREETS.
MDCCCXLV.

Henry J. Bigelow's thesis, *Manual of Orthopedic Surgery*. Library of Congress/Internet Archive.

lameness?" At the beginning of the dissertation, he stated, "It is believed that the general intention of the committee will be fulfilled, by attempt to cover the ground now occupied by *Orthopedic Surgery*" (H. J. Bigelow 1845). Interestingly, the essay included a section on strabismus and a shorter one on stammering, both of which were, at the time, treated by soft-tissue and muscle releases. Bigelow won the Boylston prize that year for his dissertation. The following year, he published its more than 200 pages as the monograph *Manual of Orthopedic Surgery Being a Dissertation Which Obtained the Boylston Prize*. Today many consider it to be "a model of excellence and one of the best of publications to illustrate the French school of orthopedic surgery, the dominant school of the time" (Bradford 1889). According to E. W. Archibald, Bigelow took an avid interest in the work of Jules Guérin, an orthopaedist working in Paris: "From him [Guérin,] very probably, came to Bigelow the impulse to write his first major thesis, 'Orthopedic Surgery'...and which may have led on to his original work on dislocation of the hip" (Archibald 1937).

In 1845, Bigelow became a surgical instructor at Tremont Street Medical School. A year later, he took a position as visiting surgeon at MGH. (Dr. Samuel Parkman and Dr. J. Mason Warren also became visiting surgeons there at that time.) In 1845, Bigelow was also made president of the Boylston Medical Society, "a society for mutual improvement, composed of students in the Harvard Medical School" (W. S. Bigelow 1894). In his presidential address that year, titled "Fragments of Medical Science and Art," "he discussed the value of the inductive method [based on a hypothesis] of applying knowledge and the use of the senses, in contradistinction to the numerical method [excluding the intellect], which, he said, made men of science statisticians" (Mayo 1921). After Bigelow concluded his speech,

> Edward Everett said to a friend, "there goes a future Professor,"–and later [he complemented] Dr. Bigelow warmly, calling the address "an honor to its author, and to the city of Boston."... Dr. Oliver Wendell Holmes [stated]: "It was not so much the originality of the thesis maintained by Dr. Bigelow, as the reasonable and forcible method by which he expounded and illustrated it, and the peculiar fitness of his choice of a subject at that particular time. He knew when to strike, as well as how to strike [; he] handled his knowledge of the great authors he cited so like an adept in book-lore that one might have thought he was born in an alcove and cradled on a book-shelf." (W. S. Bigelow 1894)

Bigelow published his address as a monograph of the same title later that year.

FASCINATION WITH ETHER AND ANESTHETICS

The year 1846 proved to be a momentous one for Bigelow. As a young surgeon in only his first or second year of practice and on the staff at MGH for only a few months, Bigelow also observed the first public operation performed with the patient anesthetized with ether in October (see chapter 3). Bigelow was just 28 years old at the time. Dr. John Collins Warren was the surgeon; Dr. William T. G. Morton, a dentist, administered the ether. The procedure greatly affected Bigelow, and he recognized the huge influence ether could have on the surgical field. He became an "enthusiastic devotee" of its use and even applied it to himself, testifying to its safety (G. H. Jackson Jr. 1943).

Early Publication and Controversy

Just a fortnight after witnessing this first use of ether at MGH, Bigelow began to prepare a presentation to the American Academy of Arts and Sciences. More than 40 years later, Oliver Wendell Holmes (1890) recalled that Bigelow had shared with him the draft of that presentation and asked his opinion on it:

> On an evening of…1846 he called upon me with a paper which he proposed reading the next evening [November 3, 1846] at the regular meeting of the American Academy of Arts and Sciences. ["In a state of excitement"] he began by telling me that a great discovery had just been made and practically demonstrated in the operating theatre of the Massachusetts General Hospital. He proceeded to read the paper, which was the first formal presentation to the world, of the successful use of artificially produced anesthesia in a capital operation. He had the sagacity to see the far-reaching prospects of the new discovery, the courage as well as the shrewdness to support the claims of the adventurous dentist's startling, at first almost incredible, announcement…Dr. Bigelow was unfolding in my library the first paper ever written on the subject, and saying to me as he did so, that within a fortnight the news of the discovery would be all over Europe.

Bigelow presented his paper to the American Academy of Arts and Sciences, but it was not published in their proceedings. Instead, his first journal article on the subject of the use of ether at MGH was published, as "Insensibility During Surgical Operations Produced by Inhalation" in the *Boston Medical and Surgical Journal* just five weeks after the operation. Although in his paper Bigelow credited various individuals for their roles—Morton for administering ether; Warren for performing the first operation (on October 16, 1846) and another, to remove part of a patient's jaw three weeks later (November 7, 1846); and Dr. George Hayward, who had done the second operation in which ether was used (October 17, 1846), and then an above-knee amputation on November 7, 1846—Bigelow was, surprisingly, listed as the sole author of the article. This young surgeon, with no previous journal publications to his name and little experience, published his paper alone, only mentioning John Collins Warren, then the chief of surgery at MGH who, at risk to his own reputation, permitted Morton to administer ether to his patient, and Morton, who did the work of delivering the ether. In the paper, Bigelow described some experiments with ether that

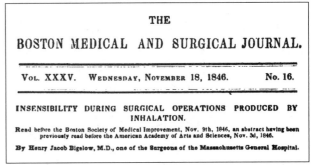

Title of Bigelow's initial publication on the first use of ether at MGH. *Boston Medical and Surgical Journal* 1846; 35: 309.

he had conducted on himself, briefly reviewed some published reports on the effects of ether, and described his observations of additional cases (surgical and dental) in which ether had been used.

On December 3, 1846, two weeks after Bigelow's article was published, in a letter to the *Boston Medical and Surgical Journal*, Warren wrote a brief history of his experience with ether at MGH. This was in response to an attorney's request, on behalf of Morton, "to furnish an account of the operations witnessed and performed by me [Warren], wherein his [Morton's] new discovery for preventing pain was employed…[with] the hope of being useful to my professional brethren."

Box 30.1. Warren's Letter Describing the First Use of Ether at MGH

"The Discovery of a mode of preventing pain in surgical operations has been an object of strong desire among surgeons from an early period. In my surgical lectures I have almost annually alluded to it, and stated the means which I have usually adopted for the attainment of this object. I have also freely declared, that notwithstanding the use of very large doses of narcotic substances, this desideratum had never been satisfactorily obtained. The successful use of any article of the materia medica for this purpose, would therefore be hailed by me as an important alleviation to human suffering. I have in consequence readily admitted the trial of plans calculated to accomplish this object, whenever they were free from danger.

"About five weeks since, Dr. Morton, dentist of this city, informed me that he had invented an apparatus for the inhalation of a vapor, the effect of which was to produce a state of total insensibility to pain, and that he had employed it successfully in a sufficient number of cases in his practice to justify him in a belief of its efficacy. He wished for an opportunity to test its power in surgical operations, and I agreed to give him such an opportunity as soon as practicable.

"Being at that time in attendance as Surgeon of the Massachusetts General Hospital, a patient presented himself in that valuable institution a few days after my conversation with Dr. Morton, who required an operation for tumor of the neck, and agreeably to my promise I requested the attendance of Dr. M.

"On October 17th [sic; this actually occurred on October 16], the patient being prepared for the operation, the apparatus was applied to his mouth by Dr. Morton for about three minutes, at the end of which time he sank into a state of insensibility. I immediately made an incision about three inches long through the skin of the neck, and began a dissection among important nerves and blood vessels without any expression of pain on the part of the patient. Soon after he began to speak incoherently, and appeared to be in an agitated state during the remainder of the operation. Been asked immediately afterwards whether he had suffered much, he said that he had felt as if his neck had been scratched; but subsequently, when inquired of by me, his statement was, that he did not experience pain at the time, although aware that the operation was proceeding.

"The effect of the gaseous inhalation in neutralizing the sentient faculty was made perfectly distinct to my mind by this experiment, although the patient during a part of its prosecution exhibited appearances indicative of suffering. Dr. Morton had apprised me, that the influence of his application would last but a few minutes after its intermission; and as the operation was necessarily protracted, I was not disappointed that its success was only partial.

"On the following day, October 18th [sic; this actually occurred on October 17], an operation was done by Dr. Hayward on a tumor of the arm, in a female patient at the Hospital. The respiration of the gas was in this case continued during the whole of the operation. There was no exhibition of pain, excepting some occasional groans during its last stage, which she subsequently stated to have arisen from a disagreeable dream. Noticing the pulse in this patient before and after operation, I found it to have risen from 80 to 120.

"Two or three days after these occurrences, on meeting with Dr. Charles T. Jackson, distinguished for his philosophical spirit of inquiry, as well as for his geological and chemical science, this gentleman informed me that he first suggested to Dr. Morton the inspiration of ether, as a means of preventing the pain of operations on the teeth. He did not claim the invention of the apparatus, nor its practical application; for these we are indebted to Dr. Morton.

Warren went on to describe his initial collaboration with Morton, the details of the first surgery and subsequent ones, and the need for more study of ether before its widespread use. The full text of his letter is reprinted in **Box 30.1**.

For several months after Bigelow's November 1846 publication, reports and letters about ether were published almost weekly in the *Boston Medical and Surgical Journal*. As Bigelow had predicted, as soon as the first boat arrived with the exciting news from MGH, the use of ether spread throughout England and Europe. By the first two weeks of March 1847, reports of the use of ether from both London and Paris appeared in the

---

"The success of this process in the prevention of pain for a certain period being quite established, I at once conceived it to be my duty to introduce the apparatus into the practice of the Hospital, but was immediately arrested by learning that the proprietor intended to obtain an exclusive patent for its use. It now became a question, whether, in accordance with that elevated principle long since introduced into the medical profession, which forbids its members to conceal any useful discovery, we could continue to encourage an application we were not allowed to use ourselves, and of the components of which we were ignorant. On discussing this matter with Dr. Hayward, my colleague in the Hospital, we came to the conclusion, that we were not justified in encouraging the further use of this new invention, until we were better satisfied on these points. Dr. Hayward thereupon had a conversation with Dr. Morton, in consequence of which Dr. M. addressed to me a letter. In this he declared his willingness to make known to us the article employed, and to supply assistance to administer the inhalation whenever called upon. These stipulations he has complied with.

"This being done, we thought ourselves justified in inviting Dr. Morton to continue his experiments at the Hospital, and elsewhere; and he directly after, Nov. 7th, attended at a painful and projected operation performed by me, of the excision of a portion of the lower jaw, in which the patient's sufferings were greatly mitigated. On the same day an amputation of the thigh of young woman was performed at the hospital by Dr. Hayward. In this case the respiration of the ethereal vapor appeared to be entirely successful in preventing the pain of operation; the patient stating, afterwards, that she did not know that anything had been done to her.

"On Nov. 12th, an operation for the removal of a tumor from the arm of a young woman was performed by Dr. J. Mason Warren. The vapor was administered for three minutes, when the patient became unconscious; the operator then proceeded, the inspiration being continued. Standing myself on one side of the patient, while the operator was on the other, so entirely tranquil was she, that I was not aware the operation had begun, until it was nearly completed...

"In all these cases there was a decided mitigation of pain; in most of them the patients on the day after the operation, and at other times, stated, that they had not been conscious of pain. All those who attended were, I think, satisfied of the efficacy of the application in preventing, or, at least, greatly diminishing the suffering usual in such cases. The phenomena presented in these operations afford grounds for many interesting reflections, but it being my principal intention at this time to give a simple statement of facts...

"All these changes soon pass off without leaving any distinct traces behind them, and the ordinary state of the functions returns. This has been the course of things in the cases I have witnessed, but I think it quite probable, that so powerful an agent may sometimes produce other and even alarming effects. I therefore would recommend, that it should never be employed except under the inspection of a judicious and competent person.

"Let me conclude by congratulating my professional brethren on the acquisition of a mode of mitigating human suffering, which may become a valuable agent in the hands of careful and well-instructed practitioners, even if it should not prove of such general application as the imagination of sanguine persons would lead them to anticipate."

(Originally published as J. C. Warren, "Inhalation of Ethereal Vapor for the Prevention of Pain During Surgical Operations," *Boston Medical and Surgical Journal* 35 (1846): 375–379)

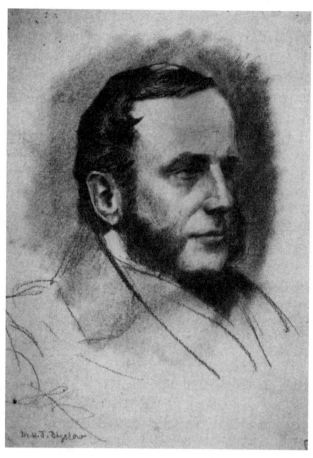

Sketch of Henry J. Bigelow by Robert Hinckley.
Harvard Medical Library in the Francis A. Countway Library of Medicine.

Boston Medical and Surgical Journal. John Collins Warren gave his last valedictory lecture at Harvard Medical School on Tuesday, March 3, 1847. He traced the history of the medical school, the type of surgical procedures commonly performed, and his efforts to bring new operations and surgical science from Europe to Boston. Surprisingly, he only briefly commented on the discovery of ether, "the invaluable means of preventing pain in surgical operations–a discovery, which every medical man, and especially every practical surgeon, must hail with unmingled satisfaction" (Warren 1847).

Pivotal Moment in his Career

During this busy time in his burgeoning career, Bigelow married Susan Sturgis, daughter of the prominent Boston merchant William Sturgis, on May 8, 1847. They began their married life at No. 5 Chauncey Place. Despite his hectic schedule, Bigelow also devoted time to the establishment of a charitable organization that year with Dr. Henry Bryant, whom Bigelow had met during his time in Paris and who was now in Boston. Together, they "established a 'Charitable Surgical Institution' in the basement of the conservative First Church on Chauncey Place, offering their gratuitous services to the poor by means of conspicuous signboards, and [they] distributed circulars among country practitioners inviting them to bring their patients to this infirmary for consultation. [T]he consternation among their confrères was both visible and audible" (W. S. Bigelow 1894). The Charitable Surgical Institution opened just a few years before Dr. John B. Brown's Orthopedic Institute closed (see chapter 7). Bigelow and Bryant held a clinic daily from 11 a.m. to noon. In addition to providing surgical advice, they also performed surgeries free of charge in the church's basement or in local boarding houses, as the patient preferred. The Charitable Surgical Institution "created a sensation, but his [Bigelow's] graceful attitude toward the members of his profession, his ability in organization, and his popularity with his clientele, made the institution a success" (Mayo 1921).

In the year after the discovery of ether, Bigelow threw himself into administrative duties at MGH. "Almost from the commencement of his connection with the hospital...[he] became one of its chief attractions to medical men and students. He was exceptionally young for a surgeon already distinguished. He was fine looking...He had... personal magnetism [and was] alert and active in every movement, full of life and animation...He was a brilliant operator" (W. S. Bigelow 1894). His forceful personality allowed him to influence numerous aspects of surgeons' role at MGH, even down to the blue blazer orthopaedic surgeons often wore during the latter half of the twentieth century and into the twenty-first: "He originated the light blue coat, the brass buttons...These and many other acts contributed to make him a

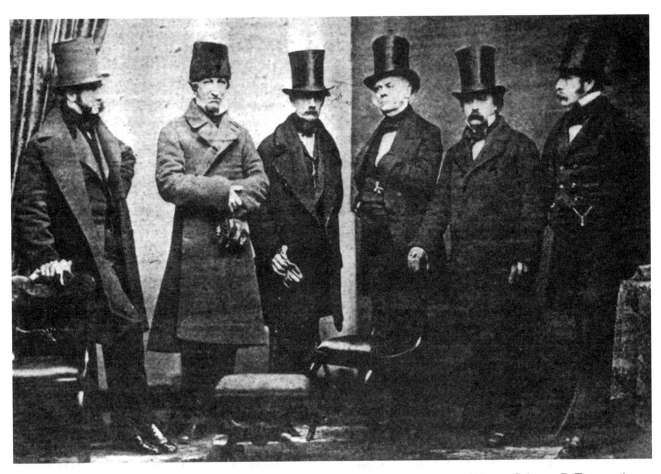

Visiting surgeons at MGH in 1855. Left to right: Henry J. Bigelow, Samuel Cabot, J. Mason Warren, Solomon D. Townsend, George H. Gay and H. G. Clark. *Every Man Our Neighbor: A Brief History of the Massachusetts General Hospital, 1811–1961* by Joseph E. Garland. Boston: Little, Brown and Company, 1961. 2nd edition, 2008 Massachusetts General Hospital, Archives and Special Collections.

marked man, and only his extraordinary ability enabled him to maintain the unusual standards he established. Yet he always searched for the truth, was always open to suggestion, even though he might dislike his informant" (Mayo 1921).

Bigelow continued to publish about ether and other anesthetics such as chloroform and nitrous oxide, producing two books and approximately 10 publications. Warren also wrote a book about each of anesthesia, ether, and chloroform. Both surgeons were quick to identify the risk of death with chloroform use. In 1849, Warren wrote, "We were soon awakened from our dreams of the delightful influence of the new agent [chloroform] by the occurrence of unfortunate and painful consequences, which had not followed in this country in the practice of etherization." Almost 25 years later, in 1872, Bigelow wrote that "death from chloroform, which has given to chloroform its doubtful reputation, is a different thing, which no human foresight can avert…no precaution yet devised by human ingenuity will prevent the insidious shock of chloroform, in even a small dose, from occasionally and abruptly killing a healthy patient…neither pulse nor breathing gives indication." After a rare reported death with ether, Bigelow (1873) responded with disbelief and reiterated its safety in his experience:

The Massachusetts General Hospital numbers more than 15,000 cases of ether inhalation, 6000 of which have been recorded within the last five years…It fell to my lot, in 1846, and for a year or two after the discovery of ether

A monument to the discovery of ether was placed in the Public Garden in Boston Common (**Box 30.2**) in 1868, more than 20 years after that momentous first surgery using ether and at a time when Bigelow was an accomplished surgeon and educator in his own right with numerous other publications. At the presentation of the monument to the city, Bigelow gave an address in the name of the recently deceased donor (Thomas Lee); notably, he did not mention Warren or Morton:

> Men had been made insensible to pain through mental excitement, or by the agency of mesmerism or hypnotism, or by the dead drunkenness of alcohol, the narcotism of opium, the inhalation of nitrous oxyde [sic] and other gasses, and even by the vapor of ether. For years all this had been known to be possible, but it attracted little attention…The question of danger from this extraordinary stance was also unsettled. No consulting board of surgeons would have dared to sanction the production of prolonged unconsciousness during an operation, before the series of consecutive experiments were made here in Tremont Street and at the Hospital…But when these consecutive experiments had been made in Boston, the discovery

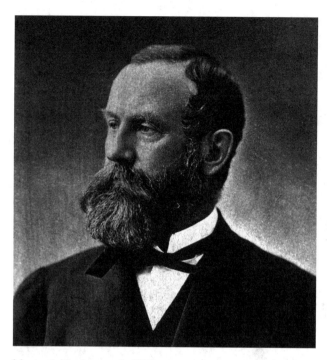

Henry J. Bigelow, early 1870s. U.S. National Library of Medicine.

> anesthesia, as junior surgeon, to administer most of the ether in that institution…I have never been satisfied of the occurrence of a single death which could be attributed to any property of ether, apart from the gradual and progressive inebriating influence which it possesses in common with other anesthetic agents.

Box 30.2. Inscriptions on the Ether Monument in Boston Common

Each of the four sides of the monument are inscribed:

I
To commemorate the discovery that the inhalation of ether causes insensibility to pain.
First proved to the world at the Mass. General Hospital in Boston.

II
Neither shall there be any more pain.

III
In gratitude for the relief of human suffering by the inhaling of ether, a citizen of Boston has erected this monument.

IV
Thus, also cometh forth from the Lord of Hosts which is wonderful in counsel and excellent in working.

had been made; and in grateful and unhesitating recognition of it the entire civilized world simultaneously rose up to hail it with acclamatory welcome. Thus, was made the discovery, and thus begun a career of anaesthetic inhalation.

John Collins Warren's grandson, Dr. Thomas Dwight, who became the Parkman Professor of Anatomy at Harvard Medical School after Holmes left the position, took issue with Bigelow's omission.

He Needs No Laurels Not His Own

Much later, after Bigelow's death in 1890, Dwight wrote a letter to the editor of the *Boston Medical and Surgical Journal*. He began by stating, "When a distinguished man dies it is but natural that many things should be said in his praise…Nevertheless, if claims are made for the departed at the expense of others no longer here, it is not only the right, but the duty, of their descendants to see that justice is done." Dwight went on to describe numerous previous claims—both by Bigelow and on his behalf—that Bigelow was "the surgeon who introduced Morton's discovery of ether." He continued by revisiting the events of that time—that "Morton brought the discovery to Dr. John C. Warren, then senior surgeon of the hospital"—noting that Bigelow himself even described Warren as such in his "History of the Discovery of Anesthesia": "'Dr. Warren was the principal New England Surgeon of the day and it was the obvious thing to do'" (Bigelow, quoted in Dwight 1890).

Although, "Great stress is laid on the fact that Bigelow was the first to announce to the world the discovery of a modern anesthesia," Dwight specified that, "The first surgical operation under ether was performed at the hospital by Dr. Warren on October 16, 1846, and the second on the next day by Dr. Hayward at Dr. Warren's invitation…Then came a pause, owing to the natural aversion of the surgeons to the use of a secret remedy of unknown composition which they were not allowed to administer themselves…" Dwight reinforced that Bigelow, at that time young (only 28), inexperienced, and new to MGH, only "announced the discovery before the Academy of Arts and Sciences on November 3d [1846]. [But] let it be noted that, so far, there had been but two operations at the hospital, neither a capital one…[and] that with neither of these Dr. Bigelow was concerned; and that besides these he had seen only some dental operations by Dr. Morton." Dwight stated that despite Bigelow's paper being presented to the Society for Medical Improvement, and then, soon after published in the *Boston Medical and Surgical Journal*, Bigelow had not been involved in any of the other new cases he described. Thus the "sober, judicial report of what had been done" that Warren published in that same journal on December 3, 1846, "may properly be called the first authoritative statement on the subject" (Dwight 1890). Dwight held to his position despite comments at a meeting of the Society for Improvement "alluding to the 'timidity or jealousy' on the part of Dr. Bigelow's seniors, declar[ing] that but for him [Bigelow] 'the primary honor of introducing the great discovery would probably have been diverted from the Massachusetts General Hospital, and from the city of Boston'" (Dwight 1890). Warren himself cited, "the slow progress of the practice of etherization in this country, beyond the vicinity of its first introduction, compared with its rapid extension on the other side of the Atlantic" (quoted in Dwight 1890) as a reason for publishing his book *Etherization* relatively soon (about a year) after the discovery.

Dwight (1890) provides further support for his claim through comments by Holmes in 1856. Just after Warren's death, during "remarks given… before the Suffolk District Medical Society," Holmes supported Warren's role in this important discovery: "He [Warren] had reached the age… when those who have labored during their days of strength are expected to repose, and when the mind is thought to have lost its aptitude for innovating knowledge…Yet nothing could surpass the eagerness with which he watched and assisted in the development of the newly discovered powers of etherization...that pain was no longer the master, but the servant of the body" (Holmes, quoted in Dwight 1890). Dwight (1890) insisted that he did not mean to "disparage the services which Dr. Bigelow rendered to the cause of anesthesia." Rather, he aimed to challenge "the claim that he [Bigelow] was practically the only surgeon who has a right to the remembrance of posterity for the introduction of ether. This, I believe, is unjust to others, indeed to several, but above all to Dr. John C. Warren. Dr. Bigelow died laden with well-won honors. He needs no laurels not his own" (Dwight 1890).

ORTHOPAEDIC CONTRIBUTIONS

In 1849, about three years after his early publication on ether, Bigelow was named professor of surgery at Harvard Medical School, replacing Dr. George Hayward. That same year, he published his first article on an orthopaedic topic: excision of the elbow. In all, Bigelow would go on to publish 15 books or monographs, five of which were on orthopaedic topics, and more than 115 articles (many brief case reports), including 28 on orthopaedic topics. His orthopaedics-related publications spanned a period of about 35 years; his last orthopaedic article was published in 1880. Notably, "His writings are almost entirely free from literary references. Until his own work was accomplished, he seldom tried to ascertain what his predecessors had done" (W. S. Bigelow). During the course of his early publications, he also experienced the heights of great joy and the depths of great sorrow. His only son, William Sturgis Bigelow, was born in April 1850. His wife, Susan Bigelow, died only a few years later, on June 9, 1853.

Hip Joint Excision

In 1852, Bigelow treated a 10-year-old boy who had a three-month history of swelling and pain, with complete dislocation of the hip. During the hip resection, a large amount of pus (suspected to be from tuberculosis) was drained, along with fragments of the femoral head. Apparently, the patient was comfortable after the operation but died 12 days later. According to Bigelow's son and biographer, W. S. Bigelow, Bigelow was the first in the United States to remove a patient's hip joint. In an 1873 letter to the editor of the *Boston Medical and Surgical Journal*, however, C. A. Wilcox wrote that this was not the case: "My brother, Oliver D. Wilcox, MD, of Easton, Pa., now deceased, performed the operation July 16, 1849...[on] a brick mason, about forty years of age...[The patient] made a good recovery in about three months' time; and, a month later, was actively engaged in his trade as a master mason. The case was never published."

Ununited Fractures

Bigelow also showed great interest in the then new field of cellular pathology and studied in detail the use of microscopes: "Since his return from Europe he had been busy with researches in surgical pathology and he was a microscopist superior to any in Boston, and second to none elsewhere in United States at that time" (W. S. Bigelow 1894). He put such knowledge to work, in 1867 publishing a case in which he removed bones from the elbow joint of a patient with an infected synovial membrane. The paper described the renewal of the humeral condyles by the periosteum. The patient's arm was later amputated, and Bigelow microscopically determined that the muscles had sufficiently attached to the new-formed condyles.

In another paper published in 1867, Bigelow described 11 ununited fractures of long bones, this time applying his research on tissue repair. Because he knew that periosteal cells can regenerate bone, he used the periosteum to form new bone and thus solid unions; he was successful in 10 of the 11 fractures. (The one nonunion resulted from a preoperative infection.) He emphasized that as much of the periosteum should be retained as possible. After visualizing the fracture, Bigelow removed the atrophic bone ends, while preserving the periosteum with its muscle attachments, and rejoined the bone ends using a tension-band technique with silver or copper wire.

Bigelow (1868) described his preferred treatment while waiting for the fractures to heal: "In all other injuries of the elbow joint [except to the olecranon], whether you are able to make an exact diagnosis or wholly unable to do so on account of the swelling, treat them as though the forearm had been dislocated backwards, and secure the arm at about right angles to an inside angular splint." He advocated for a progressive return to use of the affected limb, as the patient would regain function slowly.

Iliofemoral Ligament (Y Ligament of Bigelow)

By 1868, no longer did surgeons at MGH routinely need to use weights and pulleys to attempt an initial reduction of a dislocated hip. That year, Beach and Waterman Jr. (1868) described Bigelow's first case report on reduction of a dislocated hip:

> Upon entrance, the limb was shortened one inch, the foot inverted and the knee turned inward…Circumduction outward, consisting of flexion, abduction and eversion, was twice rapidly performed without success, owing…to the narrow laceration of the capsule. Dr. Bigelow now passed the head of the bone across to the thyroid foramen, in order to increase the laceration, and the dislocation was then reduced from the dorsum by repetition of the previous manoeuvre [sic]; the whole time consumed, from the moment of handling the limb, being one minute and forty-five seconds.

Bigelow had performed related research over eight years, which he presented separately at meetings of the American Medical Association, the

Title page of Bigelow's book, *The Mechanism of Dislocation and Fracture of the Hip*. U.S. National Library of Medicine/Internet Archive.

Massachusetts Medical Society, and the Society for Medical Improvement. Those three papers were compiled into *The Mechanism of Dislocation and Fracture of the Hip*, published in 1869 (see **Box 30.3**). According to G. H. Jackson, who wrote about Bigelow for the *Archives of Surgery* in 1943, this was the most popular of Bigelow's books. In it, Bigelow described his initial discovery of how to reduce a dislocated hip by relaxing the Y-ligament upon examining a corpse used to demonstrate a dislocated hip during autopsy to students at the Massachusetts Medical College:

In the spring 1861, having been led to expose a joint, the luxation of which had been the subject of a lecture, I was agreeably surprised to observe the simple action of the ligament, – simplicity which subsequent experience has confirmed, and which strikingly explains the phenomena observed in the living subject. The dislocated joint alluded to, presented on examination the following appearances.

1. Great laceration of the muscles about the joint.
2. The ligamentum teres broken.
3. Laceration of the inner, outer, and lower parts of the capsule.
4. The anterior and upper parts of the capsule uninjured, and presenting a strong fibrous band, fan-shaped and forked.

The remaining tendinous and muscular fibres about the joint being now completely divided, with the exception of the strong fibrous band above alluded to, it was found that the four commonly described dislocations of the hip could still be exhibited without difficulty, and that in each of them the anterior portion of the capsular ligament, which alone remained, sufficed at once to direct the limb to its appropriate position and to fix it there. (H. J. Bigelow 1868)

Bigelow noted that the iliofemoral ligament had been previously mentioned by others but until then had not received much attention. He described the anatomy of what he called the Y-ligament, which he also referred to as the ligament of Bertin, from his experience with numerous other dissections and postmortem cases of hip dislocations:

It take[s] its origin from the anterior inferior spinous process of the ilium, passing downward to the front of the femur, to be inserted fan-shaped into nearly the whole of the oblique "spiral" line which connects the two trochanters in front,–being about half an inch wide at its upper or iliac origin, and but little less than two inches and a half wide at its fan-like femoral insertion. Here it is bifurcated, having two principal fasciculi, one being inserted into the upper extremity of the anterior intertrochanteric line, and the other into the lower part of the same line, about half an inch in front of the small trochanter. The ligament thus resembles an inverted Y, which suggests a short and convenient name for it… The Y ligament is of remarkable tenacity and strength…In six…subjects [cadavers] taken at random…this ligament required for its rupture the attachment of weights to the foot varying in the several cases from two hundred and fifty to seven hundred and fifty pounds…

Bigelow described the ligament as being crucial during activities such as walking, as it keeps the femur strongly in place, thereby preventing hyperextension of the leg.

Again, Bigelow seemed to discount John Collins Warren and his work; never mentioning Warren's work with dislocated hips in his book. Warren is associated with the famous case of Charles Lowell, who had an unreduced dislocated hip (see chapter 3)—the first dislocated hip treated at MGH. Bigelow did, however, acknowledge the methods of Sir Astley Cooper, the thought leader of the time and Warren's teacher:

When the patient lies upon his back…the Y ligament becomes more and more tense as the limb approaches nearer and nearer to a state of complete extension. If, now, as is here maintained, the chief obstacle to reduction of the luxated hip is found in this ligament, it follows that the method taught by Sir Ashley Cooper, the weight of whose unquestioned authority has unfortunately availed to give it currency during many years, is based on an erroneous conception of the nature of the difficulty to be encountered. By that method the limb is placed as nearly as may be in the axis of the body, thus

Box 30.3. Bigelow's Two Main Orthopaedic Contributions

The list below, written by Bigelow in an 1869 publication, describes in his own words his two most important orthopaedic contributions: the Y-ligament of Bigelow and the flexion method for reducing a dislocated hip.

"1st. The anterior part of the capsule of the hip joint is a triangular ligament of great strength, which, when well developed, exhibits an internal and external fasciculus, diverging like the branches of the inverted letter Y. It rises from the anterior inferior spinous process of the ilium, and is inserted into nearly the entire length of the anterior intertrochanteric line.

"2nd. The Y ligament, the internal obturator muscle, and the capsule subjacent to it, are alone required to explain the unusual phenomena of the regular luxations.

"3rd. The regular dislocations are those in which one or both branches of the Y ligament are unbroken; and their signs are constant.

"4th. The irregular dislocations are those in which the Y ligament is wholly ruptured; and they offer no constant signs.

"5th. In the regular dislocations of the hip, the muscles are not essential to give position to the limb, nor desirable as aids in its reduction.

"6th. The Y ligament will alone effect reduction and explain its phenomena, a part of those connected with the dorsal dislocations excepted.

"7th. During the process of reduction, this ligament should be kept constantly in mind.

"8th. The rest of the capsule, except perhaps that portion beneath the internal obturator tendon, need not be considered in reduction, if the capsular orifice is large enough to admit the head of the femur easily.

"9th. If the capsular orifice is too small to allow easy reduction, it should be enlarged.

"10th. The capsular orifice may be enlarged at will, and with impunity, by circumduction of the flexed thigh.

"11th. Recent dislocations can be best reduced by manipulation.

"12th. The basis of this manipulation is flexion of the thigh.

"13th. This manipulation is efficient, because it relaxes the Y ligament, or because that ligament, when it remains tense, is a fixed point, around which the head of the femur revolves near the socket.

"14th. The further manipulation of the flexed thigh may be either by traction or rotation.

"15th. The dorsal dislocation owes its inversion to the external branch of the Y ligament.

"16th. The so-called ischiatic dislocation owes nothing whatever of its character, or its difficulty of reduction by horizontal extension, to the ischiatic notch.

"17th. 'The ischiatic dislocation' is better named 'dorsal below the tendon,' and is easily reduced by manipulation.

"18th. The flexion of the thyroid and downward dislocations is due to the Y ligament, which, in the first, also everts the limb, until the trochanter rests upon the pelvis.

"19th. In the pubic dislocation, the range of the bone upon the pubes is limited by this ligament, which, in the sub-spinous dislocation also, binds the neck of the femur to the pelvis.

"20th. In the dorsal dislocation with eversion, the outer branch of the Y ligament is ruptured.

"21st. In the anterior oblique luxation, the head of the bone is hooked over the entire Y ligament, the limb being then necessarily oblique, everted, and a little flexed.

"22nd. In the supra spinous luxation, the head of the femur is equally hooked over the Y ligament, the external branch of which is broken. The limb may then remain extended.

"23rd. In old luxations, the period during which reduction is possible is determined by the extent of the obliteration of the socket, the strength of the neck of the femur, and the absence of osseous excrescence.

"24th. Old luxations may possibly require the use of pulleys, in order by traction to avoid any danger which might result to the atrophied or degenerated neck of the bone from rotation.

"25th. Right-angled extension, the femur being flexed at a right angle with the pelvis, is more advantageous than that which has usually been employed.

"26th. To make such an extension most effective, a special apparatus is required."

rendering the Y ligament tense and inserting its maximum of resistance before traction is made. Hence the necessity for pulleys...By the flexion method, which dates from a remote antiquity, the Y ligament is relaxed, its resistance annulled, and reduction often accomplished with surprising facility... (H. J. Bigelow 1869)

Bigelow continued with a description of the importance of flexion to the success of the reduction. He mentioned etherization as well, indicating his continued involvement with that once-new method:

> Flexion lies at the foundation of success in the reduction of femoral dislocation, and compared with this the rest of the manipulation is of secondary importance...When the femur is flexed, reduction may be effected [sic] in either of two ways. In the first (traction), the head is drawn, or forced, at once in the desired direction. In the second (rotation), the same result is accomplished by a rotation of the femur, which, in winding the Y ligament about its neck, shortens it, and thus compels the head of the bone, as it sweeps round the socket, also to approach it. In reducing a hip, the success of rotation, adduction, abduction, and extension depends on this ligament, while the whole manipulation must be conducted with reference to it...The patient should be laid upon the floor, that the operator may command the limb to the best advantage, and should be etherized until the muscles of the hip are completely relaxed. (H. J. Bigelow 1869)

> "Dr. Bigelow's repeated and searching investigations into the anatomy of the hip-joint showed him the band which formed the chief difficulty in reducing dislocations of the thigh. What Sir Astley Cooper and all the surgeons after him had failed to see, Dr. Bigelow detected."
> —Oliver Wendell Holmes, 1883

Femoral Neck Fractures

In the last portion of his book, *The Mechanism of Dislocation and Fracture of the Hip*, Bigelow also discussed fractures of the neck of the femur; the structure of the femoral head and neck; and fractures of the pelvis, especially the acetabulum, which "may be mistaken for regular dislocation of the hip" (H. J. Bigelow 1869). He studied the bone injuries through postmortem dissections of his own patients, others who had died after fracture at MGH, and specimens in the Warren Museum of the Massachusetts Medical College.

That same year (1869), a glowing review of Bigelow's book was published in the *Boston Medical and Surgical Journal*:

> The Medical Profession in this vicinity has long been familiar with the original researches of Dr. H. J. Bigelow in regard to Dislocations of the Hip...The publication of this volume has

Dr. John Homans in the Bigelow operating room awaiting completion of ether anesthesia before attempting to reduce a patient's dislocated hip. The patient is lying on a mattress on the floor.

The Harvard Medical School: A History, Narrative, and Documentary, 1782-1905, Volume III, by Thomas F. Harrington and James G. Mumford. New York: Lewis Publishing Company, 1905. Royal College of Physicians/Internet Archive.

therefore been looked for with great interest... With the exception of the employment of anesthesia...no practical advance in the treatment of luxations of the hip has been introduced... since the time of Cooper [1842]...Pulleys and dynamometers still figure in the pages of medical journals, and patients have been pulled upon within the year, in Paris and in London, until life was threatened, when putting in their hips ought to have been the work of but a moment...

No higher praise can be awarded to Dr. Bigelow's treatise [a remarkable book], than to regard it as a successful attempt to bring under one system of explanation all the irregular and exceptional or anomalous cases of dislocation of the hip scattered through medical literature...These are deciphered and cleared from their obscurity by the simple intervention of the Y ligament. It may be safely claimed that until...this volume there was not to be found in the entire range of surgical writings any generalization of these facts...This monograph is the most original, important and exhaustive contribution to civil surgery which has been produced on this side of the Atlantic.

Before the wide availability of roentgenography, surgeons spent much time trying to identify a fracture of the femoral neck as intracapsular or extracapsular, and to ensure that fractures of the femoral head and neck and of the acetabulum were not mistaken for regular dislocations of the hip. By 1875, Bigelow had disregarded the importance of such consultation and instead brought to the fore what he considered an even larger problem: determining bone impaction in injured hips. On the basis of his study of the anatomy of the femur, he designated only two categories of fractures at the femur neck—impacted fractures at the base and unimpacted fractures anywhere above that. He stated that both required the same treatment.

In a paper titled "The True Neck of the Femur: Its Structure and Pathology," published that same year, Bigelow described a part of the femoral

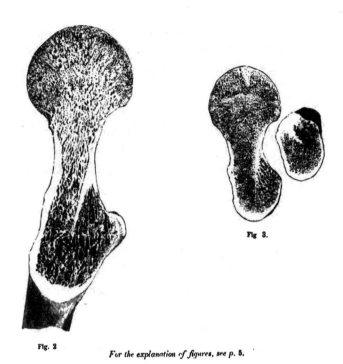

The calcar femorale as depicted in Bigelow's 1875 article.
H. J. Bigelow, "The True Neck of the Femur: Its Structure and Pathology," *Boston Medical and Surgical Journal* 1875; 92: 29.

anatomy that lends the femur neck much of its strength: the calcar femorale (also referred to as Bigelow's septum and sometimes called a femoral spur or *der Schenkelsporn*, as it was dubbed by Merkel in 1874). The calcar femorale is a thickened posteromedial plate of cancellous bone that extends distally from the distal femoral neck, anterior to the lesser trochanter, to the posteromedial aspect of the proximal femoral shaft. It is on the compression side of the proximal femur and therefore supports high compressive loads, for example, when weight bearing while walking. It is difficult to visualize.

SKILLED SURGEON AND EXPERT IN INSTRUMENTATION

Bigelow was an accomplished surgeon, one who mastered his craft. According to Dr. David W. Cheever, "To see him operate was to recognize a master" (quoted in W. S. Bigelow 1894). "To an exceptional degree he had an adroit and graceful use of his hands and fingers" (W. S. Bigelow 1894). He was ambidextrous. One of Bigelow's former students described him almost as an artist:

> He stood erect and did all his cutting at arm's length. Every stroke of the knife accomplished all and no more than he intended it to accomplish. He used the belly of the knife rather than the point, drawing it with swift strokes as a violin bow is drawn. His hands never fumbled or made uncertain motions; all were direct, unerring, firm, yet delicate. He displayed perfect coordination of mind, eye and hand. Many of his operations were performed with such swiftiness [sic] and unswerving strokes as to suggest legerdemain...His delicacy of touch was remarkable. Sometimes, by merely placing his fingers on a diseased or injured part a correct diagnosis was made. (Mayo 1921)

> "A surgeon ought to be young, or at most middle aged; to have a strong and sturdy hand, never subject to tremble, and to be no less dexterous with his left hand than with his right hand; to have a quick and clear sight; to be bold, and so far devoid of pity that he may have only in view the cure of him whom he has taken in hand, and not in compassion to his cries, either make more haste than the case requires, or cut less than is necessary, but to do it all as if he was not moved by the shrieks of his patient."
> —Celsus, quoted in Bigelow's "Introductory Lecture," delivered to the Massachusetts Medical College, November 6, 1849

Mayo (1921) noted that during Bigelow's career, "surgery was almost wholly confined to the outside of the body, and thus comparatively limited in scope," but Bigelow was highly charismatic and would arrange the amphitheater to dramatic effect, enjoying "the applause of colleagues and students." According to W. S. Bigelow (1894), "As a surgical operator Dr. Bigelow possessed, unequivocally, what may be called 'style.'"

He did experience one early occupational injury that could have derailed his ability to use any instrument, and even to continue performing surgical procedures. In 1850, the same year Bigelow's son was born and when he was 32 years old, Dr. John W. Webster was on trial for the murder of Dr. George Parkman (see chapter 13). Bigelow had been with investigators when they opened the brick wall surrounding Webster's privy and had identified the body parts found there as human. However, during the trial he "was dangerously ill from a dissecting wound, –the result of an insignificant prick on the back of his hand by a scissor point, –which culminated in a severe palmar abscess. The scars of the incisions requisite for relief, and the contractions which followed, remained permanent evidence of the intensity and extent of the suppuration, though they in no degree interfered with the flexibility of his fingers, or the use of his hand" (W. S. Bigelow 1894). Had it not been for that wound, he "would have been an important witness" at Webster's trial (W. S. Bigelow 1894).

Mastery and Modification of Surgical Instruments

Bigelow's mastery seemed to extend to all surgical equipment. "He was habituated to the use of tools, and at home with every surgical instrument. He never fumbled...He always knew what he intended to do, and accomplished it with neatness...He was precise, confident, deliberate and sometimes original in method...Dr. Bigelow had the faculty of instant decision. He knew every phase of anesthesia, and if emergencies arose he was prepared for them" (W. S. Bigelow 1894). His abilities using equipment translated to finding different and better ways of applying them: "In the routine of surgical work...[he] was the originator of many better methods...His improvements of surgeon's tools were countless" (W. S. Bigelow 1894). According to Dr. Henry H. A. Beach, "There is hardly an instrument in the operating cases of the Massachusetts General Hospital which does not show some advantage gained from his [Bigelow's] working with it" (quoted in W. S. Bigelow 1894). His work with the lithotrite, which he published in the late 1870s, "reveals Bigelow's extraordinary inventive genius and mechanical conceptions" (Mayo 1921).

W. S. Bigelow (1894) listed some of the more notable instruments modified or originated by his father:

- tourniquets for thigh, arm, and wrist
- needle holders
- a sinus dilator
- handles for drills and other handheld equipment
- mouth gags
- a urethral divulsor
- retractors for amputations
- polypus forceps
- a compressor for aneurysms
- torsion instruments
- artery forceps, with a device for discharging ligatures
- autopsy tables
- an operating chair
- an apparatus for angular extension

A SURGEON NOT LIMITED IN SCOPE

Bigelow did not limit what patients he cared for or what conditions he treated, and "he was what he called a 'practicing doctor,' as well as an accoucheur and a surgeon, operating 'from one end of the body to the other, –from cataract and strabismus to club-foot and stone in the bladder'" (W. S. Bigelow 1894). His reputation—not only in surgery but in dealing with "traumatic emergencies"—throughout the Northeast brought with it many requests from other physicians and hospitals to consult on cases.

> "Given one well trained physician of the highest type and he will do better work for a thousand people than ten specialists. One tenth of each patient will be treated better by the specialist, but the nine tenths would have little or no treatment... Dr. Bigelow belonged to generation of men who developed a keen power of observation, and who with the history of a case, and their highly trained special senses accomplished wonders."
> —William J. Mayo, MD
> "In the time of Henry Jacob Bigelow" *Journal of the American Medical Association*, 1921

Treatment of Bladder Stones

In addition to his orthopaedic contributions, Bigelow published more than 25 articles on the treatment of bladder stones. For 10 years, he "worked on a method for crushing stones in the urinary bladder...eventually publishing the description of the operation in 1878" (Mayo 1921). This procedure used a lithotrite, an instrument first used by the French urologist Jean Civale in 1832 to crush bladder stones. Originally the lithotrite was small because "it was supposed that the bladder was intolerant of all instruments...the shortest possible time was occupied at a sitting, the smallest instruments used, and the fragments were left to be evacuated naturally" ("Litholopaxy and a New Lithotrite" 1896). Bigelow's redesign of the instrument "startled the medical profession and started a revolution in the surgery of the bladder" ("Litholopaxy and a New Lithotrite" 1896). Bigelow stated, "the bladder was far more tolerant of prolonged manipulation than was previously supposed, and that the temporary presence of smooth instruments in the bladder caused much less irritation than the prolonged lodgment of sharp fragments of a calculus...He used larger and stronger lithotrites...and introduced an entirely new evacuating apparatus...to remove all the calculi at one sitting" ("Litholopaxy and a New Lithotrite" 1896). This single procedure, litholapaxy, took the place of two others (lithotrity and lithotomy).

In 1883, for his discovery of this procedure, he was awarded part (6,000 francs) of the Argenteuil prize (a total of 10,000 francs) from France for the "most important improvement made in that period in the treatment of diseases of the urinary passages" (W. S. Bigelow 1894).

AN INFLUENTIAL EDUCATOR

In September 1838, four clinicians—Jacob Bigelow (Henry's father), O. W. Holmes, D. Humphries Storer, and Edward Reynolds—formed and taught at a private medical school known as the Tremont Street Medical School. It was here that Henry Bigelow "began his long career as a public teacher, being appointed its Instructor in Surgery and Chemistry in 1844"—the same year that he had begun his practice and presented his dissertation at HMS—and a year before his appointment as surgical instructor there (W. S. Bigelow 1894).

The first course he had taught was on hernias. However, "the location of the school [was] unsuited to this project, [so] Dr. Bigelow hired a small house contiguous to the Harvard Medical College in North Grove Street...The disturbing popularity of this new enterprise, beneath the very eaves of the Medical School, seemed likely to interfere with the friendly occurrence of some members of the Medical Faculty in his preferment" to succeed Dr. Hayward as professor of surgery at Harvard Medical School (W. S. Bigelow 1894). Because of this conflict, he moved the course again, this time to the Chauncey Place Infirmary. The Tremont Street Medical School closed in 1858, just 10 years after it opened.

Bigelow had been appointed professor of surgery at Harvard Medical School in 1849, though at that time he was "hardly more than established as a practitioner and hospital surgeon" (W. S. Bigelow 1894). However, "his capacity as a teacher had already been manifested...He was without a competitor for the high and honorable position...

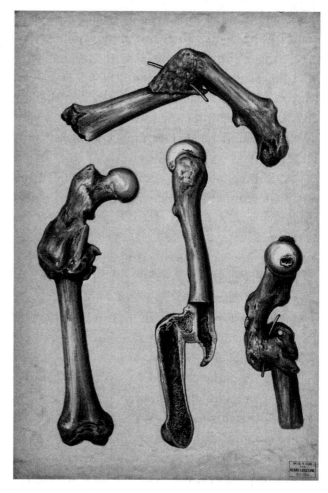

Drawing in Bigelow's illustrations, unpublished, demonstrating several different malunions of the femur. Warren Anatomical Museum in the Francis A. Countway Library of Medicine.

at the early age of thirty-one years" (W. S. Bigelow 1894). For Bigelow, nothing "is more essential to the medical student than pathologic anatomy, the cornerstone of medicine" (W. S. Bigelow 1894). When teaching, he instilled in his students the "principles underlying surgery" (W. S. Bigelow 1894). He was a compelling teacher, and hordes of students packed his lecture halls. His "power as a teacher was nowhere better exemplified than in clinical lectures...Beginning with 1845–55, Dr. Bigelow had been in the habit of demonstrating annually before his class...the usual dislocations of the hip, using...one and the same dead body for all the demonstrations" (W. S. Bigelow 1894).

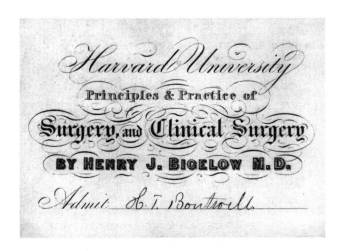

Admission ticket for Bigelow's lectures on surgery.
Courtesy of Dr. Douglas Arbitier/MedicalAntiques.com.

His lectures covered an exhaustive list of subjects, including "ligation of all the principal arteries, every form of amputation, fractures, dislocations, gun-shot and other wounds, to diseases peculiar to armies…important hygienic precautions…the peculiar duties of surgeons in the field, the professional status of the military surgeon and his relations to other departments of the service" (W. S. Bigelow 1894). Because he was speaking to practicing physicians, rather than students, he could shorten his lectures and focus on the most relevant information. For example, his lecture on wounds "was made peculiarly interesting by experiments performed in the presence of the audience…Furnished by the Adjuvant General with the various kinds of arms likely to be used, Dr. Bigelow inflicted bloodless and painless wounds on the dead body before the class…for example, of witnessing the fearful effects of the Minié ball upon the bones, crushing and completely disorganizing the large joints, where a common musket ball made a simple direct perforation" (W. S. Bigelow 1894).

At one point, Bigelow's role as teacher drew him into the theater of war. The Civil War began in 1861, and Bigelow was asked to present a course on operative surgery at MGH. Using corpses, Bigelow provided:

an exceptional wealth of demonstration [of] the peculiarities of wounds from different kinds of bullets and muskets, and the operations belonging to military surgery, were illustrated upon dead objects, and discussed in the effective way which always made his teaching noticeable…"Each lecture being from an hour and a half to two hours long…two hundred or more eager listeners…could not be drawn day after day to the college by any ordinary attraction… [but] the interest in them was sustained to the end." (W. S. Bigelow 1894)

On another occasion, General George McClellan visited MGH and attended one of Bigelow's lectures:

Few of us will forget the scene in the operating-room in the rotunda, when Dr. Bigelow introduced the popular General to the students then filling the seats, and called his attention to many interesting circumstances…As the Professor, with his native elegance of form and bearing, brightened by his enthusiasm, stood side by side with the uniformed General, who had attracted to himself the honor and hopes of a nation, one could not but compare the services to mankind rendered by the two men, and in the widely extending relief of suffering, and the rescue of thousands of lives through the brilliant far-reaching work of the Professor, find reason to accord him honors even greater than those won by the Commander-in-Chief of the Union armies. ("Reports of Societies" 1891)

In summer 1862, Bigelow briefly stepped away from his teaching endeavors when the US Secretary of War, Edwin Stanton, sent him "on a private mission…to observe and report upon the state of the medical department of General McClellan's army, then in front of Richmond [Virginia]…The nature of the report is unknown" (W. S. Bigelow 1894). While Bigelow was at McClellan's headquarters, the army began to move "from

Chickahominy [between Richmond and Williamsburg] to the James River, just previous to the Seven Days' Battle...and obliged him to fall back to the White House, which he reached barely in time to take passage on the last boat...the rebels being already at Tunstall's [Station], three miles distant...Dr. Bigelow arrived at Harrison's Landing...to hear the thunder of the battle of Malvern Hill, on June 30...After a week of desperate fighting...he returned home by way of Washington" (W. S. Bigelow 1894). As soon as he returned to Boston, he fell ill with "Chickahominy fever, a typho-malarial affection prevalent in the Army of the Peninsula, by which he was practically disabled for a year" (W. S. Bigelow 1894). The next year, in the summer of 1863, men in Massachusetts became subject to the military draft. "Bigelow's name was among those drawn. [However,] having reached the age of forty-five years in the preceding March, he was...exempt from service" (W. S. Bigelow 1894).

R. M. Hodges, speaking at a meeting of the Boston Society for Medical Improvement in 1890, listed six reasons why Bigelow had been such a successful instructor: "his graphic modes of expression, his felicitous illustrations, his clear perception of essential realities, his self-reliant audacity and indifference to conventional rules, the peculiarity of his abundant humor, and his skill in blackboard drawing." At that same meeting, David Cheever said that as "a terse, clear and epigrammatic teacher, he [Bigelow] possessed peculiar powers in extracting the wheat from the chaff of learning." W. J. Mayo (1921) remarked on Bigelow's "remarkable" ability to "[put] a subject in a nutshell": "'Gentleman,' said Dr. Bigelow, 'many pages have been written describing various more or less complicated ways of treating the shoulder after a dislocation...has been reduced. The whole thing consists of: pad in the axilla, elbow to the side, arm in a sling.'"

Bigelow took on a larger role at Harvard Medical School than only that of professor: "He was a power in its administration...Almost from the moment he entered the faculty, in 1849, he took his place as foremost in its counsels" (W. S. Bigelow 1894). He remained in that capacity throughout his time there. He resigned as professor of surgery at Harvard in 1882. Upon his retirement:

> "In recognition of his eminent services to the University and the public, Dr. Bigelow was chosen, in May last, Emeritus Professor of Surgery, and the degree Doctor of Laws was conferred upon him at the last Commencement [that of 1882]"...In parting with their colleague of thirty-three years, the Medical Faculty entered upon their records, the following minute: –
>
> "Resolved, that we recognize the great loss which this Faculty has sustained in the retirement from the Chair of Surgery of Professor Henry J. Bigelow, whose keen observation, accurate research, and rare genius in devising new and improved methods of operative procedure have done so much to render this School conspicuous, and to make American surgery illustrious throughout the world." (quoted in W. S. Bigelow 1894)

CONTROVERSY ABOUNDS

Some controversies continued to surround Bigelow throughout his career, even after his early publication on ether. He was forcefully against both women attending the medical school and vivisection, though his reasons for these oppositions are unknown. He also opposed the staff at MGH accepting fees for treating patients.

Two other main areas of contention involved Bigelow. The first was medical education reform, started at Harvard in 1869 by its new president, Dr. Charles Eliot:

> Previous to 1871 the Medical Faculty was independent as to its policy, its finances, and practically as to its official appointments. The changes introduced in that year relieved it of

these responsibilities, which were thereafter assumed by the Corporation of University. An entrance examination was instituted...a graded course was established, requiring three full years of study, with a satisfactory examination at the end of each of these years as a prerequisite...for a degree (W. S. Bigelow 1894).

Bigelow greatly influenced discussions of medical education at "a frequent succession of faculty meetings, often lasting until after midnight...His efforts to bring the President and those who followed the President to his own way of looking upon the questions at issue were determined and unrelenting" (W. S. Bigelow 1894).

> "Much of the extraordinary success of Bigelow is expressed in his happy saying, 'the wit of science,' namely, the application of the special senses, in obtaining knowledge and acting with wisdom. The wit of science not only expresses but actually reveals the science and art of medicine."
> —William J. Mayo, MD
> "In the time of Henry Jacob Bigelow"
> *Journal of the American Medical Association*, 1921

Notably, Oliver Wendell Holmes joined him in objecting to any change in medical education:

In devising a plan to raise...standard[s], he agreed with [Thomas Henry] Huxley in preferring regulations which would open to the medical student a most liberal scientific opportunity, and insist upon a competency strictly medical. He did not agree with the details of the plan drawn by his colleagues, since, in his opinion, too much stress was laid by them upon the less applicable sciences [including laboratory exercises], instead of giving more time to the study of medical sciences, especially to medical art. He anticipated that such a plan would result in a diminished attendance and diminished receipts; the immediate usefulness of the school would be impaired in accordance with the loss of numbers, and its life might be imperiled. He was ready to raise the standard of medical education, but preferred to do so gradually and with certainty, giving the best appointments to the largest numbers. (Fitz 1890)

Despite his protests, his colleagues' plan was accepted. As a result, Harvard experienced a "diminution of the number of students, [but] the finances of the school...improved" (Fitz 1890). And despite his disagreement with these changes, "Bigelow continued to labor in the Harvard Medical School with unabated devotion for ten more years" (W. S. Bigelow 1894).

The second main area of contention occurred with the development of antisepsis by Joseph Lister, which John Collins (Coll) Warren brought to MGH in 1869 (see chapter 4). In an article about Bigelow's surgical contributions published in *Clinical Anatomy* in 2011, Malenfant et al. note that Bigelow did not immediately acknowledge the benefits of aseptic techniques, nor did he use them during surgical procedures. In his article "Orthopedic Surgery and Other Medical Papers," Bigelow reiterated his original disbelief in antisepsis: "It flatters neither the vanity nor the scientific sense to exorcise an invisible enemy with something like a censer" (quoted in Malenfant et al. 2011). It took him seven years to fully "[accept] the new doctrine with most of its details" (quoted in Malenfant et al. 2011).

LEGACY

Bigelow was appointed as the first surgeon emeritus at MGH when he retired in 1882, and he was able to continue treating patients there. He accepted the position particularly because the board of trustees assured him he would retain his voting rights at staff meetings (likely related to topics such as physician payments for patient care at MGH, ethical obligations of doctors to patients and colleagues, admission policies, equipment needs, hospital obligations to patients and

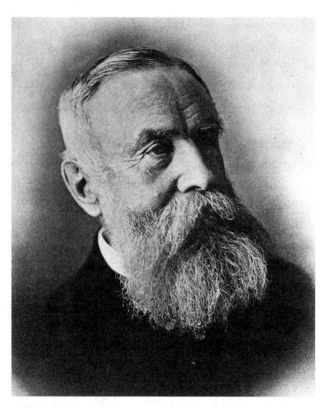

Henry J. Bigelow, age 70. *A Memoir of Henry Jacob Bigelow* by William Sturgis Bigelow. Boston: Little, Brown, and Company, 1894.

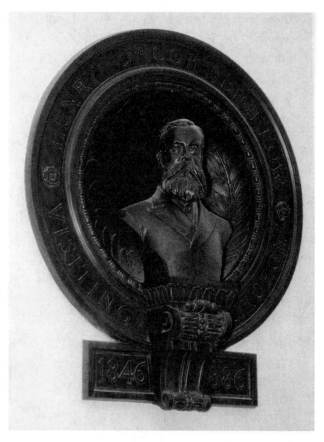

Bust of Henry J. Bigelow. Massachusetts General Hospital, Archives and Special Collections.

physicians, and staff privileges for women and minorities). However, just before making the title official, "the trustees reneged, omitting the right to attend and vote at staff meetings...This turn soured Bigelow's feelings toward MGH" (Bull and Bull 2011). He believed they did so because he was still strongly opposed to the trustees' approval of a new policy that allowed doctors to collect fees from their hospital patients.

In 1883, Bigelow was one of two emeritus professors (the other was Oliver Wendell Holmes) recognized at a dedication of a new, larger building housing five student laboratories. On behalf of ~50 donors—surgeons from MGH and Children's Hospital, close friends of Bigelow, women who had once been his patients, and numerous "surgical house-pupils" Bigelow had taught—Dr. Samuel A. Green gifted a bust of Bigelow:

> The bust is given on the condition that it shall be placed permanently in the new surgical lecture room which corresponds to the scene of Dr. Bigelow's long labors in the old building... He has taught, through his lectures, probably not fewer than 1800 students who have graduated at the School, and perhaps 7500 more who have taken their degrees elsewhere; and by these thousands of physicians now scattered throughout the land...Dr. Bigelow is remembered as most eminently a practical teacher... he always had the happy faculty of imparting to his students a kindred spirit and zeal. *Haud inexpertus loquor*. (Green quoted in "The Celebration" 1883)

According to the biography written by his son, Bigelow remained a busy man during his retirement:

> He could do nothing important without putting his whole heart into it...He was not a

great talker, but he was companionable and humorous, and had a lively disposition, which made people like to listen to him…[He] was seldom unoccupied or idle…The extraordinary, the eccentric, and above all the surprising, had a peculiar fascination for Dr. Bigelow.

These were the elements which made jugglery attractive, and…the secret of his fondness for the amusing, ingenious, but never malicious, practical jokes which he occasionally perpetrated on some intimate friend…
(W. S. Bigelow 1894)

Box 30.4. Bigelow, The Man

In his father's biography, William Sturgis Bigelow (1894), described his father's personal code of conduct, his passion for collecting, his deep fascination with not only the sciences but also the arts, and his love of the outdoors.

Code of Conduct

As a physician, Bigelow followed a code of conduct—"To obey the Golden Rule and to be a gentleman" (quoted in W. S. Bigelow 1894)—in relation to science, his patients, and his colleagues:

1. "The Relation of the Physician to Medical Science. –A physician should lend his influence to encourage sound medical education, and then uphold in the community correct views of the power and the limitation of medical science and art.
2. "The Relation of the Physician to his Patients. –The first duty of the practicing physician is to his patient, who has a right to expect that his disease will be thoroughly investigated and skillfully treated, with charitable consideration for his mental peculiarities or infirmities, and in a relation strictly confidential.
3. "The Relation of the Physician to other Practitioners and to their Patients. –In his relations with other medical practitioners and his patients, a physician should be governed by strict rules of honor and courtesy. His conduct should be such as, if universally imitated, would insure the mutual confidence of all medical practitioners."

Bigelow as Collector

Bigelow also was a collector:

"[He] amused himself with a study of ants…[and] possessed a superb collection of them…He converted the attic of his home in Chauncey Place into a pigeon loft, where he raised the choicest of fancy breeds…A superb talking Myna bird was long an ornament and a curiosity in Dr. Bigelow's consulting-room…[He] kept a collection of monkeys, so large that he had to hire special quarters for them…Dr. Bigelow was the owner of choice bric-à-brac and many curiosities."

Passion for the Arts

Bigelow appreciated not only science but also art:

"He was extremely fond of music [and had in his collection Edison's first phonograph]…[His] most of abiding and enthusiastic delight, however, came from pictures…[especially] in the works of the old masters [even though he was color blind]…As an expert in the art of picture restoration, and for the mere pleasure of cleaning them, Dr. Bigelow liked to buy old and dingy pictures at auction…[This knowledge] led to his appointment as one of the first trustees of the Boston Museum of Fine Arts, an office which he held until his death."

Devoted to the Outdoors

Bigelow spent much of his time outdoors, particularly in the sport of shooting, which he loved:

"Except during the latter part of his life, he devoted several weeks of every year to this sport…[He] made his own decoys…[and] constructed an instrument to imitate the quacking of ducks…He bred shooting dogs, –pointers, and especially the famous breed of Currituck retrievers, commonly known as "Chesapeakes" [sic]…The sheep commons of Nantucket had long been familiar to Dr. Bigelow…[He became] the owner of a considerable part of Tuckernuck, an island West of Nantucket [which was] inhabited…only by a few families of fisherman…[He] built himself a rough house on the extreme Western point [where] he usually spent eight or ten weeks of unconventional outdoor life."

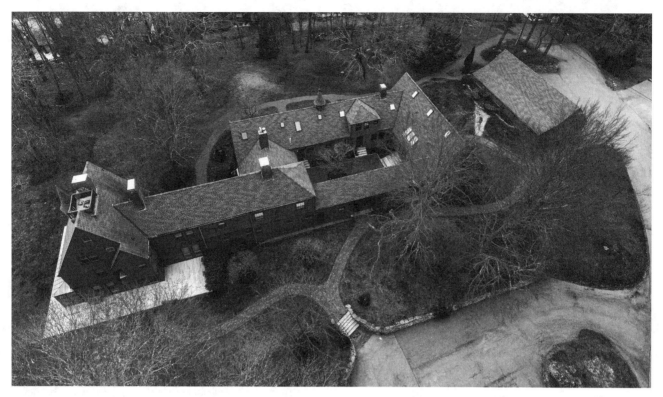

Bigelow's home at 72-80 Ober Road. Oak Hill Village, Newton, MA. Listed in National Register of Historic Places in 1976.
Kael E. Randall/Kael Randall Images.

He had led a rich life occupied by diverse interests and guided by his own highly articulated moral philosophy (see **Box 30.4**). Bigelow continued to be active in his pursuit of such learning and experiences well into his retirement years. He slowly began giving up his practice, and he retreated to his "country seat," called Oak Hill, in Newton, Massachusetts. However, he was not a vigorous man—having overcome several early illnesses—or known "to be watchful to keep himself well" (W. S. Bigelow 1894). According to his son, he "had been deeply afflicted by the circumstances attending his resignation at the Massachusetts General Hospital and was never the same afterward. They…aged him in the eyes of his friends" (W. S. Bigelow 1894).

Throughout his career, Bigelow had been an active member of the Massachusetts Medical Society, serving as its treasurer from 1823 to 1828 and its president from 1842 to 1847. Bigelow's son, William Sturgis Bigelow, mentioned in his father's biography that the elder Bigelow also was a member of a committee of the councilors of that society that prepared a code of ethics for its members. He was a long-time member of the Boylston Medical Society, serving as its president in 1845, and of the American Academy of Arts and Sciences and the Boston Society for Medical Improvement. He also held membership in the American Medical Association and in 1865 chaired its committee on arrangements; in that role he gave the welcoming address at the end of the Civil War.

Bigelow gave his last public presentation, "An Old Portrait of a Surgeon," to the Boston Society for Medical Improvement in 1889. In it, he discussed a painting that had been on display at the Boston Society for Medical Improvement for almost 40 years. Bigelow believed the portrait was of Ambrose Paré, a sixteenth-century surgeon who treated kings of France, but extensive investigation revealed that the man in the portrait was actually "Françoise Hérard, a French surgeon of eminence who died in the year 1862" (W. S. Bigelow 1894).

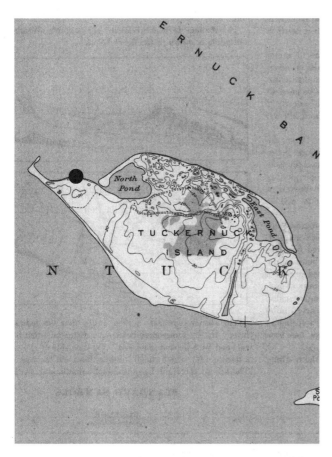

Map of Tuckernuck Island. Ca. 1944. Dot represents location of Bigelow's House.
U.S. Geological Survey, 1944, USGS 1:31680-scale Quadrangle for Tuckernuck Island, MA 1944: U.S. Geological Survey.

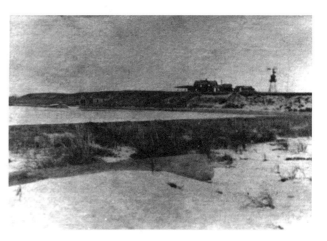

Henry J. Bigelow's house on Tuckernuck Island. Courtesy of the Nantucket Historical Association, P11853.

In 1890, while returning to Oak Hill, the carriage in which he rode overturned. He sustained a head injury, which caused "a long sickness," though he did not die from it. Instead, after the accident, "a bad cold was succeeded by an attack of gastric pain from which he never recovered… For several days before he died he took nothing but water" (W. S. Bigelow 1894). Bigelow's son notes that his father was convinced he had pyloric stenosis; this self-diagnosis was proof that "his

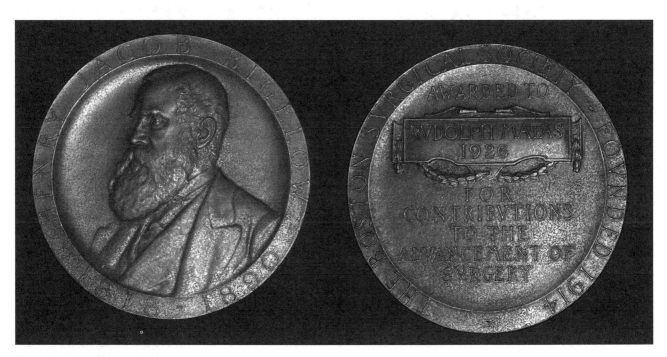

Example of the Bigelow Medal. B. Bernard Weinstein Medal Collection, Tulane University Digital Library.

mind remained bright and clear until very near the close of life" (W. S. Bigelow 1894). Bigelow died on Thursday, October 30, 1890. Autopsy revealed that Bigelow had correctly identified his condition: "a non-malignant thickening of the pyloric orifice of the stomach" (W. S. Bigelow 1894). He was buried in Middlesex County, Massachusetts, at Mount Auburn Cemetery. Many heartfelt memorials were written about Bigelow after his death. Six such remembrances are included in **Box 30.5**.

In 1921, the Boston Surgical Society, with funds donated by Bigelow's son, William Sturgis Bigelow, began to award a solid gold medal embossed with Bigelow's likeness in honor of an internationally recognized leading surgeon. The first recipient was Dr. William J. Mayo, cofounder of the Mayo Clinic. (As of the year 2019, the Boston Surgical Society had awarded 33 Bigelow medals.) In 1937, after receiving his Bigelow Medal, Dr. Edward W. Archibald, of Montreal,

Box 30.5. Posthumous Commemorations of Bigelow's Life

From the Medical Board of MGH

"It was resolved, that the hospital has lost a friend, whose interest in its success as a great charity was ever active and devoted; that through his extraordinary skill in operating and teaching, and the rare, judicial character of his investigations in weighing the evidence of disease, standards of work have been established at the hospital that have contributed much to the advancement of the art of surgery and the comfort of the afflicted; that his accomplishments in the art of treating hip-joint dislocations and stone, now adopted throughout the civilized world, distinguish his name among the leading surgeons of his time; that the entire surgical staff, who have without exception been his pupils, tender this acknowledgment in grateful remembrance of one whose first instinct was to save. '*Si monumentum quaeris circumspice.*' Resolved, that a copy of the resolutions be transmitted to the family of Dr. Bigelow, and to the *Boston Medical and Surgical Journal*"

("Dr. Henry J. Bigelow" 1890).

From the Faculty of Harvard University Medical School

"The Medical Faculty of Harvard University desires to enter into the Records its appreciation of the eminent services rendered by the late Henry Jacob Bigelow to the Medical School, with which he was connected as Professor of Surgery and Professor of Surgery, Emeritus, for more than forty years. Remarkably gifted by nature, his talents were made unusually productive and useful by his intense devotion to the work of the moment, only ceasing with the successful accomplishment of the task. His lectures were models of condensed thought and applied knowledge, and were delivered with an aptness of diction and a richness of illustration which made them ever memorable. As a member of the Faculty he was distinguished for the ripeness of his judgment, the wisdom of his conclusions, and the clearness and force of his arguments. Whether as advocate or opponent he was sure to add new light to the subjects under discussion, and was always to be recognized as a leader of men. His late and last communication to this Faculty showed a benevolent and beneficient [sic] interest in the continued welfare of the School"

("Memorial" 1890).

From the Boston Society for Medical Improvement

"Resolved, that the Boston Society for Medical Improvement desires to record its sense of the loss sustained in the death of its most distinguish member, HENRY JACOB BIGELOW. Possessed of unusual surgical perception, quick insight, great technical skill and dexterity, clearness and directness as a teacher and writer, he added to these the qualities of leadership, an unusual intelligence, and an indomitable persistency in whatever investigations he undertook. His achievements have won for him a place among the foremost surgeons of his time, and his works have benefited humanity. Resolved, that a copy of this record be sent to the family of Dr. Bigelow and to the *Boston Medical Journal*"

("Henry J. Bigelow, M.D., L.L.D." 1890).

said a few words to honor Bigelow: "His two great qualities…were untiring devotion to his patients and his reluctance to give pain. Dr. [Richard M.] Hodges said that his tenderness toward children was always noticeable, while his gentleness with dumb animals found its complete expression in a 'strenuous opposition to repetitive, unavailing or incompetent vivisection…No suffering invalid ever found him rough or thought him brusque'" (E. W. Archibald 1937).

> "It belongs to the members of the Medical Profession who have specially devoted themselves to surgery to tell the story of achievements of one whom all have recognized as a great master in that branch of the healing art. The name of H. J. Bigelow is identified with two most important innovations in surgical practice."
>
> —Oliver Wendell Holmes
> "Manuscript of the Tribute to the Memory of Dr. Henry Jacob Bigelow," November 4, 1890

From the Surgical Section of the Suffolk District Medical Society

"Resolved, that we feel that by the death of Dr. Henry Jacob Bigelow the surgical profession in America has lost its brightest star. His acute discernment and inventive genius made contributions to the surgical art which have put mankind deeply in his debt, and have won the undisguised admiration of his peers through all countries. We, his associates and scholars, know, too, his inspiration is a teacher, whose genius so illuminated his subject, that what might have been dry detail was endowed with interest and fixed indelibly in the memory. Conscious of the high gifts and genius of Dr. Bigelow, we wish to place upon our records a mark of our appreciation of what he was, and what we owe him"

("Memorial" 1890).

From the Trustees of MGH:

"The brilliant contributions of the late Dr. Henry J. Bigelow to surgical science entitle him to rank with the great surgeons of the world, and it is especially appropriate that the Massachusetts General Hospital should perpetuate the remembrance of his service of forty years upon its surgical staff, a service which contributed so much to the relief of human suffering, and gave the hospital a wide-spread renown. It was here, in 1846, that, with enthusiasm and courage, he took a leading part in the first demonstration of the anaesthetic property of sulfuric ether, a discovery which later made possible his method of reducing the dislocation of the hip-joint, and again his ingenious treatment by litholapaxy. It is no exaggeration to say that these improvements in surgery have made his name illustrious among the benefactors of mankind. It is therefore, voted: (1) That in the operating-room of the hospital be hereafter designated as "Henry J. Bigelow Operating Theatre," and the resident physician is instructed to have this name inscribed upon its walls. (2) That the Secretary be instructed to communicate the foregoing vote to Dr. William S. Bigelow, with the request that he will allow the trustees to have made a copy of one of the portraits of his father, to be placed in the Henry J. Bigelow Operating Theatre, in order that the pupils of the medical school in coming years may be stimulated by his achievements to a more thorough devotion to the noble profession which they have chosen to make their own"

("Report" 1890).

From the Indian Medical Gazette:

"India is under a special debt of gratitude to this great American surgeon. "It is to Bigelow, and to him alone, that we owe the great beneficent innovation of litholapaxy, or lithotrity at one sitting, and India, in many parts of which stone is so prevalent, promises to profit by it in a very special manner…Those who have read this Journal for the last ten years need not be told how great and good an intervention this was"

("A Tribute" 1891).

CHAPTER 31

Charles L. Scudder

Strong Advocate for Accurate Open Reduction and Internal Fixation of Fractures

Charles "Charlie" Locke Scudder was born to the Reverend Evarts Scudder and Sarah Patch Lamson Scudder on August 7, 1860, in Kent, Connecticut. He was named after both his father's father (Charles) and his mother's maternal family name (Locke). He was raised an only child in an idyllic neighborhood in Great Barrington, Massachusetts. An industrious child, he won a silver spoon for his chickens at the cattle show at 10 years of age and studiously learned Greek, Latin, French, and German at Williston Academy in Easthampton, Massachusetts, after he transferred from the local public school. He went on to study classical and religious studies at Yale, establishing an interest in medicine and participating in the Kappa Sigma Epsilon fraternity and the track team. After completing an additional year at Yale, he received his bachelor of philosophy in 1883 in addition to his bachelor of arts. He delivered the commencement speech and was elected into the Kappa Delta Epsilon honorary society.

Scudder continued to pursue his interest in medicine and went on to attend Harvard Medical School (HMS), where he showed an early fascination with orthopaedics and wrote a detailed study on congenital club foot. His father passed away in 1886, forcing him to borrow money and to work part-time as an assistant to Dr. Arthur Tracy Cabot, who specialized in urology but who also devised a wire splint for leg fractures. His mother

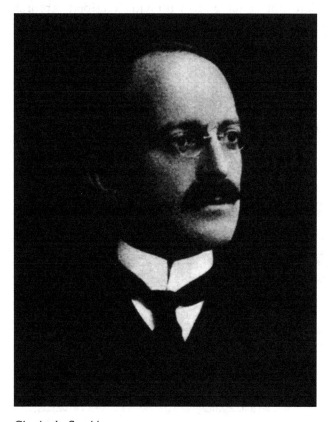

Charles L. Scudder. U.S. National Library of Medicine

Physician Snapshot

Charles L. Scudder
BORN: 1860
DIED: 1949
SIGNIFICANT CONTRIBUTIONS: Author of the seminal work *The Treatment of Fractures*; established at MGH the first fracture clinic in the United States; first chairman of the Committee on Fractures of the American College of Surgeons

was also forced to work as a house-mother in the girl's dormitory at Smith College. The following year, he received the Boylston Prize from the Boylston Medical Society of Harvard University for his research and published his article in two parts in the prestigious *Boston Medical and Surgical Journal*. In the first, he described the pathological findings that he found while dissecting three club feet in two fetuses (one bilateral), comparing his findings with those reported by previous surgeons, including Dr. William Little, a British surgeon with an equinovarus foot deformity after polio who had described cerebral palsy or spastic diplegia. Scudder also attempted a reduction of a third case of an adult club foot preserved in the Warren Museum stating, "I found it impossible…movement between the bones was blocked, and all the ligaments on the inner side of the foot were rendered tense" (Scudder 1887). In the second part of his article, he described the pathological changes in the bones in five cases:

> and in every case [he] found a marked inclination inward of the neck of the astragalus [using] the method of Parker and Shattock, of London (Scudder 1887).

He wrote:

> it is at once seen that decided differences exist at the foetal and adult extremes of life…My conclusions are: (1) The obliquity of the neck of the astragalus is greatest in cases of varus… least in adult feet. (2) A change in the obliquity of the neck of the astragalus is a part of the development of that bone…in a normal or varus foot. (3) In all probability, this obliquity of the neck of the astragalus offers greater resistance to the reduction of the deformity in [a] congenital varus or equino-varus past the first few years of life than has hitherto been supposed. (Scudder 1887)

Scudder graduated from HMS in 1888.

EARLY LIFE AND CAREER

From 1888 to 1889, Scudder was a house officer at MGH on the East Surgical Service. Because of his early interest in pediatric surgery, he worked at Boston Children's Hospital in 1889 as an assistant in clinical surgery, a position he held until 1893. Scudder quickly established a successful practice at MGH beginning in 1891 and soon confidently wrote to his creditor that "When this is paid I shall be the happiest man in Boston… free from all indebtedness and stand[ing] on my own feet" (quoted in Clark 2017). A pivotal year, Scudder was appointed surgeon to the outpatient department at Massachusetts General Hospital (MGH), where he would remain until 1903. He was described by colleagues at MGH as careful, energetic, and ubiquitously busy, never smiling or having time for banter. He would go on to become known as a meticulous surgeon who always wore white cotton gloves during every operation.

He established a relationship with Dr. John Collins (Coll) Warren at MGH, and it was both Warren and Cabot who would further influence his interest in orthopaedics. Scudder remembered "watching with awe" when Warren relieved a

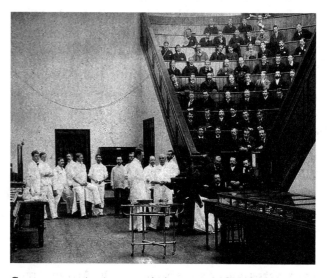

Case presentation in an amphitheater at MGH. Scudder is seated alone in first row. Ca. early twentieth century.
Massachusetts General Hospital, Archives and Special Collections.

compartment syndrome in a patient by surgically opening a closed leg fracture (quoted in Clark 2017). During the five years after graduation from HMS, Scudder published 40 articles, seven of which were on orthopaedics (six on pediatric orthoapedics and one on trauma). In 1894, he published a description of Warren's 24 abdominal operations, during which time Scudder had worked as Warren's assistant. Scudder's first major publication related to trauma was published in 1895 and included descriptions of three cases of laparotomy for penetrating abdominal injuries. He had also quickly developed an interest and expertise in general surgery—much like other surgeons of the time—as demonstrated by his first successful removal of a carotid body tumor and his advocacy for early surgical repair of pyloric stenosis.

During this transformative period of his life, he also married Abigail Taylor Seelye, who was the daughter of the president of Smith College (where his mother had worked as a house mother). Abigail was a musician and an amateur singer. She would eventually have to decrease her performances after developing a severely disabling cardiac condition. They had two children together and frequented a summer home on Little Cranberry Island near Mount Desert Island, Maine.

TREATMENT OF FRACTURES

By 1898, Dr. Scudder had begun to speak authoritatively on fractures, and he published a report on the surgical treatment of bilateral patellar fractures (see **Case 31.1**). In 1889, he was appointed demonstrator in clinical apparatus at HMS, which he held until 1893. He was also appointed assistant in clinical surgery from 1890 until 1903.

The chairman of the Surgical Section of the Suffolk District Medical Society asked Scudder to discuss the new concept of open treatment of fractures in 1900. During his presentation, Scudder said:

With permission of the visiting surgeons of the Massachusetts General Hospital, I have obtained the results of fractures [153 cases] of the bones of the lower extremity, after varying periods of time have elapsed [2-½ years –24-½ years]…In conclusion, the ideal result to be aimed at after fracture is union…without deformity and without impairment of the function of the limb, either immediately or remotely. The generally accepted methods of treating fractures do not give satisfactory results in many cases [as also shown by Frank Hamilton in 1855; see chapter 3]. There is need for a radical departure in the treatment of closed fractures [and] under [current] circumstances [with anesthesia, use of x-rays and antisepsis], it is fair to state that closed fractures should be treated by open incision and internal fixation, when other methods failed to secure reduction and immobilization. The open method will then be used more and more in oblique fractures of the diaphysis of long bones; in complicated fractures about joints; in all fractures associated with injury to nerve trunks, with injury to great blood-vessels, and associated with threatening gangrene. (C.L. Scudder 1900)

Later that same year, he published his most important and influential work, *The Treatment*

Original Articles.

THE OPEN OR OPERATIVE TREATMENT OF FRESH FRACTURES; IS IT EVER JUSTIFIABLE?[1]

WITH AN ANALYSIS OF THE RESULTS OF THE PRESENT METHODS OF TREATMENT IN ONE HUNDRED AND FIFTY-THREE FRACTURES OF THE LOWER EXTREMITY.

BY CHARLES L. SCUDDER, M.D., BOSTON.
Surgeon to the Massachusetts General Hospital, Out-Patient Department; Assistant in Clinical and Operative Surgery, Harvard University.

Title of Scudder's article in which he argues for open reduction and internal fixation of fractures if closed methods fail to maintain a stable and satisfactory reduction. *Boston Medical and Surgical Journal* 1900; 142: 289.

Case 31.1. Bilateral Comminuted Patellar Fractures

1. "B. B., male, forty-four years old, married, fell September 23, 1896, to the sidewalk from a second-story window. An examination immediately afterward found a compound comminuted fracture of the right patella, with wide separation of the fragments. The wound in the soft parts was about one-third of an inch long. The knee-joint was distended by much fluid. The left patella was also comminuted, but there was no wound of the soft parts. The fragments were small, numerous and widely separated. There was comparatively little fluid in this joint.

"Under ether anesthesia the following operation was done.

"Left Knee. —A four-inch transverse incision, made below the patella, opened the joint. The patella was broken into so many small pieces that all the fragments were removed. Little fluid was found in the joint, there having been a very slight hemorrhage following the fracture. The patella tendon and the quadriceps fascia were sutured across the front of the joint with six silk-worm-gut sutures. A small wick of gauze was left in each side of the joint, and the skin was sutured with silkworm gut. The joint, before being closed, was flushed with sterile water.

"Right Knee. —The compound wound was enlarged each way to the sides of the joint. The fragments were exposed, the joint opened and thoroughly flushed with 1 to 10,000 corrosive-sublimate solution and then with boiled water. Three of the fragments were of such size and so well attached that they were sutured with silk sutures. The other smaller fragments were removed. The skin was sutured with silkworm gut. One small wick of gauze was left at one end of the incision.

"After Treatment. —Both knees were immobilized upon posterior wires splints, with wooden side splints and straps, and aseptic-dressings applied. Three days later all wicks were removed. One week later all sutures in the skin were removed. Plaster-of-Paris splints were applied to each leg. Four weeks later the plaster was removed from the right leg. A flannel bandage was applied from the toes to the groin. A few days later the plaster was removed from the left leg and a flannel bandage was applied.

"About seven weeks from the operation, passive motion was gently made at both knees. Union was firm of the sutured fragment of the right knee. Nine weeks from the operation the patient was discharged from the hospital with crutches, wearing flannel bandages upon both knees.

"One year and four months after the operation the condition of the knees is as follows: Firm union of the right-knee fragments. Useful motion to a right angle. No pain. Practically no disability. As strong as ever. The left knee presents, in the entire absence of the left patella, a curiously flattened appearance. Motion of the left knee is slightly beyond a right angle. There are two little nodules of bone just under the skin near the outer side of the left knee. These are probably bits of bone left at the time of the operation, which if pressed upon are slightly sensitive. Otherwise the left knee is functionally as strong as if there were present a natural and normal patella."

(Charles L. Scudder 1898)

of Fractures, which he dedicated to Cabot. In the preface, he wrote that "anesthesia, antisepsis, and the Röntgen ray are making the knowledge of fractures more exact and their treatment less complicated." He was assisted by two recent HMS graduates in the writing of the book, Dr. Ernest Amory Codman (see chapter 34) and Dr. Frederic Jay Cotton (see chapter 59), the first took an early interest in imaging and the second was a talented medical illustrator. Codman's chapter, titled "The Röntgen Ray and Its Relation to Fractures," was included in all editions of Scudder's book except the 10th and 11th editions, published in 1926 and 1938, because Scudder believed that an introduction to the use and benefits of the use of x-rays was no longer needed. X-rays had become such a necessary element in the management of fractures that its use was included in all chapters. Codman, who was the first skiagrapher for Boston Children's Hospital, had produced an unpublished

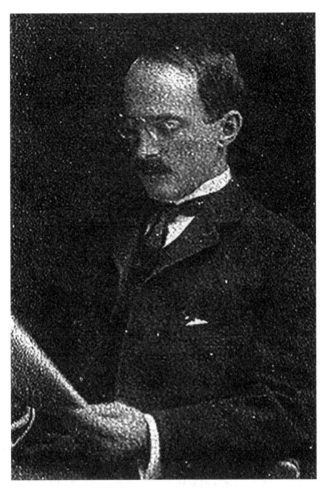

Charles L. Scudder. Courtesy of Charles S. K. Scudder and the Scudder Association.

Title page of Scudder's book, *The Treatment of Fractures*. Photo by the author.

book of photographs of x-rays of all bones in the skeleton which is kept in the archives of the Countway Medical Library. He wrote:

> On January 23, 1896, Röntgen read his announcement of the discovery of the x-rays before the Physico–medical Society at Wurzburg. The extraordinary news fled over the world in an incredibly short time. Within a few months skiagraphs of the bones of the hands appeared in every newspaper that could afford an illustration…The X-ray department has become a necessity in every large general hospital…
>
> Many people confuse an x-ray picture with a photograph. They take it to be a photograph by x-ray light. It is not a photograph, but a shadow-picture…made by the light that has passed through the hand, and shows a chart of the different densities of the different constituents of the hand, as bone, muscle, fat, and skin…As far as we know, the effects of the x-rays are only obtainable in the immediate neighborhood of their course…It is commonly said that the x-ray is dangerous to the patient and burns the skin and destroys the hair. This is true as a possibility, but nowadays is only to be feared in connection with gross ignorance and carelessness…Danger to the hands of the operator of the apparatus is quite another matter, for repeated exposure may produce the same condition…Physicians who are called upon to use the fluoroscope often should wear rubber gloves to protect the hands…

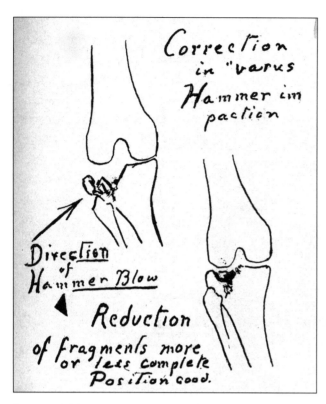

Example of Cotton's drawing in Scudder's book. Impaction of a displaced lateral tibial plateau fracture with a rubber mallet.
The Treatment of Fractures, 11th ed., by Charles L. Scudder. Philadelphia and London: W. B. Saunders, 1938. Courtesy of Charles S. K. Scudder and the Scudder Association.

Conclusions expressing the views of the American Surgical Association upon the medicolegal relations of x-rays; adopted in May, 1900.

1. The routine employment of the x-ray in cases of fracture is not at present (1900) of sufficient definite advantage to justify the teaching that it should be used in every case…

2. In the regions of the base of the skull, the spine, the pelvis and the hips, the x-ray results have not as yet been thoroughly satisfactory…

3. As to the questions of deformity, skiagraphs alone, without expert surgical interpretation, are generally useless and frequently misleading…

4. It is not possible to distinguish after recent fractures between cases in which perfectly satisfactory callus has formed and cases which will go on to nonunion…

5. The evidence as to x-ray burns seems to show that in the majority of cases they are easily and certainly preventable…

6. In the recognition of foreign bodies, the skiagraph is of the greatest value…

7. It has not seemed worth while to attempt a review of the situation from the strictly legal standpoint…

8. The technicalities of its production, the manipulation of the apparatus, etc., are already in the hands of specialists, and with that subject also it has not seemed worth while to deal. But it is earnestly recommended that the surgeon should so familiarize himself with the appearance of skiagraphs, with their distortions, with the relative values of their shadows and outlines, as to be himself the judge of their teachings, and not to depend upon the interpretation of others. (E. A. Codman 1902)

After 12 years as surgeon in the outpatient department at MGH, Scudder was appointed visiting surgeon at MGH where he served 1903–1914. In 1907, he had been appointed lecturer in surgery at HMS, where he taught until 1913, and later associate in surgery from 1913 until 1916. He also served as chief of service (fracture) on the East Surgical Service at MGH from 1914 to 1920. Scudder was asked to give the "Oration in Surgery" to the Ohio State Medical Association in 1915, "The Operative Treatment of Fractures." In this lecture, Scudder argued strongly for open reduction and internal fixation of fractures to prevent limb deformities and to provide fracture stability. This approach would allow for early motion and muscle function. He wrote:

Charles L. Scudder

Several important events have profoundly influenced the treatment of fractures. The introduction of ether in 1846 made possible painless attempts at the setting of fractures. About twenty-five years later the development of asepsis assured the safe care of compound fractures. Still twenty-five years after this the Roentgen ray demonstrated...that the supposed complete reduction of a fracture was in many cases but a caricature of reduction. And again, after twenty-five years, autogenous bone grafting is affording a sure treatment for ununited fractures.

Thus, these four general factors–anesthesia ...asepsis...x-ray...and bone grafting...have had a direct bearing upon the development of fracture treatment during the past seventy years...

Why are present methods of treating fractures unsatisfactory? The answer is—Because the functional results are so often poor... functional results were so poor...[because of] the faulty setting. Surgeons were not acutely aroused by this disclosure of the x-ray...[but] occupied during recent years with other problems [i.e. abdominal surgery]...The study of methods for...improvement of fracture results has therefore been postponed...[with] little real interest...[by] the profession. Consequently, the results have continued poor.

Certain events have directed attention to fractures...Familiarity of the layman with x-ray plate interpretations has led the fracture patient, often improperly, to demand a better setting of the fractured bone. The admission of the x-ray plate as evidence in court has undoubtedly had a compelling influence. The Workmen's Compensation Act has directed attention to the financial loss due to fractured bone. It is necessary under the law to determine the elapsed time between the accident and the return to normal work...the economic measure of the efficiency of fracture treatment.

The esthetic standard of the past...must give place to the economic standard of early functional usefulness...the accurate record of events and conditions from...the injury to the resumption of full time work...a demand has been made upon the surgeon by the laborer and the employer...for better results following all fractures...

What are the methods available for the treatment of fractures today...the nonoperative and the operative...Few men in this country appreciate what can be accomplished by the non-operative method...it has not been employed consistently and persistently in any large group of cases...Mr. Lane, on the contrary...makes it apparent that the way to secure an anatomically perfect bone...is by operation and direct fixation of the fragments by a steel plate and screws...

I believe everything that is good and effective in both methods should be employed in the treatment of fractures...The pendulum has swung away from the traction treatment to the frequent employment of operation in fractures. Improper and unnecessary operations are being done by incompetent men...Operations upon fractured bone should only be done by surgeons of very considerable general surgery experience...

I believe that non-union of fractures, the malunion of fractures, infections with osteomyelitis associated with compound fractures, disabling and painful static conditions, stiff and painful joints near to fractures of the shafts of the long bones, –I believe that these are terminal conditions usually following an appropriate non-operative treatment... Properly applied primary operative treatment will surely eliminate many of these disastrous terminal conditions. (C. L. Scudder 1915)

Scudder believed this method of treatment was essential to avoid malfunction and deformity as well as malpractice suits, and he would devote his entire career to advocacy for accurate reduction and firm fixation of fractures.

FRACTURE CLINIC AT MGH

Scudder established The Fracture Clinic at MGH in 1917, which was the first of its kind in the United States. Scudder served as its first Chief (see **Box 31.1** for a list of other clinic chiefs), and other initial appointments included Henry C. Marble, George A. Leland, Torr W. Harmer, and Richard H. Miller. Before 1917, surgeons had treated almost all fractures with traction, manipulation, and splinting in plaster-of-Paris bandages, but this work was often shoddy or not custom fitted, and fractures were often not adequately stabilized. There was a high mortality rate as a result and remaining joint stiffness and muscle weakness in those who survived. Fracture admissions were rotated among the MGH wards (East and West Surgical Services as well as the Orthopaedic Service).

In London, England, Sir Arbuthnot Lane led the way in the consideration of surgical treatment as a primary treatment method for long-bone fractures. His most significant setback (infection) was due to "dirty surgery," which Scudder rectified by always wearing white cotton gloves over the top of his surgical gloves and using Lane's "no touch" technique. Meanwhile, Dr. William O'Neill Sherman pioneered the surgical approach

Box 31.1. Fracture Clinic Chiefs and Associate Chiefs at MGH

Fracture Chiefs
- Dr. Charles L. Scudder (1917–1920)
- Dr. Daniel F. Jones, general surgeon (1920–1929)
- Dr. Henry C. Marble, general surgeon (chief 1929–1940)
- Dr. Arthur W. Allen, general surgeon (1940–1947)
- Dr. Edwin F. Cave (1947–1957)
- Dr. Otto E. Aufranc (1957–1967)

Associate Fracture Chiefs
- Dr. Nathaniel Allison, orthopaedic surgeon (1924–1930)
- Dr. Philip D. Wilson (1930–1934)
- Dr. George W. Van Gorder 1934–1940)
- Dr. Marius Smith-Petersen (1940–1947)

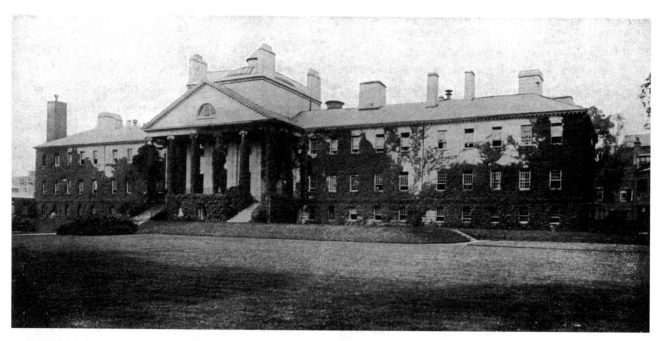

MGH—Bulfinch with East and West Wings, 1938. Massachusetts General Hospital, Archives and Special Collections.

for long-bone fractures in the United States. Prior to his work and until approximately 1915, fracture management had followed conservative techniques. Sherman was opinioned and had a great deal of experience from his work as surgeon to the Carnegie Steel Company in Pittsburgh, Pennsylvania. He shared his knowledge of surgical treatment at MGH during visits to Wards E and A thanks to the efforts of Scudder, who had established the Fracture Committee of the American College of Surgeons in 1922 which promoted knowledge sharing—improving fracture care throughout the United States.

In his book, *Lest We Forget*, Dr. Carter Rowe stated that Dr. Robert Osgood assisted Scudder in establishing the fracture clinic. However, Osgood had traveled to Europe in the US Army Medical Corps that same year in May of 1917. He didn't return to MGH until 1919, when he was promoted to chief of the orthopaedic service (see chapter 19). Osgood would later lead the effort in end-result studies of fractures and assist in postgraduate teaching of fracture management with general surgeons and Drs. Z. B. Adams, and Philip D. Wilson from the orthopaedic service.

Before stepping down as chief, Scudder kept to a busy schedule. He was asked to serve on the MGH Board of Consultants (a position he held from 1920 until 1931), appointed assistant professor of surgery and member of the advisory board of graduate instruction at HMS between 1916 and 1920, and appointed acting dean of the School of Graduate Medicine at HMS between 1918 and 1919. He stepped down as fracture chief in 1920, but he continued to practice, revise his book, and remain active in professional organizations. His guidance and recommendations for fracture care—as learned in the fracture clinic and from his professional commitments—was continually improved and updated in his frequent book revisions. We can gain deeper insight into his vision and leadership from his presentation to the American surgical Association in 1921. He was a strong advocate for accurate open reduction and internal fixation of fractures and argued that the treatment of fractures may be improved:

1. By an organized fracture service in each of the large hospitals of the country;

    (a) Special wards should be used for men, women and children, and only fracture cases admitted…

    (b) A special fracture personnel should be in charge of these fracture wards…

    (c) This continuous control should include the Out-Patient Service, where the ambulatory cases are received and treated…

    (d) The emergency ward or accident service, in so far as fractures are concerned, should likewise be under the direct care of the Chief of the Fracture Service…

    (e) An operating plant in connection with the House Service is essential. The operative fractures must be kept apart from septic operations. Separate instruments must be employed. (f) A lecture room with easy access to the wards is necessary…

2. By adequate instruction of the undergraduate medical student.

3. By instituting smaller hospital units in towns adjacent to and remote from large centres…

4. By the graduate instruction of the general practitioner interested in fractures.

5. Through the formal instruction of medical students intending to specialize in this branch of surgery…

6. By encouraging the specialization within general surgery of the surgery of fractures…The establishing of a specialty of fracture surgery or of traumatic surgery in our larger centres should conduce to (a)

better service to the community and (b) a more rapid advance in the knowledge of the treatment of special fractures.

7. By the organization of a Clinical Surgical Fracture Society meeting once a year for the sole discussion of fracture problems. The membership in such an organization should be carefully safeguarded. (C. L. Scudder 1921)

Many important advancements occurred at the clinic. In 1925, Dr. Marius Smith-Petersen designed the thin, triflanged nail there, which was used to treat femoral neck fractures. It initially caused some reactions due to corrosion of the nails, but this was later improved upon by developments both in surgical technique and in the metals used. The hospital supported the clinic by providing free annual follow-up examinations and x-rays on all patients at one year following injury. This support for the fracture clinic was discontinued after about 10 years and was replaced by tuition raised from future fracture courses.

In 1928, the first Fracture Course was instituted at MGH, which would become an annual signature aspect of the clinic until World War II. It was originally two weeks in duration but later reduced to a single week. The first course was well attended by 134 physicians. Although it ceased during World War II, it resumed:

in 1947 under Dr. Cave's inspiration and continued for several years...An interesting and unusual result of the concentration on fractures and orthopaedics at the General was Dr. Philip Wilson's book, Management of Fractures and Dislocations, published in 1938 after he went to New York, based on 4,390 fractures treated in the Fracture Clinic while he was on the staff at the MGH. It was a remarkable exposition of the treatment of trauma between the years 1923–1930 with follow-up study on patients, one year or more, according to Dr. Codman's recommendations.

A second textbook (Cave) was produced by the request of the post-graduate students who had taken the fracture courses (over 1500 from every state in the union and from ten foreign countries). Dr. Cave completed this text in 1958 (Fractures and Other Injuries) with the help of thirty-nine contributors [at MGH]. (C. R. Rowe 1996)

That book was revised in 1974 by Drs. Cave, John Burke, and Robert Boyd; titled *Trauma Management*. The editors dedicated the book to the senior editor, Dr. Cave, who had continued to serve an integral role despite personal struggle with illness. An additional educational product from the Fracture Clinic was the "Fracture of the Month" series published in the *Journal of the American Medical Association* (ca. 1960–1971). (See Aufranc, chapter 40.)

After World War II, all fractures except those in the skull were treated by the Orthopaedic Service rather than the East or West Surgical Wards. The Fracture Ward Service was discontinued in 1967, and all patients with fractures have since been treated in the orthopaedic clinics and on the hospital's orthopaedic wards.

LEADERSHIP WITH THE AMERICAN COLLEGE OF SURGEONS BOARD OF REGENTS

In May 1922, not long after Scudder's retirement as chief from the fracture clinic, he reported the improved outcomes of patients with fractures treated operatively at MGH. He presented these outcomes at a meeting of the American College of Surgeons Board of Regents. In response, the regents formed its first fracture committee to be led by Dr. Scudder. The board declared:

Be it resolved that a committee be appointed to formulate a plan of action [fracture management] to present to the Board of Regents...that this committee shall be comprised of the following: Dr. Charles L. Scudder [chairman], Dr. Joseph A. Blake, Dr. William Darrach, Dr. William O'Neill Sherman, Dr. Robert B. Osgood, Dr. Kellogg Speed, Dr. Ashley F. C. Ashurst, Dr. William L. Estes, Dr. George W. Hawley.

(quoted in M. J. Wayne 2017)

In the Committee on Fracture's first report the following year, Scudder declared the state of fracture treatment in the United States and Canada to be subpar and in need of drastic improvement. The committee continued to meet annually, and its greatest accomplishment was its many publications. The original committee eventually merged with the Committee on Industrial Injuries to form the Committee on Trauma in 1949. Scudder's early committee work included detailing their efforts to standardize equipment, documentation, and education at the New England Surgical Society's meeting in 1925. He stated there that fractures were "the most neglected subject in surgery today...a disgrace...surprisingly shocking" At the time, over 60 percent of all malpractice cases across the United States were for fracture cases.

> The results of fracture treatment in the United States and Canada are deplorably bad.
> —Charles L. Scudder, 1923

Each year at the annual meeting of the American College of Surgeons there is the Scudder Oration on Trauma (initially named the Oration on Fractures). Philip D. Wilson gave the oration in 1932, Henry C. Marble in 1948, Otto J. Hermann (Boston City Hospital) in 1949, and Edwin F. Cave in 1963. In the first of these orations in 1929, Scudder described the current state of practice stating:

- patient records were often incomplete or inaccurate
- there was a lack of understanding about the risks and types of possible workplace injuries
- surgeons increasingly saw complex and often comminuted fractures, especially around joints
- there was a lack of education on bone healing even while the art of orthopaedic surgery advanced
- there was a dearth of education on the biomechanics of fractures, the effect of muscles deforming the fracture site, and methods to reduce certain fracture
- advocacy for open reduction and internal fixation of fractures by surgeons trained in the treatment of fractures was important

In 1931, Scudder was named Honorary Surgeon at MGH and his committee published, "The

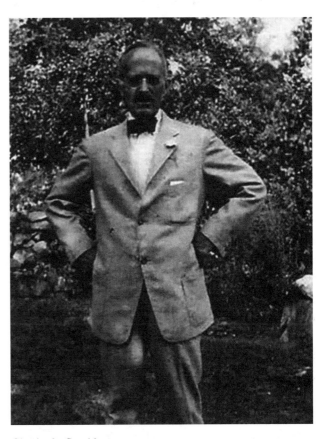

Charles L. Scudder. Courtesy of Charles S. K. Scudder and the Scudder Association.

Principles and Outline of Fracture Treatment" in the *Bulletin of the American College of Surgeons.* After reviewing the normal process of bone repair, the committee outlined the general principles of the treatment of fractures, from initial first aid to conservative measures of early closed reduction by manipulation or traction and cast immobilization to open reduction and internal fixation if necessary, i.e., satisfactory reduction not obtained. The committee emphasized the need for active motion to regain function and briefly reviewed the principles of treating compound fractures. In 1933, Scudder retired from leading the ACS Fracture Committee at age 72, but he continued as honorary chairman to advocate for fracture education and improved treatment outcomes.

Continuing to work as honorary chairman, Scudder worked with the committee in 1938 to organize 66 regional fracture committees within the ACS Committee on Fractures. They included 1,172 members, whose purpose was to educate surgeons and advance the care of patients with fractures. Scudder believed the efforts of these regional committees had achieved increased interest in and dedication to fracture treatment in the larger medical community, with a significant decrease in the formerly existing apathy. Examples of surgeons who were members of the Massachusetts Regional Fracture Committee included: Augustus Thorndike Jr. (CH and MGH), John D. Adams (BCH), Alexander P. Aiken (BCH), George K. Coonse (BCH), Frederic J. Cotton (BCH), Otto J. Hermann (BCH), William E. Ladd (CH), Henry C. Marble (MGH), Gordon M. Morrison (BCH), Frank R. Ober (CH), Mark H. Rodgers (MGH & BIH), James W. Sever (CH), and Joseph H. Shortell (BCH).

Scudder wasn't the same after his wife died in 1939. She had been deteriorating for several years, and he felt her loss keenly. They had shared an apple farm in Sherborn, Massachusetts, during their rich life together, but he never returned to it after her death. However, he resumed work in the outpatient department at MGH at 81 when younger surgeons were called to military service for World War II. In 1941, he published an editorial, "Compound Fractures and Wounds in War." The ACS Committee on Fractures and Other Traumas adopted several resolutions in response, including the use of appropriate debridement, early splinting and fixed traction when treating acute compound fractures. They advised against the use of tight-fitting plaster casts.

LEGACY

During Scudder's more than 50-year career, he published approximately 153 papers, of which 61 (40%) were on orthopaedics, fracture care, or reports about organizational/regional plans for fracture care. Only seven articles were about pediatric orthopaedics (in addition to his article on club feet): caries of the ankle joint and congenital dislocation of the shoulder. In addition, he published two books: *The Treatment of Fractures* and *Tumors of the Jaws.* Prior to 1900, when he published his book on fractures, Scudder had published only four articles on fractures or dislocations. From 1900 until 1915, when he published his first article on the operative treatment of fractures, he published only two articles on orthopaedic trauma (dislocation of the distal clavicle and radial nerve paralysis with humerus fractures). Most of his orthopaedic publications covered bone metastases or arthroplasty of the elbow; he spent the majority of his efforts on publishing new editions of his book on fractures.

Scudder became an enthusiastic supporter of open reduction with fixation of fractures, publishing numerous papers on operative treatment and indications for operative treatment of fractures after 1915, and then multiple reports about his efforts, as chairman of the Committee on Fractures of the American College of surgeons, on the regionalization and improvement of fracture management throughout the United States. Dr. Scudder published his last paper in 1944 at age

84, following his last presentation to the Massachusetts Medical Society, "How to Improve the Treatment of Fractures." He wrote:

> When the war is over and the younger men return from the active war front…[he urged] a real war effort [for physicians to get better results with fracture treatment]…By treating a fracture instantly, one treats the fracture alone; by treating it after delay, one treats the fracture together with its complications…Delayed treatment is dangerous, and late treatment is lamentable.

He continued by listing a series of recommendations to improve the results of fracture treatment.

Scudder was highly active in many professional organizations. In addition to those discussed, he helped found the Boston Surgical Society in 1914 (and was its first vice president), was a charter member of the New England Surgical Society, and along with Dr. Codman was made an honorary member of the American Association for the Surgery of Trauma when it was organized in 1938. He was a member of the American Medical Association, the American Board of Surgery, the American Academy of Orthopaedic Surgeons, the Society for Clinical Surgery and the American Surgical Association. Shortly before his death, he developed pneumonia from prescribed mandatory recumbency after cataract surgery. Bed rest was required after that particular surgery at the time. Ever devoted to his field, he was working on a revision of his book when he died at 89 years old on August 19, 1949.

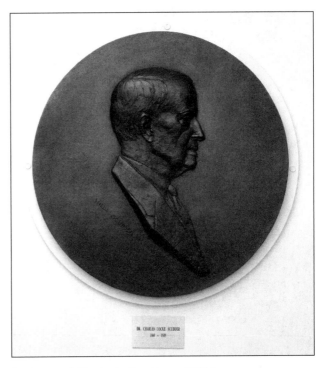

Sculpture of Charles L. Scudder at MGH. Massachusetts General Hospital, Archives and Special Collections.

CHAPTER 32

Orthopaedics Becomes a Department at MGH
Ward I

By the turn of the twentieth century, health care institutions in Boston were at the forefront of providing specialty training in orthopaedics-related knowledge and surgical techniques. The Massachusetts General Hospital (MGH) trustees had first considered creating separate departments in 1897—at that time for "nervous diseases" (see chapter 29). As the 1900s began, physician leaders at MGH began to recognize the need for another department that focused on orthopaedics and orthopaedic surgery (and that would be separate from general surgery).

The administration at MGH, however, was slower to admit this need than that at Children's Hospital, which had established its orthopaedic department in 1903. Staff at MGH began taking steps to create such a department as early as 1900. In that year, the medical board recommended to the trustees that the position of "consulting orthopaedic surgeon" be created. This was done, and Dr. Joel E. Goldthwait was duly appointed. In 1903, shortly after the opening of the new Out-Patient Department Building, the trustees voted:

> That an Out-Patient Orthopaedic Department is hereby created. That the committee on Buildings and Repairs be authorized to arrange for the establishment of the same in the new Out-Patient Building, and that the Visiting Staff be requested to transmit to the Trustees their recommendations as to the number of surgeons to be appointed and the names of suitable candidates for the position. (Washburn 1939)

Dr. Goldthwait was appointed surgeon of this Out-Patient Department on February 3, 1904. Dr. Robert B. Osgood was made assistant surgeon to outpatients, and Dr. Elisha Flagg, Dr. Max Bohm (also in charge of the Zander Room), Dr. Harry F.

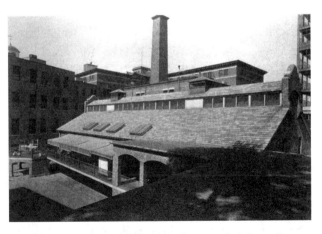

Ward I (East exposure). The veranda extended along the length of the building and was used frequently by the patients for fresh air and sunshine.

Lest We Forget: Orthopaedics at the Massachusetts General Hospital, 1900-1995 by Carter R. Rowe. Dublin, New Hampshire: William L. Bauhan, 1996. Courtesy of Bauhan Publishing.

Hartwell and Dr. Warren F. Gay were appointed assistants to the surgeon.

The new Department of Orthopaedic Surgery, however, in addition to an outpatient department or clinic, would need its own space, including patient beds, treatment rooms, and offices. After much planning, building, and fundraising—about $2 million in today's value—Goldthwait presided over the opening of this new orthopaedic ward in the newly created hospital's orthopaedic department in 1907:

> Out-Patient examining rooms, booths, and operating and waiting rooms were partitioned off in the basement on the Fruit Street end of the new [outpatient] building. Dr. Goldthwait was given permission to raise a fund for the erection of an orthopedic ward, and did raise about $70,000.
>
> This ward, called Ward I, was open November 6, 1907...The building cost approximately $40,000. The balance of the money raised was turned over to the hospital as an orthopaedic fund, the income to be used in part for research problems of the department, and the remainder for maintenance. (Washburn 1939)

As the initial funds were spent, the hospital had to begin supporting the orthopaedic ward: "The maintenance of this ward [Ward I] must be met...almost entirely by the income from the General Fund of the Hospital, as very little can be collected for board of patients because of the chronic character of the cases; for, as a rule, these patients have no earning capacity for a long period before their admission to the Hospital, and have none for some time after their discharge" ("The Resident Physician's Report for 1907," quoted in Washburn 1939). The orthopaedic ward was built new, a one-story brick building. It held 18 beds, 9 for men and 9 for women; the head of each bed was against the wall, and each bed could be surrounded by a curtain to afford some privacy. Men and women

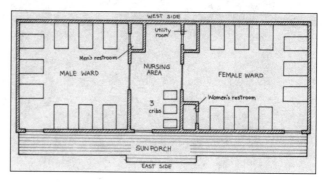

Ward I. First floor plan (1907–1940). Two wards (male and female), each contained 9 beds and were separated by the nurses' station.

Lest We Forget: Orthopaedics at the Massachusetts General Hospital, 1900-1995 by Carter R. Rowe. Dublin, New Hampshire: William L. Bauhan, 1996. Courtesy of Bauhan Publishing.

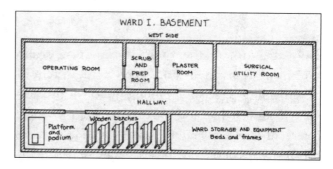

Ward I. Basement floor plan. Single operating room and a cast room were on the west side. A long conference room with wooden benches was on the east side.

Lest We Forget: Orthopaedics at the Massachusetts General Hospital, 1900-1995 by Carter R. Rowe. Dublin, New Hampshire: William L. Bauhan, 1996. Courtesy of Bauhan Publishing.

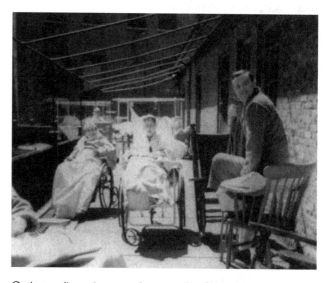

Orthopaedic patients on the veranda of Ward I.

Lest We Forget: Orthopaedics at the Massachusetts General Hospital, 1900-1995 by Carter R. Rowe. Dublin, New Hampshire: William L. Bauhan, 1996. Courtesy of Bauhan Publishing.

were treated in opposite wings. The main wings were large and well-ventilated, with high windows letting in light and air. It provided many state-of-the-art features:

- A nurse's station connecting the two treatment wings
- Four cribs for infant patients
- Lavatories
- A utility room
- A porch, where patients would sit to get fresh air
- A basement, separated into (1) a conference room with a speaker podium, seating, and demonstration tables; (2) an operating room; (3) a sterilization room; and (4) a plaster room

(**Box 32.1** describes Dr. Carter Rowe's personal experience as a resident on Ward I.)

All plasters were applied in a room in the basement of Ward I, but in 1922 the hospital

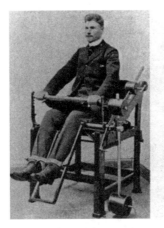
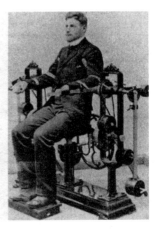

Gustav Zander's medico-mechanical equipment used to strengthen both upper and lower extremities.
Lest We Forget: Orthopaedics at the Massachusetts General Hospital, 1900-1995 by Carter R. Rowe. Dublin, New Hampshire: William L. Bauhan, 1996. Courtesy of Bauhan Publishing.

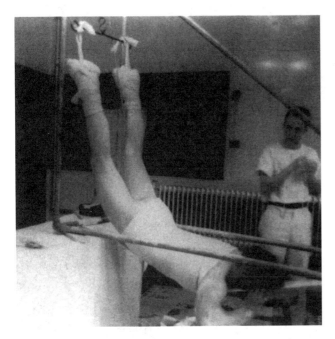

Carter Rowe (background) applying a hyperextension cast (method of Arthur G. Davis) on a patient with a fractured spine in the cast room on Ward I.
Lest We Forget: Orthopaedics at the Massachusetts General Hospital, 1900-1995 by Carter R. Rowe. Dublin, New Hampshire: William L. Bauhan, 1996. Courtesy of Bauhan Publishing.

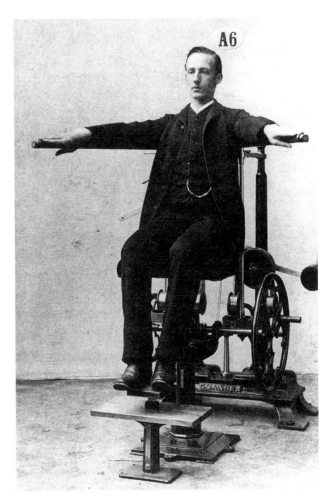

Zander's equipment was used at MGH from 1907 until the end of WWI.
Dr. G. Zander's medico-mechanische Gymnastik by Dr. Alfred Levertin. Königl. Buchdruckerei: P. A. Norstedt & Söner, 1892. Smithsonian Libraries and Archives/Internet Archive.

Box 32.1. Experiences of a Resident on Ward I

In his book *Lest We Forget*, Dr. Carter Rowe (1996) described his experience as a resident on Ward I:

"Rounds were held each Wednesday morning in the conference room in the basement of Ward I. The first half hour was taken up with fractures, in which the general surgical residents also participated. All fractures were followed and were evaluated one year after treatment [started by Robert Osgood], and graded by means of a simple and very effective rating system of E4, F4, A4 (0 = poor result, 4 = excellent result).

"E-Economic-the patient's ability to return to his original work, or to a gainful activity.

"F-Functional-range of motion, strength, and agility.

"A-Anatomic-anatomy, alignment, degree of healing by x-ray, cosmetic appearance, atrophy, motor and sensory deficits, and circulation...

"Shortly after World War II, when the surgical house officers were still assigned for a period to the fracture service... Rounds...[were] moved to the Bigelow amphitheater...

"The second half of rounds was confined to orthopaedic problems...All the house officers wore white uniforms and clean white shoes...Jackets were made without pockets [to stop house officers standing around with their hands in their pockets; Hospital Director Frederic Washburn's edict]. When Nathaniel W. Faxon became director 1935, the residents fortunately got their pockets back.

"As marriage of the house staff prior to World War II was strictly forbidden and there was little or no pay, we were satisfied to be housed in the handsome Moseley Building and to be supplied with uniforms and meals. We ate in the Domestic Building. On the second floor, there were two dining rooms around a central serving area which connected with the kitchen. One dining room served male house officers and employees; the other served nurses and women employees...In the '30s this did not seem unusual as, at the time, there were only a few women doctors and separation of male and female was generally accepted in colleges and in the workplace. Breakfast consisted of an orange, a few pieces of toast, and an occasional egg, while lunch was usually a hot dog and potato salad. I do not recall any overweight residents or nurses in those days.

"My introduction to Ward I in 1937 was to assist Dr. Paul Norton in removing an adult plaster hip spica... At that time, the only way we could remove a plaster cast was to bivalve it with a Murphy knife (a beaked-blade knife somewhat similar to the knife used to open oysters). To soften the plaster, we used a syringe with water. As I remember, it took over an hour with both of us vigorously chipping away...

"For the residents or 'house officers', the day began with early walk-rounds, after which we went to the operating room or saw patients in the OPD...Dr. Lewis Cozen's letter concerning the OPD [stated] 'At the MGH, I'll never forget the long lines of patients waiting around the corner of the street while we were seeing them in the clinic. We would start at 7:30 or 8:00 in the morning and work right through without any lunch until 4:00 or 4:30, when we would go up to the dining room and lunch. In the dining room, I remember well that it was the center for discussion of interesting medical orthopaedic problems. None of us had any money, so we did not discuss stocks, or where we would build a house, or really have any interest in anything but medicine...'

"The Moseley Building, four stories high, served as the center of our off-duty activities and as sleeping quarters. It was located on the east side of the entrance to the hospital. The emergency ward, as previously noted, was in the basement of the North end of the Moseley Building, from which we had a good view of the Bulfinch Building. The first floor the Moseley Building contained a spacious auditorium excellent for meetings and gatherings, surrounded by various administrative offices. The Treadwell Library on the second floor was a dignified, quiet area, a receptive place to study or read. Book stacks lined its east wall. The third and fourth floors were the house officer's quarters...When the resident's day was over, he returned to the Moseley for reading, rest or relaxing.

"In the center of the fourth floor was a large pool table which was the focus for pool, food, demonstrations of physical examination, and a variety of other activities...The sleeping quarters were not always peaceful and orderly, especially on Saturday nights...Reasonable requests to forgo...Saturday night escapades [often] proved fruitless."

Orthopaedics Becomes a Department at MGH

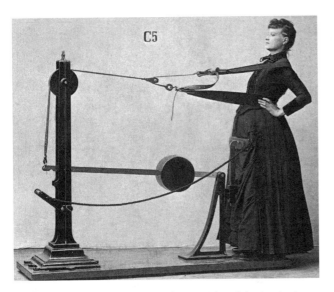

Use of Zander's equipment can be considered the beginning of modern physical therapy.

Dr. G. Zander's medico-mechanische Gymnastik by Dr. Alfred Levertin. Königl. Buchdruckerei: P. A. Norstedt & Söner, 1892. Smithsonian Libraries and Archives/Internet Archive.

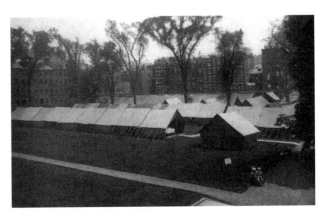

Children's Ward set up in tents in the hospital yard during remodeling of the Centre and West Wing of Bulfinch during hot summer months, 1925.

The Massachusetts General Hospital: Its Development, 1900-1935 by Frederic A. Washburn. Boston: Houghton Mifflin, 1939. Massachusetts General Hospital, Archives and Special Collections.

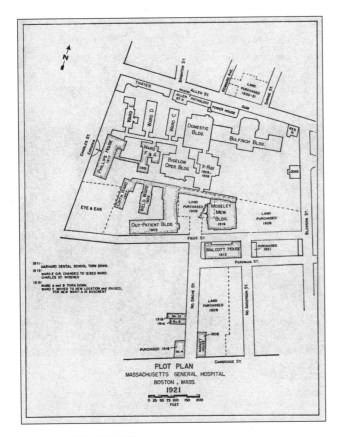

Plot plan of MGH, 1921.

The Massachusetts General Hospital, 1935-1955 by Nathaniel W. Faxon. Cambridge: Harvard University Press, 1959. Massachusetts General Hospital, Archives and Special Collections.)

administration gave orthopaedic staff an operating room in the general surgical building. The orthopaedic department added "facilities for hydro-therapy and for the application of heat and massage" (Washburn 1939) to the Zander Room (Medico-Mechanical Department) in the outpatient building, which had been "in use since 1904 with its many machines for mechano-therapy, and to the apparatus for electro-therapy" (Washburn 1939). The room was near the orthopaedic clinic and headed by an orthopaedic surgeon. It became a prototype of the modern physical therapy clinic. To create the Zander Room originally, "in 1903 the seats had been removed from the large 1867 Operating Theatre…[for] a corridor to the Gay Ward…The remaining floor space and a gallery formed by the roof of this corridor was used to house the fifty-four machines invented by Dr. Zander…imported from Stockholm. Dr. Max Bohm, a young German, was at first in charge of this treatment, and then Dr. C. Hermann Bucholz, another German trained in physio-therapy" (Washburn 1939). Its use ended "in 1917, after the outbreak of the War" (Washburn 1939), and hasn't been used since.

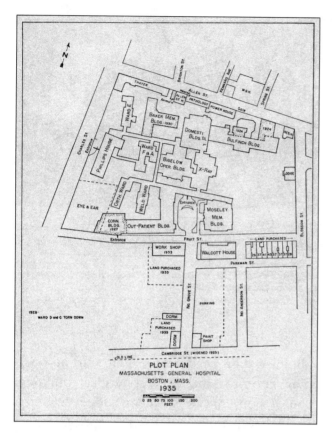

Plot plan of MGH, 1935.

The Massachusetts General Hospital, 1935–1955 by Nathaniel W. Faxon. Cambridge: Harvard University Press, 1959. Massachusetts General Hospital, Archives and Special Collections.

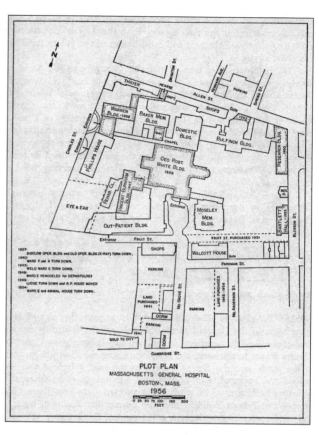

Plot plan of MGH, 1956.

The Massachusetts General Hospital, 1935–1955 by Nathaniel W. Faxon. Cambridge: Harvard University Press, 1959. Massachusetts General Hospital, Archives and Special Collections.

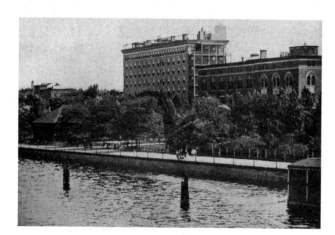

Phillips House, 1917. Donated by the William Phillips family. Charles River in the foreground.

Massachusetts General Hospital: Memorial and Historical Volume. Boston: Griffith-Stillings Press, 1921. Massachusetts General Hospital, Archives and Special Collections.

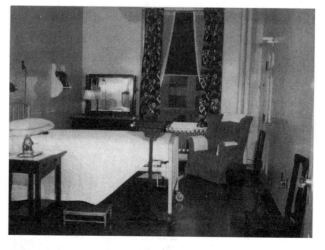

Patient room in the Phillips House.

Something in the Ether: A Bicentennial History of Massachusetts General Hospital, 1811 to 2011 by Webster Bull and Martha Bull. Memoirs Unlimited, 2010. Massachusetts General Hospital, Archives and Special Collections.

Orthopaedics Becomes a Department at MGH

Another significant element of the orthopaedics department was the surgical appliance shop [that] was set up in the basement of the 1900 Surgical Building [in 1905]. In 1916 the shop consisted of four divisions or rooms, the smitty, leather room, finishing room, and nickel-plating room. Four men, a blacksmith, a harness-maker, and two "finishers" were in charge. Measurements were taken in the wards when necessary. This shop made to order all the orthopaedic and surgical apparatus such as flat-foot plates, leather jackets, leather spicas and collars, leg and foot braces, etc., and did much hospital repair work. Some appliances, also, were made for physicians not connected with the staff…[who were] unable to receive special apparatus elsewhere. In 1937 the shop was moved to one of the old brick buildings on North Grove Street. (Washburn 1939)

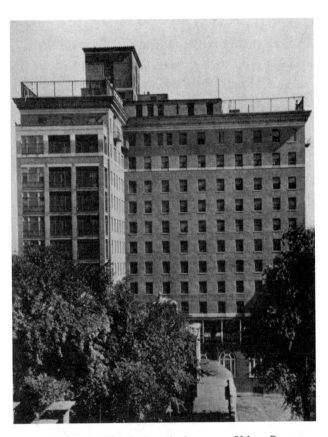

Baker Memorial, 1930. Built at the bequest of Mary R. Richardson in memory of her parents. Massachusetts General Hospital, Archives and Special Collections.

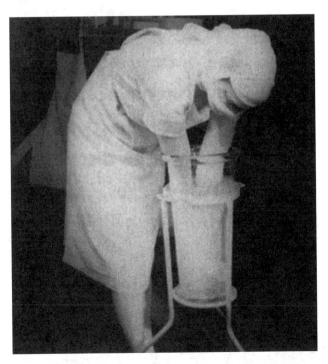

Alcohol dip. I still remember as a resident, in the late 1960s, having to dip my hands up to the elbows in alcohol after scrubbing and before entering the Phillips operating room.

Lest We Forget: Orthopaedics at the Massachusetts General Hospital, 1900-1995 by Carter R. Rowe. Dublin, New Hampshire: William L. Bauhan, 1996. Courtesy of Bauhan Publishing.

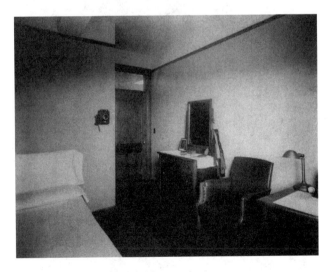

Patient room in the Baker Memorial.

Something in the Ether: A Bicentennial History of Massachusetts General Hospital, 1811 to 2011 by Webster Bull and Martha Bull. Memoirs Unlimited, 2010. Massachusetts General Hospital, Archives and Special Collections.

The last orthopaedic residents to work on Ward I, in 1938 and 1939, were Otto E. Aufranc, Carroll B. Larson, John A. Reidy, O. Sherwin Staples, William J. Tobin, Frederic W. Rhinelander, Lewis Cozen, Leo J. McDermott, Clyde W. Dawson, Russell Fuldner, Charles L. Sturdevant, and Carter R. Rowe. These 12 surgeons went on to have extensive and influential careers:

> One was elected president of the American Academy of Orthopaedic Surgeons in 1966; one was elected president of the American Orthopaedic Association in 1970; one was elected vice-president with the American Academy of Orthopaedic Surgeons in 1967; one was selected president of the American Shoulder and Elbow Surgeons in 1984; five became full professors and chairmen of their departments; three became clinical associate professors; six served in World War II, four of them overseas; three edited orthopaedic surgical text books; [and] four have created research laboratories. (Rowe 1996)

MGH continued to change and expand its physical footprint along the Charles River in Boston. In 1916, the family of William Moseley, a former "house pupil" who had died, donated a building used as a dormitory; it

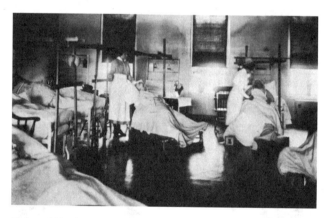

Patient Ward. Massachusetts General Hospital, Archives and Special Collections.

George Robert White Building (The White Building). 1940. Built by George Robert White, a successful Boston merchant. Massachusetts General Hospital, Archives and Special Collections.

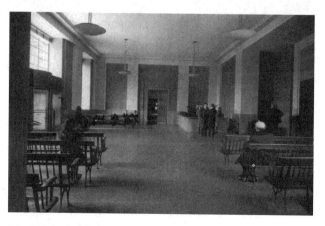

The White Lobby.

Something in the Ether: A Bicentennial History of Massachusetts General Hospital, 1811 to 2011 by Webster Bull and Martha Bull. Memoirs Unlimited, 2010. Massachusetts General Hospital, Archives and Special Collections.

was knocked down in 1981 and replaced by the Wang ACC building. In 1917, the family of William Phillips, a Massachusetts governor and an MGH donor, donated the Phillips House, with its large private rooms, and operating rooms on the top floor with windows overlooking the Charles River. Today it houses the radiology offices and various laboratories.

In 1930 came the Baker Memorial Building, funded by Mary R. Richardson. In this building "patients of moderate means"—annual incomes around $20,000 to $80,000 in 2020 values—were cared for. Patients who earned more money than that were cared for in the Phillips House; if less than that, they were cared for in the general wards.

The White Building, constructed in 1940, was funded by a donation from George Robert White. This building was a hub, where procedures were performed on patients from the general ward and where managerial and educational offices were housed. The orthopaedic service moved there from Ward I when it opened. "This relocation ended thirty-three years of use of Ward I by the Orthopaedic Service. The building, however, continued to house the physical therapy department until 1990, when it was razed to make room for the Ellison Tower. Thus, ended eighty-three years of service to the MGH by this little brick ward" (Rowe 1996).

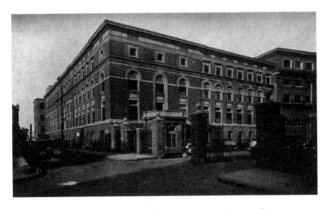

Out-Patient Department (OPD) on North Grove Street, ca. 1930.
Lest We Forget: Orthopaedics at the Massachusetts General Hospital, 1900-1995 by Carter R. Rowe. Dublin, New Hampshire: William L. Bauhan, 1996. Courtesy of Bauhan Publishing.

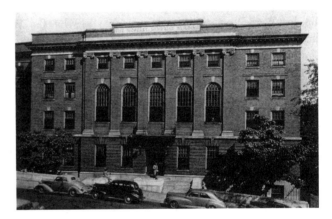

Moseley Memorial Building, 1916. Razed in 1979 for the Wang Ambulatory Center.
Lest We Forget: Orthopaedics at the Massachusetts General Hospital, 1900-1995 by Carter R. Rowe. Dublin, New Hampshire: William L. Bauhan, 1996. Courtesy of Bauhan Publishing.

CHAPTER 33

Joel E. Goldthwait

First Chief of the Department of Orthopaedic Surgery at MGH

Joel Ernest Goldthwait was born in Marblehead, Massachusetts, on June 18, 1866, to William Johnson Goldthwait, a real estate developer, and Mary Lydia (Pitman) Goldthwait. His English ancestor Thomas Goldthwait had come to America in 1630, settling in Salem, and the family had remained in the area since that time. Joel Goldthwait "received his early education in the schools of Marblehead. He then entered the Massachusetts Agricultural College," originally a land-grant college that became the Massachusetts State College in 1931 and then the University of Massachusetts in 1947 (Kuhns 1961). He had planned "to spend his life in scientific agriculture. While in college he was influenced greatly by Dr. Charles Bull, who was Professor of Botany and also physician to the students. Dr. Goldthwait assisted both in the laboratory and in the care of students. This aroused his first interest in medicine" (Kuhns 1961).

Goldthwait graduated in 1885 with a BS degree. He began his medical training almost immediately after graduation, that is, after:

> one unhappy day in business convinced him that the marketplace was not for him. He entered the Harvard Medical School, graduating in 1890. He became an intern at the Boston Children's Hospital [1890–1891], followed by [a second] internship at the Boston City Hospital [1891–1892] where he came under the influence

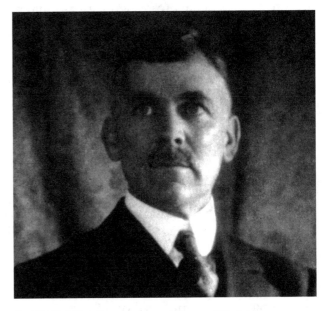

Joel E. Goldthwait. U.S. National Library of Medicine.

Physician Snapshot

Joel E. Goldthwait
BORN: 1866
DIED: 1961

SIGNIFICANT CONTRIBUTIONS: Started movement to care for the chronically disabled; coined the term "faulty body mechanics"; influential leader at the Robert Breck Brigham Hospital; responsible for the first orthopaedic inpatient service at MGH (Ward I); originator of the Goldthwait procedure; designed the Goldthwait irons, a frame with which to apply a hyperextension body cast; cowrote two major textbooks in the field, *Diseases of the Bones and Joints* (1910) and *Body Mechanics in Health and Disease* (1934) of Dr. Edward H. Bradford, who was the leading orthopaedic surgeon in Boston. After completing his [second] internship, he engaged in general practice [but soon specialized in orthopaedic surgery]. (Kuhns 1961)

Goldthwait's research had begun while he was still in medical school. As a medical student, he published two orthopaedic papers in the *Boston Medical and Surgical Journal*, and he published another four papers during his internships. In one classic article, he argued against the generally accepted use of splints to realign leg deformities. He reported "good" results with early surgical treatment (osteotomy and osteoclasis, before the discovery of radiographs) at Boston Children's Hospital; those patients were, on average, four years old. He provided illustrations of patients' legs so readers could visualize the legs before treatment and the results.

Early Research and a Burgeoning Career

In 1892, Goldthwait took a position as assistant surgeon at Boston Children's Hospital, a role he excelled in for four years. During those years he also worked as a visiting orthopaedic surgeon at both the House of the Good Samaritan and the New England Deaconess Hospital. In recalling his early experience at Boston Children's Hospital and its connection with Harvard Medical School, Goldthwait (1900) wrote:

> that came long afterwards, after the hospital was moved out to its present location. In the early days a certain amount of teaching was done there, but not much. Just what time the definite orthopaedic teaching started at the Medical School I am not quite sure, but Bradford, of course, for many years was considered a general surgeon with a leaning toward orthopaedics, and was a member of the General Surgical Staff at the Boston City Hospital where I had a service under him in General Surgery after I had completed my house officer service at the Children's Hospital.

Goldthwait developed an early interest in the care of patients with physical disabilities. In the late 1800s, no facilities were available anywhere—not just at Children's Hospital but at any hospital in Boston—for teenage or adult patients with physical disabilities. "[Goldthwait's] pleas for the continued care of these unfortunates for a long time went unheard" (Kuhns 1961). However, his strong academic credentials and his powers of persuasion eventually convinced the administration at Carney Hospital to provide him with a room on the third floor "where [in 1893] he started the first clinic for adult cripples in America...Many [patients] became better and returned to lives of usefulness" (Kuhns 1961). By the end of the first year, the clinic was at full capacity, and the hospital increased the size of the facility with support from the Massachusetts legislature, which provided $10,000 for continued maintenance and expansion of the clinic.

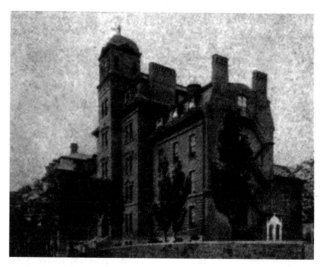

Carney Hospital. Founded in South Boston, 1863.
"From Our Field Editors' Notebooks: A Hospital Situated in Historic Surroundings—Home for Incurables Characterized by Atmosphere of Cheer—Institution for Wounded 'Dough-boys' Club-house Rather than Hospital," *The Modern Hospital* 1919; 12: 354. University of Michigan/Google Books.

> "My apology for presenting a subject in which there is so little general interest is that the impression made upon me by seeing so many of these helpless cripples has been most profound; and it is my chief desire and hope that by the discussion of the subject here a more definite understanding of the disease may be obtained, and that it may be possible to hold out more encouragement to those afflicted with diseases than which none that are non-mortal can be worse."
> —Joel E. Goldthwait
> Read at the Surgical Section of the Suffolk District Medical Society. Published in the *Boston Medical and Surgical Journal*, 1897

Also, during that time he "married Jessie [Sophia] Rand [in 1894]. At first, [they] lived at 398 Marlborough Street, where he used the first floor of the residence as his office" (Kuhns 1955). Three years later, they "moved to Milton[,] where his 3 children, 2 sons and a daughter, grew to maturity. His office was moved to 372 Marlborough Street" (Kuhns 1955), where it remained until his death.

> "I remember very vividly the first appearance with Dr. Joel E. Goldthwait, then a house officer at the Boston City Hospital. He came, I think, to demonstrate some of the newer surgical appliances. He spoke in the same earnest and enthusiastic way that he does now, and his unusual ability and force impressed us even at that time."
> —David W. Cheever
> *History of the Boylston Medical Society*, December 1906

He continued to publish prolifically, and by 1895 he reported "a fine study of the anterior arch of the foot by means of frozen sections" (Mayer 1950). In 1896, he reported a patient who had been living with chronic dislocation of the patella for 20 years (see **Case 33.1**). He published a follow-up three years later:

As soon as the patient was able to go about, even though one patella was in place and the action of the knee improved, the difficulty in completely extending the knee remained, so that the lordosis was not lessened. To correct this an osteotomy of the femur above the condyles was performed on both legs and the limbs

Case 33.1. Dislocation of the Patella

> "A woman who came to the Orthopedic Clinic of the Carney Hospital, in Boston, having had a dislocation of both patellae for twenty years. They slipped out, as she says, when she was ten years of age. She was an old rachitic subject. She is a seamstress by occupation and uses a sewing-machine all day long. She had gotten along until the present time with moderate comfort… The operation consisted in making a long oblique cut across the knee, exposing the capsule, which was so much concentrated upon the outer side that without dividing this it was impossible to slip the patella over into the trochlear groove. The capsule was slit on the outer side, the wound being about three inches long. With this it was possible to get the patella back in its place, but the attachment of the patellar tendon was so far cut on the tibia that it slipped out again as soon as it was let go. The tendon was then cut entirely off, periosteum over the inner side of the tibia freed, and the tendon was sewed to this periosteum. The loose capsule on the inner side was then taken up by a through-and-through quilting suture. To relieve the strain, the attachment of the quadriceps muscle to the patella was cut off almost entirely, leaving a little aponeurosis at the back. The wound was closed without drainage. It was a first-intention wound. The patient was up and about in five or six weeks. She wore a knee-cap, or rather a leather leg-splint, to confine the joint for four or five months. She is able to walk around now perfectly. Only one leg has been operated upon. I did not think it advisable to operate on the two legs at the same time. There is a free motion at a right angle…the patella is in its normal place, and the attachment of the patellar tendon seems to be strong enough."
> (Joel E. Goldthwait 1896)

straightened...eight weeks [later] the [opposite] left knee was operated upon to correct the position of the patella. The operation was similar to that which was used in the other joint, except that, instead of cutting off the patella tendon and reattaching it [later called the Goldthwait procedure], the whole tubercle of the tibia was chiseled off and...nailed to a depression which was made on the inner side of the bone...

The other knee had shown no signs of weakness [, but] it was my feeling that a bony attachment would probably be more secure... The functional result in this case is...not as good as the right...While complete extension is possible, there is only about 70 degrees of motion in flexion...Even though the right knee is the better of the two, the operation which was performed on the [left] knee is the better, in my opinion...In transplanting the piece of bone, instead of freeing the fragment entirely, it would be better to save the attachment of the periosteum...and to swing the bone around without completely separating it. (Goldthwait 1899)

In 1899, the leadership at Massachusetts General Hospital (MGH) asked Goldthwait to organize an orthopaedic outpatient service, and, in 1900, the trustees there appointed him consulting orthopaedic surgeon. He was just 35 years old. That same year, at the 14th annual meeting of the American Orthopedic Association, Goldthwait presented a paper on knee joint surgery in 38 cases, stating that his "personal feeling [was] that there is no more danger in opening the knee or any other large joints than in opening the peritoneum" (Goldthwait 1900).

During this time, Goldthwait began his teaching career as well. He was appointed assistant instructor at Harvard Medical School in 1902 and eventually promoted to instructor in orthopaedic surgery. In 1903, soon after the opening of the new outpatient department building at MGH, the first outpatient orthopaedic department

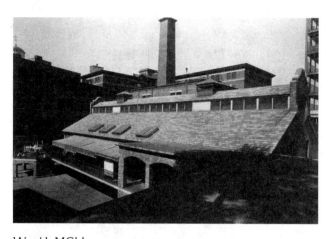

Ward I, MGH.

Lest We Forget: Orthopaedics at the Massachusetts General Hospital, 1900-1995 by Carter R. Rowe. Dublin, New Hampshire: William L. Bauhan, 1996. Courtesy of Bauhan Publishing.

was created there (see chapter 32). Goldthwait quickly recognized that facilities in which to provide inpatient care would also be required. He raised approximately $70,000 to fund Ward I, which opened in 1907 (chapter 32). In 1904, he resigned from the staff at Carney Hospital and became the first orthopedic service chief at MGH. During his approximately 10 years on staff at Carney Hospital, Goldthwait had published ~35 papers on a wide range of orthopaedic problems: patellar dislocation, muscle/tendon transplantation (he was among the first in the US to perform this procedure), inflammatory arthritis, osteoarthritis of the spine, internal derangement of the knee, and Pott's disease (tuberculosis of the spine).

During his eight years on the staff and four years as chief of the orthopaedic service at MGH, Goldthwait published almost 20 papers, including five on the diagnosis and treatment of rheumatoid arthritis and two on a field of study in which he was developing an increasing interest—posture and the support and functioning of the viscera. In total, Goldthwait published 3 books and about 105 articles—more than 40 on general orthopaedics, 15 on disability, 8 on posture, 7 on visceroptosis, 7 on orthopaedics in World War I, and others. I found only

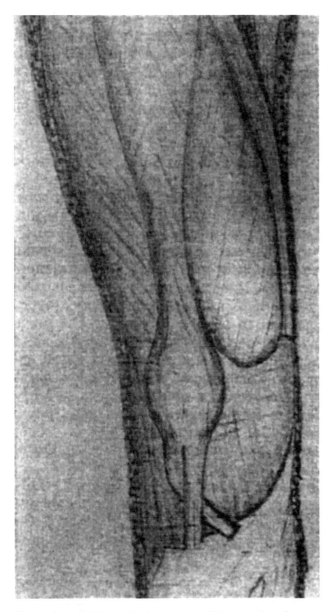

Sketch from Goldthwait's description of his procedure for a dislocating patella.

J. E. Goldthwait, "Slipping or Recurrent Dislocation of the Patella; With the Report of Eleven Cases," *Boston Medical and Surgical Journal* 1904; 150: 171.

three articles on dislocation of the patella, two of which described the same case. In the third and last article, published in 1904, Goldthwait described the procedure he used in 7 of 11 cases that he had operated upon. He observed that "in the majority of cases...the attachment of the patella tendon is distinctly farther to the outside than normal, making less direct the pull of the anterior thigh muscles...The treatment which has been most satisfactory...is an operation in which the outer half of the patellar tendon is reattached to the tibia well to the inside of the tubercle" (Goldthwait 1904).

A Focus on Body Mechanics and Chronic Disease

In 1908, less than one year after Ward I opened, Goldthwait resigned from his position as chief of the orthopaedic service at MGH after some conflicts with the director of the hospital (though he was on the consulting staff there from 1922 to 1937, and he was named honorary surgeon in 1937). He resigned ostensibly to help design the Robert Breck Brigham Hospital, and he focused on caring for those with chronic diseases or diseases that, at that time, had no cure (see chapter 45). Goldthwait had previously been appointed a trustee for the corporation in 1907.

As his career progressed, Goldthwait began to focus his efforts on identifying the etiology of orthopaedic impairments and diseases. "Goldthwait, who had at one time been particularly interested in surgery...swung away from operative orthopaedics because of an overpowering interest in posture and derangements of the lumbosacral region" (Mayer 1955). In 1910, Goldthwait, along with Drs. Charles Painter and Robert Osgood, published the book *Diseases of the Bones and Joints*. They dedicated it "to those whose patient suffering under the burden of deformity, disability and disease has furnished the incentive for investigation" (Goldthwait, Painter, and Osgood 1910). In the preface they wrote:

> One of the chief difficulties which has opposed itself to the understanding of chronic joint problems has been the paucity of clinical, and the fragmentary character of pathological, data. Sufferers from these conditions rarely afford one the opportunity to study their lesions at a time when they are clinically significant...It is

to those practitioners of medicine...to whom sufferers from joint disease make their first appeal that these Studies are offered...The writers have endeavored to present some one fundamental principle, whether it concerns etiology or treatment, rather than to offer a large number of suggestions, many of which have had no adequate trial...The very nature of these processes renders them abhorrent to the busy general practitioner and the surgeon. Their lesions are apparently not even interesting to the average consulting internist. There is no one therefore to whom these unfortunates may turn except to a comparatively small group of medical men who by the training are fitting themselves to grapple with just such problems...If those of us who have the opportunity will preserve in patience, we shall realize that no reward can be greater than that of having contributed to the relief of this large class of humanity, which until recently has been so largely ignored. (Goldthwait, Painter, and Osgood 1910)

Goldthwait, Painter, and Osgood aimed to focus on the most common conditions that nonetheless "for many years have been neglected." Many of these conditions are listed in **Box 33.1**.

> "If we are to see only the operation, leaving the after-care to the slightly trained house staff with the physiotherapy given by an entirely different department...we cease to be true orthopaedic surgeons, but just surgeons doing bone and joint work."
>
> —Joel E. Goldthwait
> "The Backgrounds and Foregrounds of Orthopaedics"
> *Journal of Bone and Joint Surgery*, 1933

Dr. John G. Kuhns wrote in 1955 that Goldthwait's work "was often misunderstood by the medical profession." However, physicians

Box 33.1. Conditions of Interest in Diseases of the Bones and Joints (1910)

- Tuberculosis of bones and joints
- Nontuberculous diseases of the joints, including infectious arthritis
- Rheumatoid arthritis
- Osteoarthritis
- Lipomata
- Neoplasms
- Hysteric and functional joints
- Lues of bones and joints
- Osteomyelitis
- Rachitis
- Osteogenesis imperfecta
- Chondrodystrophia foetalis
- Osteitis deformans
- Pelvic articulations
- Villous arthritis
- Gout
- Hemophiliac joints
- Intermittent hydrops
- Weak and flat feet
- Aneurysm
- Tabes mesenterica
- Subdeltoid bursitis
- Round or stoop shoulder
- Congenital elevation of scapula
- Fixed scapula
- Recurrent dislocation of shoulder
- Brachial neuritis or neuralgia
- Use of plaster of Paris in orthopaedic surgery

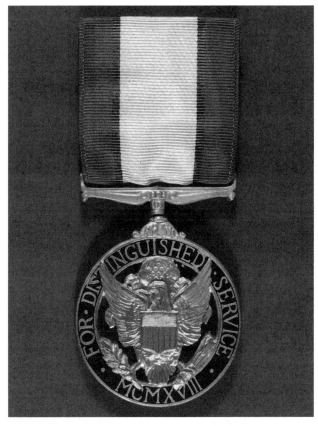

US Army Distinguished Service Medal. Smithsonian National Air and Space Museum.

from MGH traveled extensively to discuss the importance of posture, and others traveled to Boston to learn from Goldthwait. During Goldthwait's extensive observational and anatomical studies of poor posture and body mechanics in relation to medical problems, he observed improvements in various "abnormalities" after exercise and mechanical methods. He began publishing his findings in 1913 and continued to do so over two decades. His efforts illustrate a shift in his methods—from correcting orthopaedic problems through surgery in his early career to emphasizing treatment of the whole person through mechanical means in his later work. Eventually, recognition of the importance of posture expanded among nurses and even nonprofessionals. J. T. Sullivan, in 1927, noted that the shift from pharmaceutical remedies to exercise in order to cure such problems was likely a surprise for patients.

Sullivan also described the effect of Goldthwait's postural treatments on soldiers during World War I, when men who had been drafted were rejected from service because of poor posture, and when some soldiers who did go overseas to serve were unable to perform their physical duties. Goldthwait treated such soldiers, many of whom were able to return to active duty and performed well afterward. For this major contribution, Goldthwait received the US Army's Distinguished Service Medal in 1919 (see chapter 63).

Many physicians today don't know about the historical conflict around posture within the medical community. In 1998, Yosifon and Stearns reviewed the history of posture-related trends in their article "The Rise and Fall of American Posture." In the mid-nineteenth century, before Goldthwait's interest, posture was considered a way to identify both illness and faulty character. Relaxed and even slouched body presentations spread particularly rapidly among youth as the century progressed. The twentieth century brought with it professional interest from physicians such as Goldthwait. Grade schools began to check students for scoliosis and taught "good" posture during gym classes. Even colleges jumped on the bandwagon of assessing and correcting their students' posture. By mid-century, however, such a focus had begun to wane among both educational institutions and the medical community, for various reasons. One of these was the reduced prevalence of diseases such as rickets and polio. Another was its connotations for formality and restraint. Visceroptosis as a cause of—or a concept to explain—disease entities also fell out of favor, mainly because of a lack of supportive research.

At the same time he began publishing his findings on posture in 1913, Goldthwait also published a paper titled "Orthopedic Principles in the Treatment of Abdominal Visceroptosis and Chronic Intestinal Stasis." In it, he listed six reasons why orthopaedists should be interested in such a subject; these are explained in **Box 33.2**. Goldthwait wrote that:

> both from general reasoning as well as from extensive experience...a good prognosis is usually possible if the acquired features of disturbance of poise and visceral sag can be overcome...The first step is to rest the parts which have been overstrained and to stimulate the parts which have been weakened from disuse. This at times can be accomplished by the use of a brace. While this apparatus is being worn, massage, stimulating bathing, etc., are all of advantage in hastening the repair. As soon as... muscle fatigue [has] passed, active exercises should be started. In the severer cases recumbency is absolutely necessary...To prevent the sag of the organs a leather jacket should be used which is molded from a cast of the body taken when the body is fully extended [on Goldthwait irons] and with the ribs fully raised. Such a jacket is worn during the night. In the severe cases recumbency is insisted upon both day and night at times for periods of many weeks. When it is considered wise for the patient to go about, a brace is worn at first [with] special exercises. As the strength increases the brace is omitted...Supervision...should naturally be continued for a long time for the purpose of preventing relapses...Teamwork between the physician, the surgeon, and the orthopedist... shows our profession at its best.

Goldthwait was busy in 1914. Not only did he help to open the Brigham Hospital and become chairman of the board of trustees (a position he held for 19 years), he also helped to establish the American College of Surgeons and was listed as an "owner" of the *Boston Medical and Surgical Journal*. That same year, he founded the Boston School of Physical Education, furnishing equipment and supplies. He owned and ran the school until the mid-1930s. During this period, he had continued to teach at Harvard Medical School, and he was appointed lecturer in orthopaedic surgery in the school's graduate program in 1912 and, in 1916, associate in orthopaedic surgery, a position he held for 16 years.

In 1915, Goldthwait delivered the 26th Annual Shattuck Lecture before the Massachusetts Medical Society. The lecture, titled "An Anatomic and Mechanistic Conception of

---

Box 33.2. Reasons for Orthopaedists' Interest in Visceroptosis

- "Abdominal visceroptosis is invariably associated with disturbances of poise, which must result in weakness of the muscles and strain of the joints.

- "The imperfect poise associated with visceroptosis results in a gradual weakening of the trunk muscles [lessening] support for the trunk as well as for the viscera.

- "The imperfect poise, commonly showing as the droop of the shoulders and flattening of the chest, must of itself cause downward displacement of the abdominal organs.

- "Many of the chronic joint diseases are probably due to the disturbed physiology resulting from the malposition of the viscera as well as possibly to absorption from the gastrointestinal tract.

- "Treatment of the joint strains resulting from postures associated with visceroptosis, as well as the treatment of the joint diseases due to disturbances of the abdominal viscera is incomplete, and many times hopeless unless the viscera are properly treated so that undue strain is relieved.

- "The best health and greatest efficiency of the individual is possible only when the body is used in such poise that there is no undue strain or interference with any of the structures."

(Goldthwait. "Orthopedic Principles in the Treatment of Abdominal Visceroptosis and Chronic Intestinal Stasis." *Surgery, Gynecology and Obstetrics*, 1913)

Massachusetts Medical Society.

THE SHATTUCK LECTURE.

AN ANATOMIC AND MECHANISTIC CONCEPTION OF DISEASE.*

By Joel E. Goldthwait, M.D., Boston.

Goldthwait's Shattuck Lecture in which he described anatomic variations he observed in chronic diseases, 1915. *Boston Medical and Surgical Journal* 1915; 172: 881.

Disease," was published in the *Boston Medical and Surgical Journal* (1915). He chose the topic because of its broad general interest to physicians and because he could cover fundamentals of medical knowledge. He noted that his search for the causes of orthopaedic chronic diseases—an endeavor already spanning years—led him to return his focus to the basic study of anatomy: "A fairly exhaustive pathologic investigation failing to show more than the nature of the lesion, with similar experience from the bacteriologic and the biochemical investigations, led to the study of the fundamental anatomic conditions existing in patients afflicted with the diseases, with results which have been increasingly more suggestive the farther the study has been carried."

Goldthwait had published previous articles on the varieties of the skeleton, posture, and formation of the viscera. On the basis of those studies, in his Shattuck Lecture, he noted that people with chronic disease do not usually have "normal" anatomy as described in textbooks. Although the data he obtained from his studies are piecemeal, through independent verification and a review of the literature he believed that his observations, taken together, represent the truth about human anatomy. Overall, Goldthwait described "two well-marked types" of variation in human anatomy that can be easily distinguished (though he noted that variation also occurs within these types):

1. Splanchnoptotic (Glennard); Congenital Visceroptotic (Goldthwait, Smith); Carnivorus (Treves, Werner, Bryant); Hyper-ontomorph (Bean); Macroscelous (Montessori); "Narrow-Backed" (Industrial)

2. Herbvorus (Treves, Werner, Bryant); "Broad-Backed" (Industrial); Meso-ontomorph (Bean); Brachyscelous (Montessori)

In what must have been a very long lecture, Goldthwait then described in detail the mechanical, physiological, and functional differences between each of these variations of human anatomy (**Table 33.1**). Goldthwait explained that although these vary quite a bit, the parts work together to function cohesively in each, although malalignment or poor posture could affect organ function:

When the body is used rightly all of the structures are in such adjustment that there is no particular strain on any part. [However,] If the body is drooped...so that the shoulders drag forward and downward the whole body suffers...The chest is necessarily lowered, the lungs...less fully expanded...the diaphragm is depressed [and] the abdominal organs are necessarily forced downward and forward. When this occurs the possibility of mechanical interference with the function of the organs is not difficult to imagine...The postures...assumed by the other anatomic types are perfectly characteristic, so that once they are appreciated, the posture itself...indicates the type of anatomy to be found in the individual.

He concluded his lecture with high-level reasoning for the study of orthopaedics and the benefit of such study to the human race:

If the physician and teacher recognize these facts and apply the natural principles for the proper development of...individuals, the result

Table 33.1. Two Main Human Types, According to Goldthwait

	Carnivorus [sic]	**Herbvorus** [sic]
Size	"Tall and slender or small and delicate"	"Heavily built, broad-backed"
Skeleton	Light, slender Longer, mainly in the lumbar region	Large, heavy Broad spine, especially in lumbar region
Thorax and abdomen	"Fair size"	Large chest, high diaphragm Broad/deep abdominal cavity
Extremities	Long, slender	Heavy Large legs, straight knees, broad feet Heavy arms, broad and "chubby" hands
Fat	Less than in broad-backed figure Sometimes "much accumulation of fat [that is] always soft with very little connective tissue" Not much retroperitoneal fat	Excess fat with much connective tissue Much retroperitoneal and abdominal fat
Muscles	Long, slender fibers	Large, coarse fibers
Joints	More flexible	Less flexible
Organs		
Lungs and heart	Smaller than in broad-backed figure	Larger than in narrow-backed figure
Stomach	Long, tubular	Large, pear-shaped
Small intestine	Shorter than normal (only 10–15 ft)	Longer than normal (25–39 ft)
Large intestine	Shorter than normal	Larger and longer than normal (5–8.5 ft)

Adapted from Goldthwait's "An Anatomic and Mechanistic Conception of Disease," a recount of his Shattuck Lecture published in the *Boston Medical and Surgical Journal*, 1915.

must be an inevitable—a stronger and finer race. What higher incentive can there be for work than that which benefits the individual and at the same time by helping him gradually removes the weaker elements, which if perpetuated would surely lower the vitality of the race as a whole...In the moral choice man is given great responsibility and in the physical the responsibility is none the less great, unless the development of the human family is to be governed by the same law of survival of the fittest and natural selection which has governed the development of the lower forms of life.

In 1916 the *American Journal of Orthopedic Surgery* published a "Symposium on Visceroptosis as a Factor in the Causation of Orthopedic and Other Lesions." Five authors contributed, referring to Goldthwait's previous work and recognizing the importance of his research in doing so. W. E. Sullivan, PhD, from Tufts Medical School, described the anatomy of visceroptosis, limiting his discussion to the position of the diaphragm and the abdominal viscera. He concluded:

> that the most effective agent in the support of the abdominal viscera is the shape of the abdominal cavity as determined by the 'shelves' [muscles, other organs, ligaments, hepatic veins and renal vessels] and by the degree of contraction or tonicity of the abdominal musculature, together with the tonicity of the viscera themselves... supplemented by the blood vessels and ligaments in some cases and by the retroperitoneal position of the organs in others.

Dr. Henry Wald Bettman (1916), professor of medicine at the University Cincinnati, in his paper on the medical aspects of visceroptosis wrote:

> In 1914 Goldthwait hesitated to suggest that... mechanical conditions [bad posture] could lead

to these diseases [chronic kidney disease, arteriosclerosis, diabetes, high blood pressure, sclerosis of the liver, gall stones, acid indigestion]... Yet in the Shattuck lecture for 1915 he suggests that the position of the spleen may induce profound anemias...a kink in the bowel may cause an eye infection...glycosuria [may] be caused by mechanical pressure on the pancreas...epilepsy [may] be the result of enteroptosis...No! a mechanistic conception of disease is helpful only so far as it clings to facts which can be established by observation. It becomes fantastic and leads far afield when it outstrips fact and gives rein to imagination...The position of the colon teaches us nothing regarding its function.

Dr. Fred H. Baetzer (1916), of Baltimore, wrote his viewpoint as a radiologist:

Sometime ago I received a communication from the president of the American Orthopedic Association asking me for a definition of visceroptosis...I neglected replying...because I could not give a definition of visceroptosis...In conclusion, we believe visceroptosis is incidental and plays practically no part in spinal lesions.

Dr. David Silver (1916), an orthopaedic surgeon in Pittsburgh, in a paper on visceroptosis' possible role in causing arthritis deformans (rheumatoid arthritis) concluded:

It seems to have been demonstrated that the active agent in arthritis deformans may enter through the intestinal tract. This active agent is undoubtedly bacterial, probably most commonly streptococcic...Through the production of stasis...visceroptosis acts to cause increased intestinal infection, and so favors systemic invasion; thus, in an individual with lessened joint resistance it may be the deciding factor in the development of arthritis. How frequently arthritis develops in visceroptotic subjects, and what the proportion is between the number of cases of arthritis due to this cause and that arising from other intestinal infections, cannot now be stated.

The final paper in the symposium, ""What Evidence can be Brought," was by Dr. Osgood (1916). He began by stating:

Whether it [visceroptosis] is "anything more" [than a departure from an anatomic norm] or whether it is of frequent causative clinical significance is the important part of the question before us...visceroptosis which we would define as a departure from the normal position of the viscera throughout the abdomen...which is accompanied by changes in the posture, which may be said to be typical.

In reviewing the anatomic variations reported, Osgood referred to Goldthwait's study of frozen sections:

Goldthwait...clearly [demonstrates] that certain definite types of posture and relaxed abdominal walls must favor a sagging of the viscera. Whether we consider these changes to be the frequent cause of symptoms, or whether we do not, we can hardly doubt the anatomic facts, and they are impressive. It would certainly seem that derangements of this sort must predispose in time to faulty action of the viscera...

After reviewing the physiologic and roentgenological evidence Osgood summarized the clinical evidence stating:

The medical evidence is found in the very general conviction among medical men...born of clinical experience, —that visceroptosis and poor health are...frequently inseparable...so close as to have one now causal and now the other...The most striking evidence may be built up concerning the causal relationship of tuberculosis and visceroptosis...No one familiar with surgical literature can for a moment doubt that surgeons and the medical men who refer these cases have believed that many of the symptoms for which their digestive patients sought relief were caused by the coexisting visceroptosis. Relief has by no means always followed the surgical procedure...to cure of the gastroptosis or splanchnoptosis, to anchor the kidney or straighten the uterine canal. The many failures may have shaken faith in the method of relief, not in the cause of the symptoms."

Osgood then wrote of his personal experience with Dr. Goldthwait:

We all see these medical and surgical derelicts and many of us pass them on as derelicts still. It has been my good fortune to be closely associated with a man whose enthusiasm abhors derelicts, one of whose chief concerns is the repair of imperfectly used and abused human machines. Many...of these machines which have come to him have been in other men's hands, and have had the stimulation of good medicine, of good surgery, and of suggestion. It has been to me surprising, for I have maintained a scepticism which I hope has been honest, to observe the return to health of these patients when their bodies have been remodeled, their postures corrected, and their ptoses thereby relieved. Accompanying this orthopaedic treatment of visceroptosis and seemingly as a result, I have seen attacks of epilepsy cease, lateral sclerosis and progressive muscular atrophy, diagnosed...by careful and able neurologists, markedly improve over a period of years, certain cases of chronic arthritis grow steadily better, operations for...gastric ulcer and appendicitis become unnecessary, sterility turn into pregnancy, cardiospasm disappear, habitual constipation give way...One cannot fail to be impressed. I cannot fail to be persuaded, that visceroptosis, from an orthopaedic point of view, is of frequent causative clinical significance...

That the incidence of visceroptosis is great as shown by the statistics of Sever as regards children...the recent observation of Lewis...among the high school boys of Worcester...sixty per cent...were of the so-called carnivorous class...They represented bad posture, poor muscles, poor nutrition, poor teeth, prominent abdomens and ptosis...The problem is a serious one...visceroptotic patients crowd our sanitoria. Swaim declared that he saw hardly more than 20 well-postured individuals among 3000 patients at Clifton Springs...Certain surgeons and medical men are realizing that the orthopaedic possibilities of relief should be sought first, and not last.

In the discussion following this symposium Dr. Goldthwait stated:

There is one thing upon which we must all agree, that the body used fully erect is better than the body drooped. Why does the army train men to hold themselves erect? It is because the body or the human machine, will run with less friction if it is so trained. The Shattuck Lecture was written because an anatomic basis for our work [two years given to

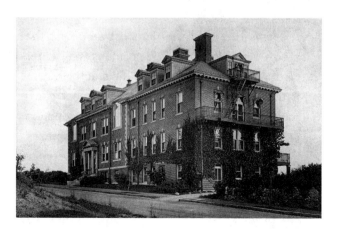

Corey Hill Hospital, 1918. Brookline Historical Society.

anatomical study] seemed reasonable…There are all sorts of complex conditions…which are not to be treated by medicine or controlled by surgery. My plea is to stop long enough to find out how the patient is made and how parts should be placed in that condition…In these cases the work of the surgeon, the neurologist, the medical man, and the orthopedic man, is needed, the orthopedist having his part and the others their part.

Goldthwait had strong ties to yet another hospital in the Boston area—Corey Hill Hospital in Brookline. Goldthwait bankrolled the construction of Corey Hill in the early 1920s, and the hospital was well equipped with supplies and equipment, and cared only for private patients. In fact, some considered Corey Hill to be the ideal such hospital and used it as a model for others. Goldthwait owned Corey Hill until 1932, when he sold it.

At some point, Goldthwait also designed a frame of curved iron bars—the so-called Goldthwait irons—upon which a patient was placed supine to apply a hyperextension body cast. I remember using these iron bars while I was a resident at Children's Hospital, but I could not find any remaining there now, nor could I identify when Goldthwait may have initially introduced this method.

Following World War I, in 1923, Goldthwait was promoted to brigadier general in the US

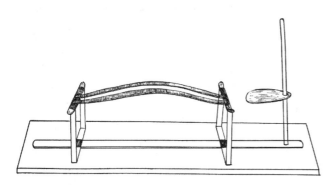

Drawing of Goldthwait irons. *Text Book of Orthopedic Surgery for Students of Medicine* by J.W. Sever. New York: Macmillan, 1925.

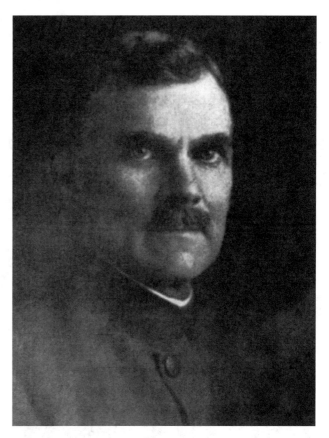

Joel E. Goldthwait in uniform, WWI.
D. P. Green and J. C. Delee, "American Orthopaedic Surgeons in World War I," *Journal of Bone and Joint Surgery* 2017; 99: e32.

Medical Reserve Corps. For many years he was an instructor at the US Army War College, at its Washington Barracks in Washington, DC. Upon leaving the army he had a large role in instituting the Bouvé-Boston School of Physical Education and the Boston School of Occupational Therapy. "His interest in young people induced him to accept a professorship at Smith College where he organized the department of physical education. He gave inspiration, instruction, and counsel to a large number of younger orthopaedic surgeons" (Kuhns 1961). At Smith College, Goldthwait spent 14 years as a visiting lecturer in the Department of Hygiene.

In January of 1932, Goldthwait's wife Jessie died. (Four years later he married Francis A. F. [Sherwood] Saltonstall, herself a widow.) During this difficult period in his life, Goldthwait went on to reemphasize his observations and recommendations for understanding and treating chronic disease in his Robert Jones Lecture, given at the Hospital for Joint Diseases in New York City in 1932. Titled "The Backgrounds and Foregrounds of Orthopaedics," he began by reviewing Nicholas Andry's book *L'orthopédie*, published in 1741, and drawing attention to the idea that physicians were generalists, serving as physicians, surgeons, and mental health caregivers in order to meet a patient's every need. Then he moved on to criticizing the process of care—that is, junior staff initially evaluate patients, house staff provide postoperative care, and the chief does the surgeries. He believed the process should be reversed, with the chief, who has more experience, examining patients in the clinic, making a diagnosis, and prescribing nonoperative treatment when indicated. Goldthwait believed that these tasks were far more difficult than operating, which he felt should be left to the junior staff.

> "Good surgery without proper care before and after the operation [can result] in too many cripples."
> —Joel E. Goldthwait
> Robert Jones Lecture, October 27, 1932

He noted that chronic diseases, e.g., back pain, arthritis, paralysis, average foot problems:

> are uninteresting because the average person does not understand them...The endless putting on of plaster jackets or braces, of strapping feet or knees, without first correcting the mechanical features that are at fault, is purposeless, and not only means waste of material and time, but, with so little gained, causes discouragement to both patient and physician. The greatest need today for those of us who call ourselves orthopaedic surgeons, it seems to me, is to train ourselves so that what is involved in the 'prevention' part of Andry's work is better understood; with the expectation that the increased knowledge of these two continues will, if properly used make it possible to carry the work in this line farther than was possible by Andry, just as it is true with the purely operative part...The great need seems to be to carry our studies farther along the two lines emphasized by Andry, –first, the body types of varying anatomical structures, and, secondly, the function to be expected of the body in all its parts once the peculiar structure is known. (Goldthwait 1933)

Goldthwait then reviewed his previously published concepts of posture and visceroptosis.

Shortly thereafter, he helped to establish the American Academy of Orthopaedic Surgeons in

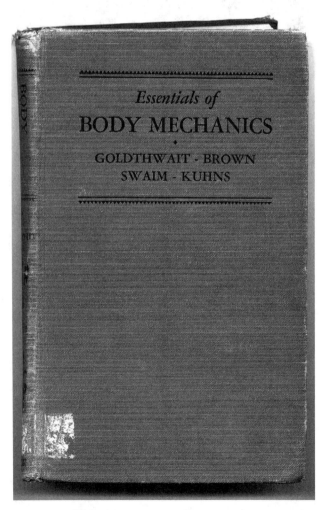

Cover of Goldthwait, Brown, Swaim, and Kuhns book on body mechanics. Photo by the author.

1933. The following year, he published his book *Body Mechanics in Health and Disease* in 1934, a culmination of his 1915 lecture "An Anatomic and Mechanistic Conception of Disease," a paper published in 1922 titled "The Challenge of the Chronic Patient to the Medical Profession," and 13 other publications about posture and his mechanistic concepts of chronic disease (in one of which he coined the term *faulty body mechanics*)—all published before 1924. His coauthors included Drs. Lloyd T. Brown, Loring T. Swaim, and John G. Kuhns, all of whom were Goldthwait's colleagues at the Robert Breck Brigham Hospital. The second edition was published in 1937, the third in 1941. It remained popular, moving into a fourth edition—now titled *Essentials of Body Mechanics in Health and Disease*—in 1945 and a fifth edition in 1953.

> "Today rapid recovery from the special symptom for which admission to our hospital is sought is expected, with the result that a certain rivalry exists with our hospitals and practitioners in the endeavor to show the smallest number of hospital days per patient, with less and less attention to treatment after the primary suggestions. This naturally leaves very little place or time for the cases that do not react promptly or for which there are no specific lines of attack."
> —Joel E. Goldthwait
> "The Challenge of the Chronic Patient to the Medical Profession" *Boston Medical and Surgical Journal,* 1922

In the preface to the 1st edition, the authors concluded that chronic diseases will only be redressed when physicians gain insight into anatomy and physiology, and understand how physiology and mechanics change as a result of such diseases. Twenty years later, in the preface to the 5th edition, they wrote that an understanding of the fundamentals of body mechanics is useful to physicians treating numerous conditions—a fact proved by the continued demand for their textbook.

Legacy

Throughout Dr. Joel Goldthwait's extensive career, he also "gave generously of his time and money to numerous civic projects" (Kuhns 1961), including the *Jessie Goldthwait*, a 76-foot schooner given to his friend and patient Sir Wilfred Grenfell, to be used as a hospital ship by the Labrador Mission. He gave to Berea College, where he was a longtime trustee, a building that has since its construction in 1930 been used as the Agricultural Building.

In the 1920s, Goldthwait had purchased 200 acres in Medfield, Massachusetts, where he had lived at various times and where he enjoyed outdoor activities and dairy farming. In 1942, he donated a stretch of woods from his acreage to the Trustees of Reservations, who created from it the Rocky Woods Reservation. In 1958, he received the annual award for distinguished

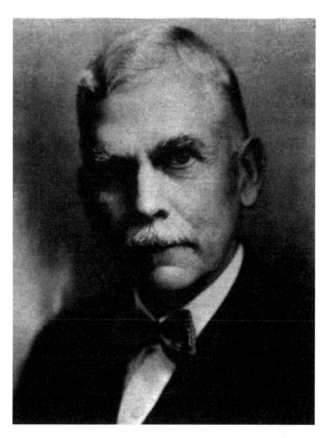

Joel E. Goldthwait. J.G.K., "Joel Ernest Goldthwait 1866–1961," *Journal of Bone and Joint Surgery* 1961; 43: 463.

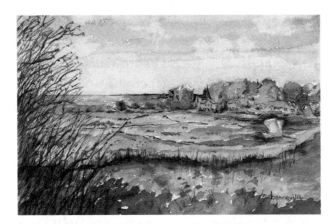

Watercolor of the Goldthwait Reservation, Marblehead, MA.
Artist: Ben Strohecker. Courtesy of the Goldthwait Reservation.

service from the Trustees of Reservations in appreciation of that donation.

In 1947, Goldthwait, who had lived in Marblehead as a child, donated to the town 12 acres of coastal land, thereby creating the Goldthwait Reservation land trust. The reservation is considered private property and is maintained by the trust through donations and membership dues rather than the town, but Goldthwait intended it for all Marblehead citizens to enjoy. Such largesse was common from Goldthwait. His generosity is also well-illustrated by yet another example: "For a number of years, [Goldthwait] provided space in his office for the *American Journal of Orthopedic Surgery* and also underwrote its deficits" (Kuhns 1961).

He was a member of other professional organizations as well, including the American Board of Orthopaedic Surgery; the American Medical Association; the Massachusetts Medical Society; the Warren Club in Boston; the Dedham Polo and Country Club in Dedham, Massachusetts; and the Harvard Clubs of Boston and New York City. Around 1919, "he was given honorary membership in the British Orthopaedic Association [and] the British Government made him a Comrade of the Order of St. Michael and St. George" (Kuhns 1961). Goldthwait received two honorary degrees: a doctor of law (LLD) degree from the University of Massachusetts in 1934, and a doctor of science (DSc) degree from Berea College in 1941.

He continued caring for patients at the Robert Breck Brigham Hospital until 1957—he was 90 years old. About four years later, on January 15, 1961, after a three-month illness, Goldthwait died of a heart attack at the hospital where he had cared for so many. He was 94 years old. His funeral was held in Medfield, and he was buried in Marblehead. J. G. Kuhns (1961), who wrote an obituary for Goldthwait for the *Journal of Bone and Joint Surgery*, encapsulated Goldthwait's career simply: "Rarely has one individual had the opportunity to observe, to contribute to, and to influence the progress of orthopaedic surgery so greatly and for such a long period of time as did Joel Ernest Goldthwait."

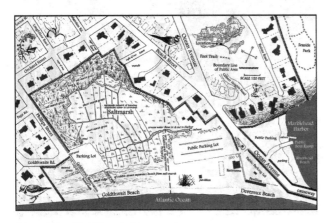

Map of the Goldthwait Reservation. Courtesy of Jay J. Johnson.

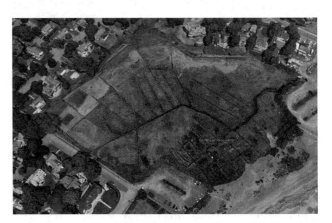

Aerial view of the Goldthwait Reservation. © Google 2021.

CHAPTER 34

Ernest A. Codman
Father of the "End-Result Idea" Movement

A descendent of early Puritan colonists, Ernest Amory (pronounced "Emmery") Codman was born in Boston, Massachusetts on December 30, 1869, to Elizabeth Hand Codman and William Combs Codman, who participated first in the East India trade (as an importer) and later worked in Boston real estate and insurance. Ernest was raised the youngest of four children—three boys and one girl—at 23 West Cedar Street.

Codman attended Fay School, founded in 1866 as the first junior boarding school in the country. Traditionally, students at the Fay were prepared to attend the nearby St. Mark's School

Physician Snapshot

Ernest A. Codman

BORN: 1869

DIED: 1940

SIGNIFICANT CONTRIBUTIONS: Recorded the first examples of charting in anesthesia with Dr. Harvey Cushing; the first skiagrapher (radiologist) at Boston Children's Hospital; the first to use x-rays for physiologic research; an early advocate for the use of x-ray to establish early diagnosis and to aid in surgical planning; author of the seminal text *The Shoulder* (in which he describes what came to be known as Codman's Paradox); champion for the End-Result Idea (now known as treatment outcomes); a founder of the American College of Surgeons and the Committee on Standardization of Hospitals; established the Codman Hospital; author of *A Study in Hospital Efficiency*; co-developer of a Registry of Bone Sarcoma; described Codman's sign, Codman's exercises, Codman's triangle and Codman's tumor; received the 1940 Gold Medal from the American Academy of Orthopaedic Surgeons

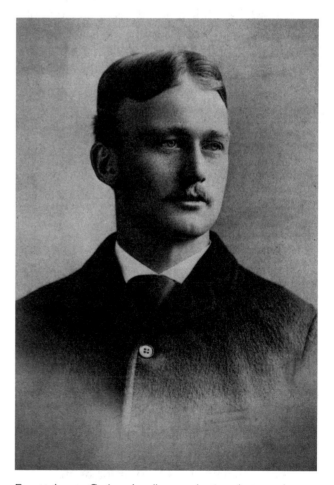

Ernest Amory Codman's college graduation photograph.
Boston Medical Library in the Francis A. Countway Library of Medicine.

93

(opened 1865), an Episcopal preparatory school. Both were located in Southboro, Massachusetts. Codman attended St. Mark's from grade 8 through 12, graduating in 1887. At St. Marks he was active in sports—including baseball, football, and tennis—despite problems with his left knee that would continue through his adult life. He also developed a passion for hunting and fishing. At graduation he received the Founder's Award, given to the best overall student in the school, including in academics. Nick Noble, communications manager and school historian at St. Mark's School reviewed Codman's record at St. Mark's and wrote the following in 1997:

> Based on my reading of the record and experience with several [records] from the late 19th Century...my assessment of the young Codman [is]: Very bright, fastidious to the point of obsessiveness (neat, punctual, precise), independent, something of a loner, not a joiner. Marches to his own drummer...congenial and popular despite (or perhaps because of) this. Perhaps some of his decorum difficulties stem from constant questioning and challenging... not uncommon in a mind like Codman's, but frustrating as hell for the typical teacher of the 1880s. A bit mischievous, and not reluctant to accept a challenge (this might also account for his popularity.) (Noble 1997)

Codman continued his studies at Harvard College, graduating with an AB degree, cum laude, in 1891. Although there is no record of where he lived at the time, he most likely remained in his house on West Cedar Street. In the Fifth Report of the Class of 1891, he wrote, "There are many men in the class of '91 who make more money, but they are very few who really enjoyed their work as much as I do, and I know of no one who has sense enough to go fishing and shooting as much"; he obviously maintained his passion for hunting and fishing ("Harvard College, Class of 1891. Secretary's Report, No. 5" 1911).

By 1891, Harvard Medical School (HMS) had been located on Boylston Street for eight years. It was there that Codman completed his medical school education, within walking distance from his brother John's home at 104 Mount Vernon Street, where he rented a room. Harvey W. Cushing, soon to be one of Codman's closest friends, enrolled in HMS in September, the same year as Codman. Cushing lived at 32 West Cedar Street as a medical student, close to both Codman's room on Mount Vernon and even closer to Codman's birthplace at the foot of Beacon Hill. On occasion, while in medical school, Codman would invite Cushing to Nahant to his brother's house during the warm summer months; both would attend a concert or have dinner in Codman's home.

At the time of their enrollment, HMS had been transformed through President Charles Eliot's leadership and foresight. Codman and Cushing received clinical instruction from illustrious teachers such as John Collins Warren, Reginald Heber Fitz, David Williams Cheever, Frederick Cheever Shattuck, Maurice Howe Richardson, and John Homans. They also benefited from the instruction of faculty such as Thomas Dwight (anatomy), Charles Sedgwick Minot (histology and embryology), Henry Pickering Bowditch (physiology), and Edward Stickney Wood (medical chemistry).

Codman and Harvey Cushing were honored early; both were selected for the Boylston Medical Society in April of their first year. During their second year, both were prosectors for Dr. Maurice Richardson's anatomy demonstrations. Codman described his medical school experience:

> I was a conventional enough Boston-Harvard boy, with relatives and acquaintances among the well-to-do, and took two years in the Harvard Medical School with success, and in the third winter had the opportunity to travel in Europe and Egypt with a friend, on the understanding that I could spend as much time as I wished at the Clinics in the various cities we visited, London, Paris, Berlin, Vienna, Cairo

and others. This experience and some study on the way enabled me to pass my third-year examinations and to get my degree on my return.

It was in Vienna that my attention was first attracted to the subdeltoid bursa, because it was mentioned in a little book by Dr. E. Albert [*Diagnostik der Chirugisher Krankheiten*, by Alfred Holder, Wein 1893]. I had never heard this bursa spoken of at home by my teachers, nor do I think it was mentioned in American medical literature at that time. (Codman 1934)

Upon his return, Codman received his medical degree on June 26, 1895. He then interned in surgery with Cushing at the Massachusetts General Hospital from 1894 to 1895. He remembered that "during this period, [I] sometimes made diagnoses of subdeltoid bursitis, which were ignored by my seniors" (Codman 1934). It was there that he also learned to give anesthesia, and he and Cushing would strive to see who could achieve the best outcomes. Codman had to grapple with losing a patient early on when his first anesthetized patient died, but their friendly competition furthered their knowledge, technique, and innovation and led them to maintain the first anesthesia records. They made note of respirations, pulse, operation performed, and the surgeon. It's unclear who won the competition, but 25 years later Codman wrote to Cushing and said:

> Katie [Codman's wife], after my departure dumped all the accumulations of years into one pile...One of the things that I cannot bear to dump in the wastebasket is a collection of ether charts which we made 30 years ago! In connection therewith, I find a long unpublished paper on "Etherization," in which I described vividly...the process as we then knew it. I must say I have never read anything better on the subject. I recall the reason for not publishing

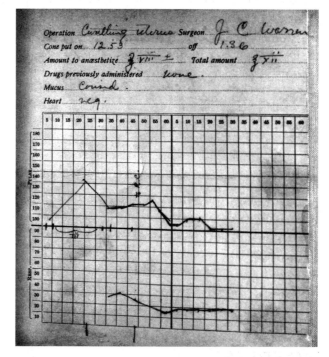

Early anesthesia record by Codman, November 30, 1894. Front of card.

H. K. Beecher, "The First Anesthesia Records (Codman, Cushing)," *Surgery, Gynecology and Obstetrics* 1940; 71: 690. Massachusetts General Hospital, Archives and Special Collections.

Early anesthesia record by Codman, November 30, 1894. Back of card.

H. K. Beecher, "The First Anesthesia Records (Codman, Cushing)," *Surgery, Gynecology and Obstetrics* 1940; 71: 690. Massachusetts General Hospital, Archives and Special Collections.

it was, that I took it to "Coll" Warren, who regarded it as too frank for the good of the hospital, for it described in detail the case which I lost in the A.R. [accident room] because I was paying attention to some tomfoolery which you...were entertaining us with, while the poor devil was inhaling vomitus. I also spoke of the case which stopped breathing under ether and interested you in brain surgery. So, I send you these charts to destroy some solemnity for you and I are the only persons that give a ____ for them. (quoted in Beecher 1940)

Dr. Henry K. Beecher wrote to both Codman and Cushing in 1939 asking permission to publish their records as the first examples of charting in anesthesia, which formally began at MGH in 1915. Codman replied:

I do not wish to take credit for starting the charts because of my recollection the keeping of these charts was suggested by my chief, Dr. F. B. Harrington. I, of course, did the work, but it was Dr. Harrington who thought that such a study would be valuable. If I recollect correctly, Dr. Cushing took up the work after I had finished my work as etherizer for I am quite sure that Dr. Cushing got his appointment about eight months later than I did, although we were in the same class in medical school. (quoted in Beecher 1940)

Ultimately, the winner of the friendly competition was to receive a dinner, but neither Cushing nor Codman were forthcoming in who won the competition.

FIRST SKIAGRAPHER AT BOSTON CHILDREN'S HOSPITAL

Codman began his practice and an appointment as assistant in anatomy at HMS in 1895, the same year he completed his training at MGH. His office was at 104 Mount Vernon Street, Boston. He noted:

It so happened that Röntgen made his announcement of the discovery of X-ray in December...Believing in its importance to surgery, I at once started to learn the technique and sought the help of Professor Trowbridge of Harvard, and also that of Professor Elihu Thomson of the General Electric Company at Lynn...[The] apparatus similar to that which Röntgen worked had existed for a number of years in many other laboratories...Trowbridge and Thomson were among the first in this city to [repeat Röntgen's experiment], and I had their most kindly, personal, instruction. (Codman 1934)

Immediately after Roentgen's discovery physicians and scientists in the United States and around the world began experimenting with and developing x-rays using different devices. Edison explored rates of fluorescing using different chemicals and finally developed a radiological scan—the fluoroscope—that could show moving images of the inside of the human body. Walter Dodd, apothecary and photographer at the MGH, also began experimenting with production of x-rays. (I was unable to discover if Codman and Dodd ever collaborated; it appears they did not. Eventually Dodd was appointed as the first radiologist at the MGH in 1908 and appointed instructor in roentgenology at HMS.) Codman remembered:

Having learned the essential points, I found at the laboratory of Harvard Medical School [a] similar apparatus [Crookes tube] and began clinical work in 1896. For five years I devoted most of my time to the x-ray, although still continuing to work in the Surgical Out-Patient Department of the MGH and to assist the late F. B. Harrington in the practice of surgery." (Codman 1934)

In February 1896, x-rays were used in a clinical setting. Gilbert Frost, professor of medicine at Dartmouth Medical School, performed a diagnostic x-ray of the wrist of Eddie McCarthy, a 14-year-old, using a battery of seven Grove cells, a Puling tube, and an Apps coil. Edwin Frost took the images. He published the case in the February 4, 1896, issue of *Science*. Almost as soon as the x-ray was developed, popular misperception was that x-rays could cure diseases—even cancer. This misperception was perpetuated by American newspapers for 20 years. For example, the *Chicago Daily Tribune* published an article asserting this in April 1896. However, Codman worked with x-rays for seven years before responding that objective review did not support this misperception and that patient outcomes in his private practice and at Massachusetts General Hospital showed that x-rays were not an effective treatment modality.

Codman followed Frost's February 1896 case shortly thereafter with his first publication of an x-ray. In a March 1896 correspondence to the *Boston Medical and Surgical Journal*, he showed a radiograph of a fetal arm. He produced an x-ray of the arm of a deceased full-term infant using a Crooke's tube with a four-inch spark induction coil and a battery. He later remembered: "[It] is interesting as showing the degree of ossification of the fetal bones at birth...Only the shafts of the long bones are ossified, while the wrist bones and epiphyses are still cartilaginous" (Codman 1896). During this period Codman simultaneously worked in Professor Henry P. Bowditch's research lab at HMS where he collaborated with Walter W. Cannon to study the physiology of swallowing in animals. Together, they were the first to use x-rays for physiologic research. Codman managed the fluoroscopy x-ray machine toward that pursuit.

By December 1896, after less than one year of producing x-rays along with many others in the United States, Codman raised the issue of skin injury secondary to exposure to x-rays with Professor Elihu Thomson. Codman wrote that he

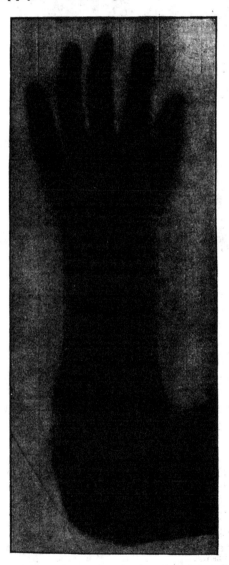

First x-Ray by Codman: Fetal arm, March 1896.

E. A. Codman, "Radiograph of Fetal Arm," Boston Medical and Surgical Journal 1896; 134: 327.

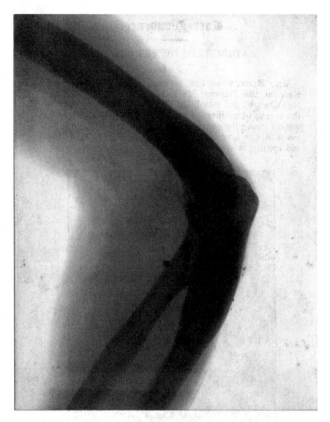

X-Ray of Dr. Henry P. Bowditch's elbow revealing retained bullet fragments from the Civil War. It was taken by Codman. Bowditch was surprised when he learned that he had these fragments remaining in his arm, when shown the x-ray taken by Codman. Boston Medical Library in the Francis A. Countway Library of Medicine.

had no skin reactions. However, Thomson, after hearing about such injuries, purposely exposed his left fifth finger very close (1-¼ inch) to the source of the x-rays for a half an hour. Thomson (1896) wrote that:

> for about nine days very little effect was noticed, then the finger became hypersensitive to the touch, dark red, somewhat swollen, stiff, and soon after… began to blister… [which] spread in all directions… [with] formation of purulent matter…escap[ing] through a crack in the blister…[After] three weeks…the healing process seems to be…slow…while the pain and sensitiveness have largely left…the last day or two…I assure you that I will make shorter exposures hereafter.

In the three years that followed, Codman recorded that he:

> studied the joints and bursae injected with non-radiable material. In 1898, after two years of these anatomic studies I presented to the Warren Museum an album, which contained standard X-ray anatomic pictures of each joint of the body in flexion, extension, etc. It was a tremendous piece of work, and for me at that time, a very expensive one. Recently, in poking around the museum I came across this album covered with dust. It probably had not been opened since left there. However, the experience had been valuable, for, after completing the study of the normal joints, I became interested in their pathology, especially in that of the wrist, knee and shoulder. Furthermore, the fact that my atlas of the normal joints was not used by my colleagues, was a good lesson to my personal sensitiveness and taught me…to postpone hope of recognition of labor.
> (Codman 1934)

Dr. Codman's album of x-rays included all the joints in the body in flexion, extension, and other positions; it remains in the Center for the History of Medicine at the Countway Medical Library. It was never published.

In 1898, however, he did publish a series of x-rays similar to a section of his album. Included were x-rays taken of a single cadaver: the wrist in various positions, with observations on carpal bone position changes, x-rays after injection of the joints with metallic mercury and some following injection of the arteries with a mixture of starch and red mercury salt (an early arteriogram). Over the next eight years, Codman published about 12 articles on x-rays.

In 1899, Codman was appointed the first skiagrapher (radiologist) at Boston Children's Hospital, and he was promoted to surgeon to outpatients at MGH from his former position as assistant surgeon to outpatients. The following

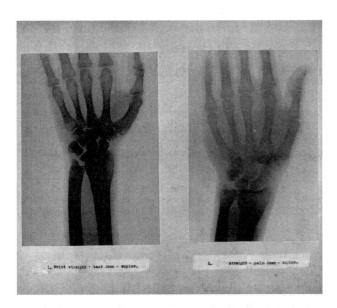

Example of x-rays (hand) contained in Codman's unpublished album of x-rays. Boston Medical Library in the Francis A. Countway Library of Medicine.

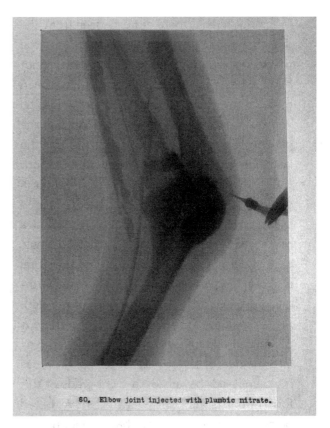

Early example of an arthrogram (elbow) by Codman using plumbic (lead) nitrate. Contained in his unpublished album of x-rays. Boston Medical Library in the Francis A. Countway Library of Medicine.

year, he also changed his HMS appointment from assistant in anatomy to assistant in clinical operative surgery. In his new role, Codman presented a paper that same year to the Boston Society for Medical Improvement. He illustrated the use of x-rays with lantern slides of clinical cases to diagnose a series of 23 cases of different diseases or infections of bone. He explained how x-rays could be used to establish an early diagnosis and aid in the surgical planning by defining the exact limits of the diseased area. In the major portion of this paper he reviewed 140 cases of fractures of the distal radius. He selected: "Colles fracture as an illustration, hoping that I may show of what value the x-ray has been in this troublesome lesion. I am indebted to the outpatient surgeons of the Massachusetts General Hospital for the cases and to Mr. Dodd for most of the skiagrams" (Codman 1900). Codman then classified the variations in fracture patterns of the distal radius into 10 categories.

Charles Scudder's (see chapter 31) groundbreaking book *The Treatment of Fractures* also published in 1900, and Codman had contributed a chapter on x-rays titled, "The Rontgen Ray and Its Relation to Fractures." Codman's chapter was included in the first several editions of Scudder's book. In only four years after Roentgen's discovery, "the X-ray department has become a necessity in every general hospital" (Codman 1905).

Codman's interest in x-rays continued throughout his career, but he left his position as part-time skiagrapher at Boston Children's Hospital in about 1901 and directed his efforts to surgery at MGH. He was succeeded for the next two years at Boston Children's Hospital by Dr. Robert Osgood (see chapter 19). In 1903, Dr. Percy E. Brown was appointed radiologist there. Following Codman's initiative, Brown continued to produce roentgenograms on glass plates, and in 1905 coauthored an article with Dr. Robert Lovett on the "radiology of hip disease" (see chapter 16.) In a letter to the *Boston Medical and Surgical Journal* in 1901, on the safety of x-rays Codman wrote:

In careful hands, there is no danger from the use of the x-ray to the patient and very little to the operator...In the last five years about 8000 exposures in over 3000 cases have been made at the Massachusetts General Hospital without a single case of x-ray dermatitis in the patient. That at the Children's Hospital, in the last eighteen months, we have made about 1000 exposures and over 300 cases, without a single case of dermatitis in the patient. That in the last five years, in my private patients, I have made nearly 1000 exposures without a single case of dermatitis in the patient. The sum total is about 10,000 exposures in 4000 cases without one case of loss of hair or burn of the skin. As far as danger to the operator goes, there is no question that a serious dermatitis extending into the deeper layers may be set up. At times my own hands have had...a slight grade of this form of burn, but they have...never excoriated or cracked, nor so severe that I could not go through the ordinary permaganate preparation for surgical operations. I attribute this...to my habit of never exposing myself near the tube if I can possibly help it. (Codman 1901)

The following year, Codman published a study on accidental x-ray burns. He reviewed the small amount of literature available in an attempt to locate every reported case. From 1896 through 1901, he found a decline in the total cases each year concluding: "The main reasons for such a decrease have been the bitter teachings of experience and the fact that the introduction of better apparatus has done away with long exposures and the close approximation of the tube" (Codman 1902). He classified the injuries into five types, completed a detailed analysis of the causative factors, and reported these factors—if known—in 171 cases. He concluded that "more than two-thirds of these injuries occurred in the first two years of the use of the X-ray...The important factors which contribute to the production of X-ray burns are: the intensity of the current used to stimulate the tube; the quality of the tube; the distance and time of exposure; the idiosyncrasy of the patient" (Codman 1902). Years later, he reflected:

> There were many amusing, exciting and tragic episodes in those days, for we all had burns and some of us gave them. Many of my old friends are now dead from X-ray cancer. It was fortunate for me that my interest in surgery was greater than in Röntgen's discovery. (Codman 1934)

Codman had an interest in common problems that he observed in the MGH clinic: sprains and fractures of the wrist, shoulder, and ankle. He found that he could more accurately differentiate a sprain from a fracture through the combined use of x-rays and his increasing clinical skills, and he reported this experience with cases. Codman published an interesting article in 1904, "Some Points on the Diagnosis and Treatment of Certain Neglected Minor Surgical Lesions." He had originally prepared it for presentation at the Worcester District Medical Society, but the meeting did not have time for his presentation, so he published it in the *Boston Medical and Surgical Journal*, the predecessor of the *New England Journal of Medicine*. He discussed the use of x-rays in the diagnosis of scaphoid fractures, lunate dislocations, tuberculosis of the wrist and other wrist entities and their value in diagnosing shoulder problems as well as ankle injuries. He wrote, "The material which I

SOME POINTS ON THE DIAGNOSIS AND TREATMENT OF CERTAIN NEGLECTED MINOR SURGICAL LESIONS.[1]

BY E. A. CODMAN, M.D., BOSTON.

BOSTON MEDICAL AND SURGICAL JOURNAL

APRIL 7, 1904

VOL. CI, No. 14

Title of Codman's article in which he stresses the importance of x-rays to differentiate sprains from fractures or dislocations.
Boston Medical and Surgical Journal 1904; 150: 371.

have used for this paper I have obtained from my service in the Surgical Out-Patient Department of the Massachusetts General Hospital...Among the lesions which have been most troublesome, are certain unrecognized fractures which we have only lately learned to distinguish from sprains" (Codman 1904).

The following year, Codman coauthored an extensive review of these common problems—especially the scaphoid fracture and a lunate dislocation—with Henry Chase. They published a two-part article in the *Annals of Surgery*, providing examples that demonstrated the benefit of x-rays when establishing the diagnosis. They also discussed the treatment of injuries. They wrote:

> The first case of simple fracture of the scaphoid bone of the wrist...was considered a sprain, but the continued symptoms led us...to examine the wrist with the fluoroscope, and the fracture was then easily recognized...During the next four years occasional examples of this lesion presented themselves at the Clinic, but it was not until a private case...came to me in December 1901, that I fully appreciated the importance of this fracture. The failure of rest, time, massage, and, finally, a forcible manipulation to restore the perfect functions of this young man's wrist, has led me to study with great care all the other cases of carpal injuries which I have met in my hospital work. As result of the study, I now recommend excision of one or both portions of the broken scaphoid...We have [reported] cases...which we have...been able to observe for some months or years after their original injury...I considered these lesions as entirely due to trauma...That error in diagnosis and treatment of these injuries is frequent as well illustrated by four articles which have appeared in this Journal during the last four years. (Codman and Chase 1905)

After discussions of the development of the carpal bones, symptoms of simple fracture of the scaphoid bone, diagnosis of simple fracture of the scaphoid, the use of x-ray in the diagnosis, and treatment of fracture of the scaphoid, the authors described the details in treatment of 18 cases. They concluded:

> I. Cases which had not been treated or have been treated as sprains...seldom, if ever, have union of the fragments. II. If the joint is kept fixed for a number of weeks immediately after the injury, union may occur, but the functional result is not perfect... III. It is too late to obtain union if fixation

Two-part article by Codman and Chase demonstrating the importance of x-rays to diagnose and treat carpal scaphoid fractures and lunate dislocations. *Annals of Surgery* 1905; 41: 863.

is not attempted within a few weeks after the injury. IV. Excision of the proximal half of the broken scaphoid promises a better ultimate result than any other form of treatment. V. Since operation…is an undesirable risk, reasonable attempt should be made to obtain union by fixation [splints], if the case is seen soon after the injury…
(Codman and Chase 1905)

In their second article, Codman and Chase discussed dislocation of the lunate with or without fracture of the scaphoid and carpal injuries in general with additional brief case reports. They summarized their important points:

1. "Sprains" of the wrist which do not promptly recover are in many cases fractures or dislocations of the carpal bones.
2. The large majority of such carpal injuries are either simple fractures of the scaphoid or anterior dislocations of the semilunar bone.
3. These two injuries are frequently combined…
4. Simple fracture of the scaphoid gives a definite clinical picture…with (a) the history of a fall on the extended hand; (b) localized swelling in the radial half of the wrist-joint; (c) acute tenderness in the anatomical snuff-box when the hand is adducted; (d) limitation extension by muscle spasm…causes unbearable pain.
5. A broken scaphoid has a little power of repair…
6. Fractures of the scaphoid which remain untreated or are treated by massage and active and passive motion generally… remain ununited…
7. Cases of fracture of the scaphoid may unite if motion of the wrist is prevented during the first four weeks after the injury, but if by this time no union has occurred, future union is unlikely.
8. Excision of the proximal half of the fractured scaphoid gives a somewhat better result than conservative treatment.
9. A posterior incision to the outer side of the tendons of the extensor communis digitorum gives an easy and safe access to the proximal half of the scaphoid.
10. Passive motion of the wrist-joint and active motion of the fingers should be begun within a week after this operation.
11. The possibility of the existence of a bipartite scaphoid should be considered in interpreting x-rays…but its occurrence must be very rare in comparison with fracture.
12. Anterior dislocation of the semilunar bone should be recognized clinically, even without the x-ray by…the following symptoms…(a) history of an injury…to the extended or twisted wrist; (b) a silver-fork deformity…(c) a tumor under the flexor tendons…(d) a shortened appearance of the palm…(e) stiffness of the partially flexed fingers, motion of which…is painful; (f)…normal relation of the styloid process of the ulna and radius [and] shortening of the distance from the radial styloid to the base of the first metacarpal.
13. Recent dislocations of the semilunar may be reduced with good result even after the fifth week by hyperextension followed by hyperflexion over the thumbs of an assistant held firmly in the flexure of the wrist on the semilunar.
14. Irreducible dislocations demand excision of the semilunar and the whole or a portion of the scaphoid if there is a coincident fracture of the latter. (Codman and Chase 1905)

That same year, Codman had submitted a monograph with associated images on "The Use of the X-ray in the Diagnosis of Bone Diseases" for consideration for the Samuel W. Gross Prize. He did not win the award, and he noted "busy surgeons had no idea of the practical value of the X-ray in the diagnosis of bone diseases, and that the pictures which I presented to this committee were to them unintelligible" (Codman 1934). He remembered he didn't feel the full import of his rejection until five years later when one of the committee members for the prize (Dr. William W. Keen) "asked me to write a chapter on 'The Use of the X-ray in Surgery'" (Codman 1934). He remembered, "I could make up my mind to the shock it gave me to feel that my essay had been discarded, for I felt absolutely sure that it was worthy of the prize...I had great satisfaction in pulling out from a closet the unpublished paper...and with practically no changes, presented it to [Dr. Keen] for his book" (Codman 1934). Codman emphasized:

> It should be stated, however, that when the limits of error are kept clearly in mind, the actual value of the discovery [of x-ray] to surgical science is very great. When there is doubt of the diagnosis of fracture, no physician has done his full duty by his patient if he can command a skiagraph examination and has not used it. This is particularly true in medicolegal cases when there is a question of liability. (Codman 1905)

Keen's textbook, *Surgery: Its Principles and Practices*, was a popular book on surgery for many years (1909–1919). Codman wrote two chapters for Keen's textbooks, including "Use of X-ray and Radium in Surgery" and in a subsequent edition, "The X-ray in Surgery." In the latter chapter Codman emphasized:

> that the data furnished by the x-ray are always accurate and that the interpretation only offers a chance of error [and therefore] we realized the importance of looking for the interpretation from a person whose fundamental knowledge of anatomy, physiology, pathology, and clinical medicine is of the best...Röentgenology has become a legitimate specialty, i.e., a branch of the science of medicine a knowledge of which sufficiently thorough to justify practice requires more time than can be accorded to it by the general practitioner. (Codman 1909)

THE SHOULDER

Codman remembered that beginning with his 1899 appointment as surgeon to outpatients at MGH, he "began to have a great clinical opportunity, and treated many patients on the diagnosis of bursitis" ("Harvard College Class of 1891. Secretary's Report No.3" 1899). As his time as a skiagrapher drew to a close and after "having

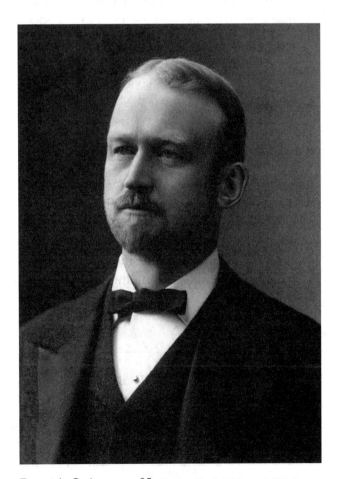

Ernest A. Codman, age 35. Boston Medical Library in the Francis A. Countway Library of Medicine.

written a number of articles on X-ray subjects, including one on X-ray burns," he "saw that I must choose between surgery and roentgenology" (Codman 1934). Codman published his first article on the shoulder in April 1904. He recalled:

> I [previously] had presented a résumé of my work, demonstrating many anatomic specimens and some patients. This attracted the attention of Dr. George Crile of Cleveland, who invited me to read a paper on the subject before the Medical Society of that city...During the discussion Dr. Carl A. Hamann of Cleveland mentioned a paper by Küster published in 1902. I had, at the time, never seen this article, and, though I am frequently quoted as having been the first to describe subdeltoid bursitis, this paper clearly shows that I was not. After seeing Küster's paper, I adopted his name of subacromial bursitis as better than the term subdeltoid. My work was original so far as I knew at the time, and it was pleasant rather than the reverse, to find that the great surgeon, Küster, had also thought it worthwhile to write...a short paper on the subject. ("Harvard College Class of 1891. Secretary's Report No.3" 1899)

Codman published his presentation to the Academy of Medicine of Cleveland in 1906, "On Stiff and Painful Shoulders: The Anatomy of the Subdeltoid or Subacromial Bursa and Its Clinical Importance. Subdeltoid Bursitis." Based upon his cadaver dissections and findings at surgery, he wrote:

ON STIFF AND PAINFUL SHOULDERS.
THE ANATOMY OF THE SUBDELTOID OR SUBACROMIAL BURSA AND ITS CLINICAL IMPORTANCE.* SUBDELTOID BURSITIS.
BY E. A. CODMAN, M.D., BOSTON.

Codman's first publication on the shoulder and bursitis, 1906. *Boston Medical and Surgical Journal* 1906; 154: 613.

> I do not know of any book on anatomy [with] a fair description of this bursa. You must go to the cadaver and demonstrate it for yourselves. Anatomists have devoted little attention to it...It has been claimed that there is a normal communication between the subdeltoid bursa and the true joint. This has not been my experience...I believe that it will be found that most minor lesions of the shoulder joint involve the bursa, and few involve the true joint...As far as I have been able to find yet, I may claim that my anatomical observation that external rotation of the humerus is necessary for complete elevation of the arm is original. (Codman 1906)

Two years later, Codman published a series of seven articles over approximately six weeks on subdeltoid bursitis in the *Boston Medical and Surgical Journal* which were also published together as one paper in the *Communication of the Massachusetts Medical Society*, also in 1908, and in the *Publication of the Massachusetts General Hospital* in 1909. He recorded:

> During the summer of 1906 [after his May 1906 article on subdeltoid bursitis] my colleagues at the Massachusetts General Hospital, not only in the surgical, but in the orthopedic, nerve and medical departments, were kind enough to turn over their shoulder cases for me to study... Thanks to their kindness and from cases in my private practice I now have complete notes on 75 lesions of the subdeltoid or subacromial bursa. (Codman 1908)

He begins his articles by describing the anatomy of the shoulder and motion of the humerus: "The ligamentous capsule of the shoulder joint is a very insignificant structure and that the real capsule of the joint is a muscular one formed by the subscapularis, the supra-and-infra-spinatus and the teres minor. These muscles have tendinous expansions at their insertions" (Codman 1908). He also described motion of the humerus: "By elevation of the arm I mean...that elevation implies a departure toward the frontal plane. As far as I know, there is no anatomical name for this motion. It is really a combination of abduction and external rotation" (Codman 1908). Some 25 years later, with the publication of his book, *The Shoulder*, Codman devoted a whole chapter (chapter 2) on normal motions of the shoulder. In it he describes what is known as Codman's Paradox:

> And now we come to a curious paradox which I have only recently observed, although I have studied the motion of the shoulder for years. You can prove that the completely elevated arm is in either extreme external rotation or in extreme internal rotation...[and] the range of rotation of the humerus diminishes as it is elevated...
>
> [It is] difficult to explain the paradox of the ability of the elevated arm to descend without rotating and come at will to the side in either external rotation or internal rotation. (Codman 1934)

In a brief section on pathology, Dr. Codman adds one observation to supplement his previous paper on the pathology of subacromial bursitis:

> The only point worth speaking of is...that the spot on the greater tuberosity where the tendon of the supraspinatus is usually found damaged...I am more convinced...that partial ruptures at the insertion of this tendon may occur from muscle violence alone...during abduction...when the burden of overcoming inertia is suddenly thrown on the supraspinatus [and with] the deltoid...jams the tendinous expansion of the supraspinatus between the two bones [tuberosity and acromion]...It is surprising how large a proportion of subjects [dissecting room specimens] show evidence of chronic or healed lesions at this point. (Codman 1909)

In his next section, he discusses symptoms in acute, subacute, and chronic cases. In his acute classification, he discussed the findings of localized tenderness in the shoulder. He wrote: "just below the acromion process and...the outer side of the bicipital groove...this tender point being on the base of the bursa will disappear beneath the acromion when the arm is abducted [Dawbarn's sign]" (Codman 1909). In a letter to the editor of the *Boston Medical and Surgical Journal*, Dr. Codman disagreed with Dr. Robert H. M. Dawbarn, who apparently had suggested that his sign was pathognomonic of subdeltoid bursitis. He pointed out that the sign is positive in only acute cases where glenohumeral motion is not restricted stating, "I must submit...that it [Dawbarn's sign] is not 'pathognomonic' and that a large majority of

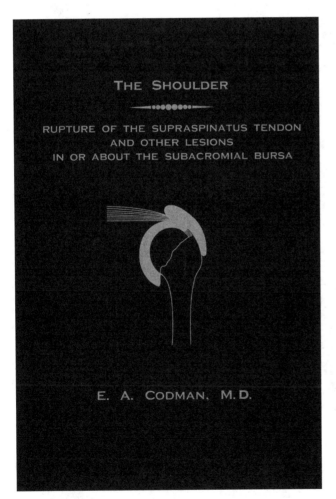

ASES reprint cover of Codman's book *The Shoulder*, originally published 1934. Courtesy of ASES.

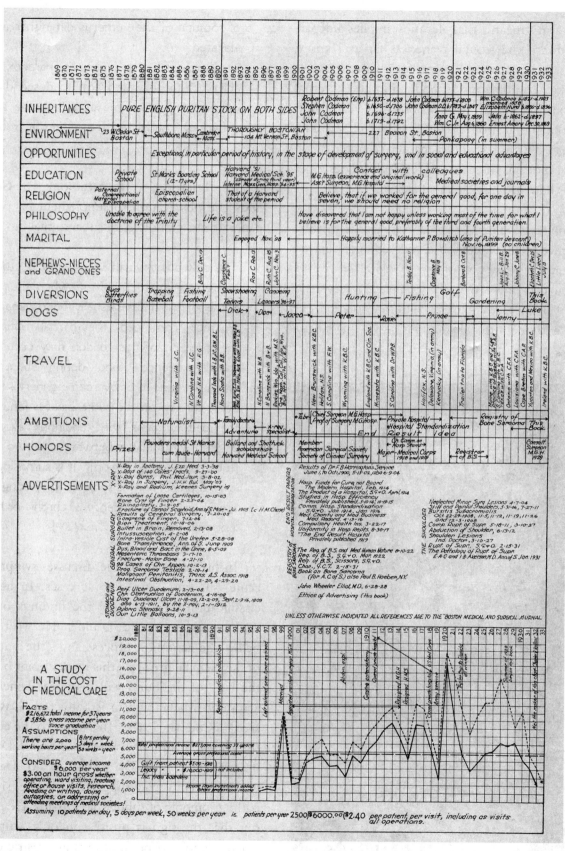

Dr. Codman reduced his life history to this chart.

The Shoulder: Rupture of the Supraspinatus Tendon and other Lesions in or about the Subacromial Bursa by Ernest A. Codman. Boston: Thomas Todd, 1934.

the cases do not exhibit this sign, because muscular spasm or actual adhesions prevent the passage of the tender point under the acromion" (Codman 1906).

After discussing differential diagnosis, Codman concludes with a discussion of treatment and brief summaries of 26 cases. For acute cases he treated the patient's pain with rest using a pillow splint with the arm abducted (preferable), or a sling with occasional swinging the arm at the patient's side (to avoid adhesions) combined with aspirin, morphine or other pain-relieving drugs. For severe cases he recommended:

treatment according to one of these three general plans:

Group A. Gradual stretching.

1. Leaving improvement to natural use.
2. Massage, passive and active exercises.
3. Manipulations by physician without anesthetic.
4. Xander exercises.
5. Baking, electric light, baths, etc.

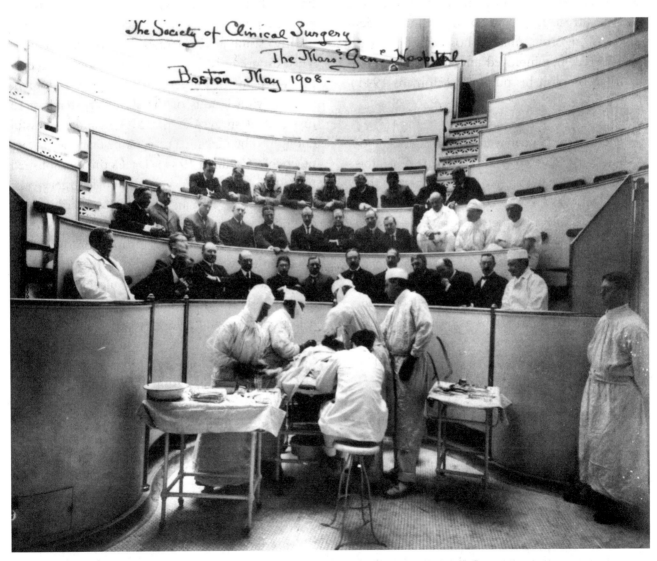

Codman operating in the Bigelow Amphitheatre during the meeting of the Society of Clinical Surgery, May 1908. Massachusetts General Hospital, Archives and Special Collections.

Group B. Rupture under an anesthetic.

1. Manipulation under an anesthetic without incision.
2. Manipulation followed by fixation in abduction.

Group C. Division.

1. Incision into the bursa and direct division of adhesions.
2. Excision of the subdeltoid portion of the bursa (Codman 1909)

Codman was known as a crusader. To him it was critical "to ensure for all in need of surgery...[the] ideal treatment" and "being an independent thinker of vigorous mind, whose emotions were easily stirred, he employed unconventional methods to accomplish his purpos"" (Homans 1941). He may have:

> inherited this tendency from his militant grandfather, the Reverend John Codman. When this Congregational minister became aware that his flock was likely to be contaminated by the teachings of his brother preachers, he refused to allow any other than his own discourses in his church in Dorchester. A hostile element placed another minister in the pulpit and protected him there by a guard. But John Codman climbed up the steps as high as he could, addressed the congregation and walked out with a large majority of those in church. The opposition soon gave in. (Homans 1941)

So too was Codman unwavering in his work and endeavors. In addition to and following his numerous publications on subacromial bursitis, Codman remembered that:

> We younger surgeons at that time did most of the night emergency operations, and in one such case I was able to make a preoperative diagnosis of perforated duodenal ulcer and to successfully operate on the patient. This took my mind from the shoulder to the duodenum... This led me to study chronic duodenal ulcer, and the shoulder remained displaced behind the duodenum and stomach for the next two years...I think I was among the first to appreciate its [duodenum] importance. (Codman 1934)

Dr. Codman suffered for many years himself with a duodenal ulcer. During the summer 1910, after attending a meeting of British surgeons in London, he recorded, "I spent several weeks after our official meeting was over. Part of this time I was a patient, and thanks to his [Mr. Moynihan] skill and a gastrojejunostomy, I was greatly relieved physically, and my zeal for surgery was greatly stimulated mentally" (Codman 1934). This experience led to him becoming "deeply interested in the surgery of the upper abdomen, still studying lesions of the shoulder, steadfast to my general surgery at the MGH, and successful enough to be making a reasonable living in private practice" (Codman 1934). Dr. Codman published more than 10 articles on abdominal surgery over the next three years. In addition to describing the diagnosis and successful surgical treatment of duodenal ulcers, he wrote classic papers on the differentiation of symptoms of ulcers in the duodenum versus ulcers above the pylorus, ulcer perforation, intussusception, chronic appendicitis, and intestinal obstruction and pyloric stenosis.

He devoted five chapters in his book on the supraspinatus tendon beginning with chapter 5, "Rupture of the Supraspinatus Tendon." Following a "Chart Contrasting Four Common Causes of Painful Shoulders," he opens the chapter with a reprint of his classic article of 1911, "Complete Ruptures of the Supraspinatus Tendon. Operative Treatment with Report of Two Successful Cases," stating:

> I have had two cases of complete rupture of the supraspinatus tendon on which I have operated, and in both of which I was able not only

to demonstrate the existence of the anatomical lesion in conjunction with the above symptoms, but succeeded by suturing the tendon to the tuberosity in bringing about complete restoration of the function of abduction. I have also, in a number of cases, verified the clinical diagnosis of partial rupture...a common lesion. (Codman 1934)

In addition to these five chapters, he published three articles on rupture of the supraspinatus in 1911 and 1912, but he did not publish another article on the supraspinatus for another 14 years.

From 1926 until 1938 (his last publication was on the supraspinatus), he published another six articles on ruptures of the supraspinatus. In addition, Dr. Codman left an unpublished paper describing the 89 cases that he had operated upon for supraspinatus tears and subacromial bursitis between 1902 and 1914. It was titled, "Abstracts and References to Hospital Records of the Cases Hitherto Operated on by Dr. Codman for Lesions About the Shoulder Joint. Bibliography." Codman concluded, "This list is offered to the surgical staff of Massachusetts General Hospital as a Standard in shoulder surgery, with the hopes the staff may assign this class of surgery to someone of their number...that he may raise the Standard by further contributions to the knowledge of the subject...demonstrated by improved results of the patients" (Harvard Medical School Archives, n.d.). Following the repair of the supraspinatus and other shoulder lesions Codman described his postoperative treatment:

After the first night...[I] let the patient put the arm in any comfortable position which he can find. Each day I exercise [the arm with] the general purpose...to let the patient bend his body from the hips with the arm relaxed [for] stooping exercises [later called Codman's pendulum exercises]...When in the stooping position, either lateral or antero-posterior motions can be done with pendulum-like movement without great muscular effort. In this position the humerus not only tends to avoid a fulcrum, but actually the weight of the arm helps to stretch the contracted tissue of the joint. (Codman 1934)

After chapters on nonadherent subacromial bursitis—which he believed was a tendinitis and called frozen shoulder—and dislocations and fractures involving the shoulder joint including his original description of the four-part fracture of the proximal humerus and humeral head which he described later in more detail, Codman included a chapter written by Dr. James H. Stevens, "Brachial Plexus Paralysis." Other than this chapter, Codman was the sole author of all other chapters in this book. Stevens, a neighbor of Codman, had completed 92 dissections of the brachial plexus (see chapter 17). At Codman's request, Stevens analyzed 16 cases for a chapter in the book, but Stevens died suddenly of a heart attack before completing his manuscript. Codman, in an introduction to the chapter, stated that he had edited Steven's paper and published it as chapter 11 in his book.

Chapter 13, "Hysteria Neurasthenia, Neurosis, Traumatic Neuritis, Malingering" covers a variety of complex issues that Codman correctly stated:

The line between organic and functional lesions is difficult to draw...Yet the distinction should be made...Every surgeon and practitioner unavoidably see cases in which the hysterical or nervous element is involved...Unavoidably, the question of the nervous element is frequently presented in cases of lesions of the shoulder...It would seem to me that a twenty-five per cent allowance for exaggeration might be fairly given to any normal patient when there are Medico-Legal questions involved. Furthermore, it is true that the longer a patient is laid up as the result of an injury, the more his mental state is involved in relation to the physical side...One of the strongest arguments against our Workmen's Compensation Laws is, that they so often result in producing this state [hysterical or malingering] of mind…[However] I do think that there is usually a physical basis for complaints of pain after shoulder injuries, and that injuries of the supraspinatus should be carefully considered in every case. (Codman 1934)

Following chapters on tumors (see Sarcoma Registry in this chapter) and other rare lesions of the shoulder, and before his epilogue, Codman, in his thoughtful and detailed way, included an index that on the left side included 33 diagnostic points and across the top 51 clinical entities, with the page numbers identified and where each of the diagnostic points and clinical entities are described in his book. He noted:

> The chart is capable of presenting a whole chapter on differential diagnosis…by writing out…the information contained in all the vertical and transverse columns…Unsatisfactory as this list may be, I challenge any student or professor to produce a better one…It offers a form of mental exercise for in the one who may be interested in lesions in and about the subacromial bursa. (Codman 1934)

END-RESULT IDEA

Early in his practice—as early as 1900—Codman became intrigued by "the common sense notion that every hospital should follow every patient it treats, long enough to determine whether or not the treatment has been successful, and then to inquire 'if not, why not'? with a view to preventing similar failures in future" (Codman 1934). He called this the End-Result Idea, which in today's terms is understood as treatment outcomes. He recorded: "My chief, Dr. F. B. Harrington, and I had been applying this plan practically to our service since 1900" (Codman 1934). For example, in 1902 and again in 1904, Codman reported in the *Boston Medical and Surgical Journal* a summary of the one year or longer results of cases treated from January 1 to October 1, 1900 and then again from January 1 to October 1, 1902. He stated:

> Last May, with Dr. Harrington's approval, postals were sent to many of the patients who had been in the East service of the previous year, asking them to call at the hospital on any morning during the first two weeks of June at about eleven. More than half of those…responded by letter or in person…were examined, and the results were noted in the records. These results were…so interesting and instructive to us that we…present them briefly to you in the following table…hoping that they may give some idea of a one–ninth of the surgical work of the hospital. (Codman 1902)

Codman then listed, in a table, the diseases treated and the results in the following categories: number traced, perfect result, good result, no improvement, bad result, died, died after leaving hospital, and total number treated. For example, in cases of bone and joint disease, there were eight cases traced with three perfect results and five good results with a total of 13 cases treated. In cases of fracture, there were 11 cases treated with three perfect results and eight good results with a total of 40 cases treated. Dr. Harrington concluded:

> I think the examination and tabulation of the results a year after operation is of great value. Certainly, it is of great interest to the operator. I was pleased and surprised at the number of cases which reported. Results are sometimes less successful than they seem to promise when the cases leave the hospital…Some of the other surgeons are in the habit of making this yearly examination of cases. I think all services should do so…I believe that a discharge card should be given to each patient, requesting them, when they leave the hospital, to report at the end of

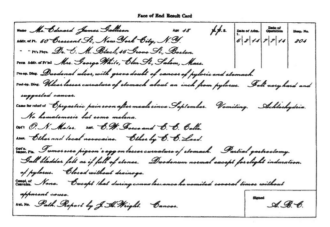

End-Result Card. Front of card (5-by-8-inches).
A Study in Hospital Efficiency: As Demonstrated by the Case Report of the First Five Years of a Private Hospital by Ernest A. Codman. Privately printed, 1918.

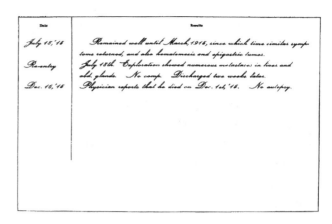

End-Result Card. Back of card.
A Study in Hospital Efficiency: As Demonstrated by the Case Report of the First Five Years of a Private Hospital by Ernest A. Codman. Privately printed, 1918.

the year during a certain period. To examine these cases does not require much time, and certainly is of great value, not only to the surgeons but to the house officers, who are thus enabled to see end results. (Codman 1902)

In the 1902 publication the patients were examined at one year by Codman or Harrington. Codman personally viewed the results in the 1904 publication, except for "a few who replied by letter (Codman 1904). In the latter cases:

> even if they reported that they were well, [they] are not classed 'as perfect' because they were not examined, for it is found that patients frequently consider themselves well...when they have...undesirable after-results...Perfect results are not discussed in the remarks... because they...speak for themselves. Good results include those cases which, while they showed some benefit from the operation, were nevertheless not completely relieved. (Codman 1904)

A few examples of Codman's remarks on bone and joint diseases included:

Perfect Results. One each of tuberculosis of the patella (excision...and drainage of joint...); "mice" in knee joint; displacement of semilunar cartilage; chronic synovitis of the knee... excision of shoulder for tuberculosis; excision of tubercular sequestra from humerus...excision septic bursa of olecranon; excision of necrosis of bone and amputation stump...Good results. One each of: excision of knee...excision of metatarsal and proximal phalanx of the great toe for tuberculosis...caries of ilium...reduction of semilunar bone of wrist and excision of portion of fractured scaphoid–somewhat sore and easily strained, some limitation of motion... No improvement. Periostitis of femur; chronic

Codman's report of the one-year results of patients treated on Harrington's service in 1900. *Boston Medical and Surgical Journal* 1902; 146: 513.

synovitis of the knee (probable tubercular). (Codman 1904)

Codman's concept of the End-Result Idea was not original, but he expanded and enhanced the concept, stressed its importance and spearheaded, to the objection of many, a major movement for both hospitals and surgeons to report their end results of treatment at one year or after the treatment. In Europe, some hospitals had been disseminating outcome reports as early as the 1760s. For example, starting in the late 1700s, the Edinburgh Infirmary published annual statistics in newspapers. Patients were designated as "incurable," "dismissed" (by decision of the hospital or patient, or for "irregularities"), "died," "cured," or "relieved." By the 1800s, British hospitals disseminated these outcome reports as a matter of routine.

The Massachusetts General Hospital also had previously published reported outcomes. For example, in 1838, Dr. Hayward, who replaced Dr. John Collins Warren while he was on vacation in Europe (see chapter 3), published the diagnoses and results at discharge of 222 patients treated on the surgical service. The category of discharge status included: well, much relieved, relieved, not relieved, died, unfit, or eloped. Dr. Codman expanded the concept of end results to include an analysis of the outcomes at one year after treatment. **Box 34.1** records Codman's memories of a plan he formed in 1910 with Dr. Edward Martin to organize the American College of Surgeons and a Committee on Standardization of Hospitals as a means to introduce the End-Result Idea to hospitals.

After formulating this clear vision for the future, Codman opened his own private hospital (12 beds) at 15 Pickney Street in Beacon Hill—just a few blocks from the Boston Common and six to eight blocks from MGH—in 1911. The ideals of the hospital are set forth in **Box 34.2**. He was concerned that the End-Result System would not be fully implemented at the MGH and, to some extent, it was a protest against the seniority system at the MGH. The End-Result Idea upheld the ideal that every patient would be evaluated at one year after surgery to determine their outcome or result of treatment. The End-Result System entailed a process in which the results of treatment at one year after surgery would be recorded on a card and kept in a file for all patients. Codman kept the cards in boxes in a dedicated room, and outcomes were reported by surgeon and by hospital. He remained on the staff at MGH while

Clinical Department.

A RÉSUMÉ OF THE RESULTS OF DR. F. B HARRINGTON'S SERVICE, MASSACHUSETTS GENERAL HOSPITAL, FROM JUNE 1 TO OCT. 1, 1902, AS SEEN IN THE FOLLOWING JUNE OR LATER.

BY E. A. CODMAN, M.D., BOSTON.

Codman's second article reporting the one-year results of patients treated on Harrington's service in 1902. *Boston Medical and Surgical Journal* 1904; 150: 618.

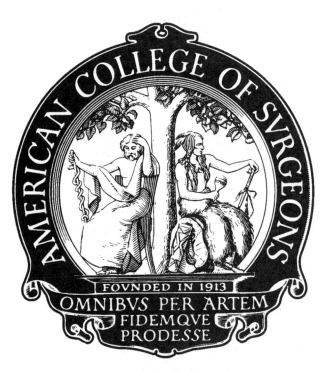

Seal of the American College of Surgeons. Courtesy of the American College of Surgeons.

Box 34.1. Introducing the American College of Surgeons and the Committee on Standardization of Hospitals

"From the day in the summer 1910 on which Dr. Edward Martin of Philadelphia and I drove back to London in a… cab from the Tuberculosis Sanatorium at Firmly, this End Result Idea has taken the major share of my intellectual efforts. Martin at once recognized that the idea was practical, and took advantage of my monomania to make me the servant of his own ideas about Hospital Standardization. We were visiting the British Surgeons as members of a small American Association called the Society of Clinical Surgery…Our little society was composed of very active-minded members [where] talk of an American College was inevitable [and] by the end of that meeting, the American College of Surgeons was underway…

"Edward Martin, after hearing me…caught at it as the catalyst to crystallize the College Idea. An American College would be a fine thing if it could be the instrument with which to introduce the End Result Idea into hospitals; in other words, to standardize them on a basis of service to the individual patient…As Martin remarked, "the tail is more important than the dog, but we shall have to have the dog to wag the tail"…I was only an assistant at home, had never had a hospital service entirely on my own, owing to the seniority system then in vogue, apparently very unlikely ever to have one…I returned [to Boston] in September 1910, full of enthusiasm and determined to undertake the following things: First: To proceed with my work on the shoulder…Second:…I wanted the opportunity to demonstrate what he [Mr. Moynihan] had taught me [about lesions of the upper abdomen], and…to progress still further in this kind of work. Third:…My talk with Edward Martin and the discussions…about an American College of Surgeons, took a dominant part of my mind.

"I determined that, as any increased opportunity at the MGH was most unlikely since the addition of a seniority system was so firmly fixed, I would start a small hospital where I would be my own master and could work out my own ideas. I especially wished to make it an example of the End Result Idea. There would be no trustees to consult, or other members of the staff to plicate, if I wished to state publicly the actual results of the treatment which the patients received…I would make this small hospital an example of the advantage of an organization based on actual efficiency analyses of the results of treatment…

"I had two assignments at the MGH, one to study shoulder cases, and the other to treat 100 successive cases of ulcers of the stomach and duodenum…Necessarily, if all our eighteen operators, who shared a service of only 180 beds, were to have a sufficient number of relatively rare occasions, each of us must agree to give his major attention to one field.

"In search of a convincing argument, I took great pain to look up the end results of our cases of stomach surgery, a total of about 600 in the previous ten years. I tabulated these…according to the lesions [and] to the results of each individual operator. These tables offered overwhelming evidence that good results had not been obtained by the eighteen surgeons…I naturally earned by this campaign a certain amount of hard feeling. My colleagues were very glad to have me attend the shoulder cases, for nobody else was interested in them…

"Meantime, I was stressing the End Result Idea and urging the staff and…the trustees, to make our clinic the pioneer in the movement. Through private donations, I obtained the money to provide an 'End Result Clerk', whose duty it was to…trace each patient a year from the date of discharge from the hospital and enter the result… on an End Result Card…

"[In 1910 Dr. Franklin Martin organized] the great meeting of surgeons…known as the Clinical Congress of Surgeons of North America [later named the American College of Surgeons] which held its first informal meeting in October 1910, in Chicago. [In its second meeting] in New York [in] (1912)…Dr. Edward Martin's [President] first act was to appoint two committees; one to organize an American College of Surgeons…the second a Committee on Standardization of Hospitals which I [Codman] was appointed Chairman with Dr. W. W. Chipman…Dr. J. G. Clarke…Dr. Allan B. Kanavel…and Dr. W. J. Mayo as the other members of the committee."

(Codman 1934)

also operating at his own private hospital. His goal was to:

> devote himself to his own hospital in future with the hope of setting up a practical and successful example to prove that...[his principles] are capable of actual demonstration. Even if a small fraction of the numbers of the profession of this community will help support this small hospital...to make it a practical success the big hospitals [especially the MGH] will be forced to accept these ideas, or else see capitalized institutions take up their work...If it is supported by the profession half the earnings will be devoted to increasing the equipment in diagnostic apparatus and the other to the salaries of myself and other young physicians...will be offered an opportunity to develop special skill in the different branches of diagnosis [specialists]... The hospital is open for the use of other surgeons [approximately twenty-four] under the same conditions as those under which we use it ourselves, namely strict observance of the End Result System. When we know that any surgeon has demonstrated at any recognized public institution results in any branch of surgery which are superior to ours [i.e. a specialist], we shall refer the case to him...Cases requiring expert diagnosis will be referred in the same way. (Harvard Medical School Archives, n.d.)

Box 34.2. The Ideals of the Codman Hospital

> "This hospital stands for the following ideals which it desires to help to introduce into modern medical and surgical practice.
>
> 1. The best possible modern diagnosis should precede any form of treatment.
> 2. Diagnosis should be made impersonally for large numbers of patients for relatively small fees, whereas personal care and the friendly attention of the private physician should command relatively large fees, for it necessarily can be well given to but few people.
> 3. Skilled treatment, especially surgical treatment, should also be given to large numbers for small fees, for the attainment of skill necessitates constant practice.
> 4. Large fees are only justifiable when the profession has recognized the skill of the operator from the published reports of a recognized institution where his unexcelled ability in some particular kind of work has been demonstrated.
> 5. The prime function of the large charitable hospitals is the treatment of patients too poor to employ a physician, not to give diagnosis to physicians. Their secondary function is to contribute to medical science and to train doctors and nurses to serve the community.
> 6. It is an abuse of their function to allow men who neither contribute to science nor medical education, to serve on their staff, unless these men can demonstrate superior skill by their results.
> 7. It is in abuse of the confidence of a patient for a physician or surgeon to undertake his treatment unless the diagnosis is obvious or has been made authoritatively, or the need is urgent.
> 8. It is an abuse of the confidence of the patient for any physician or surgeon to undertake treatment which he knows he is not well qualified to give, even if the patient thinks he is.
> 9. Successful treatment is justifiable but the physician or surgeon who undertakes treatment which proves unsuccessful should be liable to the law to show that his diagnosis was authoritative and his experience justified his undertaking the treatment."
>
> (Harvard Medical School Archive, n.d.)

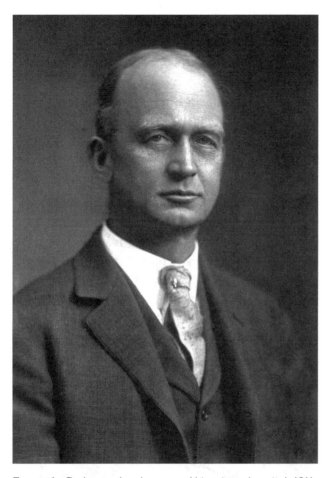

Ernest A. Codman when he opened his private hospital, 1911.
U.S. National Library of Medicine.

Codman argued that quality control was important for charitable hospitals, indicating that efficiency committees should publish results and that funding of hospital infrastructure, such as equipment or physical plant, should be conditioned on the quality of care.

Codman presented his first report from his Committee on Standardization of Hospitals to the annual meeting of the Clinical Congress of Surgeons in Chicago on November 11, 1913. It was an appeal to surgeons to participate in determining the end results of all cases operated upon at one year after surgery by both the hospitals and the individual surgeons. In his report, he stated:

> Further personal investigation of a number of the best institutions in the country developed the astounding fact that no effort is made to trace the patient beyond the gate of the hospital except such investigation as is individually made by members of the staff for their own interest...We have a paradox that neither the hospital trustees, the physician nor surgeon nor administrator consider it their business to make sure that the result to the patient is good.
>
> A factory which sells its product takes pains to assure itself that the product is a good one, but a hospital which gives away its product seems to regard the quality of that product as not worthy of investigation. In a way, trustees of hospitals who did not investigate the results to their patients do not audit their accounts. We believe it is the duty of every hospital to establish a follow-up system, so that...the result of every case will be available at all times for investigation by...the staff, the trustees... administration, [and] by other authorized investigators or statisticians...A method such as suggested is at present in use at the Massachusetts General Hospital...and other similar plans are being tried by a few other institutions...
>
> Your committee has been in touch [with committees in the American Medical Association and the American Hospital Association and] has approached the Carnegie Foundation with a petition that it should investigate the efficiency of American hospitals after a similar manner to that in which they recently investigated medical education [Flexner Report]...It is safe to assume that those employed by the Carnegie Foundation will thoroughly investigate such matters as business efficiency... (Codman et al. 1913)

> "Every hospital should follow every patient it treats long enough to determine whether or not the treatment was successful, and to inquire if not, why not, with a view to preventing similar failures in the future."
> —E. A. Codman, *The Shoulder*, 1934

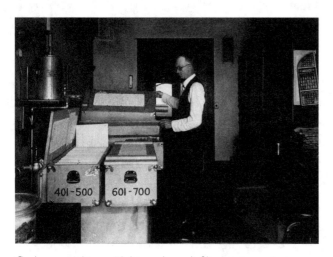

Codman working with his end-result filing system. Boston Medical Library in the Francis A. Countway Library of Medicine.

Some years later the Carnegie Foundation did partially finance the Hospital Standardization Program.

Prior to opening his private hospital in 1911, Codman had published four articles on patient outcomes. After his "Committee on Standardization of Hospitals" report in 1913, he published another 10 articles within four years. It was during the period of 1913 through 1917 that he passionately pursued the acceptance of his concepts concerning his End-Result Idea and Standardization of Hospitals. Codman read an address (see **Box 34.3**) to the Philadelphia County Medical Society on May 14, 1913, "The Product of a Hospital" which he published the following year.

In 1914, the leadership of the Clinical Congress of Surgeons in North America contacted Dr. Frederic J. Cotton for his assistance in arranging for their annual meeting to be held in Boston the following year. Dean Bradford invited Dr. Codman to a meeting on July 14, 1914, to discuss such a possibility and the hospitals' interest in a meeting of surgeons; and he learned that 184 notices had already been sent out by Dr. John T. Bottomly and Dr. Charles A. Porter asking surgeons to attend the meeting. Twenty-four surgeons attended; fourteen opposed the proposition for two reasons: they did not approve of the membership of the Clinical Congress of Surgeons or their leadership and they believed the meeting, where patients were operated upon with a general audience of surgeons, would be a danger to the patients. Codman, in a letter to the members of the Harvard Medical Association in Massachusetts, agreed with both arguments, but felt that both could be avoided (see **Box 34.4**).

Codman supported the clinical congress meeting in Boston. Following his request in his letter, there were numerous correspondences, both for and against the meeting; many letters were addressed to "Dear Amory." Codman kept a record of the votes and listed the names of Boston surgeons on both sides of the question. Some examples of those voting in favor included Drs. Charles Painter, Albert Ehrenfried, Elliott Brackett, Frederic Cotton, James Sever, Augustus

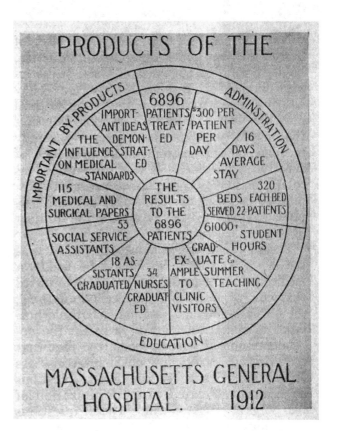

Graphic demonstration by Codman of various facts that depend on the central idea of the final results of 6,896 patients treated at MGH in 1912. E. A. Codman, "The Product of a Hospital," *Surgery, Gynecology and Obstetrics* 1914; 14: 496.

Box 34.3. Codman's Address to the Philadelphia Medical Society (May 14, 1913)

"The object of this address is to stimulate thought on and discussion of the standardization of hospitals. I take it that the word standardization implies a general movement toward improving the quality of the products for which the hospital funds are expended. As a rule, standards are raised by stimulating the best–not by whipping up the laggards… In various manufacturing businesses…it is not difficult to render an exact account of the product of a factory…With educational institutions and hospitals the problem is very different…It would be supposed that in the annual reports of hospitals some account of their products would be found [After comparing the annual reports of several large hospitals] I am proud to say that the report of…the Massachusetts General Hospital…I find to be as full and instructive as the report of any hospital in the country; but it is not wholly satisfactory…I will briefly attempt to give an account of the products of this hospital for the year 1912…from the annual report, and mentioning some of the more important things… accomplished but which are not stated in the report.

"The Massachusetts General Hospital has 320 beds and a large outpatient department…Six thousand eight hundred and ninety-six were treated in the wards and 22,639 in the outpatient department…The number of patients treated, and the per capita expense are some indisputable facts which appeal to minds trained for business problems, as those of…hospital trustees…The question of cure or benefit is entirely in the hands of their medical brethren, and of little consequence to them or to those who support the hospital. Really the whole hospital problem rests on this one question: What happens to the cases?…

"Leaving aside the number of patients treated and the question of whether or not these patients were benefited, there are certain products of the institution which are of great value…irrespective of the result to the patient… instruction of medical students receiving clinical experience…At the Massachusetts General Hospital, 61,000 student-hours of instruction were given to 163 students… Clinical treatment, as well as clinical instruction, requires time [and] is by no means proportionate to the number of patients. There are much larger hospitals at which no such enormous amount of time is utilized for medical instruction…Personally, I believe that the system of paying the instructors…by giving them an opportunity to do advertising as consultants is a vicious and false system. It puts too great a strain on weak human nature…

"But let suppose, in surgery…that all the operations which have been watched by these students have been misdirected…the students have learned to do something which is not worth while and does not really improve the patient. The product of the hospital in this case…as regards student instruction, would be nil—even worse than nil…The product of the hospital in medical education, like the product in the number of cases treated, depends on whether or not the cases are well treated.

"Another product is a number of nurses graduating… number [and quality]…The Massachusetts Hospital also furnished the community with the product of 18 trained house surgeons and physicians…Will they do good…if the basis of their education was founded on opinion which ignored the real results of the treatment of their cases?

"In 1912, 53 ladies were either paid or voluntary helpers in the social service department. The social service worker is really a therapeutic agent—she forces the prescriptions of physicians down the throat of the careless or refractory patient. She blindly believes the prescription will do good…I must confess I have doubts…whether the actual treatment…by these social workers…has given real benefit, and yet I consider Dr. Cabot's exploitation of the social-service idea one of the most important products of our institution in the last decade…'If the medical diagnosis is faulty, the social work based on it may do serious harm'…

"In 1912, 115 papers were printed by the staff at the Massachusetts General Hospital…Dividends of honor are still coming to the hospital from Bigelow's work on the hip-joint and Fitz's work on appendicitis, and we may hope that other epoch-making papers are now in progress of construction…Such epoch–making contributions, however, are not the ordinary products of our hospital factories. The ordinary paper is merely an additional stone thrown to swell the progress of the wave…

"There remain many other by-products to a hospital, some of which are important. To my mind the influence of the hospital on the standards of medical practice in the community is of greatest importance…[I] place the

> raising of the standard of professional honor—or shall I say accuracy—in a community as one of the most important by-products of a great hospital…Does a community get the best service by allowing as many as possible of its busy practitioners to brush themselves up by superficial work at the hospital [unpaid staffs on a seniority system], or by putting the hospital in the hands of a few paid men who shall set an example for the practitioners to follow?…
>
> "We must formulate some hospital report showing… what are the results of the treatment obtained at different institutions. This report must be made out and published by each hospital in a uniform manner, so a comparison will be possible. With such report as a starting point, those interested can begin to ask questions as to management and efficiency."
>
> (Codman 1914)

Thorndike, and Joel Goldthwait. Those opposed included Drs. Charles Scudder, John Dane, John Homans, and Robert B. Greenough. In his letter to Dr. Robert Greenough, who opposed his End-Result System, Codman wrote:

> Dear Bob,
> …It is your nature to oppose innovation and publicity…you ought to realize the responsible position in which you now stand [Director of the Harvard Cancer Commission] in the Medical School and MGH…I feel you were blind in opposing this Congress [in reference to a planned surgical meeting at the Boston Medical Library the following year, Codman continued] I hope that you standpatters at the MGH will jump in and help instead of being rebellious about little Amory Codman's suggestions as you have in the past. Try to think up any one of my previous foolish sounding prophecies which have not come true! Then step in to help in future. (Codman, n.d.)

In Greenough's reply to Codman, he defended his position and stated his feelings about Codman: "You have taken up the agitation in favor of the coming of the Clinical Congress chiefly because you see in it an opportunity to popularize and advertise your cherished scheme [End-Result Idea] I for one, am glad to support your publication of end-results, as a general plan, but I differ with you…of such detailed plans as you have…adopted in the case of your own hospital" (Codman, n.d.). Greenough did not think that Codman's plan for his hospital was feasible for the MGH because there were too many insignificant and unimportant details.

Throughout these endeavors and as discussions regarding the meeting of the Clinical Congress continued, Codman had simultaneously been on staff at both the MGH and his own hospital, Codman Hospital. In 1914, he resigned from the staff at MGH "as a protest against the seniority system of promotion" which he found "incompatible with the End Result Idea" and as a means "to attract the attention of the trustees" (Codman 1934). He remembered:

> It became apparent to me that the medical profession of Boston, its great hospitals and the Harvard Medical School, must be made to pull together with real strength of will, if Boston was to set the example in this movement…It seemed to me that Boston had the best opportunity, for the Harvard influence extended not only through the medical schools and hospitals, but into the banks and into every branch of business, philanthropy or social endeavor. There were two ways open to unite the wills of the various branches of our community, leadership on my part, or a defense-reaction on theirs [Since leadership would take] many years and I was only a junior surgeon who must also earn a living. I had, on the other hand, observed that the defense reactions of our social forces were fairly prompt and forceful. Harvard is sensitive to ridicule and…to presentation of facts. If I could awake the steam roller of Harvard public

Ernest A. Codman

Box 34.4. Codman's Letter to the Harvard Medical Association, July 20, 1914

> Dear Doctor,
>
> If the hospitals in this city agreed that every case operated at the meeting should have a brief clinical history and "End Result Report" published after the manner suggested by the Committee on Hospital Standardization of the Clinical Congress. This report to be printed and mailed over a year later to everyone who registers. This plan would necessarily protect the patient because every individual operator would expose himself to public criticism if he was in any way careless or otherwise influenced by the presence of an audience. I condemned public amphitheater operations as they are conducted today where no such report is made, and the audience obtains no authoritative information about the outcome of the case. I instanced two cases which had occurred within recent years at a prominent hospital, in one of which a patient who died on the table was smuggled out of the amphitheater and the audience was not informed that death had occurred. In another case, a surgeon who had not examined the patient did a hysterectomy for supposed fibroid tumor. The specimen when examined in the laboratory proved to be a full-term pregnancy. The audience was not informed that such was the case and the surgeon gave as an excuse to his colleagues, to whom the fact was known, "that he had taken his house officer's diagnosis." These two apparently wrong impressions were given by two surgeons who have held the respect of the entire community and these men are no more to be held guilty than the rest of us who tacitly allow such things to occur.
>
> I claim that if the Congress of Surgeons came to Boston and we insisted that all cases operated upon before it should be reported, Boston would have the credit of beginning a new era in clinical science, and that it is a pity that Harvard University and the Massachusetts General and other hospitals affiliated with Harvard should not rise to this opportunity.
>
> To those who oppose this invitation on the ground of objecting to public operations…the Congress will simply meet in another city. There will always be public operating—what we need is publicity of Results…In his [Dean Bradford's] remarks he intimated that the reason for not having this Congress was that there was no man whom they could rely on to put it through…Although not connected with Harvard University [Codman was not reappointed recently] or the Massachusetts General Hospital [Codman had resigned in 1914], I personally am ready to accept this challenge and to undertake to put this meeting of the Congress successfully through, merely for the sake of personal advertising. I regard the principle involved in it as so important that I do not in the slightest fear the criticism of being supposed to work for my own interests…My own sense of duty enters only so far as I am involved as Chairman of the Committee on Hospital Standardization of the Clinical Congress…As I see it, the principal involved means an enormous amount to the whole medical profession and it would be a great gratification to see Harvard and the Boston Hospitals do their share in it. The men who take the trouble to come from a distance to this Congress are as a rule earnest men who want facts, and many of them do far more surgery than the average Boston operator. What we can teach them is our respect for scientific fact rather than showy technique…If of the results to this letter two thirds favor the coming of the Congress, Dr. Bradford has agreed to call another meeting at once to try to see whether we cannot get together on the subject…We can establish the great principal that Public Operating should also mean Public Record of the Result to the patient.
>
> —Ernest A. Codman
>
> (Harvard Medical Alumni Association, 1914 [Countway Medical Library, Box 1, Folder 17])

opinion, either by a clear presentation of facts or by well-advertise ridicule, I felt sure I could get at least a united defense-reaction and some inquiry into existing conditions. I was confident that the End-Result Idea would become an intellectual landmark of which any university would be proud and…Harvard would claim as a jewel in her crown [along] with the diamonds of ether anesthesia and social service. (Codman 1934)

After he resigned at MGH, he acknowledged the End-Result Idea—specifically the requirement that all hospital should publicly report their end results of treatment at one year—was an experiment. He arranged a meeting in his capacity as chairman of the local Suffolk District Medical Society "for the discussion of Hospital Efficiency at the Boston Medical Library, Wednesday January 6th, 1915, at 8:15 p.m" (Codman 1934). He noted:

> In most hospitals there has been no official or department whose duty it has been to ascertain the results of treatment at all, much less to compare the results attained by different members of the staff in any one institution, or even to make a collective comparison of the results attained by the whole staff, with those of another similar institution...Obviously, if there is any difference in the value of services of one surgeon or physician and another—which the public...[will] pay large fees—this difference must be capable of demonstration by some comparative test, so that the distribution of cases may be made more rationally than by calendar or seniority. No physician or surgeon nowadays can be expected to be proficient in all the branches of even a single specialty... Comparisons are odious, but comparison is necessary in science. Until we freely make therapeutic comparisons, we cannot claim that a hospital is efficient...The meeting on January 6th is to stimulate thought on these questions.
> (Codman 1934)

Dr. Codman arranged for the following speakers at his meeting: Boston Mayor James M. Curley; two hospital trustees (Dr. Joel E. Goldthwaite [sic] at the RBBH and Dr. Walter Wesselhoeft of the Massachusetts Homeopathic Hospital); Dr. Herbert B. Howard, superintendent of the PBBH; Dr. Robert L. Dickinson, surgeon at the Brooklyn Hospital in New York; and Mr. Frank B. Gilbreth, an efficiency expert from Providence, Rhode Island. He remembered:

Nobody in any position of authority in our [Harvard] medical school cared to take the responsibility answering...questions. They all knew the answer...nobody was responsible for examining the results of treatment at hospitals, and that the reason was money...The staffs are not paid, and therefore cannot be held accountable...

To make sure that the questions should be answered, I had prepared beforehand, secretly, a cartoon about eight feet long and concealed... at the back of the stage, ready for use at the end of the discussion...The large hall in the Medical Library was packed. There was hardly standing room...When I rose to close the meeting...I said that I would present my own answers to the questions in the form of a painting which had...been made for me by a friend—the late Philip L. Hale, the artist. No one but Mr. Hale and myself had seen this cartoon, not even... my own wife, who was in the audience. I did not wish anyone to share the responsibility for the shock I knew it would give the audience... The audience held its mouth open while I explained the meaning of the picture, and... after I had finished, continued to be aghast for a minute or two. Then there was...an uproar as ever I have seen at a Medical Meeting. Some five old men...walked out with both bowed heads...Other younger ones...rose together to seek the floor, with anger, but with nothing practical to say. The great majority, however, were amused more than they were shocked... For weeks some of my friends did not speak to me, and if I entered the room where other doctors gathered, the party broke up from embarrassment or changed their subject. I was asked to resign as Chairman of the local Medical Society. For some months I was in disgrace, but the publicity obtained...in our local papers [and] those of all the other large cities, fulfilled my expectations...Soon after, I was dropped from the position of "Instructor in Surgery," which I then held at Harvard...I had already resigned from the M.G.H....and therefore had only my own hospital for clinical opportunity. (Codman 1934)

Within two weeks of the meeting of the Suffolk District Medical Society, Dr. Codman's presentation was extensively covered by the press; the *Boston Globe*, the *Boston Post*, and the *Boston Herald*:

In the cartoon Dr. Codman showed an ostrich, the Back Bay people, with its head buried in the "hill of humbug, laying golden eggs for the Back Bay medical ring and afraid to raise his head for fear some one might cure it." In his description of the Back Bay ring...Dr. Codman named a number of leading institutions and men, including President Lowell of Harvard, the Harvard Medical School, the Massachusetts General Hospital and the Peter Bent Brigham Hospital.

Dr. Codman, when he cartooned the Back Bay public paying undue sums for unnecessary operations offended only part of the Suffolk Society...Many in the audience...thoroughly sided with his attitude on the matter. Today the society is divided...one [faction] is with Dr. Codman, who urges education of the public as to the simplicity of certain operations which are now generally believed to be dangerous and difficult, while the other faction defends the action of the supervisory committee, which accepted Dr. Codman's resignation from the chairmanship of the surgical section of the society. (*Boston Globe* 1915)

After the event, in the article "Doctor-Critic Stirs Wrath," Codman apparently stated, "that the cartoon was intended to be humorous and that his criticism of men and institutions was friendly[and that] 'There was no head hit by the cartoon, which was not a high one, and abundantly able to bear my friendly, if impudent, criticism'...Dr. Codman said that he had resigned as chairman of the surgical section because he found his attempted humor was taken too seriously by the audience and he felt that, having called the attention of the medical public to hospital efficiency, he could safely leave future efforts to effect improvement to the Massachusetts

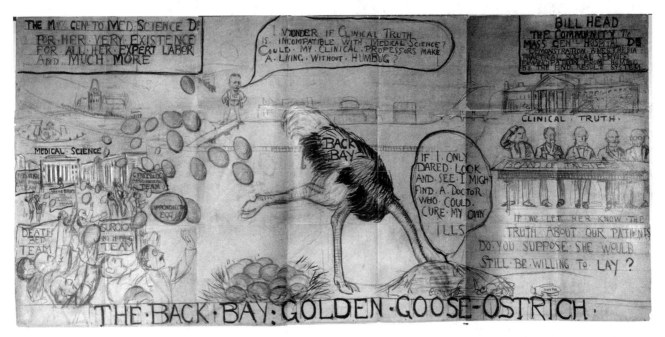

The famous cartoon (six feet long) that Codman presented to the Surgical Section of the Suffolk District Medical Society in the Boston Medical Library on January 6, 1915. Boston Medical Library in the Francis A. Countway Library of Medicine.

Medical Society" (*Boston Globe* 1915). Dr. Horace D. Arnold, president of the Suffolk District Medical Society, in an interview with the *Boston Daily Globe* "expressed a hope that the public will not miss understand [*sic*] the situation."

Dr. John G. Clark later wrote to Codman stating that he did not approve of his (Codman's) personal vendetta against anyone opposed to his End-Result Idea. Dr. Shattuck also responded negatively, writing to Codman the following day:

> I told your wife downstairs last night, before the meeting that I came to applaud. I am sorry that I left the meeting in a very different frame of mind. Your cause is good, and as you know had my sympathy. That fire that possessed you to damage your cause by personalities, insults, and a picture on the level with yellow journal Sunday editions, I do not know. I am awfully sorry. Is it not conceivable that a person should differ from you without being a knave or a fool? Your cause is too good to fail, but, as it seems to me, you retarded instead of advancing it last night. (Harvard Medical School Archives, n.d.)

Despite the controversy that ensued, Codman arranged for the cartoon to be preserved in the Boston Medical Library. It is now in the Center for the History of Medicine in the Countway Medical Library. He later published the cartoon in his book *The Shoulder* and explained the meaning of the cartoon:

> I published this cartoon now, because, having been condemned by a previous generation on its account, I hope that I may be judged by a future one to whom the subject will appear less serious. It depicts President Lowell standing on the Cambridge Bridge, wondering whether it would be possible for the professors of the Medical School to support themselves on their salaries, if they had no opportunity to practice among the rich people of the Back Bay (the residential portion of Boston). The Back Bay is represented as an ostrich with her head in a pile of sand, devouring humbugs and kicking out her golden eggs blindly to the professors who show more interest in the golden eggs than they do Medical Science. On the right is the Massachusetts General Hospital with its board of trustees deliberating as to whether, if they really used the End Result System, and let the Back Bay know how many mistakes were made on the hospital patients, she would still be willing to give her golden eggs to support the hospital, and would employ members of their staff and thus save the expense of salaries. Across the river and over the hill are seen armies of medical students coming to Harvard because they

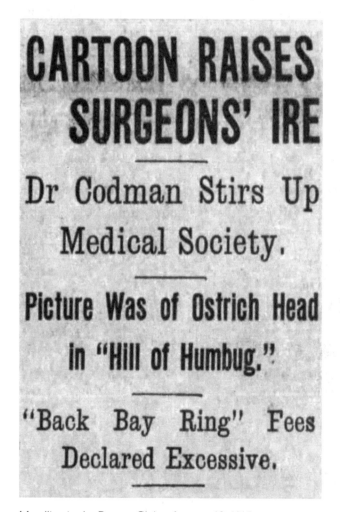

Headline in the Boston Globe, January 18, 1915. *Daily Boston Globe*, Evening Edition, January 18, 1915 (1: 5).

have heard that the End Result System will be installed in her affiliated hospitals.

A few of my contemporaries have credited me with "moral courage," but I deserve no such credit for I have merely reacted to stimuli... Whatever credit I may deserve from my tirades should not be for moral courage, but it seems to me that I deserve some credit for restraining myself as well as I have done, having once started on the campaign. To see our hospitals turn their forces away from evident facts is... repulsive to me...It is not...physicians I attack, but the lack of logical organization in our profession where, as students, we get instruction by example. (Codman 1934)

Despite a measure of animosity from his peers, Codman continued in his unshakeable faith in the End-Result System and his belief that promotions and credentialing should be a function of outcomes, not years in practice. Codman wrote to Mr. Charles H. W. Foster—an MGH trustee with particular influence—attempting to persuade him to his ideas about seniority, credentialing, and the End-Result System. Mr. Foster responded that surgical outcomes were beyond the control of the practitioner and that tying patient outcome to quality of care was impossible as a sole indicator of success because the outcomes were beyond the surgeon's control. Foster replied by letter: "Personally, I have very little sympathy with your idea of reducing results to figures as to regard medical efforts...The results of a surgical operation depends so much upon matters beyond the control of the surgeon and is such an inexact science, so to speak, that it is improper to me to use figures for any other purpose than as one of the indicators of success..." (quoted in Maguire 1993). Codman responded:

> while each member of your staff knows that if he does nothing utterly disgraceful that he will be borne along by the seniority system, can you expect him to exert himself in favor of an analysis of results which may bring to the knowledge of the efficiency committee his own laziness or incapacity...Mr. Foster, I am confident that I am right in feeling that the seniority system has outlived its usefulness and that you are wrong in supporting that the information... to a trustee in the way of praise and criticism and general gossip is the sort of information on which a trustee can base a sound estimate of the attainments of his staff... (quoted in Maguire 1993)

On January 15, 1915, Codman wrote to his colleague Robert L. Dickinson that seniority based on time in practice and general unsupported opinions could not serve as a basis for evaluating performance. He wrote, "The future surgeon should be pushed to the top of his accomplishments instead of elbowing his way to the top by concealing his failures and exaggerating his successes" (quoted in Maguire 1993). Codman's unwavering determination won out, and MGH eventually delivered a public statement in 1916 upholding his idea that appointments and promotions should be based on performance and not seniority. The statement read that "in making appointments the trustees will consider the fitness of the appointment for special services which [the physician] will be called on to perform, and will seek to secure the best service available, without being found by any custom or promotion by seniority" (quoted in Maguire 1993).

About nine months later, the fifth annual meeting of the Clinical Congress of Surgeons of North America was approved to take place in Boston from October 25 through October 29, 1915. Surgical demonstrations were held daily in most of the Boston hospitals including the MGH, Boston Children's Hospital, the Peter Bent Brigham Hospital, the Robert Breck Brigham Hospital, and the Codman Hospital. The evenings were devoted to clinical and organizational talks.

Codman, during one of these evening sessions, presented his report of the Committee on Hospital

Standardization. He wrote, "Your committee... has stated its belief that a fair standardization of a hospital is impractical unless the hospital...has some method of following up its end-results...[We have] succeeded in bringing this idea to the attention of most of the hospitals...[We have] been content to try to interest the medical public in the end-result system and to leave each hospital its chance [to participate] for another year" (Codman 1916). Codman went on to say:

> Fortunately, the Committee on Arrangements of this meeting in Boston has come to our aid in the matter of giving further publicity to the end-result idea. A year hence a report will be sent out to each of you of the "end-results" to date of each case operated on before you during the week of this Congress. You only have to note the number of the case...to refresh your memory of the operation by looking at the abstract in the report together with the note of the success or failure of the operator to relieve the symptoms from which the patient suffered. We believe that the adoption of this method in all teaching clinics will be of the greatest service both in graduate and undergraduate instruction...Our policy of advocating the use of the result to each individual patient [is] the most important unit in the standardization of hospitals. (Codman et al. 1916)

Codman also drew attention to the MGH in his report:

> The Massachusetts General Hospital...gives us an example of a hospital whose organization is strong enough and whose esprit de corps vigorous enough, to permit the use of a "surgeons card" on which each member of the surgical staff authoritatively records his own errors in diagnosis, skill, judgment, and care. At this hospital, too, the policy of the assignment of special groups of cases [to specialists] has been successfully carried out. This plan assures the efficiency committee of a weapon to use in dealing with any class of cases which by the end-result cards is shown to have a low percentage of successful results [and] that in making appointments the trustees will consider the fitness of the applicant for the special services which he will be called on to perform, and will seek to secure the best service available, without being bound by any custom of promotion by seniority...However, we cannot help regretting that the trustees at this great hospital have not shown a willingness to bear part of the burden of the professional staff by appointing one of their members on the Efficiency Committee. (Codman et al. 1916)

Apparently, George Wigglesworth, a trustee of the MGH, believed that the "liability of a hospital to law suits would be too much increased" if there was a policy for an end-result system (Codman 1914).

Two months later, in December 1915, Codman resigned as Chairman of the Hospital Standardization Committee for the following two reasons:

> First, Harvard University and the Massachusetts General Hospital, —my own Alma Mater and Pater—have shown no enthusiasm in backing me up. In fact, they have sat on me and obviously intend to suppress me...The second reason is that my hospital is a financial failure. The public do not care for ideas from a man who is a self-confessed failure, as far as money is concerned...I believe that the American College of Surgeons will degenerate into a "union" unless it takes hold of some big truth like this End Result Work and pushes it along.

In Finney's return letter, he acknowledged that Codman was correct that "the Boston crowd have not backed you up and this fact is fairly generally known throughout the country [and asked Codman to continue leading the End Result Work with the American College of Surgeons because]... you, more than anyone else, deserve the credit for its real discovery and the bona fide attempt to put it in operation..." (Codman 1915).

The End-Result Idea and the concept of Hospital Standardization continued to spread around the country in spite of Codman's personal failure at the Massachusetts General Hospital. Codman recorded: "The Surgical Staff at the Massachusetts General Hospital unanimously voted in favor of the adoption of the whole plan, but it was discountenanced by the General Executive Committee and the Board of Trustees so far as the making of a report was concerned" (Codman 1914).

Codman had continued to write about the End-Result Idea during this time, and he summarized his thoughts and previous publications in the monograph, *A Study in Hospital Efficiency*, which published the same year he stepped down from MGH in 1914. He reprinted the monograph in 1915 and again in about 1918. The foreword to the last printing states:

> It is idle to Consider the Standardization of Hospitals without considering the Standard of the Product of each Hospital, the part which the Professional Staff plays in raising the Standard of the Product, and the Compensation which the Hospital grants the Staff in return for their services.
>
> This Hospital has for sale a Product of the Standard found on pages 12-63 [337 case reports]. It aims to be a Hundred Dollar Hospital with a Hundred Dollar Surgeon. (Codman 1918)

The first two printings included patient case reports from the first two years of his private hospital; the third included case reports of the first five years from his hospital. **Box 34.5** provides an extract from part 1 ("The Case Report"), in which he provides a detailed explanation of the End-Result System. In the book, he used abstracts from the End-Result Cards in 337 patients treated in his private hospital that would be presented weekly to the chief of the surgical service. In part 1, he wrote:

> To the thoughtful person it will be at once apparent that the Chief of Service who criticizes the results of his juniors or colleagues... would soon lose the esprit de corps which is necessary in successful work. Successful leadership always requires tact... To most men it is enough to know that the work is observed and measured, and if found of value, will be appreciated. If the Chief has the gift of leadership, he will praise here and condemn there... Results accomplished must be better than one by which they are ignored...

Codman's book, *A Study in Hospital Efficiency*. Internet Archive/Columbia University Libraries.

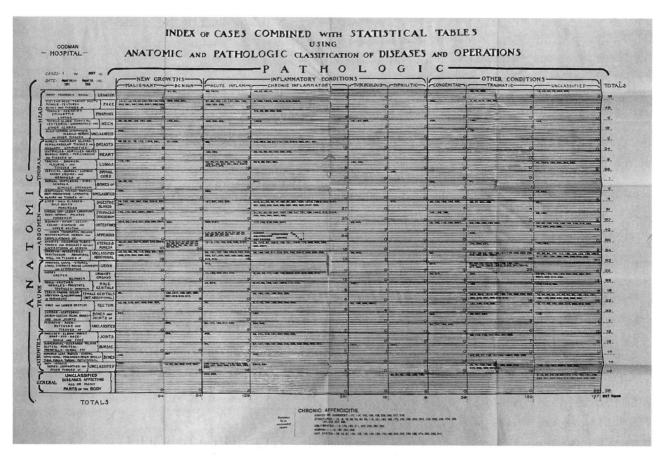

Example of the database of end-results of cases treated at Codman's Hospital. Contained in an envelope attached to the back cover of Codman's book, *A Study in Hospital Efficiency*. Privately printed, 1918.

All results of surgical treatment which lack perfection may be explained by one or more of the following causes.

Errors due to lack of technical knowledge or skill.

Errors due to the lack of surgical judgment.

Errors due to lack of care or equipment.

Errors due to lack of diagnostic skill.

These are partially controlled by organization.

The patient's unconquerable disease.

The patient's refusal of treatment.

These are practically controllable by public education.

The calamities of surgery or those accidents and complications over which we have no known control. These should be acknowledged to ourselves and to the public, and study directed to their prevention.

The practice of medicine and surgery will always be to a certain extent experimental. Every operation...is an experiment... The public is entitled to know the results of the experiments it must endure...Let the hospital do the advertising of good and bad alike, and the public will respond. (Codman 1918)

Dr. Codman continued in part 1 with his previous reports on the advantages to his End-Result System and essential steps using his cards and a card catalog cabinet. In the third and final printing, he reviewed his own personal cases operated upon in his hospital over a five-year period. Regarding errors due to lack of technical

Box 34.5. Extract from Part 1 of A Study in Hospital Efficiency: An Explanation of the End-Result System

"The argument in our previous reports has been somewhat as follows: That the Trustees of our Charitable Hospitals do not consider it their duty to see that good results are obtained in the treatment of their patients. They see to it that their financial accounts are audited, but they take no inventory of the Product for which their money is expended. Since the Product is given away, they do not bother to standardize it and to see whether it is good enough to be sold. It is against the individual interests of the medical and surgical staffs…to follow-up, compare, analyze, and standardize all their results, because:

1. It is seldom that any single individual's results have been so strikingly better than…his colleagues, that he would desire such comparison and analysis…

2. An effort to…analyze is difficult, time-consuming, and troublesome, and…pointing out lines for improvement [leads] to much onerous committee work by… the staff…

3. Neither Trustees of Hospitals nor the Public are as yet willing to pay for this kind of work.

"Although the staff would admit that such follow-up and analysis was a good thing for all, yet each…man…would wait for someone else to do the work. The superintendent would lose his position, if he undertook to insist on "good results"…Therefore, if the trustees, the staff, and the superintendent all avoid the analysis of results, and it is only for the interest of the patients, the public, and medical science, —why bother about it? The truth is, the patients and the public do not yet understand the problem. They suppose that of course somebody is looking into this important matter…As for Medical Science's not caring, —this is the consequence of our medical schools' paying their teachers by giving them the opportunity to advertise…As unpaid or partially paid medical teaching is the custom in most parts of the world, we have become used to it…

"We have not offered this destructive criticism without a construct the remedy:

The End Result System

"We have advocated a simple system of hospital organization [by the Committee on Standardization]…That the Trustees of Hospitals should see to it that an effort is made to follow-up each patient they treat, long enough to determine if the treatment…has permanently relieved the condition or symptoms…That they should give…the Staff credit for taking the responsibility of successful treatment and promote them accordingly [and eliminate the seniority system]…They should see that all cases in which the treatment is found to be unsuccessful or unsatisfactory are carefully analyzed, in order to fix the responsibility for failure on:

1. The physician or surgeon responsible for the treatment.

2. The organization carrying out the…treatment.

3. The disease or condition of the patient.

4. The personal or social conditions preventing the cooperation of the patient…

"Technically to start this system in a hospital, it is necessary to introduce the use of an 'End Result Card' which is kept for each patient [card catalog system; the foundation of Codman's concept]: The symptoms or condition… The general plan…of treatment given. The complications…before the patient left the hospital. The diagnosis which proved correct…at discharge. The result each year afterward…

"Undoubtedly a layman could not enter authoritatively into the details…but could insist that the End Result System should be used…and that an efficiency committee be appointed for that purpose. At present, in most hospitals, no such investigation is made by any one. There is no standard of results to go by, but we are sending standards in this Report…In our Charitable Hospitals…it is a disagreeable Duty which neither the Staff or the Board of Trustees nor the superintendent has the strength to assume alone. An Efficiency Committee composed of members of each of these departments should assume this burden…When this step is taken by our Great Hospitals, True Clinical Science will begin…

"A hospital that has an End Result System has an authoritative method of admitting and recording its failures in diagnosis and treatment."

(Codman 1918)

knowledge or skill, he mentioned five trivial cases and nine cases of minor problems such as "surgical hernias or bulging scars...[stating] I am perfectly willing to admit that I am not a rapid or skillful operator, but I insist that my analysis does not convict me of lack of skill" (Codman 1918). Regarding errors due to lack of judgment, he cites seven cases of trivial errors with good results and another four cases, one in an asymptomatic patient and three in whom treatment was "perhaps too conservative...My judgment may be questioned for carrying the End Result Idea so far that I publish my own errors, but I defy any public or private hospital in Boston to show a consecutive series of results which will prove better surgical judgment" (Codman 1918). Codman mentioned 25 cases of minor complications due to lack of care or equipment. In conclusion, he stated, "in five years there has been no death from sepsis or even a serious consequence...There has been no other bad consequence which we can attribute to lack of care or equipment" (Codman 1918).

> "My idea is that the Hospital is a place for mutual help. The Patient, the Student, the Professor, the Chief of Service, the Trustee, the Hospital, the Community, and World-Wide Medical Science—each part owners of 'the case.' We must all be willing to learn from, to teach from, to study, to be trusted by, to contribute to, to record, and to analyze each 'case' and all 'cases'."
> —Ernest A. Codman
> "A Study in Hospital Efficiency" (1918) in *Index Medicus*, (n.d.)

Under his category of errors due to incorrect diagnosis, Codman listed 22 of academic importance only. He noted, "If we had had superhuman diagnostic ability, we should have been saved 19 errors of academic importance only; four cases would perhaps not have had exploratory operations; and four patients might have been saved some time and trouble. Would this have justified our employing a diagnostician...Certainly not from a business point of view" (Codman 1918).

However, he then proceeded to offer a place in his hospital for a young diagnostician.

Codman then identified a number of cases where the nature and extent of the disease was the main cause of failure, stating: "We do not want to undertake the treatment of cases of advanced cancer; ptosis and neurasthenia; Banti's disease; anteflexion, oblique fractures of the clavicle in young [ladies] who wear low-neck gowns; chronic nephritis; neglected empyema; pulmonary tuberculosis; epilepsy; endocarditis; bacteriuria; diabetes; or enlarged seminal vesicles. We know we cannot have success with these conditions..." (Codman 1918). He went on to say:

> In five years, we find very few, if any, real errors due to the lack of coöperation of the patients while in this hospital, and these errors were most cases, perhaps, due to our lack of conviction and the advice we gave...What can we do, in the future, to diminish the number of errors due to patients' not seeking operation in time? Reduce the price of our consultation fee for thorough examination by precise methods, such as the X-ray and laboratory tests...to a low enough figure, so that the patients and their physicians will not be withheld from seeking our advice...This we are doing in the grouping of specialists [to] let every one in the community know that they can obtain a high standard diagnosis at a certain fixed sum...to compete with the Massachusetts General Hospital clinic, which already performs this service to a certain extent. We plan to show the Community that we can do the work better...at a low enough [charge] to compete with that of the Massachusetts General Hospital. (Codman 1918)

Regarding deaths (a calamity of surgery), Codman reported that he had five deaths in the hospital during this five-year period. He explained:

> All were necessarily errors of judgment, because they resulted in failure. In each case

I knew that the chance for the patient was very small, but as all of the patients suffered so intensely...it seemed only fair to give each of them the chance of cure by operation... What can we do about these "bad risks" in the future?...Shall I say...1. You are too bad a risk; go to a first-class surgeon. 2. You are bad risk; I must double my usual fee. 3. You are a bad risk; you need not pay me unless you live. All are logical. I like the last best. (Codman 1918)

For other calamities (pulmonary embolism, heart failure, etc.), he asked:

what can we do to prevent [them] in the future? By a constant review of the literature... devote research to the question...review... cases [such as those] published reports of the causes of death in the Annual Reports of the Peter Bent Brigham, Boston City, and Massachusetts General Hospital...Before Trustees vote more funds for new buildings and equipment, let them appoint Efficiency Committees to make analyses of the results they are getting now. They can then decide whether to spend their money for improvement in quality or quantity, —for products or waste products. (Codman 1918)

Part 2 of Codman's book, *A Study in Hospital Efficiency*, is a review of his thoughts about the monetary value of a surgeon's services, specialization, the seniority system, and the influence of the charitable hospitals. He described his personal experiences:

I started my practice of surgery primarily to make an honest living...It was [my teachers] custom, and of their teachers before them, to undertake treatment because the patient sought their aid, even though they knew that other available colleagues were more competent to obtain a good result for that particular disease...It was the custom in the hospitals [led by Harvard University] for the visiting staffs to give treatment or to operate by the ward, by the calendar, or by the time of day, seldom because of...demonstrated ability to succeed in relieving the condition in hand. Again, and again I have seen surgeons who have given special study [specialist] to some particular group of cases stand by and watch some colleague do what they knew was the wrong operation...I saw cases relatively neglected in the wards of surgeons who took no interest in that particular disease, and at the same time other surgeons, who were interested in, and had made special study of such cases [specialist], standing idle because of the calendar [seniority system]... As a young surgeon I did at night the most serious and difficult operations, and in the day-time watched the great surgeons hurriedly do trivial and simple ones...Sometimes sixty patients were visited, and several patients operated on by a man with "reputation" in an hour...Thus, I was taught by eminent examples that these abuses were necessary in the practice of surgery, just as "business methods" are necessary in successful business...

When I entered private practice...I found I must take whatever cases came to me; and that as I had my living to earn, I could not be expected to refer to those more competent...I must make my errors just as those before me had...I must obtain a hospital appointment or... take advantage of every patient that came to me, and let him think that I was as competent a surgeon as he could get. (Codman 1918)

Dr. Codman continues this section describing his beliefs about the unfair competition between the surgeon in private practice versus the surgeon in a charitable institution, the estimates of profits and potential losses of surgical cases, the financial estimates of running his own hospital, and finally some comments about his own experiences after resigning from the staff at MGH and operating in his private hospital. He asked:

If [one] does resign, it will mean the loss of prestige, loss of practice, and the end of his career as a surgeon. I have been through part of this experience during the last two years, but by assuming the financial burden of this hospital [Codman's Hospital], I have been able to cling to my ambition to be a good surgeon. My opportunity to be a great surgeon has gone, unless some large hospital will give me the opportunity for manual practice. If I can make such an analysis of my cases, why could they not at a Charitable Hospital when there is a question of a promotion? (Codman 1918)

The last part of part 2 includes a brief summary of the diagnoses of the 114 cases of Dr. Codman's who died after surgery at the Massachusetts General Hospital from 1900 to 1914. It included the following orthopaedic injuries: seven cases of extremity amputations (both upper and lower extremities), three multiple injuries with fracture, three hand and one foot with infected wounds, and two fractured spines. The final part is his bibliography; a list of 44 publications. He wrote:

I do not boast when I state that these [papers on the shoulder] have been accepted in Surgical Literature. I have received credit from foreign writers, from the text-books, and from practically every writer on the "shoulder." But the Massachusetts General, the hospital for whose cases I did the work, has given me no credit for it, in spite of the fact that every case I treated was benefited. Was I asked to continue to treat the shoulder cases? Are such cases ever referred to me now by the hospital? Or are these cases simply neglected in the hurry of the Out-Patient work? Who cares whether they are relieved? Are the trustees, the Chiefs of Staff, or any one else held accountable for them? Have my results ever been improved upon?...

Why did I write these articles? As I look back to analyze my intentions...I find the following reasons: 1. Advertisement for personal business. 2. Hope of recognition of ability by my own hospital, the Massachusetts General, by my colleagues and friends, by my distant readers, by the rising generation. 3. A real desire to use the best that lies in me to do my bit for humanity, recognition or no recognition. I always had all three in mind and...believe most men who write have also...In my own case the desire to be recognized by my own hospital weighed the strongest. I thought that if I could do well, I should receive recognition and be promoted...But no [the Trustees] expected me to go on accumulating a good private practice, in order to make a good living and a reputation...If Trustees had an End Result System, they could tell whether to promote scholars or operators, and both... might know their own deficiencies and be able to proportion their work. (Codman 1918)

In part 3, "The New Organization," Codman provides an example of "how a group of earnest men may compete with the cliques who dominate the charitable hospitals in any city" (Codman 1918). After discussing his ideas concerning the new position of a general practitioner, fee-splitting, the business value of a consultant, new financial plans for a practitioner, preferred sources for loans, how to obtain a staff of specialists, duties of the consulting staff and discussions regarding cutting or raising prices, he concludes with advice on how a young surgeon can start under the End-Result System. He explains:

It is clear...that I do not want to give [a new young surgeon] a chance to learn surgery by making mistakes on my patients [in Codman's hospital]. I shall have to pay an assistant...for I must fix responsibility on him. At present, at the Charitable Hospital, he is usually not paid, for he receives his reward in the opportunity to learn by his own mistakes. He has the appearance of taking responsibility, but is not really held accountable for his errors. If he is to be held accountable, he should be paid… The End Result System would ultimately oblige Trustees to pay for much of their professional labor…It is not possible to conceive of a charitable hospital which makes it a rule not to except for treatment any cases which its Staff cannot relieve? A business organization which started…on this basis would insist on its Staff becoming competent, or it would seek men who were competent…At present, anyone with an M.D. will do, for he does not have to be competent.

To express it plainly, —if the End Result System were in common use all hospital work would have to be done so much more thoroughly than it is today, that competent assistance would be a great demand…If a young surgeon devoted his time and brains to studying some difficult class of cases, and [developed] a satisfactory method of treatment, his services would be in immediate demand. If his methods were really good, they would be advertised in the End Result Report of his hospital. Others would come from distant hospitals to learn from him. His work would be a credit to the hospital and a cause for his promotion…The result of this would be a…rational diffusion of new…successful forms of treatment, instead of scattered instances of experiments performed by individuals…aimlessly, and without adequate record [of success]…

We should find, as is shown in our analysis in part I, that our failures result from errors… The young surgeon's education should be developed with regard to these facts. We should… make the young surgeon qualify by demonstrating that he can exhibit constant care in doing what he has been taught to do. He can then attain skill by assisting, by dissecting, by operating on animals, and by doing routine operations. He can acquire knowledge by study, travel, observation and by following the End Result of cases he has helped to operate on, so that he can learn by his superiors' errors as well as by their successes. Judgment must come by experience, as well as by training and an inborn balance of mind…Finally, having qualified at these tests [selecting cases he is competent to treat rather than be assigned cases as a record for assisting his senior in private practice] he may qualify as a great surgeon…

Truth is Right and Science is but a synonym of Truth…Individual leaders can never read the future clearly enough to justify their employing secrecy to increase Efficiency…Secrecy… produces suspicion and distrust…and victory depends on…superior integrity. Publicity is the cure of the disease, Secrecy. Publicity acknowledges not only the importance of Truth, but the fact that it is difficult to obtain, even when we earnestly try for it… (Codman 1918)

Codman continued to participate in the American College of Surgeons program on Hospital Standardization and the qualifications required for admitting fellows into the college. He received many letters of support for his End-Result Idea and the concept of Hospital Standardization from physicians and hospitals throughout the country. He never stopped speaking about these two issues. Hospital standardization was inaugurated and financed by the American College of Surgeons in 1918, which eventually became the Joint Commission on Hospital Accreditation (a freestanding organization to inspect and certify hospitals). Candidates for admission into the American College of Surgeons had to submit the 100 cases for review to demonstrate a certain level of surgical judgment and technical ability. The American Medical Association also established state advisory committees on the Standardization of Hospitals. In Massachusetts, Codman headed the committee that graded hospitals with an "A" or "B."

WORLD WAR I

World War I had begun in July of 1914, while Codman pursued his End-Result Idea. He remembered, "When the war broke out I was contently carrying out my numerous plans" (Codman 1934). He said:

> By 1917 the American College of Surgeons had taken over the Hospital Standardization work, and it has flourished under the able leadership of Dr. MacEachern. I was enlarging my little hospital as fast as I could make, or borrow money. The MGH was maintaining its End Results cards; the follow-up system and the special assignment policy were flourishing. Other hospitals were following suit…I heard more and more signs of appreciation of what I was trying to do. I often think that had not been for the war, my plans would have reached fruition, but when the war came, the thoughts of men, my own included, left their jobs. My appeals for improvement fell on deaf ears…No one was interested in avoidable improvements in hospitals or in ideals…I, too, wanted to volunteer and be with other friends who were joining British units. However, my hospital was holding me fast…I felt that I could do more for my country by making a demonstration of the End Result Idea than by doing what other surgeons could do as well in the Army… (Codman 1934).

Codman remembered, "[but] then came the great disaster at Halifax" in Nova Scotia, Canada (Codman 1934). On December 6, 1917, a catastrophe occurred when the French munition ship *SS Mont-Blanc* collided with the Norwegian-operated Belgian Relief Commission ship, the *SS Imo*. The *Mont-Blanc*—heavily loaded with explosives for the war effort in Europe—exploded, leveling large sections of the city, killing roughly 2,000 people, and injuring an estimated 9,000 others. Codman said, "I telegraphed my good friend, Dr. Thomas Walker of St. John, New

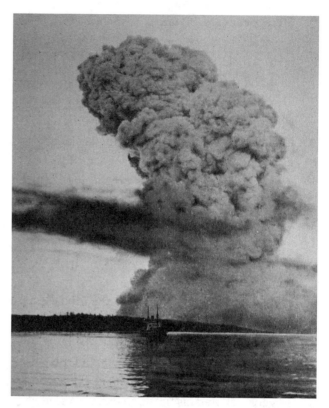

Massive explosion in Halifax Harbor, December 6, 1917. National Archives and Records Administration.

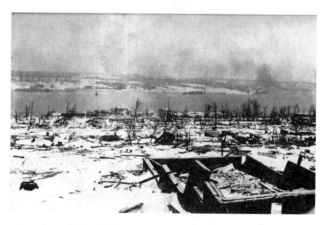

Aftermath of the Halifax explosion. Nova Scotia Archives and Records Management/Wikimedia Commons.

Brunswick, offering the help of my hospital staff and in a few hours later we were on our way" (Codman 1934). The destruction of the northern portion of the city had left another 25,000 in need of shelter.

Codman left for Halifax the next day on Friday, December 7, on the 7:30 AM train, along with staff from the Codman Hospital: Dr. H. V. Andrews (surgeon), Miss W. L. Stevens (nurse), and Miss M. Adams (nurse). His team was joined by two other surgeons, Dr. L. M. Crosby and Dr. C. W. DeWolfe, and a nurse, Miss L. Allen, as well as an assistant, Miss Bridges. Codman remembered:

> When I arrived in Halifax early Sunday morning, I reported as directed by Dr. Walker of St. John to Victoria General Hospital. At the suggestion of Dr. McDougall…of Victoria…I accordingly went to the Y.M.C.A. building [hospital] and since have continued to direct the hospital without any further written authority but with the consent of the directors of the institution and the various emergency committees. [Other physicians, surgeons and nurses also served under Dr. Codman during his two weeks at the Y.M.C.A. hospital]. This

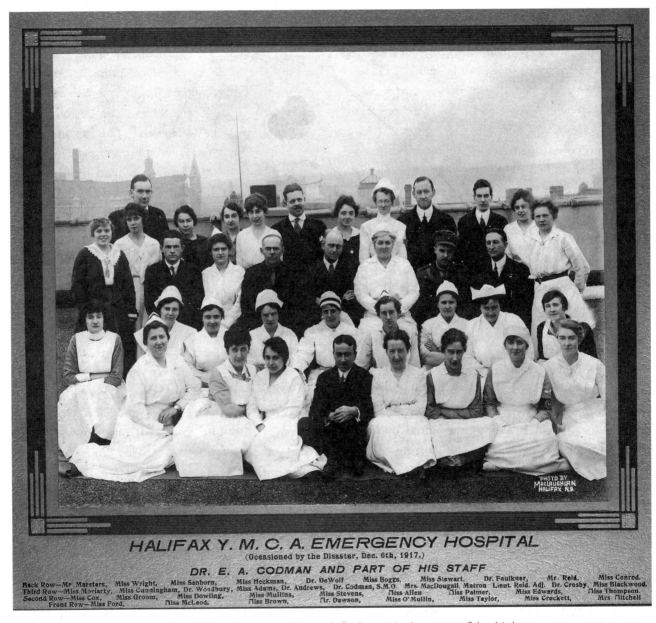

Codman and his staff at the Halifax YMCA Emergency Hospital. Codman is in the center of the third row. Boston Medical Library in the Francis A. Countway Library of Medicine.

staff has to care for fifty-eight patients, eight of whom are obstetrics, nine are eye, and the rest surgical or trivial...In addition...we have now fifty empty beds [on December 14, 1917]...The whole hospital is now in fairly good order and can go on expanding or contracting according to the wishes of the Medical Committee...We have a card catalog of the important facts about each patient received since I took charge...I feel that the work that I have done so far...has been the best that I could give it, but my own office at home renders it necessary for me to return unless it is very clear that there is no one to take my place as administrator.

It seems to me that...this hospital should be a proper-going military institution or...it should be taken over by some of the local surgeons and doctors as a civil hospital...Dr. Andrews, Miss Stevens, Miss Adams and Miss Trombley should return when I do...Up to the present time they are in my own employ, but...I need them in my work at home...Dr. DeWolfe, Dr. Crosby and the other nurses, are thoroughly independent of my part, and it is time that some definite arrangements should be made with them, (Public Archives of Novia Scotia, n.d.).

Responders also came from New York, Toronto, and Montreal in addition to Boston. Abraham Captain "Cap" Ratshesky—who helped found Beth Israel Hospital and led the disaster efforts in 1908 to two large cities destroyed by fire, Salem and Chelsea—was appointed by Governor Samuel W. McCall to lead a group of first responders from Boston to the Halifax disaster. These responders:

arrived at about 3 a.m. [Saturday morning to] "a gruesome start. Debris had not been removed from the streets...buildings shattered on all sides; chaos apparent; no order existed." A contingency of surgeons and nurses accompanied him. In addition, a third group from Boston, arrived "the next day, Sunday December 9th [the same day of Codman's arrival]...Unit No.5 with the American Red Cross commanded by the surgeon, Dr. W. E. Ladd [later to become chief of surgery at Boston Children's Hospital]. This group brought 750 cots, more than 7000 blankets, and $10,000 worth of medical supplies. Dr. Ladd and his group took over Saint Mary's College...Carpenters and plumbers transformed the school in twenty-four hours from a wrecked, snow-filled building to a warm comfortable hospital of 138 beds. This large unit worked there until January 5th with it staff of 105 personnel: 22 army surgeons, 69 nurses, and 14 civilians...In the months following the explosion the local press commented on the brave support from the American physicians..."the local doctors...also helped materially with the wounded." This inflamed an already irritated medical community [who] responded in...[a] letter published in the *Herald* on February 16, 1918: "the splendid work done by the American surgeons is hereby not in the least minimized, the local practitioners naturally resent being described merely as helpers during a period in which, unquestionably, they and their provincial brethren were the chief performers." (Sullivan 2017)

Codman left Halifax on Wednesday, December 19, 1917. He noted, "When we left [the Y.M.C.A. emergency hospital] was running smoothly with an End Result Card for every patient. Although these cards may now be...scattered...they served to keep my finger on every pulse in the hospital and to illustrate the simplicity of installing the plan, even in a city paralyzed by a calamity" (Codman 1934). In addition, the relationship between the cities of Boston and Halifax grew stronger after Boston provided aid to Halifax. They had previously established strong ties with many native Nova Scotians living in Massachusetts and supporting union with New England rather than the Dominion of Canada, and many Boston businesses were involved with shipping

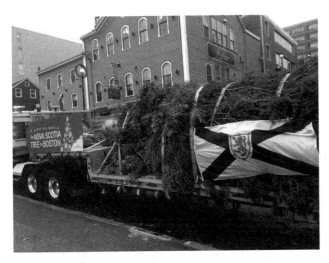

Annual Christmas Tree (either balsam fir, white spruce, or red spruce) gift: "The Nova Scotia Tree for Boston."
The Canadian Press/Alison Auld.

and fish trade in Halifax. In 1918, Halifax sent a large (40–50-foot) Christmas tree to Boston as thanks, beginning a tradition that continues to this day. This annual tradition was directly inspired by the work of Ratshesky and his colleagues, most likely including Codman and Ladd.

Although Codman closed his hospital on the day he left for Halifax, I was unable to discover if he ever reopened it. Dr. William Mellon states he did not. Codman recorded, "Having left with regret…an indescribable restlessness came over me, until September [1918], I find myself in our own Medical Corps, wrestling, as Senior Surgeon of the Coast Defenses of the Delaware, with the impossible 'paperwork' of our Army, in the midst of the influenza" (Codman 1934). It is also unclear where Codman worked, if at all, during the period between leaving Halifax and being in the army in September 1918; a period of about nine months.

While Codman served in the army, tens of millions of people died from influenza between 1918 and 1919; approximately 500,000 people died in the United States alone. During this time, about 20% of all soldiers stationed in the United States were sick with the flu. He recorded:

In November, as Regimental Surgeon in the Artillery, I had a card for every one of 1,800 men, and enjoyed the new duty of studying how to keep men well, and getting rid of them when sick…At this camp in Virginia, after the Armistice, I received an honorary appointment as Fish and Game Officer for the General in Command, and my Christmas leave was spent in camp with daily expeditions after pike and bass, duck, quail and wild turkey, with my agreeable superior.

In January 1919, not having applied for discharge, because [of] the need for medical officers…I was transferred to be Surgeon-in-Chief to the Base Hospital at Camp Taylor, and again had a chance to test the working of my record system. Five hundred beds and some 300 convalescent soldiers in barracks gave an excellent opportunity. An orderly carrying my box of cards attended all visits or operations…My cards were of the greatest help, for I could talk over his cases with each ward officer as often as seemed desirable…In June 1919, I returned to my closed hospital, in debt, with no borrowing capacity, and somewhat disillusioned as to the possibility of altering the ways of human nature by my intellectual efforts. (Codman 1934)

Codman was a forward and innovative thinker whose contributions proved invaluable. More than 50 years later, in an acceptance speech for the Henry Jacob Bigelow Medal in 1973, Dr. Francis D. Moore (chief of surgery at BWH) said:

In the light of present day events, it is an easy matter for us to appreciate the remarkable foresight of this iconoclastic man. Today's concepts of the problem-oriented record, peer review panels, Professional Service Review Organizations, the Bennett Amendment, HR–1, Medical Foundations, Manpower Surveys, and the whole concept of upgrading the quality of medical and surgical care by having doctors examine each other's work in a realistic and objective way, traces back to Codman. Only a few persons today recognize the fact that the Joint Commission on Accreditation of Hospitals [now named Joint Commission] owes its origin to Ernest Amory Codman. When we use the words "Peer Review," "Quality Control," "Hospital Accreditation," "PSRO," or "JCAH" we are merely nodding in the direction of that thorny Bostonian. (*Harvard Medical Alumni Bulletin* 1975)

BONE SARCOMA

As early as 1904, Codman had published a case report of a bone cyst in the middle phalanx of the long finger in a 40-year-old woman. Fearing a bone sarcoma, Codman removed the entire middle phalanx with its periosteum in order to avoid an amputation. From the gross appearance of the lesion after opening the phalanx, Codman believed the lesion was an enchondroma that had undergone myxomatous degeneration. The decalcified preparations of sections of the bone were lost and therefore he was unable to provide a valid histologic diagnosis. It would be another 18 years before he published any article about bone lesions or tumors.

> "A good deal of this end-result discussion has emanated from the community in which we are now meeting [Boston], and not a little of it through the expectations of one person [Amory Codman], who finally under the auspices of the College has undertaken, as a type-study, the investigation of the operative results of a single pathological lesion—the sarcomata of bone. It is not a question of how many legs or arms have been amputated for osteosarcomata, nor how many seconds it took to 'drop the limb', a matter which chiefly interested our forbears, nor indeed, by what particular method the operation was performed. The important questions are whether the amputation should have been done at all in view of the pathology of the lesion, and, granting an immediate recovery,

> whether the individual's expectation of life has been augmented...Does [a] survival mean good surgery or an erroneous diagnosis?...
>
> "Only by the whole-hearted co-operation of a large body of surgeons, we have kept detailed and reliable records, can a reasonably exact answer be given."
> —Harvey Cushing, MD
> "Surgical End-Results in General" (*Surgery Gynecology and Obstetrics* 1923; 36: 305.

Codman had returned from the army in the summer of 1919 to a closed hospital broke and in debt. He reopened his private practice in his home on the first floor at 227 Beacon Street and—in order to pay off his debts—"charged most of [his] patients three times as much as formerly" for about two years (Codman 1934). As a result, he remembered:

> I subtly drifted into the organization of the Registry of Bone Sarcoma, because one of my best patients had a bone tumor. My dream was that this one disease could be used as an example of the inadequacy of our present methods, and that some day records would serve to demonstrate the value of the End Result System in hospital organization...I have probably spent more time over this Registry, during the last thirteen years, than the average medical student requires to get his degree, yet, in all this time, I have had the actual care of not more than a half dozen patients with this disease... Many consultations, of course, but the patients are not turned over to me, although one may live next door. What is the reason? The hardest thing in my Quixotic career to explain to my colleagues is my plan for free consultation in cases of bone sarcoma. (Codman 1934)

In order to support his plan to use bone sarcomas as a means to demonstrate the value of his End-Result System and in the light of his few personal cases and a small number of consultations, he reached out to the two leading experts in bone tumors at the time: Dr. James Ewing (Cornell) and Dr. Joseph C. Bloodgood (Johns Hopkins). He wrote a letter to each member of the American College of Surgeons in August 1920 asking for a list of their patients who had survived for five years after being diagnosed with a bone sarcoma. In response he received the data in **Table 34.1**. He noted:

> It will no doubt be a surprise to many [that] we know of only four cases of true bone (osteogenic) sarcoma which are alive in this country today, who were treated over 5 years ago [by amputation]…Concerning 454 cases… reported to us…it seems surprising that they have boiled down to so few…most have not preserved slides or tissues of their cases… many hospitals do not preserve tissue or slides [or x-rays] of their cases for more than a few years…Another great reason why we have not been successful in finding more living cases is because hospitals, as a rule, have no follow-up systems [no end result documentation]. (Codman 1922)

Table 34.1. Patients who Survived for 5 Years after Diagnosis with Bone Sarcoma

Total cases about which we have had correspondence	454
Cases excluded for lack of X-rays, slides or tissue or obviously incorrect diagnosis	317
Cases which we have little doubt are cases of osteogenic sarcoma	41
Cases of giant-cell tumor	43
Cases still undetermined or other tumors	53
Cases of osteogenic sarcoma living over 5 years	4

Codman 1922.

The following year the American College of Surgeons approved their (Codman, Ewing, and Bloodgood) request to form a committee to develop a Registry of Bone Sarcoma. In February 1922 Codman, in a letter to the Editor of the *Boston Medical and Surgical Journal* stated:

> I wonder if you would give me your help in obtaining some statistics for the Registry of Bone Sarcoma. It is desirable to know the frequency of occurrence of cases of this lesion and there are no statistics by which we can obtain it…
>
> According to the directory of the AMA the population of Massachusetts is 3,662,329 and the number of physicians 5,494. If each one of these physicians should drop me a postal saying, either, 'I do know, or I do not know a case of bone sarcoma at present alive in Massachusetts', we should have…The best information in the world on the percentage of this disease per capita of population…
>
> I believe that every doctor in Massachusetts would be glad to contribute his bit to medical science, if the doing so did not involve too much time and expense…but a minute of time and a cent apiece…
>
> The Registry of Bone Sarcoma…organized independently by Dr. Bloodgood…Dr. Ewing… and the writer…is now a Committee of the American College of Surgeons. Our object is to register every case of bone sarcoma and by following the cases…to learn what the result of each is and what, if any, forms of treatment are effective. At present these cases are too rare for any one surgeon or clinic to obtain a sufficient number for study…In fact, during the year and a half in which we have been collecting cases, we have only found four five-year cures by amputation, and altogether only under one hundred cases which are now living…
>
> The American College of Surgeons holds its Clinical Congress in Boston next October. I hope we shall then be able to state the exact number of cases of bone sarcoma in Massachusetts with pathologic proof of each case if it is obtainable… (Codman 1922)

Over the next three months Dr. Codman would make another four appeals through the Editor of the *Boston Medical and Surgical Journal*. In August, with a limited response (less than 100 cases; four alive five years after amputation) to his questionnaire, he wrote to the editor again and listed some of the reasons for not participating that physicians had sent to him. He wrote:

> Undoubtedly in sending the questionnaire I have added to the many annoyances which affect the modern practitioner…We are beset by telephone, by mail, by interviews by social service sleuths, family welfarers, accident and health insurance certificates, workman's compensation documents, lawyer's letters, etc. These time-consuming, insistent nuisances have multiplied most horribly in the last ten years…Another wrote that he was no more interested in bone sarcoma than I was in knowing "how many flies could light on a golf ball"… There were other interesting replies, but none were so depressing as those who did not reply at all, for they spoiled the statistics…
>
> My motives…were in fact to interest the practitioner in this study, so that when the American College of Surgeons meets in Boston next fall I can state that…every case in Massachusetts is being put on record for the benefit of future sufferers with this disease. Financially I have nothing to gain for no charge is made for the services of the registry. Personally, I should gain…success in a difficult task [and] I shall have an example to set before the world…
>
> My objective was twofold. First, to let every physician in Massachusetts know of the registry…and what help it could be to patients with this lesion. Second, to locate every case of bone sarcoma in the state…How far we succeeded?…Of [5,420 physicians]…we have heard from 2,230…[and] have located only 71 cases of possible bone sarcoma…Now with regard to the other questions on the card which have no relation to bone sarcoma, but to medical human nature…only 56 bothered to answer the first two letters. Only 2,230 bothered to answer the postal [of which] only 658… read the letter and [gave]…their reasons for not answering it…This leaves still in doubt the state of mind of 3,190 who did not bother to apply at all. Certainly, the opposition cannot be strong if only six bothered to express it…
>
> So far as I know no one has ever attempted to gather statistics in this way before…As chairman of the committee I have expended $135.25 in this effort…to my mind the importance of making the study complete can hardly be measured in dollars… Will some wise man show me (not tell me) how to reach the other 3,190 necessary to complete my statistics? I have expended all the money I think it is right to expend for the college on this questionnaire, but I believe I could obtain from private sources a like amount to be spent on a better method.
> (Codman 1922)

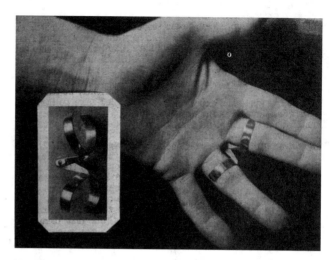

Unique surgical scissors designed by Codman for cutting sutures with "sleight of hand." "Miscellany," *Boston Medical and Surgical Journal* 1924; 190: 709.

In October 1922, before the meeting in Boston of the American College of Surgeons Codman stated, "The registry collection is at the disposal of anyone [of those] who wish to study the collection so as to be fore-armed should do so before the meeting of the College...because after that it is to be sent about to other cities for the opinions of other pathologists. If there are other cases now in Massachusetts we should be very grateful for their registration" (Codman 1922). He then briefly listed nine living cases of malignant osteogenic sarcoma and 22 cases of living patients with giant-cell tumors in Massachusetts. He said:

> There are four practical points brought out by the investigation thus far:
>
> 1. That the diagnosis should be made with great caution [often diagnosed as osteitis fibrosa, syphilis, non-suppurative osteomyelitis, metastatic cancer, myositis ossificans and ordinary callus based on insufficient evidence].
>
> 2. That Bloodgood's claim of the benign character of giant-cell tumors (erroneously called sarcoma) is confirmed by experience in Massachusetts.
>
> 3. That true osteogenic sarcoma is almost always fatal (the rare exceptions being cases where early amputation is performed).
>
> 4. That since only nine living cases could be located in a population of 4,000,000 there are probably only 225 in the whole United States (10,000,000). It certainly is not likely that there are more than double this number at any rate. We...will now plan our campaign to study the disease in other states...Another point of considerable interest...is the frequency with which amputation has been performed for giant-cell tumor. It should be possible by early diagnosis and complete local excision to save the limb in all such cases. (Codman 1922)

Codman maintained his interest in bone tumors for the rest of his career, commenting on it in the preface of his book, *The Shoulder* (see Box 34.6). Over the next 15 years, he published another seven articles and one book on tumors. In 1924, as chairman of the Registry of Bone Sarcoma for the American College of Surgeons, Codman published the article, "The Method of Procedure of the Registry of Bone Sarcoma." In this article, Codman described the contents of a box containing the data on an individual case being registered by a physician or hospital clinic. In addition to x-rays (or prints) of the bone lesion, photographs of the patient or gross specimen, slides of the histology, and a brief history with a diagnosis and the latest condition of the patient. The list of clinical entities included:

1. Metastatic Tumors
2. Periosteal Fibrosarcoma
3. Osteogenic Tumors

    Benign

    a. Exostosis

    b. Osteoma

    c. Chondroma

    d. Fibroma

    Malignant (Osteogenic Sarcoma)

    a. Anatomic types

    Medullary and subperiosteal

    Periosteal

    Sclerosing

    Telangiectatic

    b. Undifferentiated sarcoma

4. Inflammatory Conditions that may stimulate bone tumors

    Myositis ossificans, e.g., Osteoperiostitis

    a. Traumatic

    b. Syphilitic

    c. Infectious

    Osteitis fibrosa

5. Benign Giant Cell Tumor

6. Angioma

    Benign

    Malignant (angio-sarcoma)

7. Ewing's tumor

8. Myeloma (Codman 1924)

The Committee's policy was "to send the series of cases in similar boxes to each of the laboratories which are helping in the research so that many different surgeons and pathologists [and radiologists] may see the same cases and each express in his own writing the name [diagnosis] which he prefers for each particular case" (Codman 1924). The registry was started in the summer of 1920, supported by a grant of $8,000 from the American College of Surgeons. By 1924, Codman reported, "The Registry is now well started. Nearly 450 cases are already registered. Twenty-odd laboratories are receiving and studying the boxes of cases" (Codman 1924).

In 1925 Codman published "The Nomenclature Used by the Registry of Bone Sarcoma," which he then reprinted to a large extent in a small monograph, *Bone Sarcoma*. Regarding nomenclature he wrote:

> One of the main objects of the Registry is to get a uniform classification which roentgenologists, clinicians and pathologists can use in order to have a mutual understanding of the clinical entities which are referred to. At the time the Registry was started, four years ago, there were many different terms in use and while each term was vaguely understood by all who were interested in bone tumors, yet there was a considerable amount of misunderstanding among individuals...Two years ago a committee was appointed by the Clinical Pathological Association to formulate with us as definite a nomenclature as possible. (Codman 1925)

Together, the two committees developed the following classification. Codman described it as having "eight divisions, or really ten, for the

Box 34.6. Comments on Bone Sarcomas in the Preface of Codman's seminal publication, *The Shoulder*

> "I wish to make my knowledge of Bone Sarcoma so conspicuous that my opinion would be acknowledged to be a real value, and by making no charge for consultation, clear myself forever from the imputation that I was advertising for that purpose...Bone sarcoma was a partially good illustration [of the problem of letting our patients think that 'skill in operating or general reputation are more important than knowledge about their diseases'], not only because I had no claim to special success in treatment, but because it is a rare and usually fatal disease in which accurate diagnosis and wise advice as to the choice of treatment are far more important than the slight superiority in operative dexterity which any one surgeon may possess above the average. In 1920 blunders in the diagnosis or in the choice of treatment were very common in these cases, but could always be pardoned because the most eminent surgeons made similar ones...My chief interest in all this work was to show, in epitome, an example of the End Result Idea. Could any hospital, which really aimed to do its best for its cases, permit patients with a rare disease to be cared for by members of its staff, no matter how dexterous, who were not conversant with all attainable knowledge about the disease? What incentive would there be to thoughtful young men to spend years in the study of obscure conditions, if patients were to be assigned, by the ward by the calendar, to other less studious surgeons who were too busy making money even to read the literature of the subjects?
>
> "Of course these studies of mine are unpopular with the majority of our profession who have spent their lives in the practice of the art of medicine rather than in that of the science, and, being financially successful, are able to influence the trustees of hospitals against an analysis of results...They know our results are not as brilliant as the public thinks...They vaguely, and I think correctly, fear that if we succeeded in collecting complete records of every case of bone sarcoma, the evidence would lead to radical changes in our hospital methods."
>
> (Codman 1934)

benign and malignant osteogenic tumors are different entities, and so are the benign and malignant angiomas.

1. Metastatic tumors of bone
2. Periosteal fibrosarcoma
3. Osteogenic tumors, benign and malignant
4. Inflammatory conditions
5. Benign giant cell tumor
6. Angioma (benign and malignant)
7. Ewing's sarcoma
8. Myeloma (Codman 1925)

Codman's article on bone sarcoma, 1926. In part 1, he described Codman's Triangle, and in part 2, he analyzed 5-year cures in 13 cases of osteosarcoma. *Surgery, Gynecology and Obstetrics* 1926; 42: 381.

Both HMS and the MGH allowed Codman to use their facilities for his clinical research on bone tumors and provided him with an office to conduct his clinical research. Codman remembered, "The Harvard Medical School gave me a room for five years from which to conduct the Registry of Bone Sarcoma, and the Massachusetts General Hospital, since 1929, honored me with the appointment of Consulting Surgeon, which enables me to operate on private patients whom I have referred to its various departments" (Codman 1934). He performed his research at Harvard's Countway Medical Library in the Warren Museum. Afterward, his x-rays, microscope slides, and case notes were included on display at the museum.

In 1926, Dr. Codman reviewed the expenses of the "Registry of Bone Sarcoma," which he had originally funded with the support of the family of a patient he was treating. The purpose of the registry was to identify any patients with bone sarcoma who were cured and those treatments that had proven successful. In his financial report, he noted the outcomes of his work five years into the creation of the registry. He had located 17 cases of primary and malignant bone tumors that he believed were cured, including 13 cases of osteogenic sarcoma and 4 cases of Ewing's sarcoma. Nevertheless, the patient who the registry had been founded for died despite everything Codman had tried. The patient's autopsy revealed metastatic cancer of unknown origin. Other physicians assisting with the registry and analyzing cases at MGH and Huntington Memorial Hospital found 148 cases that were believed to be sarcomas. Of those cases, only 68 were proven to be bone sarcomas. The remaining 82 included

- 29 metastatic tumors of bone
- 28 soft tissue sarcomas
- 11 inflammatory conditions
- 14 non-sarcoma tumors

Codman then listed 25 criteria for making the diagnosis of osteogenic sarcoma and brief summaries of 13 cases of five-year cures. Codman assessed five-year patient outcomes by categorizing treatment using amputation, chemotherapy, radiation, or a combination of chemotherapy and radiation.

In part 1 of this paper reviewing the results of his experience with the Registry, Codman described in detail the x-ray changes with osteogenic sarcoma, including what is now called Codman's Triangle. Codman attempted to establish diagnostic criteria for bone cancer, given that some unrelated conditions could mimic it. He described a tell-tale triangle of new bone formation bilaterally on each side of the shaft that pushes the periosteum away from the bone. He observed that as the tumor spread, healthy osteoblasts retreated in a circular manner. Malignant tumors are visible beneath the periosteum and in the intramedullary cavity, whereas benign tumors are confined to either one or the other.

Codman published three more papers on bone tumors (from 1931 to 1936). In 1931, he described what we now call chondroblastoma or Codman's Tumor in an article, "Epiphyseal Chondromatous Giant Cell Tumors of the Upper End of the Humerus." Codman defined a benign giant cell tumor that appears in adolescents at the proximal edge of the humerus at the epiphysis of the articular head. He described its distinctive cottony appearance and asserted that the name of this tumor should be simple and communicate that this form of tumor appears in adolescents.

In 1934, he served as chairman of the Memorial Hospital [New York] Conference on the Treatment of Bone Sarcoma and published a brief summary of each of the papers presented. In 1936, at age 67, just four years before he died, he was asked to speak at the American College of Surgeons Cancer Symposium in Philadelphia. He reviewed the Registry's data on giant cell tumors of the knee concluding patients with giant cell tumors at the knee can be treated by amputation or by one of a combination of resection of the tumor, radiation, or curettage. He recognized two Philadelphia physicians: Dr. Samuel W. Gross, who recommended amputation, and Dr. Pfahler, a radiologist who was successful in treating these lesions with irradiation.

On July 10, 1939, Codman was invited to present at the annual meeting of the AAOS by president Joseph S. Barr. At that meeting, he was given a gold medal in recognition of his work on sarcoma, though it excluded mention of either the publication of his book on the shoulder (which was the first in the United States) or of his ideas on quality control.

FAMILY AND OTHER INTERESTS

Dr. Codman married Katherine "Katy" Putnam Bowditch, daughter of Charles Pickering Bowditch, in Boston on November 16, 1899. It was a year of transformations in Codman's personal and professional life and the same year that he was appointed the first skiagrapher at Boston Children's Hospital and promoted to surgeon to outpatients at MGH. His early findings on the use of x-rays between 1895 and 1900 took place at HMS in the physiology lab established by Charles P. Bowditch. (Bowditch was the grandson of the famous astronomer and mathematician, Nathaniel Bowditch. He had graduated from HMS in 1868 and had studied physiology in Europe under the leaders in the field: Drs. Claude Bernard, Louis A. Ranvier, Jean-Martin Charcot and Willy Kühne. In 1871, Bowditch established the first physiology laboratory in the United States at HMS where he was an assistant professor.) There, Codman met his future wife in late 1896.

They became engaged in November 1898 and were married about a year later in Chestnut Hill. They moved into his modest home at 104 Mount Vernon Street, which he had inherited from his brother, John. In 1904, they moved to 227 Beacon Street. (Katy lived there until her death in 1961). In 1905, they also purchased a summer home in Ponkapoag, where Dr. Codman would spend much of his last decade. Katy Codman supported reforms in nursing education and was prominent in the woman's suffrage movement. Her two closest friends were Dr. Alice Hamilton and Emily Balch, both leaders of a peace movement during and after World War I. Balch later won the 1946 Nobel Peace Prize (Gunnar 1946). During the war, she was a delegate to the International Congress of Woman in 1915 at The Hague, and, also in 1915, helped found the antiwar Women's International League for Peace and Freedom. She donated funds to the Simmons School of Public Health Nursing and became secretary, and then president, of the Instructive District Nursing Association of Boston.

Dr. William Mallon, in his book, briefly described Katy and Dr. Codman's relationship. Surprisingly, neither Dr. Codman nor Katy Codman mentioned each other in their voluminous writings except in passing. They had no children. Little is known of their personal and familial life. In his writings, Codman did talk about his dogs frequently, taking them everywhere he could and even occasionally during the performance of his duties. There are many photographs of the Codmans with their dogs.

Dr. Carter Rowe recalled meeting Dr. Codman in 1937 at the bedside of a patient with a tumor of the shoulder while Rowe was a student. Dr. Codman had brought his English setter with him, who sat in the corner of the room while Dr. Codman took the patient's history, performed an examination, and reassured the patient. Rowe remembered Codman as "a quiet, gentle person, with steady, penetrating eyes. One quickly sensed integrity, intelligence, and self-confidence" (Rowe 1966). Rowe went on to write that:

> Dr. Codman spent much of this time on Ward I and in the orthopaedic OPD clinic. Dr. Paul Norton recalls that "frequently old E.A. would drop by the orthopaedic clinic to discuss problems of the shoulder, and the causes of shoulder pain"...Dr. Henry Marble, one of our early hand surgeons at the MGH and an associate of Dr. Codman's, told me the story of his summons one day to Dr. Codman's office because "Dr. Codman has a bone to pick with you." With trepidation, he arrived at Codman's office, wondering what he had done, or had not done. Within a few minutes, Dr. Codman's secretary accompanied him to Dr. Codman's office where a table had been set with two beautifully cooked partridges awaiting him. Dr. Codman said "Henry, I thought you would enjoy picking a few bones with me." Henry would tell this with delight and never-failing amusement.
> (Rowe 1966)

Throughout his life Codman was also an avid hunter and fisherman. A prolific writer, Codman kept a detailed diary and wrote many letters to friends and at least one published article about his fishing and hunting trips from 1889 to 1936. Codman remembered:

> At school I gave more thought to collecting bird's eggs, trapping rabbits, muskrat, mink and skunks, than I did to religious instruction...My attention has been riveted on so managing my life that I could get "days off," during the spring for trout fishing and a month in the fall for partridge and woodcock, that I have given little thought to morals and have substituted reasonable habits. If you are to know me, I may as well admit that I have averaged at least thirty days a year in hunting and fishing. I have tried these

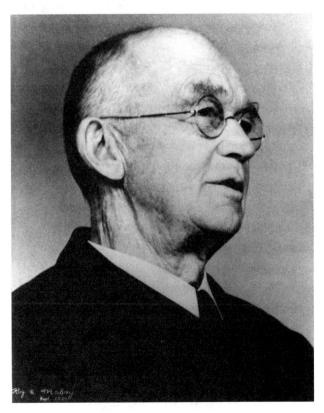

Ernest A. Codman. Massachusetts General Hospital, Archives and Special Collections.

things in thirty-six states…in England, Scotland and Ireland; in Ontario, New Brunswick, Nova Scotia, Quebec, Cape Bretton; in Egypt and in Yucatan; and in the case of at least two New England states, in every Township. Yet I have never hit ten ruffled grouse in succession. A few years ago I got six in sequence…As in my professional work, the thing I try to do consummates…in many friendships…Perhaps I have sacrificed my success as a distinguished surgeon to these pursuits. I have loved them better than teaching dozing medical students, the pride of amphitheater dexterity, or the hushed dignity of the consultant at the bedside of important persons. On many a bright October day I have been glad that my talents as a teacher were not in demand. In the spring when I dig up the first worm in my garden…I get my reward for not being an overworked "Chief of the Surgical Service." In summer as I drift about some out-of-way pond…I am grateful that I am not in demand at the bankers' bedsides. (Codman 1934)

Box 34.7. MGH Resolution Honoring Dr. Codman

The Trustees of the Massachusetts General Hospital [adopted] the following resolution…at their meeting [on December 13, 1940]:

Champion of truth; original in thought; firm in his convictions, and willing to sacrifice personal place and standing to achieve what he believed to be right. To him rightfully belongs the credit for conceiving and effecting many policies which have contributed to the improvement and advancement of surgery and to the renown of this Hospital. Through his efforts the General Executive Committee was formed, the policy of Special Assignments accepted, the practice of advancement solely upon the basis of seniority abandoned, and a Follow-up and End Result system adopted. He showed early promise of originality and energy. As a House Officer, together with Harvey Cushing, he compiled the first recordings of the administration of anesthetics and "Ground out on the old static machine the first faint x-ray picture of a hand ever taken here."

As a surgeon Dr. Codman will be remembered primarily for his work on duodenal ulcer, for his book on *The Shoulder* and for the institution of the Registry for Bone Sarcoma.

Mankind, Medicine, and the Massachusetts General Hospital are his debtors.

The Board of Regents of the American College of Surgeons, at a meeting held in Chicago on February 16, 1941, adopted the following resolution:

WHEREAS, Dr. Ernest Amory Codman of Boston, Massachusetts, a Founder of the American College of Surgeons, and a member of the Board of Governors of said College, has contributed in an extremely important manner to its work, especially through the establishment and conduct of the Registry of Bone Sarcoma, and

WHEREAS, this Registry of Bone Sarcoma not only introduced a new co-operative method of scientific study on a large-scale but made possible definite advances in the knowledge of a subject concerning which much ignorance had prevailed, and as a result of which many human lives have undoubtedly been saved, and

WHEREAS, it is recognized that the success of the Registry of Bone Sarcoma was overwhelmingly due to the scientific zeal and self-sacrificing labors of Dr. Codman, and

WHEREAS, Dr. Codman passed from this earth November 23, 1940,

THEREFORE, BE IT RESOLVED by the Regents of the American College of Surgeons at their regular meeting held in Chicago on February 16, 1941, that an expression of their appreciation of the work of Dr. Codman be spread upon the minutes of the said meeting and that a copy of this resolution be sent to his widow, Katherine Bowditch Codman, with an expression of their deepest sympathy.

(Harvard Medical School Archives 1940)

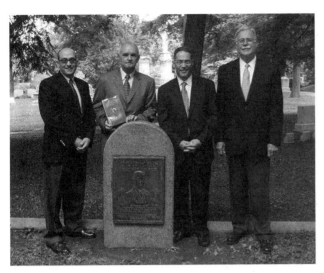

Dedication ceremony of Dr. Codman's headstone, July 22, 2014. Attendees (left to right): Jonathan B. Ticker, William J. Mallon, Jon J. P. Warner and James H. Herndon.
Courtesy of the author.

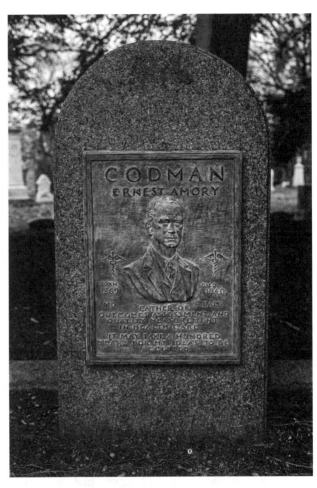

Headstone of Dr. Ernest Amory Codman. Kael E. Randall/Kael Randall Images.

LEGACY

In the last 10 years of his life, Dr. Ernest A. Codman hunted, fished, and golfed. He was a member of several elite country clubs, though he suffered from financial difficulties and the couple lived off of Katy's inheritance, which had shrunk during the Great Depression. He lived primarily at Ponkapoag, occasionally consulting at Massachusetts General Hospital, while Katy remained in their home at Beacon Street. Ten months before his death, he received the Gold Medal from the American Academy of Orthopaedic Surgeons for his contributions in the field of bone sarcoma.

> "Ernest Amory Codman, surgeon, good Bostonian, and crusader...A crusader is one who makes a difficult, dangerous campaign to save something precious, and without thought of gain for himself... [His] crusade was to ensure for all in need of surgery what he believed to be ideal treatment."
> —John Homans. *NEJM*, 1941

He developed malignant melanoma and died on November 23, 1940. His financial circumstances by that point were so dire that Katy could not afford a headstone. He was buried in Mt. Auburn Cemetery in the Bowditch family plot. He donated his medical library to Massachusetts General Hospital. Dr. John Homans, a friend of Dr. Codman, wrote Codman's obituary for the *New England Journal of Medicine* and included some personal reflections. He was:

> a crusader; one who makes a difficult, dangerous campaign to save something precious [End-Result Idea], and without thought or gain for himself...When the roentgen ray was discovered...with his characteristic thoroughness he secured from physicists at Harvard and Technology the best advice and assistance

available. It is even more characteristic that, having made complete roentgenographic studies of the important joints of the body, at considerable expense in time and money, all without being asked to do so by anyone...presented his collection to the Warren Museum where it was buried...and apparently forgotten...[This] strengthened [his] conviction which earlier experiences had created, namely, that his labors were not likely to be recognized...This attitude of mind, a sense of isolation, a feeling that others would not readily agree with his views, was a strong influence in his life, a peculiarity which in its most violent form caused him to introduce his astonishing cartoon dealing with hospital efficiency...But his self-consciousness about this matter was never morbid; he was not so introspective as all that. Indeed, he was often more than a little amused at himself...

For his too-impulsive action at the library meeting Codman had to pay in loss of dignity, prestige and professional income—a small price, he believed, considering the great result...

When he failed to save one [of his patients]—the wife of an intimate friend—he became inspired to make his great fight against bone sarcoma, for which he received no earthly reward...If one thinks of him as in any sense a disappointed man...such was by no means true. He agrees that he has had a good time in life...calls himself quixotic, but intensely dislikes being dubbed "a reformer." He certainly describes himself as, though he does not use the word, a "crusader"...He never said hard things of those who disagreed with him, only of those whose motives he felt to be unworthy. And even then, he never attacked individuals...It was impossible to resist his fundamental goodness and charm.

Amory Codman had many devoted friends in many walks of life. No one could associate with him intimately without coming under the spell of his enthusiasm, his squareness and the attractive whimsical streak which...took the sharp edge off his intensity. In everyday life he was affectionate, thoughtful, fair, a good companion. His was a strong character, remarkably free from pretense and affectation, uncompromising, of a sort much needed in this day. He should be counted one of New England's great figures, a man who has left a deep mark and has deserved well of posterity for whom he labored. (Homans 1941)

Shortly after his death the trustees of the MGH passed a resolution honoring Dr. Codman (see **Box 34.7**).

In 1997, Codman was recognized by the Joint Commission on Accreditation of Healthcare Organizations (JCAHO), now named the Joint Commission, with the annual Ernest A. Codman Award, which recognizes healthcare facilities that ensure evidence-based and quality control practice to improve quality of care. In 2002, the Department of Surgery at the Massachusetts General Hospital established the Codman Center for Clinical Effectiveness in Surgery whose mission is to provide safe and valued care as well as to furnish cutting-edge research and education.

On Tuesday, July 22, 2014, a small private ceremony was held at Mt. Auburn Cemetery at the Bowditch family plot. Dr. Andrew Warshaw, the recently retired chief of surgery at MGH and president-elect of the American College of Surgeons at the time, arranged to have an engraved granite and bronze headstone for Dr. Codman placed just behind Nathaniel Bowditch's grave. The effort by Dr. Warshaw took over two years and donations of $20,000. In addition to the leadership of the American College of Surgeons and a few distant family members of Dr. Codman, leadership from the American Academy of Orthopaedic Surgeons and the American Shoulder and Elbow Surgeons attended the brief ceremony. The headstone includes the inscription: "It may take a hundred years for my ideas to be accepted."

CHAPTER 35

Elliott G. Brackett

His Character Was a Jewel with Many Facets

Elliott Gray Brackett was born on April 6, 1860 in Newton, Massachusetts. In pursuit of his Harvard Medical School (HMS) degree, he had to work hard to overcome a disabling disease of the hip, and this personal challenge inspired a later commitment to research and charity. At one point, he was bedridden for a full year, but a classmate kept him up-to-date on his coursework while Dr. Edward Hickling Bradford treated his symptoms. Despite these obstacles, he graduated on time from HMS in 1886. Following internships at Boston City Hospital and Boston Lying-in Hospital from 1886 to 1887—where he did not miss a day of work despite requiring assistance with crutches when walking—he worked as an assistant in materia medica and therapeutics at HMS in 1887 and 1888. He had demonstrated an initial interest in psychiatry after graduating from HMS and may have pursued this interest as well but, ultimately, he specialized in orthopaedic surgery. His own health condition drove him to continue to tirelessly pursue research in chronic disabling diseases.

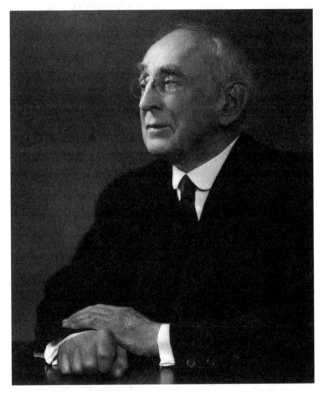

Elliott G. Brackett. "Elliott Gray Brackett, April 6, 1860—December 29, 1942," *Journal of Bone and Joint Surgery*, 1943; 25: 245.

Physician Snapshot

Elliot G. Brackett
BORN: 1860
DIED: 1942
SIGNIFICANT CONTRIBUTIONS: Contributed outstanding executive leadership, served as a distinguished editor of the *Journal of Bone and Joint Surgery*; was respected by his peers for a quiet, keen devotion, wide breadth of understanding, and deep sympathy

EARLY RESEARCH AND SERVICE

Brackett quickly joined Bradford—the same surgeon who had cared for him—in practice, and he served on the orthopaedic staffs of Children's

Hospital and the House of the Good Samaritan. While practicing at Boston Children's Hospital, Brackett began his studies of the hip, and he coauthored about 12 articles, "Recent Progress in Orthopedic Surgery" in the Medical Progress Series of the *Boston Medical and Surgical Journal*. He also published another 30 articles on a wide variety of topics ranging from clubfeet to studies of hand unsteadiness; but his primary focus included three areas: lateral curvature of the spine, Pott's disease, and hip disease.

Over time, he became a leading voice in precise, evidence-based recommendations relied upon by his peers. In 1889, he had reported early experimental findings on distraction of the hip joint:

> The value of traction in the treatment of the acute conditions of hip disease has abundant evidence, both in its relief of symptoms and its influence on the course of the disease...[However,] the occurrence of the separation of the two joint surfaces...is a matter of dispute... From the experiments [traction in a cadaver of a three-year old] and observations [traction in twelve children, ages 5 to 12 years, for hip disease] the following conclusions are drawn. The anatomy of the joint in small children does not offer any obstacle to a separation; but in older children...some opposition...is encountered [especially due to the resistance of the Y-ligament]...Experiments show that distraction is an evident anatomical possibility... [with] continual traction...a means of producing muscular exhaustion, the ability to respond [and] is overcome [and] does not pose an active counter-force to the traction...In ordinary cases a breech [sic] of contact does occur [and] affords relief to the spasmodic condition which is the source of so much suffering in the course of acute disease, and its influence is beneficial, not only by alleviating the pain but also by preventing...the mechanical injury to the diseased parts, from this condition of excessive muscular irritability. (Brackett 1889)

At the time, the effect of traction of the hip joint was controversial because results were unclear, but he successfully demonstrated that traction did indeed separate the joint surfaces of the hip in young children because of the laxity of their ligaments. In older children, however, joint separation was more difficult because the ligaments are stronger.

He continued to support the use of traction, and, 10 years later, he demonstrated its effectiveness in the treatment of children with tuberculosis of the hip. He concluded:

> The immobilization must be complete [even during] the child turning or twisting, both when awake and asleep. For this reason, it is not sufficient that a child be simply placed in bed...but must be so secured...by the use of the frame, to which the child can be properly strapped, that all injurious motion may be prevented, and attention given to the child's wants without disturbing the rest to the joint. The traction of the limb to overcome the spasm of the muscles must be sufficient to prevent the unusual pressure of the head of the femur against the acetabulum, and must be constant...This traction must be carried on in the line of deformity of the limb, must be continuous, both when it is applied by the weight during the recumbent and by the apparatus during the ambulatory treatment...The treatment by conservative methods, although it requires time and patience has the advantage that the cure is obtained with the least destruction of bone. (Brackett 1898)

Before the discovery of antibiotics in the twentieth century, Pott's disease—or tuberculosis of the spine—was a serious condition with the possibility of leading to paralysis. Brackett published his experiences treating the condition in several papers, and he also later headed a commission organized by the American Orthopaedic Association to study the results of fusion in tubercular

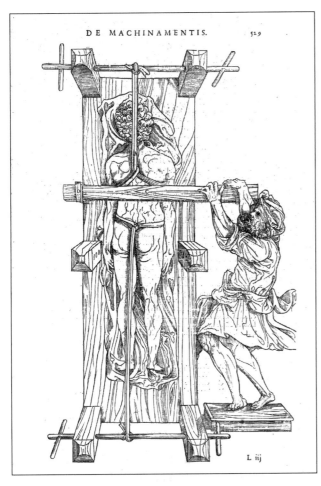

De Machinamentis of Oribasius, a medieval method to reduce the gibbus of Pott's disease.
Chirurgia by Nicetas, compiled and translated by Guido Guidi (Vidus Vidius). Paris: Excudebat Petrus Glaterius Luceciae, 1544. Getty Research Institute/Internet Archive.

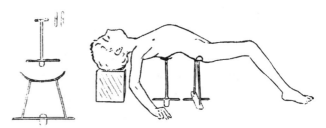

Goldthwait's method of reducing the gibbus and application of a body cast. *Deformities Including Diseases of the Bones and Joints*, Volume 2, by Alfred H. Tubby. London: Macmillan and Co., 1896.

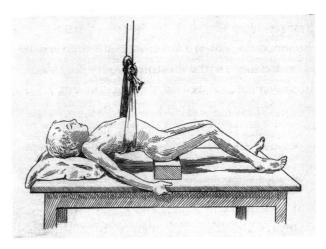

Bradford's method of reducing the gibbus and application of a body cast.
Treatise on Orthopedic Surgery, 2nd edition, by Bradford and Lovett. New York: William Wood and Company, 1899. Columbia University Libraries/Internet Archive.

spines (discussed later in this chapter). In his first paper in 1891, he discussed treatment for paralysis:

> Paralysis in Pott's disease may usually be expected to disappear in the course of several weeks, or a few months, and therefore its appearance gives no particular reason for alarm...The value of rest...will probably be acknowledged by everyone...but simple rest is apparently not always sufficient. The paralysis usually appears at a time when the bone disease is in an active stage. (Brackett 1891)

In the same paper, he reviewed four cases of Pott's disease with paralysis that had been present for between two and five months in three patients and recurrent in another each time the patient was allowed to get out of bed. To treat them, he used extension of the spine:

> particularly to both the head and feet [with] gratifying results. In two of these, when [extension was] added to the treatment which had been carried out for several months, the improvement began within two to three weeks...Strict recumbency [is required] until the course of the recovery is well established, [He concluded]: that in paralysis...recovery may be looked for even after its persistence for at least a year and a half, and with sensation as well as motion affected. That the treatment in extension...should be given a thorough

trial before resorting to other means. That the improvement, although usually early seen, may not be apparent for several weeks or a few months. That the most careful attention should be given to the details in securing a well-adapted support to the whole back, the continued and even extension, and the avoidance, as far as possible, of all motion. (Brackett 1891)

Less than a year later, on January 11, 1892, Brackett was afforded the honor of reading the esteemed Dr. Edward Bradford's prepared remarks at a meeting of the Boston Society for Medical Improvement as well as a few comments of his own. Brown had recently died, and his substantial legacy was recognized at the meeting. We do not know whether Brackett knew Brown personally since he joined the staff of the House of the Good Samaritan after Brown had retired as chief and shortly before his passing, but Brown had mentored Brackett's own mentor, Bradford. In his speech, Brackett said:

> To Dr. Buckminster Brown belongs the credit of having introduced into this country the best of the English school of orthopedic surgery [at that time the leading and most active school], and of having placed this specialty in America on a most excellent foundation. But he was in no true sense a follower, as his mind worked independently; in many of his methods he was bolder than many of his English compeers; and in thoroughness and persistency, he equaled and surpassed his teachers.
>
> Conservative by nature, too scholarly and well trained to accept without cautious reserve brilliantly announced cures and speedily successful procedures in the treatment of affections essentially chronic, he relied chiefly upon the painstaking measures which aid and cure through daily attention. Although he relied chiefly upon appliances in the treatment of deformity, he had the instincts of a surgeon and believed in operative methods whenever it was proved that operation was beneficial. He, by no means belonged to the more timid school of orthopedic surgery, which shuns operation, though his experience was chiefly limited to non-operative procedures. The methods which he worked in, have, in the progress of surgery, in some instances been superseded; but his work in clubfoot, in tenotomy, in infantile paralysis, in correction of right-angled contraction at the hip and knee-joint, and especially in the cure of congenital dislocation, by long-continued traction and manipulation will always be of value in orthopedic surgery.
>
> His tastes were essentially scientific in the best sense, and his work is characterized by a tenacity of purpose and a persistency not to be surpassed; and to whomever he was bound by the contract of professional duty he gave his whole attention and ability with untiring zeal, and that in spite of obstacles in the lack of physical vigor which none could appreciate who did not know him. He husbanded his resources carefully and spent them lavishly in his work. Besides his achievements he left as a legacy to his successors an example of loyalty to purpose, unremittent persistency, and a courage always superior to the obstacles and limitations surrounding his life. (*Boston Medical and Surgical Journal* 1892)

Brackett's remarks allow us a window into Bradford's and his own value system, their high esteem for a conservative, persistent, and evidence-based approach to practice as well as their enthusiastic commitment to the field.

C. F. Painter (1943) later described these particular traits in Brackett when he wrote that Brackett was:

> a past master in the fitting of apparatus, he used braces and other means to support to a greater extent than many present-day [1943] practitioners. He did excellent surgery when he thought surgery was indicated, but was never

hurried into it before he had reason to think it would be the opportune time…His familiarity with the literature of his specialty and his acquaintance with the ablest exponents served to make him "not the first by whom the new is tried, nor yet the last to lay the old aside"… though conservative…he was open-minded.

As someone personally affected by a chronic hip disease, he had an intimate understanding of disability, and—while busy with research and the demands of his practice—he also dedicated time to found the Industrial School for Crippled and Deformed Children in 1893 with Augustus Thorndike and Edward Bradford. It was the first school in the United States designated for children with physical disabilities, and Brackett later served as president and a consultant in orthopaedic surgery. The school continues to serve the needs of children with diverse disabilities today and is now called Cotting School.

During the latter half of his 15 active years in practice with Bradford, Brackett published eight papers on scoliosis, only four of which he coauthored with his mentor. He may have already begun to consider starting his own independent practice, and he demonstrated an increasing interest in caring for adults in addition to children—a trend in orthopaedics that increased throughout the early twentieth century. In 1896, he wrote:

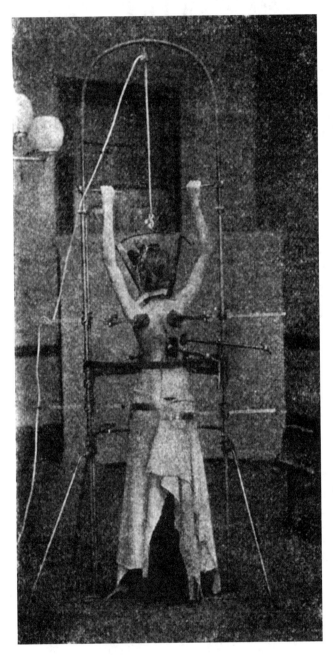

Pressure correction apparatus (Hoffa-Schede). Plates are applied to the sites of maximum deformity while the patient is standing. A body cast is made with the spine in an improved alignment.

Treatise on Orthopedic Surgery, 2nd edition, by Bradford and Lovett. New York: William Wood and Company, 1899. Columbia University Libraries/Internet Archive.

> lateral curvature cases can be divided into two classes, representing, not different types, but different stages of one condition, which is distinctly progressive…The first class includes cases of such slight degree, in which little or no bony change has occurred…postural curves… The second class includes those cases in which…definite structural changes have taken place in the bones and ligaments and muscles [that] present a distinct obstacle to the complete restoration. The first class…treatment must…be directed to overcome this asymmetrical development [with] flexibility of the spine…and second…to improve the muscle strength…
>
> In the second class…the object of treatment…is two-fold: (1) To so increase the range of flexibility…of the spine…in which the patient

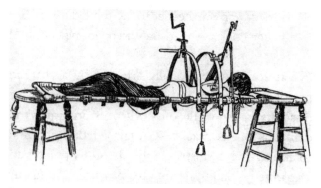

Recumbent pressure correction apparatus (Hoffa-Schede). Plates are applied to the sites of maximum deformity while the patient is recumbent on a Bradford frame. A body cast is made with the spine in an improved alignment.
E. H. Bradford and E. G. Brackett, "The Employment of Mechanical Force in Treatment of Lateral Curvature," *Boston Medical and Surgical Journal* 1895; 133: 359.

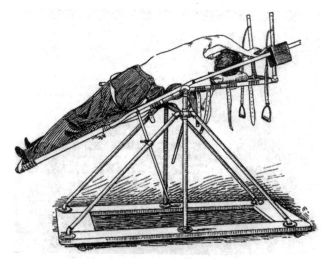

Modified Zander apparatus (tilt table) for correcting scoliosis.
E. H. Bradford and E. G. Brackett, "The Employment of Mechanical Force in Treatment of Lateral Curvature," *Boston Medical and Surgical Journal* 1895; 133: 357.

can be made straight or nearly so. (2) To then hold the spine and trunk in nearly as possible… whether by means of apparatus or by increased muscle development, or both, while the bones are being shaped and ossification is taking place. The principle used to accomplish the first of the measures…is done by forcible exercise, aided by manual pressure of an assistant…A more accurate way is by the so-called mechanical correction, by which the desired amount of force can be applied to any part of the spine and in any direction with an accurate graduation [and] precision. There have been numerous forms of apparatus used for this purpose…as examples of these can be seen the modification of Hoffa's apparatus, in which the patient is partially suspended…shoulders and hips secured by… clamps and pads, and the desired amount of rotatory force applied to the trunk…A second form is that of the rocker, in which the patient is made to lie on an oblique frame [and] bent above and below at the point where the pressure is desired to be made…This portion of the treatment must be supplemented by some method [cast, brace] by which the spine is held in the best position…during the process of growth and development. (Brackett 1896)

Two years later, by the end of the Spanish-American War in 1898, Brackett joined the Volunteer Aid Association, with his primary goal to distribute hospital and food supplies to two Massachusetts regiments—the 2nd and the 9th—in Cuba. It was here that he began to exhibit his superb executive leadership skills. When he arrived that July in Santiago, Brackett wrote that the city was:

> in much the same condition as after the surrender…under martial law…in a condition of extreme filth…and the midsummer heat was intense. There was a…great scarcity of proper food and medicines…The sickness among our troops…had become alarming…principally a pernicious form of malaria [and] some typhoid and yellow fever…During August there was but one hospital, the Nautical Club, in the city [where] the sickest of men were sent.
> (Brackett 1899)

While serving under General Wood and after initially arranging for distribution of supplies for the sick, Brackett first organized general care of the convalescents and the care of troops during their

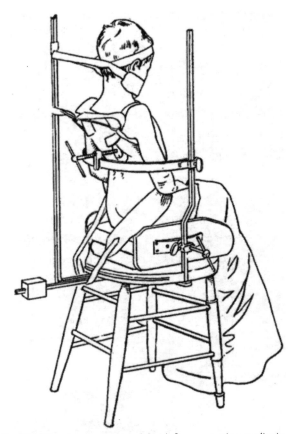

Modified Zander Apparatus (chair) for correcting scoliosis.
E. H. Bradford and E. G. Brackett, "The Employment of Mechanical Force in Treatment of Lateral Curvature," Boston Medical and Surgical Journal 1895; 133: 358.

evacuation. General Wood then appointed Brackett to oversee the Centro Benefico, a hospital in Santiago that had been closed for several months.

After returning from Cuba, Brackett continued to work at Boston Children's Hospital and the Massachusetts General Hospital. He was also on the staffs of the New England Baptist Hospital, Faulkner Hospital, and the Beth Israel Hospital. By 1899, Drs. Bradford and Brackett had published their last coauthored paper on scoliosis, "Correction in Lateral Curvature," in which they summarized their thinking about the importance of applied forces in the correction of the complex deformities of the condition. In this paper, they discussed a third class of cases:

> where resistance and flexibility of the spine exist [but] treatment by gymnastics and flexibility exercises will not be sufficient, and for these cases mechanical measures have always been attempted. They have, however, never been thoroughly successful...The important problem...is to the selection of the best possible means of exerting pressure directly upon the projecting positions of the trunk...
>
> It was supposed that the treatment by plaster jackets suggested by Sayre would be corrective, but the subsequent experience has shown that although this method is of value in caries of the spine, its value is considerably less in lateral than in anteroposterior curves from caries. The reason of this is [was] the fact that suspension as applied by Sayre does not sufficiently correct the twist of the spine seen in lateral curvature...
>
> Experience has taught that if sufficient pressure is applied properly, faulty shapes of bone in growing children can be corrected in various portions of the skeleton...and we need this pressure so severe as to be unendurable, provided it be constantly or continuously applied. Bone may be expected to grow straight, if it is prevented from growing crookedly. The softer the bone and the younger the child the more easily is the change produced...
>
> A plaster jacket...applied in lateral curvature often slips on wearing and presses on the concavity, injuring as much as it corrects... [if] at all. It is manifest that the jacket should be applied with the patient corrected as far as possible...until the plaster-of-Paris is sufficiently hard to maintain this corrected pressure... The most feasible way of straightening the spine has been found...by the recumbent position rather than by vertical suspension...If the patient is placed upon the back, with or without head and foot traction...with the weight of the trunk supported only upon certain points, where upward pressure is applied, the sag of the unsupported portions of the trunk will serve to aid in the correction of the twist of the trunk... aided by pressing upon the prominent portion

of the distorted chest and thorax...The plaster bandages are applied as usual...A correcting force should...be applied not beyond the easy endurance and the jackets should be frequently changed. The treatment should be continued as long as it is possible to obtain correction, after which a removable corset and gymnastic treatment is to be employed. (Bradford and Brackett 1896)

INDEPENDENT PRACTICE AND EARLY CONTRIBUTIONS

In 1901, Brackett married Katherine F. Pedrick and opened his independent practice at 166 Newberry Street. At the time, the specialty of orthopaedic surgery was expanding into the care of adults, and Brackett would go on to join an association with the Orthopaedic Clinic of MGH, which treated both adult and pediatric patients. He was also appointed an assistant in orthopaedics at HMS in 1903. As the field of orthopaedic surgery continued to mature and expand, there was much controversy and debate. Brackett, however, "achieved a reputation for fairness and integrity, which made him acceptable to all factions, and in 1905 he was elected president of the American Orthopaedic Association" (*Boston Medical and Surgical Journal* 1943).

As Brackett grew his own practice, he continued his research, and by 1910 he reported pathological findings in tubercular spine specimens preserved in the Warren Museum. He described two features indicating the possibility of a cure:

1. In instances of marked destruction...a solid bony union occurs throughout, forming a large wedge of bone, as a strong protective barrier toward further increase of deformity.

2. In instances of destruction of large areas... bridges of bone are...in the angle of the curve, much in the form of a buttress...as a mechanical prop...In instances where there is not a broad opposing service for firm ankylosis two methods of protection are seen:

    a. ...new bone on the anterior part of the vertebra, extending from one body to another...

    b. The most ingenious, that of fusing together of the posterior part of the vertebrae, the laminae, or even the spinous processes. In many of the specimens...the posterior wing of the laminae and of the spinous processes are found fused together into a solid mass...This acts as a kind of stay...to prevent the spine from yielding in the forward direction and also prevents

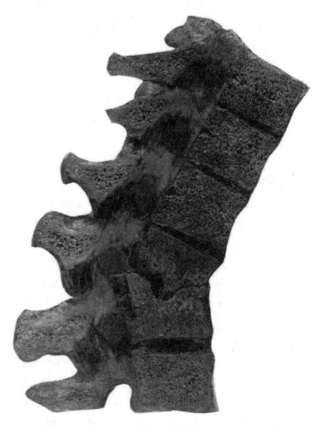

Pathological specimen of the spine with Pott's disease preserved in the Warren Museum. Note the involvement of the disease in the front of the vertebra with destruction of the disc space and adjacent vertebrae.

E. G. Brackett, "Study of the Relation Between Clinical Evidence and Pathological Conditions in Spinal Caries," *American Journal of Orthopedic Surgery*, 1910; s2-8: 367.

lateral and twisting motion in the section where the natural protection has been lost. (Brackett 1910)

Brackett's paper was published at the same time that Dr. Russell Hibbs was experimenting with spine fusion in cadavers and animals and one year before Hibbs performed his first posterior spine fusion in a child for tuberculosis of the spine. By 1911, Brackett was appointed chief of orthopaedic surgery at MGH, after Dr. Joel Goldthwait's resignation. Little information is available to us about Dr. Brackett's time as chief, but we do know there were two departments at the time: the older orthopaedics and the relatively new genito-urinary. Brackett continued to publish more than 60 articles on a variety of topics, was very active in the American Orthopaedic Association (volunteering as treasurer for a number of years and as president) and was an active member of the Interurban Orthopaedic Club.

In 1915, he published a paper with his coauthor H. W. Marshall on late results of surgery of the hip in osteoarthritis. In a long-term follow-up of nine of 20 patients (**Case 34.1**), they found:

> Two important varieties of operations [were] performed. Firstly, removal of small bony prominences around acetabula and heads of femori in hip joints still fairly normal...and secondly more extensive operations in disabled hips...(a) arthrodesis...and (b) decapitation of femoral heads. (Brackett and Marshall 1915)

Depending on the position the hip was fused, arthrodesis of the hip joint could similarly be disabling. If extended, the patient would not be able to sit easily and, if flexed, the patient might not be able to walk or stand well. He continued to publish prolifically, and, in an additional paper in 1915, he made the following remarks regarding arthrodesis:

> It is to be remembered that the walking and standing function is good—sitting giving the inconvenience, but which can be mitigated by a few degrees of flexion...But the joint is kept...fixed, the lumbar spine and knee compensating. We must therefore consider in making the choice of operation [arthrodesis versus femoral head excision]: (a) the occupation and social requirements of the individual. (b) whether sitting or labor at standing must have the greater consideration. (c) whether the necessary restriction of a decidedly handicapped joint can be carried out, for these joints require care long after they leave the surgeon's hands.
>
> (Brackett 1915)

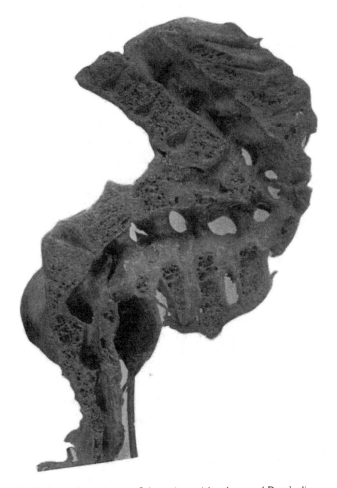

Pathological specimen of the spine with advanced Pott's disease preserved in the Warren Museum. Note the weak area of union with new bone formation at the apex of the kyphosis—acting as a prop or bridge to prevent further deformity.

E. G. Brackett, "Study of the Relation Between Clinical Evidence and Pathological Conditions in Spinal Caries," *American Journal of Orthopedic Surgery*, 1910; s2-8: 376.

No standard position had been agreed to yet.

After World War I began, he soon again pursued military medical service, and he left his position as chief at MGH to serve as a Colonel in the Division of Orthopaedic Surgery, a position he fulfilled with great distinction (see chapter 63). Brackett was appointed director of the US Army's Department for Military Orthopedics, and Major David Silver—who later became the professor and chair of orthopaedic surgery at the University of Pittsburgh (the department chair now holds the David Silver Professorship in his honor)—was his assistant director. During Brackett's tenure as director, he selected orthopaedic surgeons to serve overseas, serving himself at the front for a time (see **Box 34.8** for Brackett's thoughts on gunshot injuries). Major Goldthwait directed the newly created Military Orthopedics for the Expeditionary Forces

Case 34.1. Hip Fusion for Severe Disabling Arthritis

> In one of the long-term follow-up cases, they examined a 53-year-old male patient who was employed as a sea captain. His case was an example of an extensive operation that should be considered only in cases of severe disability:
>
> "The right hip was found at operation to have the joint capsule bound down obliterating the joint cavity; also the muscles about the joint showed evidences of chronic inflammatory process. A wedge-shaped piece of bone was removed from the head of the femur; and the acetabulum after curettage was allowed to unite firmly with the head of the femur.
>
> "Before operation the thigh was flexed at ninety degrees and adducted forty-five degrees. Muscle spasm held the hip nearly rigid, but under ether there was a relaxation to forty-five degrees of flexion and ten degrees of permanent adduction.
>
> "Three years after operation at the final observation the thigh was firmly ankylosed in fifteen degrees of flexion, ten degrees adduction, with the foot pointing nearly straight to the front. He then continued to work as captain of a steamer, had no pain, used no cane, walked with a slight limp and was in good health.
>
> "The original trouble came from septicemia which developed after an injury to the thumb. During convalescence from this poisoning the hip became involved and continued to become inflamed at intervals for a year's time until he finally came to the Massachusetts General Hospital. Six months before the hip joint was opened the adductor muscles were tenotomized and the leg held straightened in a spica, and during this period the patient gained twenty-five pounds, recovering nearly completely his healthy vigor."
>
> (Brackett and Marshall 1915)

Box 34.8. Brackett's Introduction to The Orthopaedic Treatment of Gunshot Injuries

> Dr. Brackett wrote the introduction to Leo Mayer's book on *The Orthopedic Treatment of Gunshot Injuries* published in 1918:
>
> "It is a satisfaction to give a welcome to a book that comes to us at a time when it is definitely needed… [with] many of the new problems which have come to us in the last three years of military life. It has been definitely demonstrated that early radical methods are frequently necessary for ultimate conservative results, and the final completion of full function, and that continued treatment, given as early as possible, and…that the early application of correct mechanical principles are necessary, if we are to have…the complete rehabilitation of the injured man…The need of surgeons who have a knowledge of these correct principles and of the mechanical supplements to surgery, is emphasized in this work of Dr. Mayer…
>
> This attention to mechanical features of treatment includes in many cases the fitting of artificial limbs. Too little thought and time has been given in the past by the medical profession to this important subject, not only to the proper selection…but also to the fitting and training…and to the early preparation of the stump… As much time and personal attention should be given by the surgeon to this important subject as to that of splints and apparatus for acute joint infections."

(which fell under the authority of Brackett's division) through which "all affairs related to military orthopedic surgery [passed] through [and] when bearing the signature of any of the three directors may be regarded as official and representing the policy of this department" (Brackett 1917) (see chapter 63). Major Dr. Robert B. Osgood and Captain Dr. Nathaniel Allison served as assistant directors to Goldthwait. There were a very high number of injuries incurred during the war, but 70% to 75% of patients were able to resume military duties after receiving orthopaedic treatment. An Advisory Orthopedic Board was formed, adopting classifications of orthopaedic conditions from the British that comprised early definitions of orthopaedic conditions and included:

- Derangements and disabilities of joints, including ankylosis
- Deformities and disabilities of the feet, such as hallux valgus, hallux rigidus, hammertoes, metatarsalgia, painful heels, flat- or claw-feet
- Malunited or ununited fractures
- Injuries to ligaments, muscles, and tendons
- Cases requiring tendon transplantations or other treatment for irreparable destruction of nerves
- Nerve injuries complicated with fractures or stiffness of joints
- Cases requiring surgical appliances, including artificial limbs

Dr. Robert W. Lovett (Massachusetts), Dr. Albert H. Freiberg (Ohio), Dr. G. Gwilyn Davis (Pennsylvania), Dr. F. H. Albee (New York), and Dr. John L. Porter (Illinois) were the first members of that board.

Contributions to the American Orthopaedic Association and the *Journal of Bone and Joint Surgery*

Upon his return to Boston, Brackett immediately resumed his industrious contributions to a field

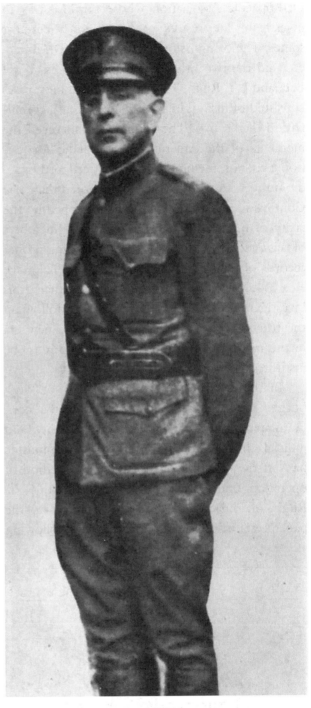

Elliott G. Brackett in uniform, WWI.
D. P. Green and J. C. Delee, "American Orthopaedic Surgeons in World War I," *Journal of Bone and Joint Surgery* 2017; 99: e32.

growing exponentially in the wake of World War I. In 1921, he was simultaneously appointed editor of the *Journal of Bone and Joint Surgery* and appointed to lead a commission by the American

Orthopaedic Association whose purpose was to investigate the results of fusion on tubercular spines. The commission was headed by Dr. Brackett, and the two other members were Drs. W. S. Baer and J. T. Rugh. They reported that most cases consisted of fusion, inlay grafts, or rarely a combination of the two. The commission surveyed the members of the American Orthopaedic Association and non-members who practiced orthopaedic surgery. In their findings, they noted that "the Commission has been greatly handicapped by the laxity of methods which the individual members of this Association have pursued in keeping proper records of their cases" (Brackett et al. 1921) (see **Box 34.9**). Ultimately, they declared that "this investigation has demonstrated...that to follow up the true-results of any group of cases, a new era in the methods of record and follow-up must be instituted."

In the discussion, Dr. David Silver, of Pittsburgh, stated, "The Committee is to be congratulated on the completeness, impartiality, and judicial character of its report...The Committee has left the question of the preferable method of operation undecided." (Silver 1921). Dr. J. T. Rugh, of Philadelphia, made a correction to the paper's statistics regarding paralysis, "following the operative procedure or the long rest combined with it...seven cases of paralysis disappeared, and one remained" (Rugh 1921).

That same year, Brackett accepted the editorship of the *Journal of Bone and Joint Surgery*, and

Report of the AOA Commission on the results of spine fusion in patients with Pott's disease. *Journal of Orthopaedic Surgery* 1921; 3: 507.

Box 34.9. Clinical Features Reported at Two Years Post Operation

Adapted from Brackett et al. 1921:

- The ankylosing operations alone, by either method, cannot be depended upon to prevent the increase of destruction or deformity...unless supplemented by thorough mechanical support...too much dependence must not be put on the protection afforded by the inlay itself...since fracture has occurred in [some of] the cases of all the operators...and has also occurred in one case of fusion...Although this experience demonstrates the value of the graft...it also suggests the necessity of a large and firm inlay...

- In the great majority of cases (80%) ankylosis of this [operative] area was found to be present, the percentage varying directly with the age of the patient...

- Ankylosing operations have had apparently little effect on the production of ankylosis of the bodies of the vertebrae...18 showed actual fusion of the vertebrae...all in younger subjects. No instance of fusion was seen in the adults...

- Although the successful ankylosing of the posterior part of the spine by either method it...does exert a favorable influence on the acute symptoms...

- The effect of the operation upon abscess or paralysis are too few to give sufficient data upon which to base an opinion...

- This operation itself is not one attended by a large mortality...In 163 cases...only three deaths occurred... [However] when a complete series is followed, and complete data obtained...the mortality assumed rather alarming proportions,–16 cases of death in 137 cases operated...The mortality among the younger children certainly shows a much larger ratio...

he followed Dr. H. Winnett Orr who had recently stepped down. The journal was independent with its own board of trustees, but it was also the official journal of the American and British Orthopaedic Associations. Brackett was their "first true editor in the modern sense" (Osgood 1943). During his tenure, he generously gave of both his own time and finances to ensure its success (the journal's financial situation was quite dire), and his faithful efforts resulted in a substantial increase in subscriptions from 779 in 1921 to 3,300 in 1942 at his retirement. According to Dr. R. B. Osgood, "[Brackett's] conduct of the *Journal* may well prove to be his most enduring monument. From a small and poorly illustrated publication of rather meager worth it has become under his strong and devoted direction a beautifully illustrated quarterly publication of over two hundred pages with a wide circulation" (*Harvard Medical School Alumni Bulletin* 1943).

Although the journal's content itself did not significantly change under his editorship, it shifted to a more data-driven focus and one that "emphasize[d] the clinical side of practice as an art, contrasting with the scientific side" (*Harvard Medical School Alumni Bulletin* 1943).

Articles began to include detailed bibliographies (rather than personally reported cases), focused discussion sections rather than what was a more biased remarks section, and an increased use of illustrations (including radiographs) and tables to more clearly and accurately present data. Nevertheless, there were few research articles until research began to receive federal funding. Brackett maintained the journal's focus on orthopaedics and emphasized clinical material; most content differences were:

> attributed to sociological changes and advances in medicine and technology…Notable…was the number of short articles and abstracts and their character. Most of them fell into either of two categories—experiments or basic science. Only rarely was there a large article…

The AOA membership and the agenda for the annual meeting remained the main source of Journal articles. (Osgood 1943)

Brackett's vision and leadership enabled the journal to assume the distinguished role it has today. By the 1930s, "*JBJS* had moved from the top floor of Brackett's home to 8 The Fenway in the Boston Medical Library [E. H. Bradford was president] [and] the Advisory Editorial Staff [included] three orthopaedic surgeons plus a small foreign group" (Osgood 1943). Brackett completed most of the editing and was assisted by Florence Daland, assistant editor and advertising manager. (See **Box 34.10** for an example of Brackett's correspondence while editor of the journal.) He became "acquainted, often quite intimately, with a leader of thought and clinical activity the world over [and they] served to keep him abreast of what was going on in the orthopedic world" (Osgood 1943). He visited various British and European orthopaedic societies during annual two-month vacations, and he obtained many foreign subscriptions for the journal at these meetings. These organizations included the British Orthopaedic Association, the Czechoslovakian Orthopaedic Society, the Deutsche Orthopadische Gesellschaft, the Dutch Orthopaedic Society, the Scandinavian Orthopaedic Society, the Société Belge d'Orthopédie, the Società Italiani di Orthopedia, and the Société Fran asie d' Orthopédie. On one such occasion:

> The Rockefeller Foundation, learning that Dr. Brackett was thinking of visiting China, invited him to give a course of lectures to the medical students at Peking Union Medical School and demonstrate the methods of treatment employed in American clinics. At Shanghai and at Shantung Christian University were located two of his former house officers. (Painter 1943)

He was especially dedicated to the time he spent in Geneva was even granted a diploma from

Box 34.10. Dr. Elliott Brackett's Correspondence as Editor of the JBJS

There are two letters that remain as a historical record in the editor's office at the *Journal of Bone and Joint Surgery*, both of which had been sent to Dr. Brackett while he was editor in 1929. The following is one example:

June 14th, 1929.
Dr. E. G. Brackett,
166 Newberry St.
Boston, Mass.

My Dear Dr. Brackett:

Please pardon me for not replying to your very kind and courteous letter of May 22nd. before this. To show you that I am not too hard boiled to listen to reason I am asking you to place my name on your subscription list. Please send me bill and will remit. At the risk of being a bore I am going to inflict a rather long letter on you.

I was born and reared on a Michigan farm. My father was a good farmer and I had a good home. However my dad was always on the verge of going to the "poor house." As I had two sisters and a brother I concluded the farm was too small for me. I used to ask my father and my grandfather, "why do they not set broken bones for animals as well as for humans?" "Because they would get feverish and die," was the reply. Why? "Get out of here and play." was the reply. I began by setting a Pott's fracture for a rooster. Result perfect. I next tackled a broken leg for a turkry [sic], (I was about eleven years old.) Result perfect leg, but toes off, because I splinted the leg too tight. I was not sued for malpractice and the hen turkey being better than human, rewarded me with a fine brood the following summer.

However I never forgot that I splinted the leg too tight. I also learned to deliver pigs and lambs when nature got stuck. In my boyhood I had the sad spectacle of my oldest sister, screaming and moaning with a tuberculous hip. After years of torture she came out with an ankylosed hip and four and a half inch shortened limb. My father employed the best surgeons in Chicago and Detroit as consultants in that day. A beautiful little girl schoolmate dropped out of school, at ten years of age to become a hideous "hunchback."

Several young men went about with a thigh off, because of "white swelling" of the knee. Several bad cripples there were from poliomyelitis. Many from congenital causes. I pondered this before entering medical school in 1883, where I matriculated in the University of Michigan. After a year I dropped out until 1887 when I went to Bellevue Hospital Medical College, where I had a great joy of being taught by Lewis A. Sayre for two years.

When I saw what he could do with cases, that hitherto had seemed to be hopeless, I found my place. After fourteen years in general country practice I spent two years in post graduate work, the last year with Albert Hoffa in the University of Berlin Germany.

For fourteen years I taught Orthopaedic Surgery at the College of Physicians and Surgeons in San Francisco. My best excuse for having taught this department is, that some of the boys I taught have made a record for themselves in the line I followed.

I am nearing the sunset of my career. I am a better student than I was forty years ago, because I have had the chance to shed some of the scales of youth and bigoted hero worship. I feel how little I know as compared with all we may know. I learn from young fellows and some of them are kind enough to listen to me.

"Standardization," that slogan, byword or what will you, that seems to have emanated from Chicago, is the stumbling block in the way of Medical and Surgical progress today. A bigoted, sterilizing, stereotyping, stagnatizing blot on modern surgery.

I am enclosing under separate cover, some reprints. If they are ridiculous, please remember they are of the past efforts of one of the old men of today. The men of tomorrow may well laugh at me. If they only laugh in kindly fashion I shall be glad to laugh with them and sit on the sideline and root for them. They will soon enough reach the seat I shall vacate when I have ceased to be.

Yours fraternally,
Ethan H. Smith

the League of Nation's; he believed strongly in the League's cause and desire for world peace.

At the 1936 annual meeting of the American Orthopaedic Association's Executive Committee, there was a discussion about providing a "memorial to Dr. Brackett to recognize his long service for the Journal of Bone and Joint Surgery" (*Journal of Bone and Joint Surgery* 1936). The committee created the Elliott G. Brackett Fund "to be used in making illustrations and in assisting authors of articles for the Journal of Bone and Joint Surgery when necessary" (*JBJS* 1936). The purpose of the memorial is "to provide for improvements in the *Journal* and for the embellishment of certain articles for which neither the author nor the *Journal* could provide the necessary expense under ordinary conditions" (*JBJS* 1936). Brackett continued in his commitment to the journal as editor through most of the 1940s, but he retired after he was beset by an additional illness. Dr. Charles Painter described Brackett as showing "few indications of any toll that advancing years and an almost lifelong handicap to his physical activities had imposed upon him" (*JBJS* 1936). Painter further said that he had "never heard [Brackett] refer to this handicap" (*JBJS* 1936).

In his final years of service to the journal, Brackett had simultaneously maintained his busy orthopaedic practice. He retired in 1942, but toward the end of his tenure, advisory editors stepped in and he was briefly followed by Murray Danforth (for four months) and then by Charles Painter, "who served pro tempore until William A. Rogers was appointed Editor in 1944" (Osgood 1943).

LEGACY

Brackett continued to practice until his death on December 29, 1942, when he was 83 years old. He had helped found the Industrial School for Crippled and Deformed Children as well as the Roxbury Clinical Record Club (R.C.R.C.), and he had chaired the Professional Committee of the International Society for Crippled Children. He had been an active member of the Society for Occupational Therapy, the Boston Orthopaedic Club, the Boston Surgical Society, the Massachusetts Medical Society, the American College of Surgeons, and the Vermont State Medical Society, the American Medical Association, the American Association for the Surgery of Trauma, the International Orthopaedic Society, the American Orthopaedic Association, and the American Academy of Orthopaedic Surgeons.

Dr. Charles F. Painter, in his obituary of Dr. Brackett, recalled some personal reflections of him:

> His character was a jewel of many facets… serenity, understanding sympathy, and quiet, tireless devotion to the tasks that were before him…His was a life of unstinted devotion of all his talent to the service of his patients. His records reveal how meticulous he was…no detail was too trivial…To any unusual degree he acquired an understanding of the bearing of seemingly wholly extraneous circumstances that often exerted a psychic influence over the purely physical complex…[To] initial care he added a 'follow-up' that left no doubt in their [his patient's] minds that he was wholeheartedly concerned with their progress toward recovery. No one who was privileged to work with him could fail to appreciate the value of this attitude toward the practice of a profession…It mattered not to him what the social status of his patients were, whether he met them in an outpatient clinic or they came to him as private patients; they commanded the complete absorption of his attention…To appreciate the esteem in which he was held by all who have been under his care, one should see the many letters that have come from his former patients…There are [also] numberless letters from physicians who, at one time or another during their student years, had come under the spell of his influence…

Here in Boston his influence has been actively felt in such organizations as the School for Crippled Children and the Society for Occupational Therapy. He was a member of the Boston Orthopaedic Club and the Boston Surgical Society. The R.C.R C. (Roxbury Clinical Record Club) had Dr. Brackett as one of its originator's. He was a member of the Massachusetts Medical Society, the American College of Surgeons and the Vermont State Medical Society. He served as chairman of the Professional Committee of the International Society for Crippled Children. (Painter 1943)

Brackett led a rich life of service and steadfast fidelity to conservative, evidence-based clinical care, and he was warmly remembered by his colleagues.

CHAPTER 36

Nathaniel Allison
A Focus on Research and Education

Nathaniel Allison was born May 22, 1876, to James Allison and Addie (Shultz) Allison, in Webster, Missouri. James Allison was a merchant, and his father—also Nathaniel Allison—was a physician in the pioneer days in mid-eastern Missouri. Allison's ancestors had immigrated from England, settling in Chambersburg, Pennsylvania, in the southcentral part of the state, which was at that time still a British colony. James Allison moved the family to St. Louis when Nathaniel was just a boy; there Nathaniel received his schooling at Smith Academy. He resigned after one year at West Point to follow in his grandfather's footsteps, deciding at age 17 to become a physician. After studying further at the Penn Charter School in Philadelphia, he was admitted to Harvard University in 1894. He spent his undergraduate years there and continued on to the medical school, from which he graduated in 1901.

After medical school, he spent two years as a house officer at Boston Children's Hospital. During that time, he also traveled and continued his studies. In 1903, he returned to St. Louis, where he practiced as an orthopaedic surgeon, taught, and began his career in research at Washington University School of Medicine. He recognized his aptitude for and interest in research, which became a focus throughout his career.

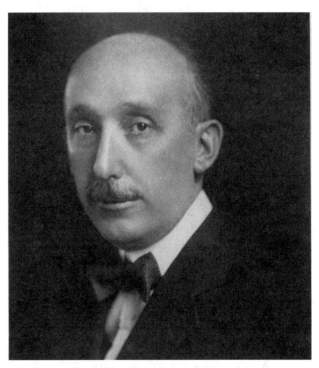

Nathaniel Allison.
Studio portrait of Nathaniel Allison, VC410-S01-ss27-i01, Bernard Becker Medical Library Archives, Washington University in St. Louis.

Physician Snapshot

Nathaniel Allison
BORN: 1876
DIED: 1932

SIGNIFICANT CONTRIBUTIONS: Performed extensive animal research on joint conditions; pushed for a closer connection between orthopaedic surgery and general surgery; helped to standardize splints and surgical dressings during World War I

A FOCUS ON ORTHOPAEDIC RESEARCH

During his time at Washington University, Allison published about one-third of the ~61 articles he wrote throughout his career. It was at Washington University that he demonstrated an interest in clinical research. From 1905 to 1921 he published eight research papers, the first a detailed anatomical study of the pathology three months after reduction (with the Lorenz technique) of bilateral congenitally dislocated hips in a seven-year-old child. She became infected with diphtheria two months after the reduction, and she later died from tuberculous meningitis. Allison (1905) summarized his findings:

- An acetabular cavity not of normal developing
- A femoral head that is more or less irregular in shape
- A changed direction in the neck of the femur
- An adductor group of muscles too short before operation, and after operation injured both as to muscular elements and nerve supply
- All the posterior muscles with the fascia lata and the ilio-tibial band much shortened
- A much-shortened group of pelvitrochanteric muscles
- An ilio-femoral band abnormally short and strong

Allison particularly emphasized his last finding regarding the iliofemoral band. He compared his findings with those described in publications by Dr. Edward Bradford and other surgeons, which contained less detail of the pathological anatomy.

In 1909, he married Marion Aldrich, from Chicago. One year later, during this time of great celebration and transition in his life, Allison, in collaboration with the neurologist Dr. Sidney I. Schwab, reported a unique experimental approach to treating spasticity and athetosis in patients with cerebral palsy and flaccid paralysis in patients with poliomyelitis; they also mentioned one case of complicated tic movements. Their first group included nine patients with cerebral palsy, in whom they injected alcohol, under direct observation, into the nerves to specific spastic muscles. This temporarily damaged the nerve(s), but then allowed the patient, or the assistants, to control the limb, thereby improving function and hygiene. (This method was later refined to include the use of phenol [alcohol] and botulism toxin [Botox].) In the discussion of their publication, Schwab stated that "he and Dr. Allison had been doing [these experiments] for the last three years... The alcohol injections in spastic cases...are not curative...[but] he and Dr. Allison had had their patients walking about the ward a few days after the operation...When they injected the nerves with alcohol the athetosis completely disappeared and did not return" (Allison and Schwab 1910).

Their second group included three patients with polio and one patient with traumatic paralysis of the radial nerve. In the latter case, using electrical stimulation, they identified the portion of the nerve that did not respond:

> It was divided in its middle for a distance of 3 inches longitudinally and the inner half cut free at the upper extremity of the longitudinal cut. This segment [was] carried under the biceps tendon and inserted into the median nerve. [Four months after injury the] patient can hold [his] wrist extended and use his crutch on that side with very little difficulty...There is definite extension movement at the wrist and fingers."
> (Allison and Schwab 1910)

Schwab commented that "by the time the nerve regenerated the antagonizing group had not regained its original strength, so that the condition was more hopeful of future cure than by any other method" (Allison and Schwab 1910). Dr. Allison's clinical and research interests varied widely, covering a broad spectrum of orthopaedic-related topics. He also performed many investigations using animals. His interest in the treatment of joint conditions continued with experimental studies of arthroplasty over at least a five-year period.

By 1912, Allison was named chairman of the Department of Orthopaedic Surgery. Numerous changes occurred at the university and its hospitals while Allison was in charge of orthopaedic surgery. Both Barnes Hospital and St. Louis Children's Hospital became affiliated with the medical school of Washington University; this partnership was influenced by a critical report of the medical school written by Abraham Flexner in 1909. Two things happened as a result of these changes: the medical school was officially renamed as the Washington University School of Medicine, and the Department of Orthopaedic Surgery merged into the Department of General Surgery, becoming a section of that department, rather than a separate department in its own right. That organization was in place until 1995—almost 80 years.

Case 36.1. Operative Treatment for Knee Derangement

> "Case I.–T. B., aged twenty-eight years, was hurt while playing basket-ball at college, she sustained a twisting knee injury of her left knee. A diagnosis of displaced internal semilunar was made by a competent surgeon. Palliative treatment was resorted to for eight years; it consisted of a heavy brace attached to the shoe and a bandage. This young woman spent her twenties practically in constant fear of a misstep, which she took on many occasions, the ordinary train of symptoms following. Arthrotomy here revealed a detached internal cartilage, except for its posterior end; it was considerably worn. It was removed, recovery was uneventful, perfect restoration of joint function has followed."
>
> (Nathaniel Allison 1912)

While continuing to further his research, Allison had described in 1912 a patient with displaced semilunar cartilage who was treated with arthrotomy (see **Case 36.1**). By 1914, Allison and his coinvestigator, Dr. Barney Brooks, reported the results of their attempts to perform arthrodesis of joints. They studied "the nature, sequence and duration of the tissue changes which lead to bony ankylosis...[using] the knee-joints of dogs" (Allison and Brooks 1914). They investigated four experimental models of infected joints, concluding that, in joints infected with tubercle bacilli or staphylococci:

> any inflammatory process...of sufficient severity to result in the formation of granulation tissue, will destroy the joint-cartilages...Experiments in which the cartilage was removed by operation, or the joint partially excised... [resulted in] ankylosis of bone...a slowly developing process which consists of the following stages: First, there is union by granulation tissue; second, there is union by dense fibrous tissue; third, there is metaplasia of fibrous tissue into fibrocartilage and a direct transformation of this tissue into bone. The shortest period of time...[to] complete ankylosis...was one hundred and eighty days...In man the duration of the process is equally prolonged...The long duration of the fibrous stage of ankylosis also shows...that any method of arthroplasty should have as its object the prevention of fibrous ankylosis rather than bony ankylosis; also that the insertion of an irritable substance into a joint should be avoided. (Allison and Brooks 1914)

The following year, Allison and Dr. Ellsworth Moody published a review of eight cases of Legg-Calvé-Perthes disease, describing Legg's and Perthes's initial ideas about the condition:

> Legg described this condition and presented his observations on five cases at the Hartford meeting of this association [American Orthopaedic Association] held in June 1909. Perthes contribution to the subject appeared in 1913. Legg...offered as a tentative explanation...it seems to be a disturbance of growth which is

started...by a slight injury and...[is] dependent upon a change in the circulation at the growing epiphyseal line. Perthes...[stated that] "the illness...we are considering...must be differentiated from arthritis deformans juvenalis [sic] as it rests only on the pathological processes inside the head of the femur without participation of the joint cartilage...We are dealing with a disease running its course in the interior of the bone with reformation of the cartilage, resulting in a deformation of the head of the femur.
(Allison and Moody 1915)

Neither Allison nor Moody believed that tuberculosis was the causative agent in Legg-Calvé-Perthes disease. Allison then briefly mentioned experiments with six rabbits in which he applied gentle pressure to the head of the femur during arthrotomy; he noted that no substantial changes developed. Legg (1915), in his discussion of Allison and Moody's paper, stated, "As regards their etiology, I believe we will come to accept this as traumatic. Of my fifty-five cases 67 per cent have a traumatic history and the preponderance in boys is very large...I believe the condition to be a circulatory disturbance [which Allison had mentioned]. There is, I believe, a blocking of the blood supply to the epiphysis..."

During the tumultuous time of World War I, Allison was also committed to his military service, which Osgood describe as "outstanding." "In 1915, [Allison] served under the French flag at the American Ambulance Hospital [with Dr. Osgood] on the outskirts of Paris [see chapter 63]. In May 1917, commissioned as Captain, he sailed with the Washington University Base Hospital No. 21 which took over a British Base Hospital [No. 12] at Rouen" (Osgood 1932). Major Osgood was serving at the British General Hospital No. 11 in Dannes Camiers, France.

One month later, Allison participated in a symposium on arthroplasty at the American Orthopaedic Association's (AOA's) annual meeting, presenting a paper titled "Arthroplasty:

Title of article by Allison and Brooks in which they reported their experimental results using absorbable and nonabsorbable tissues and materials in attempts to obtain a satisfactory arthroplasty. *American Journal of Orthopaedic Surgery* 1918; s2-16: 83.

Experimental and Clinical Methods." Other speakers there included Dr. M. S. Hendersen and Dr. William S. Baer (the first to use, in 1909, an absorbable membrane [chromatized pig bladder] in an attempt to produce a painless mobile joint). Allison and Brooks later published that paper together in 1918. In it, they noted that little experimental work had been done on the mobilization of joints in animals. They reviewed such work involving nonabsorbable and absorbable foreign bodies researchers had used as interposition materials in treating ankylosed joints. They also summarized the published research on the use of living tissues (fascia, muscle, fat, tendon, or peritoneum) in arthroplasty, noting that such interposed tissue "undergoes more or less complete degeneration or substitution by fibrous tissue...There is no evidence...of the reformation of anything like a normal joint cavity. The results...in animals [have] not differed materially from the end-results of simple destruction of the joint surfaces without the interposition of any materials..." (Allison and Brooks 1918). With regard to the small amount of work with nonabsorbable foreign bodies, "In light of present knowledge, so much discredited," they "dismissed" such treatment "with a statement that silk, plates of magnesium, silver, gutta percha and other things...[were all] tried and discarded" (Allison and Brooks 1918).

They also discussed research with absorbable animal membranes:

> The first to recommend and use extensively an absorbable foreign body as interposition material in the treatment of ankylosed joints was W.S. Baer [who used chromatized pig's bladder]...Allison and Brooks reported a series of experiments in which various substances were used...Cargyl's membrane [ox peritoneum] persisted...only for a few days, and did not prevent adhesions...[whereas] chromatized pig's bladder persisted...longer...but it was found that the reaction...was of such an intensity... [that adhesions formed] between the granulating surfaces...Fascia which had been fixed and impregnated with silver remained intact... for about thirty (30) days...[and] caused relatively little reaction...and the adhesion of the opposed joint surfaces was prevented...In our own experimental and clinical work we have used the fascia lata from the animal or patient...fixed and impregnated with silver, and later used in the arthroplasty...The commercial preparation of this fascia has been undertaken...and animal experiments are now in progress to determine the results of the use of this commercial product...At the present time...there is no longer question that the interposition method is the best method of treatment of joint ankylosis. The kind of material interposed, the operative technique, and post-operative care are still matters for discussion. (Allison and Brooks 1918)

Allison and his coinvestigator, Dr. Roland F. Fisher, studied the early stages of tuberculosis of bones in dogs. Earlier, in 1916, they had published a report of tuberculosis in 40 dogs. They introduced tubercle bacilli beneath the periosteum in 19 dogs, into the epiphysis in 11, into the diaphysis in 6, and into joint surfaces in 4. They also injected one ankylosed knee joint. On the basis of this work they believed it would be "possible to establish experimental foci of tuberculosis in any

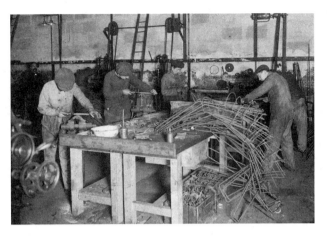

Splint factory in Paris during WWI. Splints seen are for the thigh and leg. Library of Congress, Prints & Photographs Division, American National Red Cross Collection, LC-DIG-anrc-15579.

region of the bones of dogs. Our sections show growing foci in the epiphysis, in the metaphysis, in the diaphysis, in the cortex of the shaft, and on the joint surfaces...There are no essential differences in the reaction to tuberculosis foci between spongy or cancellous bone and compact cortical bone, except, that in the latter, the element of bone proliferation plays an important rôle" (Allison and Fisher 1916).

In July of 1917, following the symposium, Allison visited Osgood, and both noted that the British general hospitals had large stores of more than 120 types of splints. Allison (1926) later wrote:

> I was struck with the clearness of his [Osgood's] vision as to what we should need in the way of splints for our Army, when we should have one, fighting in France...also, there was no uniformity in the French service as to the splinting of fractures...[and the] great majority of American surgeons coming to France with the Army would have had little or no experience with the treatment of battle casualties, especially fractures.

Recognizing mistakes in treatment when physicians use poorly designed or poorly made splints, he and Osgood agreed "to assemble the best splints from both the Allies and after eliminating the unnecessary ones, establish a standard" (Allison 1926).

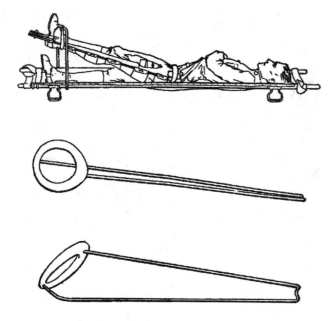

Sketch of an early Thomas traction leg splint.
R. B. Osgood, "The Transplant Splints of the American Army." *Some Essentials in Military Surgery*. Printed for the Surgeon General, United States Army. Chicago: Press of the American Medical Association, 1920.

Allison went to Paris in August 1917, where he served under Colonel William L. Keller on the US Army Board (the First Splint Board). During his time on the board, it "succeeded in standardizing the splints and surgical dressings for the American Expeditionary Forces" (Osgood 1932) (see chapter 63). After General John J. Pershing approved these new standards, Allison's focus changed:

> [His] life became for many months completely concerned with arranging for the manufacture of these splints and dressings and for their delivery to the places where they were needed. The test was a test of tact, resourcefulness and courage, splendidly met and carried out with complete success. It won him his majority and later his colonelcy. As Assistant Director of the Section of Orthopaedic Surgery, A. E. F., under General Goldthwait, he traveled through the American area of combat, arranging for adequate supplies of apparatus, consulting with surgeons, organizing and training teams of stretcher bearers, to the end that under the slogan, "Splint 'em where they lie," the great number of bone and joint casualties among our soldiers should receive the most efficient and pain-relieving "first aid" before they left "no man's land." (Osgood 1932)

In October 1917, the army ordered 28,100 splints: 22,000 from the Red Cross and 6,100 from England. They standardized splints to consist of just 10 types, both for the upper and the lower extremities. Despite such a large order, by June 1918, the army was experiencing "an absolute shortage of splints" (Allison 1926). A second order was for an additional 54,000 splints, which required 45 tons of steel-wire rods.

Allison's work with the US Army Board (the Second Splint Board) continued, and it "revised and reprinted the Manual of Splints and Dressings" (Osgood 1932). Allison remained as assistant director and consultant in orthopaedic surgery until the end of 1918, when the armistice ended the war. He "return[ed] to the United States in 1919[, where] he served for a few months as Assistant Director of the Surgical Service of the Walter Reed Hospital and was then honorably discharged with the rank of Colonel in the summer of 1919. In September of that year he was sent to Rome as representative of the Medical Department at the Inter-Allied Congress of Surgery. He later received

> VOLUME XVI NOVEMBER, 1918 No. 11
>
> *The* American Journal *of* Orthopedic Surgery
>
> THE TRANSPORTATION OF THE WOUNDED, WITH SPECIAL REFERENCE TO THE APPLICATION OF SPLINTS.
>
> BY NATHANIEL ALLISON, LIEUT.-COL., M.C., U.S.A.

Allison's article on the use and benefit of special splints to transport wounded soldiers. *American Journal of Orthopaedic Surgery* 1918; s2-16: 389.

the Distinguished Service Medal from the President of United States" (Osgood 1932).

In November 1918, Lieutenant Colonel Allison published a paper in which he described hypothetical experiences of a wounded soldier in standardized splints during transportation. He set the stage: "let it be supposed that an infantry man, engaged in the firing trench, sustains a fracture of one of his extremities or a severe wound, making his transportation to the rear in a position of recumbency necessary" (Allison 1918). Then he took the reader through the three phases of transport—from the initial stop at the Battalion Aid Station, to the Ambulance Head or Regimental Aid Post, and finally removal from the region on a hospital train—describing splinting at each stage. A more complete description from Allison's paper is provided in **Box 36.1**.

Box 36.1. Splinting of an Injured Soldier during Transport

"In order to visualize the situation as it exists, let it be supposed that an infantry man, engaged in the firing trench, sustains a fracture of one of his extremities or a severe wound, making his transportation to the rear in a position of recumbency necessary; this soldier is carried to the Battalion Aid Station, which is situated in a dug-out, where the battalion surgeon dresses his wound, administers 1500 units of antitetanic serum and places the man on some type of trench litter, splinting his fracture as well as possible… The trench litter…is of several types, i.e., bamboo poles and sacks, chair litters, etc. The difficulties of carrying a man out of the trench are…quite obvious; to meet these difficulties…[after] experiments…a type…has proved to be the best so far discovered. It has been called "the snowshoe trench litter"…made of a piece of ¾-inch iron pipe, bent in curves and covered with a light rope knotted in squares, like a rope mattress…not unlike a huge snowshoe. It is six feet long and 20 inches wide…a broad webbing tape Y goes over the shoulders and meets a webbing strap which comes up through the crotch with a buckle…a horizontal webbing tape band at the abdomen, at the knees and at the ankles…This appliance weighs in the neighborhood of eight pounds, is very durable, can be scrubbed with a broom…no loose parts or pins to be lost and is easily understood and adjusted. During a recent demonstration, a heavy man of 6 feet 2 inches was carried about and over all kinds of trench construction without discomfort to him.

"The second step in this wounded soldier's career is at the Ambulance Head or Regimental Aid Post; here in the ambulances are loaded and the wounded man is properly splinted for his trip to the hospital. A difficulty…encountered was that…[with a] small Ford ambulance…a Thomas traction leg splint…prevented the tailgate…from being closed. To offset this difficulty in a stretcher bar…[was added] which holds the splint in a flexed position, so that the tailgate of the ambulance may be closed…Each ambulance has one bar of this type…an extra Thomas leg splint, a Thomas arm splint with several modifications, extra blankets and water bottles, and surgical dressing packets…

"The next step in the transportation of the wounded will be their removal from the zone of advance to the intermediate or base zones. This will be done by hospital trains, to each of which an orthopedic surgeon, under the direction of the director of orthopedic surgery will be attached. This officer will be responsible for the proper transportation of fractures and joint injuries, and will see to it that during the journey proper splinting is maintained.

"The advance section of this scheme of supervision has been tried out and the system is taking hold in an admirable manner…The cases of fractures thus far received in evacuation hospitals have left little to desire in these details. One instance has occurred where an elbow joint injury came in poorly protected; the orthopedic surgeon on duty with the brigade went immediately to the dug-out and to the combat battalion surgeon, whose error had been discovered, and straightened out the difficulty.

"The artillery positions are…more easily reached by ambulances, and the difficulty of carrying the wounded out is much less…It is one of the functions of the Division of Orthopedic Surgery to occupy itself with these details, which are so important in the treatment of battle casualties."

(Nathaniel Allison, 1918)

Meanwhile, Allison and Brooks had continued to work together, and in 1921 they attempted to explain the "exact nature" of modifications in the bones of the extremities when they are not used. To do so, they applied three techniques to prevent dogs from using a foreleg: (1) cutting the brachial plexus (n = 13), (2) removing the upper end (the head, neck, and tuberosities) of the humerus (n = 7), and (3) ensconcing the leg in a plaster of Paris cast (n = 4). They noted that "when the experiments were terminated the bones of both forelegs were compared by X-ray examination, measurements, weights, and as to chemical composition and breaking strength…The changes observed in the bone in [each group] were the same. The degree of atrophy of the bone was directly proportional to the degree of non-use…" (Allison and Brooks 1921). Therefore, they concluded that "the process of bone atrophy is not a change in the characteristics of bone as a tissue… [nor] as a substance. The process of bone atrophy is a change in the amount of bone present. This affects the size, shape, thickness, length, weight and texture of the whole bone and accounts for its changes in gross anatomy, X-ray photographs, breaking strength, and chemical composition. The chemical composition, breaking strength, and regeneration of bone remain unchanged" (Allison and Brooks 1921).

EXPANDING ORTHOPAEDIC EDUCATION

After leaving the military, Allison had returned to practicing and teaching in St. Louis; he was chief of the Section of Orthopaedic Surgery at Washington University Medical School, and he was appointed dean there in 1920; he remained a professor and chief of orthopaedic surgery during that

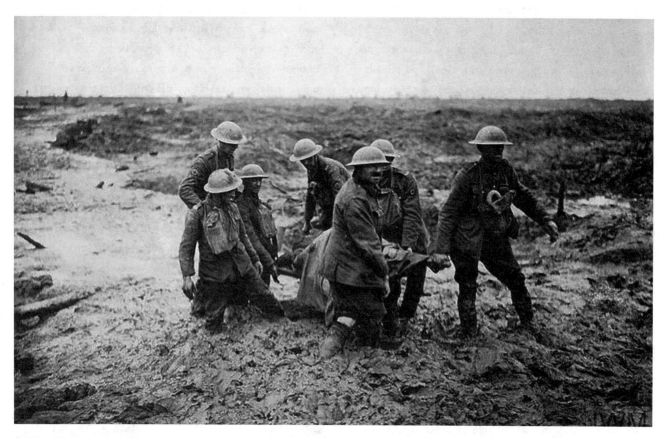

Soldiers carrying a wounded man on a stretcher through deep mud. John Warwick Brooke/the Imperial War Museums/Wikimedia Commons

Article in which Allison expressed his views on orthopaedic undergraduate and graduate education. *Journal of Orthopaedic Surgery* 1921; 9: 3448.

time. Allison began disseminating his views on orthopaedic education in 1921, spurred on by a recent report from an American Medical Association committee that defined the minimum requirements for the training of an orthopaedic surgeon (see chapter 11). He published a paper titled "The Teaching of Orthopaedic Surgery," which he had presented to the association's annual meeting. Now that the AMA committee had developed training specifications, Allison (1921) responded, "it remains for us, as teachers, simply to decide what we shall teach and how we shall teach it."

In that 1921 paper, Allison also first mentioned his belief that, at the core, "so-called orthopaedic surgery differs in none of its principles from so-called general surgery...that the part cannot be greater or more important than the whole...[and] that surgery is more important than orthopaedic surgery." Allison (1921) wrote, "The medical student is, as a rule, a surfeited listener at lectures, he is mildly bored with the demonstrations and at the operations and clinics, he is an 'onlooker in Vienna.'" Thus, he believed, undergraduates must be taught with a focus on surgical diagnosis and in a way that ensures their attention and receptiveness:

> I believe that surgery should be taught [to] the undergraduate medical student without any qualifying or hyphenated characteristics...The undergraduate should be instructed in surgery and that part of surgery which falls into the hands of orthopaedic surgeon should be taught by the orthopaedic surgeon...The surgery that concerns the undergraduate student is not surgical craftsmanship, but surgical diagnosis... It is our custom to teach orthopaedic surgery in the third and fourth years, by lectures and demonstrations...Certain students who show an interest in the subject...[are encouraged] to elect courses in orthopaedic surgery in their fourth year. A better plan would be to teach the principles of orthopaedic surgery throughout the clinical years...merged into the instruction of surgery...[so that the graduate is] one educated in principles and instructed in the methods of diagnosis. (Allison 1921)

> "The real scholar is not a man who devotes his erudition to a small thing, or who achieves eminence in paths that no one cares to read; not the man who knows all about antennae of the Paleozoic cockroach, or some Greek root; but the man who has the sharpened brain, who has developed that tool so that he can use it for any purpose for which, in life, he may hereafter desire to use that tool."
> —President Charles Lowell, Harvard University, quoting from Nathaniel Allison, "The Teaching of Orthopaedic Surgery," *Journal of Bone and Joint Surgery*, 1921

Allison (1921) went on to discuss graduate-level education in orthopaedic surgery, jumping off from the AMA committee's recommended minimum standards—which began with "an intern[ship] for one or more years...[then] one year in the orthopaedic service in an active clinic, and six months in allied work"—with the intention of making for the specialty "a man well enough versed in the craft of our specialty to start out on his own for a further development." For Allison (1921), such "scanty training for applying the label of full ability as a specialist...will suffice as a minimum, and not an ideal standard of attainment. An ideal equipment for such a man would be three years of work, with a university [graduate] degree...insuring thoroughness and breadth by the demand for a demonstration of research ability. After that, several years as an assistant to some of our ablest and best orthopaedic surgeons" would be required. Allison (1921) believed that "the training necessary to an oncoming orthopaedic surgeon" was straightforward:

> First of all, he must be by training and experience, one qualified to do surgery...After several years...he may...proclaim himself a practitioner...He must always be a surgeon plus considerable of special qualifications. He must never be a specialist with a low-grade ability as a surgeon. Much harsh criticism has come upon us from this, one of our faults in the past. Future developments must correct it.

Allison (1921) went on to describe three prevailing teaching modalities—"the didactic lecture, the demonstration, and the clinical conference"—and their respective importance in surgical education:

> The didactic lecture is used less each year in all our methods of education...The demonstration will always have a place, but it should be a demonstration of some principle rather than a demonstration of skill on the demonstrator's part...As a measure of stimulation, both to the teacher and to the student, the properly conducted clinical conference is of great value. The student is put upon his own mettle, he has an opportunity to work up the case...His omissions are as instructive as are his observations...The student must be encouraged to set out for criticism...and to defend his methods of examination and the deductions made therefrom. Above all else this method tends to develop proper thinking...The thing most needed is the realization on the part of the teacher that he himself should be a student. It is in ourselves, in our attitude toward our work, that lies the future of training and teaching better orthopaedic surgery and better surgeons to do the work.

Allison was president of the AOA in 1922. In his presidential address, "The Specialist in Surgery and His Viewpoint," he described three "tendencies" within orthopaedic surgery as it has developed and solidified as a specialty. For Allison, the most considerable was "an increasing evidence of self-satisfaction with our accomplishments," particularly advances that were once thought unattainable:

> The men who founded this Association–were concerned with the same conditions that we are now called upon to care for surgically...They felt it necessary to join together because of the mutual improvement and satisfaction gained by discussing their difficulties...The clinical conditions which gave the founders...their raison d'être including, among others, lateral curvature of the spine, congenital dislocation of the hip, infectious arthritides, and the residual paralyses that follow anterior poliomyelitis...We are entrusted with...[gaining a definite] solution both by our colleagues in medicine and by the laity. Indeed it is the chief reason for existence today as surgical specialists, and much of our future use in medicine depends on the way...we work to alleviate these and similar conditions. (Allison 1922)

A second tendency is to place limitations on what the specialty of orthopaedic surgery can encompass: "If our specialty in surgery is to become routinized and compressed with narrow boundaries, then will our specialist be a narrow man and our Association will no longer be mature, but will be old and settled" (Allison 1922). In line with this, Allison dubbed the third tendency "smug standardization." Allison (1922) noted that this started during World War I, when the military had to develop "fool-proof" methods for the "untrained men" performing "special duties." Allison (1922) decried this tendency, stating, "If our young men are to be no better than we, if our future is to be no broader than our present, then our specialty is at once old and dead."

During that presidential address, Allison (1922) mentioned a fourth tendency occurring within the specialty: "To those of us who hold dear the position of our Association in surgery, there comes another thought...We are constantly tending toward a belief that we may allow men to become surgical specialists without first being trained as surgeons, and...the idea that a special part of the surgical field may be greater than the field of surgery itself." He pushed for general surgical training for those who wished to specialize in orthopaedic surgery, allowing them greater knowledge and a more well-rounded foundation for practice:

> I would demand that the background for it be secure...one path [for future orthopaedic surgeons] leads to narrow specialization with smug standards and lack of broad vision...The other path leads to...a future of greater achievement. Men who enter this path must be broadly trained. The whole of surgery must be theirs. They shall...add to the general qualifications that of special interest...They shall not be men alike in mind and outlook...The future will hold no limitations and our Association...will continue to advance with the procession of modern surgery; not following, but leading...Some one has divided all surgeons into two classes—carpenter and plumber surgeons. Our Association should represent the best interests of the carpenter surgeons. (Allison 1922)

Dr. Frank D. Dixon, the fourth president of the American Academy of Orthopaedic Surgeons, in his 1936 presidential address, recalled Allison as being "one of the wisest of those who have served the interests of orthopaedic surgery," who "constantly cautioned against orthopaedic surgery's isolating itself, since such isolation leads to narrowness and loss of vitality and progressiveness." Dixon reiterated Allison's position: "Let us keep our contacts with general surgery and even draw them closer; it would help both the general surgeons and ourselves."

> "In 1922, Allison said that our specialty had come out of its infancy, youth, and early manhood and had gone into a vigorous maturity. Having been fully matured for over three decades, we should, theoretically, now be in our prime. We represent today one of the largest and strongest of the medical specialties. Orthopaedic surgery has attained this position not alone because it is closely affiliated with medicine and all of surgery, but also because through wise leadership and hard work on the part of its membership over the years, it has rendered good service to the public..."
> —Alfred Rives Shands Jr., MD
> "Responsibility and Research in Orthopaedic Surgery" *Clinical Orthopaedics and Related Research*, 1971

ALLISON'S LATER CONTRIBUTIONS TO ORTHOPAEDICS

In 1923, the St. Louis Shriners Hospital for Crippled Children was built next to the Washington University School of Medicine. Leadership at Shriners Hospital named Allison to be the chief surgeon, but he ceded the position before the hospital opened because he had received another offer: assistant professor of orthopaedic surgery at Harvard University and chief of the orthopaedic department at the Massachusetts General Hospital (MGH). He was offered the position just three years after he was appointed dean at Washington University Medical School, at the age of just 47. He once again returned to Boston.

When Allison arrived at MGH, Dr. Robert Osgood had just resigned as chief of orthopaedics (see chapter 19) and Dr. Mark Rogers was serving

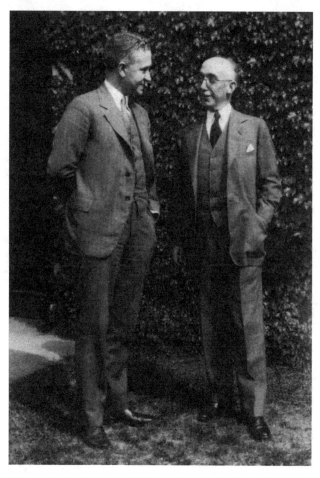

Marius Smith-Petersen (left) and Nathaniel Allison (right).
Massachusetts General Hospital, Archives and Special Collections.

During Allison's six years (1923–29) as chief of orthopaedic surgery at MGH, he published 17 papers on a variety of topics. Allison's interest in research continued, and, with his collaborators, he published in 1926 an important study on the differences between synovial fluid and plasma:

> Proteins, chloride, sugar and non-protein nitrogen have been determined in plasma and pathological synovial fluid in twenty-three instances…The protein content of the synovial fluid is less that of the plasma…The chloride content is greater…analogous to that found between plasma and peritoneal effusions, pleural effusions, and a cerebral spinal fluid… Low plasma chloride is accompanied by low chloride in the synovial fluid…The non-protein nitrogen is approximately equally distributed between plasma and synovial fluid…In fasting patients, the sugar content of non-infected synovial fluid is…slightly lower than that of the plasma…The hyperglycemia caused by anesthesia is accompanied by a rise in sugar content of the synovial fluid…In four instances of bacterially infected fluids the sugar content was markedly lowered, while in two cases of

as interim chief of the department (see chapter 53). A year later, in 1924, Allison "was made full Professor…after the death of Dr. Robert W. Lovett, in whose office he then began private practice. He also succeeded Dr. Lovett as Chief of Staff of the New England Peabody Home and became acutely interested in its heliotherapeutic service to children crippled by chronic bone and joint disease" (Osgood 1932). He also replaced Osgood as the associate chief of the Fracture Service. In 1939, Dr. Frederic Washburn, then director of the hospital, wrote that during Allison's time at MGH, "Allison had been very helpful as Chairman of the Staff Committee that drew up the plan of the limitation of fees of the professional staff in the Baker Memorial, and gave other assistance in the organization of that unit."

VOL. VIII, No. 4 · OCTOBER, 1926   Old Series: Vol. xxiv No. 4

The Journal of Bone and Joint Surgery

COMPARATIVE STUDIES BETWEEN SYNOVIAL FLUID AND PLASMA*†
PRELIMINARY REPORT
BY NATHANIEL ALLISON, M.D., FRANK FREMONT-SMITH, M.D.,**
MARY ELIZABETH DAILEY, A.B., MARGARET A. KENNARD, A.B., BOSTON

Article in which Allison and colleagues describe, probably for the first time, a method of comparing synovial fluid to plasma in order to diagnose a joint problem, such as an infection.
Journal of Bone and Joint Surgery 1926; 8: 758.

tuberculosis in the joint the sugar content was moderately lowered. This is analogous to the low sugar content of the cerebro-spinal fluid in purulent and tuberculous meningitis…It is suggested that the determination of the sugar content of synovial fluid may prove to be of diagnostic value.

Osgood (1926), in discussing that paper, stated, "I am interested in this as a new method of diagnosis. As far as I know, there has never been an attempt before to obtain from synovial fluid information which would lead to an earlier conception of the type of joint infection or joint pathological condition that we are dealing with. I congratulate Dr. Allison very much on this paper."

> "Our well-being and advancement will depend entirely upon what we do, how we do it, and the direction of our vision. Particularly will it depend upon what we do to strengthen the foundations of our specialty. This strengthening cannot take place without our devoting ourselves to the following… (1) the meeting the responsibilities, both old and new, as they arise, (2) good clinical and basic science training programs for the development of practitioners and teachers…and (3) sound basic research to provide good building material for future advances in therapy."
> —Alfred Rives Shands Jr., MD
> "Responsibility and Research in Orthopaedic Surgery" *Clinical Orthopaedics and Related Research*, 1971

Allison published two more articles on the congenitally dislocated hip in 1925 and 1928 (following on the first he had published two decades earlier in 1905). He drew two main conclusions in his last article:

1. Congenital dislocation of the hip should be reduced at the earliest possible time for two reasons: a. The reduction is more easily accomplished. b. Adaptive changes and injury to the upper femoral epiphysis are increased by function in the unreduced hip.

2. Manipulative reduction in the early years of childhood may be successful. It should be tried first. But force and resulted injury should be avoided if the hip is not easily reduced. Open operation is the better method. We are dealing, it seems to me, with an embryological defect…the hip is not normal at birth and that throughout the individuals life it is to be deformed…this abnormality of growth may develop into a change in the upper end of the femur…incompatible with normal hip function…Reduction of the dislocation does not [therefore] mean a perfect hip, no matter how reduction is accomplished. Reduction (and early reduction) does mean, however the lessening of all the secondary changes…[that] follow the faulty mechanics of the unreduced hip. Force of any kind…will add its influence to the development of the deformity in the upper end of the femur as growth is accomplished.
(Allison 1928)

He also later focused his work on low-back pain and made many attempts to resolve it, including through spinal fusion and manipulation and with spica casts. In 1927, he published a paper on backache in the *American Journal of Neurosurgery*.

Allison moved once again in 1929—this time to Chicago University, where he was appointed a professor of surgery in charge of the Division of Orthopaedic Surgery, and chief of the orthopaedic staff of the university hospitals. After he resigned from MGH that year, he was appointed to the board of consultation. Soon after leaving MGH, Allison and Dr. Ralph Ghormley (who also had just left MGH) completed their monograph, *Diagnosis in Joint Disease*, most of which they had written while at MGH. It was published in 1931.

LEGACY

Throughout his career, Allison had been "active in many organizations, including the Medical History Club of St. Louis. He served as co-editor of the *American Journal of Orthopedic Surgery* (predecessor of the *Journal of Bone and Joint Surgery*) from 1917 to 1919" (Brand 2010). Some of the more notable organizations he belonged to are listed in **Box 36.2**. He also was part of "many civic and country clubs in St. Louis, Boston, Chicago, Washington and other places" (Brand 2010).

Box 36.2. Allison's Professional Memberships

> Allison was a member of the following organizations, a partial list:
> - American Medical Association
> - Association of Military Surgeons
> - Southern Surgical Association
> - American Orthopaedic Association
> - Massachusetts Medical Society
> - Massachusetts Association for Occupational Therapy
> - St. Louis Surgical Society
> - Boston Surgical Society
>
> He also was active in other groups:
> - Honorary member, British Orthopaedic Association
> - Corresponding member, Société des Chirurgiens de Paris
> - Fellow, American College of Surgeons
> - Fellow, New England Surgical Society
> - Fellow, American Academy of Arts and Sciences
>
> Allison served as president of the Massachusetts Association for Occupational Therapy from 1925 to 1929. (Brand 2010)

Allison maintained his positions in Chicago "until illness made active work impossible in 1932" (Osgood 1932). He was 56 years old when he died. Upon Allison's death, the director of MGH wrote that "he was liberal-minded, [and his death is] a real loss to the profession" (Washburn 1939). Osgood, Allison's colleague and friend, wrote a heartfelt obituary for Allison, published by the Massachusetts Medical Society. Osgood (1932) portrayed Allison as a quiet reserved figure: "Few people besides his wife and his family knew him intimately." Because of this:

> Even close friends would find it difficult to paint a word picture of his character which would do him justice, for he was one of the most reserved of men. He was a delightful comrade in arms and in play; widely read and urbane, he yet maintained a guard over his deeper feelings which was seldom lowered. This shield, which was composed of keen intelligence and wisdom, often concealed an ultimate goal, enabling him, undisturbed, to obtain the desired objective. He rarely appeared in medical politics, yet the influence of his attitude was often felt. (Osgood 1932)

Despite his restrained and composed personality, Allison was:

> possessed of unusual organizing ability, [and] he never seemed to be hurried, or tired, or discouraged; nor did his sense of humor ever desert him. He smiled as he overcame his difficulties, laughing best because he laughed last. Conservative Boston admired his quiet strength, and he became the trusted advisor of the authorities of the Medical School, the Massachusetts General Hospital, and the New England Peabody Home. The Boston School of Occupational Therapy owes him a deep debt of gratitude for his services as a member of the Board of Directors. Medical and social clubs

valued his membership and always welcomed to him. (Osgood 1932)

Osgood (1932) ended the obituary with a glimpse into Allison's personal life and struggles, pinpointing Allison's influence on friends and colleagues alike:

Exercise he acccepted as one of his many responsibilities. He was fond of horses and for years his daily ride was a daily duty; golf was a preparation as well as a pleasure. The value of long vacations and short holidays had been learned and he was seldom ill. Those who knew him best were unaware that behind the calm and merry front which he presented to the world, there lay concealed exhausting struggles of head and heart which were draining his vitality. Under this strain, his circulatory system finally weakened to such an extent that a physical surrender became necessary in the full tide of mental victory. He died before the time that men had allotted to him but not before he gained the respect of colleagues in every branch of medicine. He has left a strong and permanent impression upon the specialty in which he won an international distinction.

CHAPTER 37

Marius N. Smith-Petersen
Prolific Inventor in Orthopaedics

Marius "Mads" Nygaard Smith-Petersen was born in the coastal town of Grimstad, Norway, on November 14, 1886. His parents were Morten Smith-Petersen, a lawyer, and Kaia (Ursin) Smith-Petersen. His ancestors "were owners and operators of a great fleet of merchant vessels which called at ports all over the world. Talented in music, patrons of the arts, cultivated, they knew the best life had to offer" ("M. N. Smith-Petersen" 1953). After his father's early death at just 34 years old, the family moved to Oslo, and in 1903 they emigrated to the United States, settling in Milwaukee, Wisconsin. Marius Smith-Petersen was just 17 at the time, and unable to speak English. His mother, an acclaimed violinist and pianist, gave violin lessons to support him and his three siblings.

Smith-Petersen had attended the gymnasium in Grimstad from 1902 to 1903. After relocating to Milwaukee, he attended West Side High School from 1904 to 1906. He then matriculated at the University of Chicago, but after just one year transferred to the University of Wisconsin, where he received a bachelor of science degree in 1910. "There, in his senior year, he became President of the Cosmopolitan Club [a student organization in the United States and abroad, first formed at the University of Wisconsin in 1903, that encouraged local community projects and promoted international cooperation and peace]. Embarrassed in that office by his lack of knowledge of

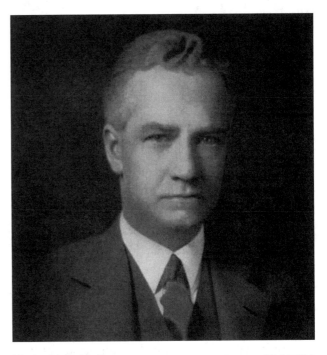

Marius N. Smith-Petersen. "Marius N. Smith-Petersen 1886–1953," *Journal of Bone and Joint Surgery* 1953; 35: 1042.

Physician Snapshot

Marius N. Smith-Petersen

BORN: 1886

DIED: 1953

SIGNIFICANT CONTRIBUTIONS: Created a tri-flanged nail for stabilizing intracapsular femoral neck fractures; developed the anterior subperiosteal iliofemoral approach to the hip joint; developed the new method of mold (cup) arthroplasty of the hip joint; created a surgical treatment for femoroacetabular impingement; developed a new approach for arthrodesis of the sacroiliac joint; developed a new (medial) approach to the wrist during arthrodesis

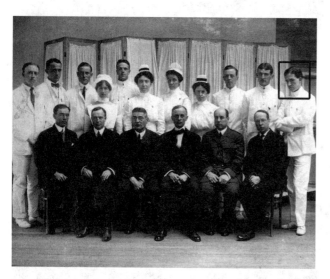

Harvard Unit at American Ambulance (17 doctors & nurses) in Paris. Ca. 1917. Smith-Petersen is standing in the back row at the far right. Boston Medical Library in the Francis A. Countway Library of Medicine.

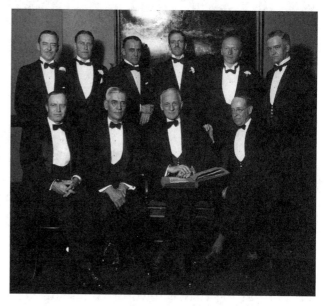

Cushing Alumni. Cushing and members of the First Harvard Medical Unit. Robert Osgood is seated at the far right. Harvey Cushing is seated next to him. Standing in the back row is Marius Smith-Petersen at the far right. Standing next to him is Philip Wilson.

P. D. Wilson, "Robert Bayley Osgood 1873–1956," *Journal of Bone and Joint Surgery* 1957; 39: 728.)

parliamentary law, he promptly mastered that procedure and even enjoyed a facility in it which few possess" ("M. N. Smith-Petersen" 1953). In addition to his involvement in student organizations there, "he was laboratory assistant to the great physiologist, [Joseph] Erlanger" ("Marius N. Smith-Petersen" 1953). His thesis was titled "Physiology of Purkinje Fibers." After completing his undergraduate education, he went to Boston to attend Harvard Medical School; he graduated in 1914.

He initially remained in Boston upon graduation, taking a "general surgical internship…at the Peter Bent Brigham Hospital…under Dr. Harvey Cushing. Undoubtedly, that distinguished surgeon and scholar strongly influenced the young surgeon, combining as he did, surgical boldness and radicalism with the most meticulous preparation, caution and technical accuracy" ("M. N. Smith-Petersen" 1953). Shortly thereafter, he served in France (stationed in Paris) for a few months during World War I between April 1 and July 1, 1915, in "the First Harvard Medical Unit at the American Ambulance Hospital [with Drs. Harvey Cushing and Philip Wilson] ("Marius N. Smith-Petersen" 1953)."

EARLY CAREER AND PUBLICATIONS

After he completed his military service, Smith-Petersen resumed his training in Boston, dedicating "2 years [as an intern to] orthopaedic surgery at the Massachusetts General Hospital under Dr. Elliott G. Brackett" ("Marius N. Smith-Petersen" 1953). This work with Brackett at MGH provided "Smith-Petersen's orthopaedic foundation… There, after the day's hospital work (which usually was completed about ten p.m.) he and his fellow orthopaedic intern, Dr. LeRoy Abbott, could go to their room and until the wee sma' hours they would read *Whitman's Orthopaedic Surgery*. At the close of their service they had mastered this weighty tome" ("M.N. Smith-Petersen" 1953). In addition to his in-hospital training with Brackett, during that internship Smith-Petersen "occasionally assisted Dr. Brackett in private practice ("M.N. Smith-Petersen" 1953)." Smith-Petersen practiced orthopaedic surgery for his entire career at MGH, and he accepted a position on January 1, 1917, as Brackett's office assistant.

Anterior Supra-articular Subperiosteal Approach to the Hip

Apparently unaware of Carl Heuter's description of a direct anterior approach to the hip (see C. Heuter 1883), while an orthopaedic intern at MGH, Smith-Petersen conceived the anterior supra-articular (iliofemoral) subperiosteal approach to the hip joint, and his first paper, published in 1917, described this new approach. He delineated the five main steps of the method:

1. Anterior incision…from the anterior superior spine along the anterior border of the tensor fascia femoris, to below…the trochanter…follows an intermuscular plane between the sartorius anteriorly, and the tensor fascia femoris posteriorly…

2. Curved incision…from the anterior superior spine along the crest of the ilium, through the origin of the gluteus medius…

3. Subperiosteal dissection: The flap outlined by the two incisions is freed from the ilium by subperiosteal dissection…By reflecting the origin of the tensor fascia femoris with the flap, the superior gluteal nerve and artery are preserved…

4. Incision of the capsule: The chief point… is the preservation of the Y-ligament of Bigelow. The incision is…made in the superior portion of the capsule…[which] is freed positively along the cotyloid ligament…

5. Closure: The capsule is sutured, the flap turned back, and the anterior limb of the incision is closed in layers. The curved limb…is closed by suturing the origin of the gluteus medius to its periosteal attachment. (Smith-Petersen 1917)

Article in which Smith-Petersen described his unique "bloodless" approach to the hip. *American Journal of Orthopedic Surgery* 1917; s2-15: 592.

Smith-Petersen's approach to the hip became the standard at MGH during hip procedures such as open reduction of congenitally dislocated hips, hip arthroplasty, femoral neck fracture, and hip fusion. Thirty years later, when he gave the Moynihan Lecture at the University of Leeds in 1947, he described his attempts to bring this new approach to light. An excerpt from his published lecture is provided in **Box 37.1**.

Mold Arthroplasty

During this period of his life, Smith-Petersen also routinely used fascia lata hip arthroplasty, but he was dissatisfied with the outcomes. In 1918, he started "work[ing] on mould arthroplasty, inspired by the perfect foreign-body cyst he exposed, which had formed around a piece of glass embedded in a boy's back" ("M.N. Smith-Petersen" 1953). The benign foreign body he removed was a piece of glass; this suggested to him:

that here was a process of repair which might be applied to arthroplasty…and [thus] the idea of the "mould" was conceived. A mould of some inert material, interposed between the newly shaped surface of the head of the femur and the acetabulum, would guide nature's repair so that

Box 37.1. Smith-Petersen Describes His New Approach to the Hip Joint

"The teachings of Dr. Harvey Cushing—respect for structure and structural planes—were directly responsible for a new approach to the hip joint. After finishing my surgical internship at the Peter Bent Brigham I started an orthopaedic internship at the Massachusetts General Hospital in January 1916. In the spring of that year, I assisted in an open reduction of a congenital dislocation of the hip. The hip was exposed through a Kocher incision; it was bloody; it was brutal. The patient survived by a very narrow margin. Being used to the technique of Cushing, I was shocked, and I said to my senior, Dr. Roy Abbot, 'There must be some other way of exposing the hip.' 'Why don't you figure one out?' was his answer. That night, frontal bone flaps, approach to the pituitary, temporal decompression, exposure of the cerebellum, kept passing through my mind. In all of them, when the periosteum was reached it was clearly incised, its edges carefully elevated, and it was reflected intact, always as a continuous structure and never in shreds.

"The cerebellum exposure, by retraction of muscle flaps with their periosteal attachments, was probably the one that gave me the idea of combining the anterior hip approach with the periosteal reflection of muscles from the lateral aspect of the ilium.

"The next day, I went to the Medical School and asked my old friend, Tom Bonney, for a hip. He gave me a nice clean one; I can still see it. It did not take long to demonstrate to my own satisfaction that the approach had merit, but would older and experienced surgeons feel the same way about it? I brought the specimen back to hospital and carefully hid it in the plaster room under Ward I. At the first opportunity I told the visiting surgeon that I thought I had a new way of exposing the hip joint. He laughed heartily and said 'I like the enthusiasm of youth; if there were a better way of getting into the hip joint, don't you think that generations of surgeons who have gone before you would have discovered it a long time ago?' This was not exactly encouraging, so I did not invite him to see the specimen.

"It was several days before the Chief of Surgery, Dr. Elliott G. Brackett, paid a visit to Ward I. At the end of Rounds, I asked him if he would be interested in seeing a specimen which I thought demonstrated a new approach to the hip. 'Why, certainly Doctor, of course I am' was his response. His reaction to the specimen was even more favorable. 'You know Doctor, I think that approach has possibilities. Would you allow me to take the specimen with me? I am going to the American Orthopaedic Association Meeting tonight and I would like to demonstrate it.' Returning from the meeting he reported a very favorable reaction on the part of the older surgeons. In less than a year after this demonstration I had a nice letter from Dr. Fred Albee telling me that he had used the approach on many occasions and that from then on, he would use no other.

"This supra-articular subperiosteal approach to the hip improved the exposure of the head and the neck of the femur, but the other side of the joint—the acetabulum remained inaccessible. It was not until 1935 that this came within reach. 'Acetabuloplasty'—excision of the anterior superior wall of the acetabulum—solved this problem. This operative procedure was developed in an attempt to relieve a patient with bilateral, intrapelvic protrusion of the acetabula. The attempt was successful and for a number of years…was used quite commonly. Because of the increasing success of complete mould arthroplasty, it is now seldom used. We do owe it credit for showing us the way to expose the anterior acetabulum by subperiosteal retraction of the sartorius and iliacus muscle from the ilium. We owe it credit for proving that the anterior acetabulum can be excised without joint instability resulting. We owe it credit for starting our thoughts in the right direction. The making of a joint demands reconstruction on both sides of the joint so that the surfaces will be congruous and work smoothly in relation to one another. The present exposure of the hip is extensive, but it is no more than adequate; and it is unaccompanied by shock because it respects structures and follows structural planes."

(M. N. Smith-Petersen
"Evolution of Mould Arthroplasty of the Hip Joint,"
Journal of Bone and Joint Surgery 1948)

defects would be eliminated. Upon completion of the repair the mould would be removed, leaving smooth, congruous surfaces mechanically suited for function. (Smith-Petersen 1948)

Despite this early work, he did not publish his findings until 1936, 18 years later, because "it was not until then that he felt the work was advanced far enough to justify publication" ("M. N. Smith-Petersen" 1953).

Sacroiliac Joint

The early 1920s were a pivotal point in Smith-Petersen's career. By 1920, he was appointed an assistant instructor in orthopaedic surgery at Harvard Medical School, he began his own practice in 1922, and he continued to specialize in orthopaedic surgery at MGH.

His next publication, "Arthrodesis of the Sacroiliac Joint: A New Method of Approach," had come in 1921. In it, he explained that because the sacroiliac joint lies so deep within the anatomy, access is precluded from the anterior or superior direction, thus making surgical procedures on this joint problematic. He described possible lateral and posterior approaches and determined which works best:

> The different methods of approach from the posterior aspect all offer great difficulties…only the case of Dr. Painter's approach is an actual exposure of the joint accomplished. Dr. Painter's approach, which consists in turning back a flap of bone from the posterior portion of the ilium, is too extensive to undertake except as a last resort…In the literature on the sacroiliac joint, no article or reference to…[the lateral approach] has been encountered, and yet it seems the most logical approach. This method has been used…during the past three years, and the experience…has been the same in every case: an anatomically easy approach with no trauma to important structures, resulting in good exposure of the cartilaginous joint surface of the ilium and the sacrum. The principle of the operation is similar to…the hip joint—a sub-periosteal approach. (Smith-Petersen 1921)

Then he outlined the six main phases of the procedure:

1. Curved incision from the posterior superior spine along the crest of the ilium…carried down to the bone and the reflection of the periosteal started.

2. Incision from the posterior superior spine in the direction of the fibers of the gluteus maximus for…three to four inches…This incision is carried down…until the junction of the ilium and sacrum…is reached…posterior branches [of the superior gluteal artery and nerve] give off posterior branches…[that] have to be sacrificed in order to get satisfactory reflection.

3. The flap…is reflected sub-periosteally…

4. A [rectangular] window is now cut through the ilium within the projected area of the joint…the entire block of bone from the outer table to the inner table of the ilium…[is] removed in one piece…[exposing] the cartilaginous surface of the sacrum…

5. After removing the cartilage and cortex from the block of bone…[it] is replaced in its original site and countersunk, so that its cancellous surface will be in contact with the cancellous bone of the sacrum…

6. The flap is now returned to its place and…sutured in layers…In cases of tuberculosis…the curette has to be used effectively to reach the parts of the joint not actually exposed. (Smith-Petersen 1921)

During the next five years, he published another four papers on the sacroiliac joint, describing the diagnosis of sacroiliac disease, end results after fusion, and fusion for tuberculosis of the sacroiliac joint.

Before Mixter and Barr's classic 1934 paper on herniated disc as a cause of sciatica, most experts believed that the lumbosacral joint and especially the sacroiliac joint were the cause of low back pain and leg pain. In 1924, Smith-Petersen described how to differentiate pain associated with each of these joints when examining a patient with low back and leg pain. For the lumbosacral joint, Smith-Petersen (1924) noted that because it receives "innervation from the fifth lumbar and the first sacral" nerves, injuries to the joint "are apt to give pain...referred along the distribution of [those nerves], that is, the dorsum of the foot, first toe, mesial aspect of the sole and heel...and anterior-lateral and posterior aspects of the lower leg...second, third, fourth and fifth toes and lateral aspect of the sole." The sacroiliac joint is innervated by numerous sources: "the lumbo-sacral cord...the first and second sacral nerves...the superior gluteal nerve...[and] the obturator nerve" (Smith-Petersen 1921). Thus, "in sacro-iliac cases we may have pain referred along the fourth and fifth lumbar, and the first and second sacral nerves...pain referred to the posterior aspect of the thigh...[and] to any part of the lower leg... posterior aspect of the thigh, antero-lateral and posterior aspects of the lower leg and lateral aspect of the ankle" (Smith-Petersen 1921). In light of these differences, he "emphasize[d] the need of careful analysis of every sign and symptom." For example, when lifting a straight leg from the hip, "in sacro-iliac cases we are able to bring the leg to a higher level without pain. In lumbo-sacral conditions, pain comes on at the same level as it does on the affected side" (Smith-Petersen 1921). He also noted that during "compression of the crests and pressure on the pubes, when the tests are positive they are definitely in favor of a sacro-iliac condition" (Smith-Petersen 1921).

Smith-Petersen continued to advocate arthrodesis of the sacroiliac joint. In 1926, he and Dr. William Rogers published an end-results study of sacroiliac joint fusion for arthritis. To begin, they stated their objective: "to offer evidence justifying the diagnosis of traumatic arthritis of the sacro-iliac joint...[S]urgeons of the opposite viewpoint in order to refute it will have to do more than simply state 'there is no such condition as traumatic sacro-iliac arthritis.' There are a great many orthopaedic surgeons who hold this latter point of view in a passive, non-aggressive way" (Smith-Petersen and Rogers 1926b). Then they described the results from 26 patients: "Four... or 15.5% [*sic*] had negative roentgenographic findings." They modified the procedure he had described five years earlier, mainly by using "a motor driven saw [to extend] the window...posteriorly into the inferior sacro-iliac ligament. [The] sacral joint surface is removed exposing cancellous bone; joint cartilage is curetted with angled curettes" (Smith-Petersen and Rogers 1926b). In the later cases, under microscopic examination Smith-Petersen and Rogers (1926b) noted alterations, including "erosion of the joint cartilage...and replacement fibrosis...at the junction of the cartilage with underlying bone, but also in the medullary spaces." Among their patients, 22 (84.6%) achieved a complete recovery; only two failures resulted. This was "a very high percentage of successful cases, [and] consequently we feel justified in concluding that the diagnosis as well as the treatment has been correct" (Smith-Petersen and Rogers 1926b).

The discussion of this paper sheds some interesting light on the opinions of orthopaedic leaders regarding sacroiliac fusion in the 1920s. Dr. Robert Osgood (1926) gave the procedure high praise: "This very fine piece of work...illustrates my own change of conception. I have watched these cases, starting with the opinion that this was rather radical surgery and that we were getting most of our cases well without it...I have come to the conclusion that this piece of work represents...not radical, but conservative, surgery...The shock [not a single death], as Dr. Smith-Petersen performs the operation is extraordinarily slight." Osgood (1926) pointed out that "The immobilization is practically nothing." Smith-Petersen (1926b) described his method of immobilization as using: "At first a double plaster spica…Now an abdominal binder while…in bed…[for] three weeks…At the end… the patient is allowed up and about, wearing a sacro-iliac belt with a pad over each gluteal region… Patient leaves the hospital four weeks from the day of the operation." Osgood (1926) proclaimed the significance of Smith-Petersen's approach: "We must accept it absolutely at its face value; that is, we have a new method of controlling low back pain in a type of case that has been to us at times very obstinate." He ended his commentary with an anecdote: "I am allowed by Dr. Smith-Petersen to say that his wife had this condition and was treated by the best orthopaedic talent we have in Boston, but did not become permanently well. Dr. Smith-Petersen was quite convinced that her lesion was in the sacro-iliac joint and we had a long discussion as to who would perform the operation on her. I told him that he was the man to do this operation. He did and after years of invalidism she is about the healthiest person in Boston."

Such praise came as well from other important orthopaedic surgeons in Boston: Smith-Petersen's mentor, Elliott Brackett (1926), commented that "in Boston we all practically advocate for this operation, certainly in select cases." Dr. Nathaniel Allison (1926) agreed with Osgood "that here we have a complete piece of work." Allison went on: "When I first became associated with Dr. Smith-Petersen at Massachusetts General Hospital I knew very little about this subject. I know very little about it now, but I have learned vastly from him in regard to the diagnosis of these cases, and one point in diagnosis I would like to emphasize: the importance of a careful physical examination… We are dealing as Dr. Smith-Petersen has shown, with an arthritis." Even physicians elsewhere in the Northeast supported Smith-Petersen's procedure. Dr. M. S. Danforth (1926), practicing in Providence, Rhode Island, reiterated the importance of examination and diagnosis:

I think we are to be very much congratulated on this piece of work by Dr. Smith-Petersen. I feel the real point of it all is the diagnosis. The question of whether low back pain with leg pain or without leg pain is due to a lumbo-sacral or a sacro-iliac lesion is what is most necessary for me to solve. I believe that every piece of work like this that is carefully carried out will help to get us to the point where we can make a reasonably positive diagnosis.

That same year, Smith-Petersen and Rogers also reported the end results of fusion of the sacroiliac joint in patients with tuberculosis. In it, they explicitly contradicted Jones and Lovett's earlier suggestion that "sacro-iliac tuberculosis, when treated by arthrodesis, is…'the most fatal of all joint affections'" (Smith-Petersen and Rogers 1926a). To support their procedure, they provided overall results from their cohort: "Sixty-nine percent of the patients have returned to…their previous occupation…[and] ninety-two percent have had no pain since the time of operation" (Smith-Petersen and Rogers 1926a), but they also reported the deaths of four patients (31%) from advanced tuberculosis.

Femoral Neck Fractures

Smith-Petersen, with Drs. Edwin F. Cave and George W. Van Gorder, were the first to use a new tri-flanged nail, which Smith-Petersen had created in 1925, in the fixation of intracapsular femoral neck fractures. "Many of his [Smith-Petersen's] colleagues believe this to be his greatest contribution" ("Marius N. Smith-Petersen" 1953). As the story goes, "the three-flanged nail occurred to his mind as he passed a sleepless night on the train. He had spent part of the previous stay in an out-of-town clinic, viewing the failure of treatment of fractures of the neck of the femur by external fixation" ("M. N. Smith-Petersen" 1953).

In their 1931 report, Smith-Petersen, Cave, and Van Gorder described the results of the first

> ## ARCHIVES OF SURGERY
> VOLUME 23   NOVEMBER, 1931   NUMBER 5
>
> INTRACAPSULAR FRACTURES OF THE NECK OF THE FEMUR
>
> TREATMENT BY INTERNAL FIXATION *
>
> M. N. SMITH-PETERSEN, M.D.
> EDWIN F. CAVE, M.D.
> AND
> GEORGE W. VANGORDER, M.D.
> BOSTON

Article describing the use of the triflanged nail for intracapsular fractures of the femoral neck, with results in 24 cases.
Archives of Surgery 1931; 23: 715.

24 cases for which they used the tri-flanged nail. They began by describing two main reasons why results were so divergent with both round and square nails that had previously been used for internal fixation. The first was because fixation was incomplete and did not last over the long-term, and a plaster cast was required to ensure the leg was completely immobilized, thus limiting function too extensively after the procedure. Another reason was the size of the nails: because they were so large, they put pressure on the adjacent bone, causing necrosis. This would, in turn, eventually loosen the nail, rendering it ineffective. Smith-Petersen's tri-flanged nail addressed these two deficiencies. It was set within the cortical bone, which disallowed rotation, and the smaller size (albeit larger surface area) also caused less necrosis. Both of these effects together provided longstanding complete fixation.

Smith-Petersen, Cave, and Van Gorder modified Smith-Petersen's extensive subperiosteal approach to the hip joint to accomplish open reduction of the fracture. After the fracture was reduced, the nail was driven through the lateral surface of the greater trochanter. Reduction was maintained with obstetrical forceps, and then, using an impactor, the bone fragments were impacted, as recommended by Frederic Cotton (chapter 59). The stability of the fracture was tested by moving the hip through a wide range of motion in all planes. The capsule was then closed.

Initially, the patient wore a plaster cast after the procedure and then ring calipers when they resumed walking. Eventually, traction (5 pounds) would be applied to the leg, and patients would wear a bivalved short plaster spica (10–15 degrees abduction) while ambulating. They would continue wearing the spica cast for another 3–6 months. The nail remained in the femur over a wide range of time—anywhere from 6 months to 4 years. Among Smith-Petersen, Cave, and Van Gorder's 24 patients, four experienced non-union over the long-term (10–30 months) and three achieved bony union. Smith-Petersen et al. highlighted the lack of pain their patients—most of whom were older (50–70 years)—felt after the procedure. As future studies and different surgeons' experiences with the procedure proved, the very high mortality and complication rates in these patients were markedly reduced.

Smith-Petersen, Cave, and Van Gorder noted that previous methods of treating a femoral neck fracture would only maintain an anatomical reduction if the patient was immobilized. Because their tri-flanged nail provided strong and continuous fixation, however, joint immobilization was not required, allowing movement—and the achievement of function—sooner. Smith-Petersen

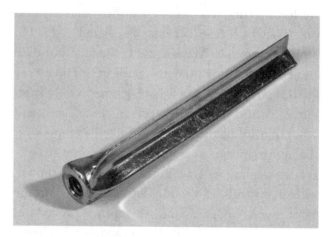

Original Smith-Petersen triflanged nail (non-cannulated).
Author's nail; photographed by Massachusetts General Hospital Photography Department.

continued to refine his tri-flanged nail throughout his later career.

CHIEF AT MGH AND LATER PUBLICATIONS

After Dr. Nathaniel Allison resigned as chief of the Orthopaedic Service in 1929, the trustees at MGH named Smith-Petersen to that position. At that time, in addition to Drs. Philip Wilson, William Rogers, and Edwin Cave, Drs. George Van Gorder, Sumner Roberts, and Joseph Barr became new members of the department. Smith-Petersen was "affectionately known" as "Pete" or "Smith-Pete" ("M.N. Smith-Petersen" 1953). His residents, colleagues, and friends also referred to him as "the Chief." About 10 years after his appointment at MGH, he was also promoted to instructor at HMS, a position he held until 1935. At that time, he was promoted to clinical professor of orthopaedic surgery.

In his book titled *Lest We Forget*, Dr. Carter Rowe wrote about his experiences with "the Chief." He specifically mentions the high expectations Smith-Petersen had of his assistants, both the house officers who prepared the surgical instruments before and anyone who assisted during the procedure. He preferred silence while operating. Any who worked with Smith-Petersen recognized what could be considered his four pillars of surgical care:

- Appropriate patient selection
- Engendering trust from the patient
- Thorough planning
- Focus on every detail during the procedure

Smith-Petersen provided excellent care to his patients outside the operating room. He always took time to explain all aspects of a procedure and to ensure that patients understood. But like his assistants, Smith-Petersen held patients to high standards, as well. He expected them to cooperate completely—both while preparing for the procedure and during postoperative recovery—in order to obtain the best results. His patients responded to this obvious personal interest from Smith-Petersen. Rowe shared a recollection from Dr. Lewis Cozen, one of Smith-Petersen's orthopaedic residents:

> [When] Dr. Smith-Petersen made rounds, as you will recall very well and the entourage that followed him was impressive. If he bent over and talked to the patients as he made rounds… [and asked] "how are you?" They would invariably say, "Oh, I'm fine. You are wonderful, Dr. Smith-Petersen." Later, when we would make our individual rounds, we'd hear the same patients complaining of pain and discomfort of various kinds. That is what I call a real bedside manner! (quoted in Rowe 1996)

According to one account, he was most adept with individual patients, and he "inspired all of them, from the poorest occupant of a ward bed to the wealthiest in the most luxurious surroundings. This cooperation from patients…was to a considerable extent responsible for his unusual success with any operation he performed" ("Marius N. Smith-Petersen" 1953).

His personality was one of Smith-Petersen's defining characteristics. A former house officer, resident, and assistant of Dr. Smith-Petersen wrote:

> Uppermost in my mind is the personal magnetism that emanated from the grand old man. This magnetism had far-reaching effects, even down to influencing the results of his arthroplasties and to making those people around him work out their hearts and souls for him without any direct demand on his past. This quality, it seems to me, is one he may have been born with perhaps but nonetheless possessed, and had no small part in his ultimate greatness.
> ("M. N. Smith-Petersen" 1953)

He was described by another as exuding life and energy, and emanating:

> love and inspiration which he gave and in turn received from a devoted family and a wide circle of friends at home and abroad gave his life balance. His tremendous capacity for work lead [sic] to extraordinary accomplishments and in turn rich satisfactions…One of his most dominant characteristics was singleness of purpose…what he asked of himself he asked of all who worked with him and lived with him—a like single-mindedness. They had to help pay the price for the profession ideal which he had set before himself. Such single-mindedness as was his is reserved only for the great. ("M. N. Smith-Petersen" 1953)

However, despite the success brought on by his caring demeanor and skillful hands, he was never satisfied, and "to some of his friends, there was something sad about 'Pete' which seemed to come from a sense of his falling short of the goal he had set for himself, and from a realization that he did not have power enough to fully satisfy his desire to be of service" ("M.N. Smith-Petersen" 1953) "He experienced periods of great inner conflict and depression. His friends described him as having moments of "an overpowering sense of possible error in professional or moral judgement. He would then seek out a trusted friend who he felt was competent to judge, tell him all, and, straightway, seemed to be relieved when it was pointed out convincingly he had actually made no error" ("M. N. Smith-Petersen" 1953).

As chief, Smith-Petersen also shared his knowledge and skill through clinics attended by colleagues, residents, students, and even patients. In this,

> there were few who were his equal. At his clinical demonstrations, case after case would be presented with much dramatic skill, force, and enthusiasm that [everyone in attendance] at once felt his outstanding ability…The basis for this power lay not alone in his personal magnetism but also in the most infinite care and pains he unsparingly took in making his diagnosis, in working out the details of his operations, in perfecting his skill and technique and in the aftercare. ("M. N. Smith-Petersen" 1953)

Despite the demands of his position and his dedication to sharing knowledge with future orthopedists and patients alike, he also continued to publish innovative research after his appointment. During his career, Smith-Petersen published about 24 articles—most of which were major contributions to orthopaedic surgery and became classic papers.

Femoroacetabular Impingement

By 1936 Smith-Petersen had reported a new surgical procedure for treating femoroacetabular impingement. This advance was brought about because of a 55-year-old patient who "was admitted [to MGH in February 1935]…with a diagnosis of 'bilateral intrapelvic protrusion of the acetabulum,'" and for whom the team determined, after discussion during ward rounds, "that nothing could be done" (Smith-Petersen 1936). Smith-Petersen (1936), however, believed that the patient's pain was being caused by "the impingement of the femoral neck on the anterior acetabular margin… [giving] rise to congestion of the synovia, synovitis, and, because of periosteal irritation, hypertrophic changes." He thought that:

> if we could eliminate this impingement, we should be able to eliminate the resultant reaction and, therefore pain. To eliminate impingement two regions may be attacked, — the neck of the femur and the anterior margin of the acetabulum…The patient was informed that the operation had never been performed before, but that it did offer a chance of success. She accepted the operation willingly (Smith-Petersen 1936).

The procedure was a success: the patient walked out of the hospital four weeks later and returned to work as a housekeeper four months after the procedure, free of pain and without a limp.

Smith-Petersen reported that he had done this procedure in eight patients with advanced arthritis and in two with an old slipped capital femoral epiphysis—all 10 with impingement. The patients reported no pain or only soreness after the procedure. Smith-Petersen admitted that not enough time had elapsed since to allow for a valid assessment of end results, but he offered this operation as a remedy for patients with severe hip pain secondary to arthritic impingement. To avoid sacrificing too much bone from the femoral neck, "he advocated removing the anterosuperior portion of the acetabulum…[and to] also remove a portion of the anterosuperior capsule, [as he was] sure it would remove a source of the innervated tissue causing symptoms" (Brand 2009).

Femoral Neck Fractures

Smith-Petersen had continued to research and finesse his tri-flanged nail. In 1937, he reviewed the use of the nail and described his current technique (**Case 37.1**). He chronicled reports from the literature that described changes by and outcomes from other surgeons worldwide—from Virginia to Sweden to Australia—during the five years after he first published the procedure. All of them simplified the use of the nail. Most important were Johansson's design of a centrally cannulated nail, which allowed the surgeon to insert a guide wire into the femoral neck and then take an x-ray to ensure the guide wire is positioned accurately before inserting the nail over the Kirschner pin. Smith-Petersen eventually used Johansson's modification. King also modified the nail (independently from Johansson) to include a central hole, through which he inserted two guide wires into the femoral neck under fluoroscopic control. As with Johansson's nail, this allowed the surgeon to check the guide wires' proper positioning before inserting the nail. Smith-Petersen emphasized the importance of retaining the cortex and using the starter correctly in order to avoid extrusion or slipping of the nail.

Case 37.1. Treatment of Fractures of the Neck of the Femur by Internal Fixation

> 1. "A young woman of 32 years entered the hospital with an ununited fracture of the neck of the femur of 19 months' standing. Roentgenograms showed a relatively dense head, but there were areas apparently undergoing Phemister's "creeping substitution"; there was slight absorption of the neck. Open reduction with nailing was done; slight bleeding from the head, good bleeding from the neck. The nail was low but good relationship between the head and distal neck was obtained. After 8 weeks' recumbency, with extremity suspended, the patient was allowed up in a leather spica; crutches with increasing weight bearing were used for 8 months, followed by a cane. The nail was removed 12 months after operation. Roentgenogram 3 years later showed slight thinning of joint cartilage and mild hypertrophic changes; at this time there was no pain and the function was excellent."
>
> (Marius N. Smith-Petersen 1937)

Smith-Petersen then described his current technique, achieved after performing open reduction in another 26 patients. First, he noted that radiographs are necessary in order to measure the length of the normal leg and thereby avoid excessive shortening. He used the well-known Leadbetter method to achieve reduction, applying traction to the limb with the hip in flexion, then abducting and extending the hip. After the reduction, the thigh must be kept parallel to the operating table; an assistant holds the leg steady, and the knee is flexed 90° and the hip internally rotated 20° with 25° of abduction. Smith-Petersen relies on radiographs again at this point to ensure the reduction is complete.

Next, after preparing and draping the patient, he makes a four- to six-inch-long incision over the greater trochanter. The vastus lateralis is reflected subperiosteally and then, using a nail starter, he used the starter to make a hole in the femur, three-fourths to one inch below the vastus lateralis attachment. Angling the nail at 40–50° cephalad and parallel to the horizontal plane (operating table), he hammers it into the femoral neck. Again, radiographs allow him to visualize the reduction, ensuring that it has been maintained and that the nail is well positioned. In a final step he impacts the fracture site and closes the incision.

After describing his surgical approach, he laid out the patient's progression to ambulation postoperatively:

- traction (5 lbs.) for 4 weeks
- bivalve spica during ambulation for 4–8 weeks
- crutches for 4–6 months (only partial weight-breaking initially)

He noted that the nail remains in place for at least a year, if not longer. For him, two of the most important factors in regaining function were gentle impaction and valgus positioning.

> "A great responsibility rests on the surgeon who introduces a new method of treatment. The desire to have a new idea published is so great that the originator is often let astray, and the method is broadcast before it has proved worthwhile, and before the technique has been perfected. The method that is the subject of this paper has been used for five years, and a sufficient series of cases has been studied to prove that it is worthwhile; the technique has been developed, and many errors eliminated."
>
> —Smith-Peterson, Cave, and Van Gorder "Anterior Intracapsular Fractures of the Neck of the Femur. Treatment by Internal Fixation" *Archives of Surgery*, 1931

Table 37.1. Experience with Femoral Neck Fractures among 100 AAOS Members as of 1939

Cases each year	
1903	1
1918	1
1925	4
1926	3
1927	5
1928	9
1929	11
1930	13
1931	7
1932	10
1933	45
1934	78
1935	183
1936	482
1937	489
1938	144
Patients	
Male	275
Female	1210
Procedure performed	
Arthroplasty	228
Closed reduction with internal fixation	1257
Implants used for internal fixation	
Smith-Petersen flanged nails	883
Moore pins	396
Knowles pins	71
Steel spikes or lugs	25
Kirschner wires	36
Screws	61
Beef-bone pegs	4
Autogenous grafts	9
Method for postoperative fixation	
None	794
Plaster cast	342
Traction	349
Results	
Nonunion	173
Union	882
Avascular necrosis of the femoral head	46
Pulmonary embolism	2
Death	127
Pneumonia	35
Congestive heart failure	19
Other	73

Data from M. N. Smith-Petersen, "Treatment of Fractures of the Neck of the Femur by Internal Fixation," *Journal of Bone and Joint Surgery* 1939; 21:483–486.

As the 1930s came to a close, Smith-Petersen was serving as chair of the American Academy of Orthopaedic Surgeons Fracture Committee. Under the leadership of Secretary Dr. H. Earle Conwell, the committee had been gathering data from academy members about their experiences with femoral neck fractures. This effort probably represents the academy's first attempt at a national registry. A total of 200 members responded, but only 100 of them reported having experience treating femoral neck fractures. The data from these members are shown in **Table 37.1**. Overall, after the procedure, patients remained in the hospital for a mean of 45 days and were allowed full weight-bearing after 5–8 months. The Fracture Committee continued to follow the remaining cases for two or more years.

> "In the hands of experienced surgeons, the end-results obtained in fractures of the neck of the femur have been greatly improved by the use of internal fixation."
> —AAOS Fracture Committee Report, 1941

Approach to the Wrist during Arthrodesis

In addition to the aforementioned original contributions, Smith-Petersen described a new medial approach to the wrist joint during arthrodesis. He resected the distal ulna (Darrach procedure) through a medial approach, exposing the radiocarpal joint, thus providing adequate exposure to complete a wrist fusion and thereby preserve forearm rotation. In an article published with Aufranc and Larson, Smith-Petersen suggested that the following resection arthroplasties: acromioplasty and removal of both the radial head and the distal ulna can be performed early. He believed that allowing too much joint destruction to occur before performing a surgical procedure could result in pain and prevent the patient from reaping any beneficial results from the procedure. It is unclear when he published his recommendations, but he most likely completed this work in the early to mid-1940s.

The Sacroiliac Joint and John F. Kennedy

Smith-Petersen had also continued as a foremost expert in treating problems of the sacroiliac joint, which was exemplified when he was called on to evaluate John F. Kennedy—then in the US Navy Reserve and not yet in congress or the presidency—in May 1942. After previous consultations at the Mayo Clinic and the Lahey Clinic, Kennedy had spent almost the whole month of April in the Charleston Naval Hospital because of severe chronic back and abdominal pain. Specialists at the teaching hospitals concurred that Kennedy had a dislocated sacroiliac joint but the doctors in Charleston couldn't agree on the diagnosis or whether a sacroiliac joint fusion was the best course of action to treat it. Because of their indecision, Kennedy traveled to Boston to see Smith-Petersen, who diagnosed a ligamentous strain of the sacroiliac joint and, with a normal neurological examination, recommended conservative treatment. Kennedy returned to the naval hospital in Chelsea, Mass., where Dr. John White, a neurosurgeon, agreed with Smith-Petersen's diagnosis and recommended against any surgical procedure. White sent Kennedy back to Charleston, South Carolina, to serve his country not on the front lines, but behind a desk.

World War II and End of an Era as Chief

During his time as chief—a position he held for almost 20 years—Smith-Petersen also provided consultation and advice to the surgeon general of the army during World War II from 1942 to 1945. One year after the war, in 1946: "He relinquished his duties as active Chief of the Service [at MGH, but he] continued to come to rounds [and operate,] and [he] gave his contributions which were received with enthusiasm and respect" ("Marius N. Smith-Petersen" 1953). That same year, he stepped down from his teaching position at Harvard Medical School. Probably because he continued in private practice, he had never received a named professorship.

CONTINUING TO ADVANCE THE FIELD

Smith-Petersen continued to contribute to research and clinical work after he retired from his appointments at MGH and HMS. His admirers were not limited to his friends and colleagues in Boston. He continued to see patients worldwide, and "in his later days he spent many of his holidays in Europe and retired to his beloved Norway as frequently as possible. On more than one visit there he did a number of arthroplasties...[leaving] a host of devoted friends and patients" ("Marius N. Smith-Petersen" 1953).

Mold Arthroplasty

During the 25-year period between the first vitallium mold arthroplasty and his 1947 Moynahan Lecture, Smith-Petersen had worked with various other physician-researchers on staff at MGH, including Drs. William Rogers, Edwin Cave, George Van Gorder, Paul Norton, Milton Thompson, Otto Aufranc, and Carroll Larson. Smith-Petersen published a total of five articles on mold arthroplasty of the hip—the first in 1939 and the others between the years 1947 and 1949.

In his Moynihan Lecture, published in 1948, Smith-Petersen described his initial work with molds:

> Glass naturally suggested itself as the inert material from which moulds could be constructed. Macalister Bicknell of Cambridge, Massachusetts, who made the first x-ray table for Dr. Water Dodd, made the first crude moulds. Looking back on these moulds now, I am amazed that I had the courage to use them... The day after constructing the first glass mould arthroplasty I received a call to see Dr. George Holmes in the old X-Ray Department, the former accident room. 'What are you up to now?' He was looking at two x-ray plates..."Here we have bony ankylosis of the hip and here, twenty-four hours later, we have what appears to be a joint lined by cartilage," I explained. George laughed and shook his head: "What will you be up to next?" This was in 1923.

Article in which Smith-Petersen described the evolution of his concept of a mold or cup interposition arthroplasty of the hip. He had used a Vitallium cup in 29 patients in the previous 10 months and published the paper without clinical results in these patients because of the "success of the method."
Journal of Bone and Joint Surgery 1939: 21: 269.

More from this publication, describing the development and implementation of the first molds, is provided in **Box 37.2**.

The same year as his Moynahan Lecture, Smith-Petersen—along with Larson, Aufranc, and Dr. W. Alexander Law from London, England—reported the results of 42 cases of complications from femoral neck fractures treated by vitallium mold arthroplasty. In treating these complications, they recognized four approaches to mold

Box 37.2. The First Molds for Arthroplasty

"Some glass moulds broke after...a matter of months. This was a disheartening experience...but the acetabulum and head of the femur were found to be covered by a firm, glistening lining...The original glass moulds were abandoned and the search went on for some other material, inert and strong enough to stand up under weight-bearing. Viscoloid, a form of celluloid, was tried first experimentally and later clinically, but it produced too much foreign body reaction and had to be given up. Eight years went by without success. In 1933 we went back to the use of glass, this time 'pyrex.' The moulds were...heavier and were tested under the polariscope for evidence of strain under compression. Theoretically, they were strong enough, but... some of them broke...[T]hey were used only in selected cases and...the majority...did well. When the moulds were removed after fifteen to twenty-five months the joint surfaces were smooth, glistening, firm, and congruous. Histologic examination...showed fibrocartilage around the periphery of the articular surfaces, and hyaline cartilage in the central portion...[I]t seems reasonable to conclude that metaplasia from fibro-cartilage to hyaline cartilage takes place in response to...physiological physical stresses. The principle involved in mould arthroplasty may be represented diagrammatically...

MOULD ARTHROPLASTY
↓
Cancellous Bone Surfaces and Blood Clot
↓
Fibroblast Invasion of Blood Clot
↓
Mould
↓
Movement = Function
Intermittent Pressure
↓
Metaplasia of Fibrocartilage
↓
Hyaline Articular Cartilage

"...In 1937 my dentist, Dr. John Cooke, suggested vitallium as the ideal material from which to make the moulds. After several unsuccessful attempts a satisfactory mould was obtained. In 1938, the first vitallium mould arthroplasty was performed [15 years after the first glass mould was used]. Since then [a period of ten years], over 500 hips have been operated upon by this method at the Massachusetts General Hospital; eighty of these were bilateral. The fact that we have been willing to perform this operation on such an extensive scale is evidence that the results have been satisfactory."

(M. N. Smith-Petersen, "Evolution of Mould Arthroplasty of the Hip Joint," *Journal of Bone and Joint Surgery* 1948)

arthroplasty: "1. Routine mold arthroplasty; 2. Modified Whitman reconstruction operation; 3. Modified Colonna reconstruction operation; 4. Intertrochanteric mold arthroplasty" (Smith-Petersen et al. 1947). Each of these is described in Smith-Petersen's (1947) words in the list below.

- *Routine mold arthroplasty*: "In aseptic necrosis of the head, limited in extent... after union of the fractured neck, a routine mold arthroplasty is indicated...reshaping the head and acetabulum so as to create two congruous surfaces...[of] bleeding bone... in cases of extensive necrosis, the...defect is packed with cancellous bone."

- *Modified Whitman reconstructive operation*: "When the aseptic necrosis involves most of the head...[and] the fracture united...the 'dead head' is discarded, reshaping the viable remaining neck, [and] covering it with a vitallium mold...[if] the viable neck is too short...osteotomy of the greater trochanter and transplantation to the subtrochanteric region are indicated."

- *Modified Colonna reconstructive operation*: "In non-union with a dead head and absorption of the neck...a deep acetabulum [is created] and freeing all muscle attachments from the greater trochanter down to the infratrochanteric region. After the

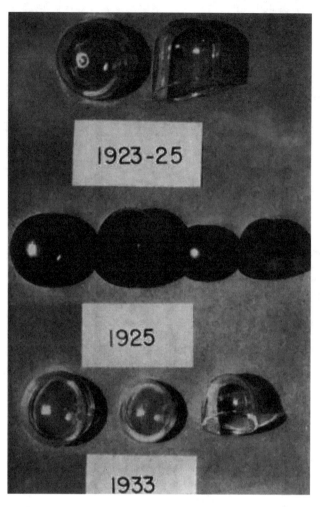

Historical evolution of Smith-Petersen's molds: glass: 1925; Viscoloid: 1925; Pyrex glass: 1933.
M. N. Smith-Petersen, "Arthroplasty of the Hip: A New Method," *Journal of Bone and Joint Surgery* 1939: 21: 270.

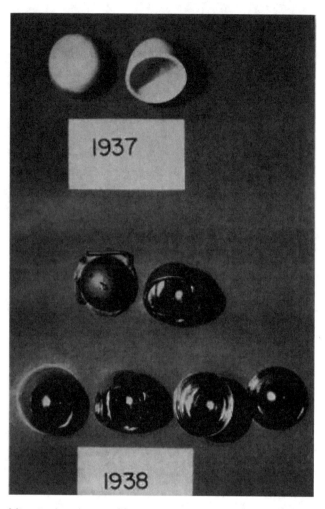

Historical evolution of Smith-Petersen's molds: Bakelite: 1937; unsuccessful and successful Vitallium molds: 1938.
M. N. Smith-Petersen, "Arthroplasty of the Hip: A New Method," *Journal of Bone and Joint Surgery* 1939: 21: 270.

trochanter has been shaped with reamers, care being taken to sacrifice a minimum amount of bone, the mold is applied, and the greater trochanter is introduced into the acetabulum. The divided muscles are transplanted to the infratrochanteric region... To prevent subluxation, the inferior ilium is osteotomized vertically...the outer cortex... sprung laterally; [iliac] bone grafts...are introduced into the cleft...[deepening] the acetabulum...by half an inch or so...Subperiosteal excision of the lesser trochanter... [may be necessary to prevent] mechanical impingement."

- *Intertrochanteric mold arthroplasty*: "In one patient, extensive degenerative changes occurred under the mold, allowing the mold to...rest on both trochanters...After subperiosteal excision of the lesser trochanter, the intertrochanteric region was reconstructed to fit the mold...the atrophied greater trochanter was transplanted to the infratrochanteric region of the shaft...but the shortening is deplorable."

Smith-Petersen (1948) described his experience with what he referred to as "encouraging" results of arthroplasties:

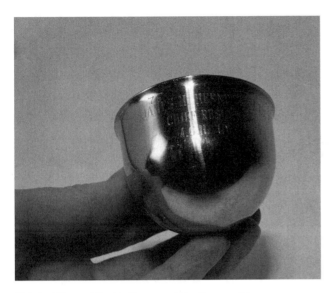

Original flanged Smith-Petersen Vitallium mold or cup. Presented (engraved) to me upon completion of my chief residency at MGH by the HCORP residents, December 1970. Author's cup; photographed by Massachusetts General Hospital Photography Department.

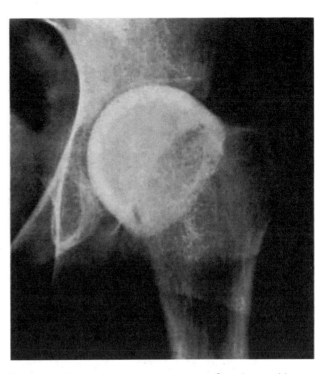

Postoperative roentgenogram, one year after glass mold arthroplasty. M. N. Smith-Petersen, "Arthroplasty of the Hip: A New Method," *Journal of Bone and Joint Surgery* 1939: 21: 271.

- [*Osteoarthritis*]—"[In] eighty-four arthroplasties, six of them bilateral...the results have been more satisfactory than those of arthrodesis. The range of movement obtained has usually been sufficient to enable the patient to put on shoes and stockings. Most...have a limp, but it is a pain-free limp which allows them to lead an active life..."
- *Rheumatoid arthritis*—"[In] seventy-eight arthroplasties, forty-nine of them bilateral... It is fair to say that the results are at least encouraging. The range of movement is not as great as in [osteoarthritis] and seldom sufficient to enable the patient to put on shoes and stockings. As a rule...general activities are increased because of relief of pain; and many...return to active, productive life..."
- *Complications of fractural hips*—"A total of fifty-seven cases have been operated for non-union, aseptic necrosis, and dead heads. The results are very satisfactory and compare favorably with those obtained in [osteoarthritis]..."

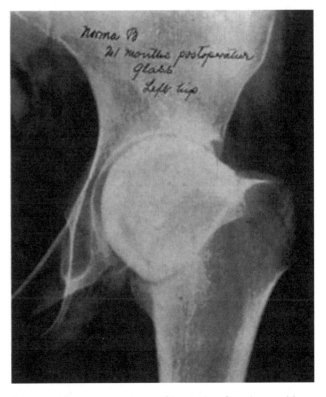

Postoperative roentgenogram, 21 months after glass mold arthroplasty. M. N. Smith-Petersen, "Arthroplasty of the Hip: A New Method," *Journal of Bone and Joint Surgery* 1939: 21: 271.

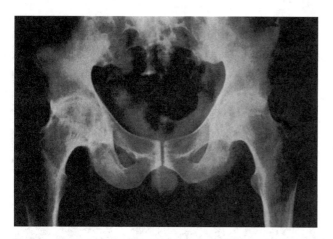

Preoperative roentgenogram of patient with bilateral bony ankylosis of the hips.
M. N. Smith-Petersen, "Arthroplasty of the Hip: A New Method," *Journal of Bone and Joint Surgery* 1939: 21: 276.

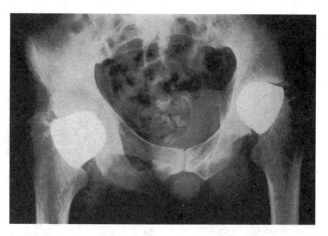

Postoperative roentgenogram of the same patient about 10 months after bilateral Vitallium cup arthroplasties.
M. N. Smith-Petersen, "Arthroplasty of the Hip: A New Method," *Journal of Bone and Joint Surgery* 1939: 21: 276.

- *Old septic hips*—"Twenty-four cases, eight of which were bilateral...The discouraging aspect...is the post-operative flare of original sepsis. This occurred in eight cases. When this complication does not occur, the results are very satisfactory...better than that obtained in rheumatoid arthritis..."
- *Congenital dislocation*—"Forty cases, ten of them bilateral...The results are most satisfactory...The Trendelenburg sign is markedly diminished..."

He also described results of: "Secondary revisions of the first arthroplasty [in] fifty-three patients...these revisions have been necessary to a great extent because of errors in technique and judgment during the early development stages of the procedure" (Smith-Petersen 1948) Complications included sepsis "in twenty cases; eight... in patients with old septic hips" (Smith-Petersen 1948). "Pulmonary embolism has occurred, but never with a fatal outcome" (Smith-Petersen 1948), and vein ligation was resorted to in one case. "In this series of approximately 500 arthroplasties there has been no operative mortality" (Smith-Petersen 1948). Dr. Leo Mayer wrote in a 1950 article published in the *Journal of Bone and Joint Surgery* that:

an intense controversy is still raging with regard to the comparative merits of arthrodesis versus arthroplasty in cases of osteoarthritis [of the hip]. Smith-Petersen in a personal communication has informed the author [Mayer] that within the past ten years he has not once been forced to resort to arthrodesis; other competent surgeons, however, prefer the more certain results of arthrodesis, even though arthrodesis unquestionably throws a severe strain on the lumbar spine.

Dr. Mather Cleveland, an orthopaedic surgeon in New York who was president of the AAOS in 1949, six years after Smith-Petersen, apparently became involved in the controversy about the value of the cup arthroplasty versus the standard accepted treatment—fusion in hip disease at the time. In an unmailed letter to Cleveland, Dr. Smith-Petersen wrote: "Your attitude toward hip arthroplasty was unfavorable...I am writing this letter to make you stop and think." Cleveland may have made some comments against the cup arthroplasty—probably at a professional meeting—and Smith-Petersen composed this letter, but had second thoughts and never mailed it.

Final Teaching and Clinical Contributions

Smith-Petersen "had been elected to all of the important societies of orthopedic surgery, both national and international" ("Marius N. Smith-Petersen" 1953); the most notable are listed in **Box 37.3**. In addition to this impressive list of associations and societies: "Perhaps he was most devoted to the Robert Jones Club to which he was elected shortly after World War I" ("Marius N. Smith-Petersen" 1953). His last clinic was held in April, before this club: "He entertained this group of 25 distinguished American and Canadian orthopedic surgeons in Boston [at MGH] shortly before he died, by operating for them during the morning, demonstrating more than 40 [Vitallium mold] hip arthroplasties in the afternoon, and presiding at a large dinner during the evening" ("Marius N. Smith-Petersen" 1953). The patients he presented at this clinic were effusively grateful

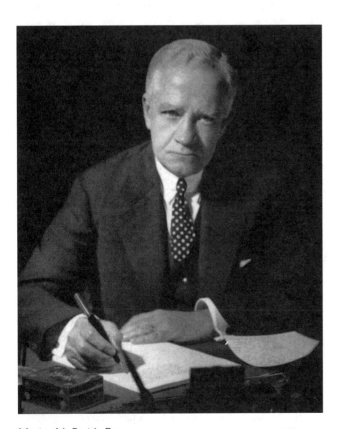

Marius N. Smith-Petersen. "Marius N. Smith-Petersen 1886–1953," *Journal of Bone and Joint Surgery* 1953; 35: 1043.

Box 37.3. Smith-Petersen's Numerous Professional Memberships

In 1953, the *Journal of Bone and Joint Surgery* stated, "Almost endless were his [Smith-Petersen's] honors." He held membership in many societies:

- American Orthopaedic Association
- American Academy of Orthopaedic Surgeons
- International Society of Orthopaedic Surgeons
- International College of Surgeons
- International Academy of Medicine
- World Medical Association
- American College of Surgeons
- American Medical Association
- New England Surgical Society
- Massachusetts Medical Society
- Boston Surgical Society
- Boston Orthopedic Club

He was bestowed honorary memberships in many others:

- Norwegian Surgical Society (1946)
- Grand Cross Royal Norwegian Order of St. Olaf (1947)
- British Orthopaedic Association (1947)
- Société Française d'Orthopédie et de Traumatologie (1948)
- Società Italiana di Orthopedic e Traumatologia (1948)
- Royal Medical Society of Edinburgh (1949)
- Canadian Orthopaedic Association (1949)

His other honors included:

- serving as president of the American Academy of Orthopaedic Surgeons (1943)
- receiving an honorary degree (MD) from the University of Oslo, Norway (1946)
- receiving an honorary fellowship with the Royal Society of Medicine (1952)
- election to Phi Beta Kappa while at the University of Wisconsin

(From "M.N. Smith-Petersen. 1886–1953," *Journal of Bone and Joint Surgery* 35 [1953].)

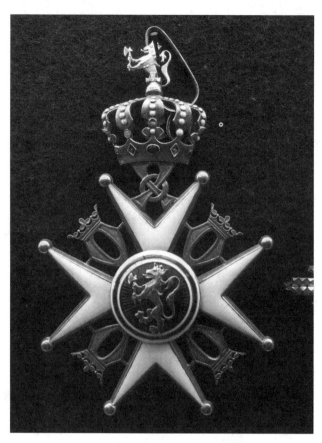

Grand Cross, Royal Norwegian Order of St. Olav.
Daderot/Wikimedia Commons.

LEGACY

Dr. Marius Smith-Petersen had a heart attack and died on June 16, 1953, leaving behind his wife, Hilda (Dickenson) Smith-Petersen, and his three children (two sons and a daughter). Shortly after his death, the Smith-Petersen Foundation was established by former patients as:

> a fund...to be used for furthering orthopedic knowledge. At the discretion of its medical committee (Dr. Otto E. Aufranc, Dr. Joseph S. Barr, and Dr. Morten Smith-Petersen) the funds can be used to care for certain types of hip conditions or indigent patients who have special problems. The funds can also be used to publish results of research in connection with orthopedics. Grateful patients have added to this fund from time to time . . . many of Dr. Smith-Petersen's old students, medical

to him for alleviating their pain and helping them to regain function. "It was his last great teaching effort—a fitting memorial to thirty years of almost ceaseless labor and devotion directed toward the perfection of hip arthroplasty" ("M. N. Smith-Petersen" 1953).

One month later, in May 1953, Smith-Petersen performed a vitallium cup arthroplasty on Arthur Godfrey, a radio-TV star whose hips had been crushed in a car accident more than two decades earlier. Soon after Godfrey's operation, Smith-Petersen became ill himself and was admitted to the Phillips House, where Godfrey was recuperating. Smith-Petersen remained at Phillips House for three-and-a-half weeks.

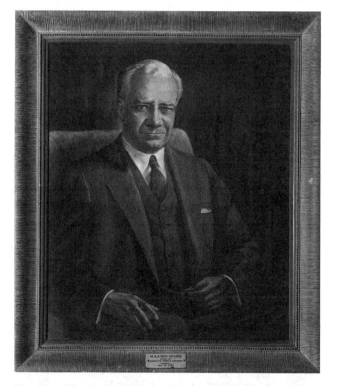

Portrait of Smith-Petersen, by Frankie Aufranc (wife of Otto Aufranc). The portrait hangs in the Smith-Petersen Conference Room, 6th floor of the White Memorial Building.
Massachusetts General Hospital, Archives and Special Collections.

associates, and other friends have also contributed. ("The Smith-Petersen Foundation" 1953)

And about one year after his death—in April 1954—Arthur Godfrey contributed $10,000 to MGH in Smith-Petersen's honor for use in outcome studies of cup arthroplasty.

W. Alexander Law (1953), a British orthopaedist, remembered Smith-Petersen in the *British Medical Journal* and wrote:

> With the death of Dr. M.N. Smith-Petersen the world has lost not only one of its leading orthopaedic surgeons but one of the greatest thinkers in the art and science of surgery....Although he was somewhat sensitive and shy, his greatness was thrown into relief by his humility and sincerity, and he was never happier than when he was surrounded by his students and pupils. Norway, the land of his birth, always lay close to his heart, and his visits there in recent years were sources of great joy and uplift. His own kindliness and generosity matched in full the hospitality and warmth of welcome he came to receive in his native land...His work and writings will last for all time. His quiet smile and sly wink will never be forgotten by his patients and friends, but above all will stand his philosophy of life which he described in these words—written to his godson—"Derive happiness from doing for others. This is a privilege we all have at all times—no one can take it from us."

Joseph S. Barr

A "Gentle Scholar" and a Great Teacher

Joseph Seaton Barr was born October 16, 1901, in Wellsville, Ohio, where he was raised and educated. He attended the College of Wooster in Wooster, Ohio, and graduated in 1922 with a bachelor of science degree. Soon after he left Ohio for Massachusetts to attend Harvard Medical School, from which he graduated magna cum laude in 1926. A general surgical internship at the Peter Brent Brigham Hospital led him to specialize in orthopaedic surgery, for which he received further training at both Children's Hospital and Massachusetts General Hospital 1928–1929. After completing that training, he joined the staff of MGH and became an associate in practice with Dr. Frank Ober (chapter 20). During his almost 35-year career, Barr held various appointments at MGH and elsewhere (**Box 38.1**).

Barr joined the US Navy, beginning active duty on December 20, 1941, soon after Pearl Harbor. He served as chief of the orthopaedic service at the US Naval Hospital in Bethesda, Maryland, until 1946, when he was named senior orthopaedic consultant to the Boston and West Roxbury Veterans Administration Hospitals. During his time in the navy, he helped to establish the Audiovisual Division of the Bureau of Medicine and Surgery and to develop numerous films used by the navy to teach medicine (see chapter 9). He was later appointed as a rear admiral in the US Naval Reserves (Medical Corps) in 1958. He retired from that position in 1962.

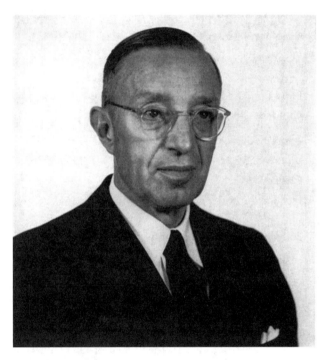

Joseph S. Barr. MGH HCORP Archives.

Physician Snapshot

Joseph S. Barr

BORN: 1901

DIED: 1964

SIGNIFICANT CONTRIBUTIONS: Identified and first described the condition of a herniated disc (along with Drs. Mixter and Kubik); responsible for the establishment of the Orthopaedic Research Laboratory at MGH; one of the founders of the Orthopaedic Research and Education Foundation and the American Academy of Orthopaedic Surgeons

Box 38.1. Barr's Appointments and Positions, 1929–1963

Massachusetts General Hospital

Assistant, Department of Orthopaedics	1929–1932
Orthopaedic Surgeon to Outpatients	1933–1936
Assistant Visiting Orthopaedic Surgeon	1937–1941
Associate Visiting Orthopaedic Surgeon	1942–1947
Chief of the Orthopaedic Service	1947–1964

Harvard Medical School

Assistant in Orthopaedic Surgery	1930–1940
Instructor in Orthopaedic Surgery	1940–1947
Clinical Professor of Orthopaedic Surgery	1947—1964
John Ball and Buckminster Brown Professor	1947–1964

New England Peabody Home for Crippled Children

Assistant Surgeon	1929–1932
Visiting Surgeon	1933–1936
Chief of Staff	1947–1961
Honorary Staff	1961–1963

Journal of Bone and Joint Surgery

Member of the Board of Associate Editors	1944–1947
Vice chairman of the Board of Associate Editors	1948–1955
Shriner's Hospital for Crippled Children, member of Advisory Board of Orthopaedic Surgeons	1949–1963
Children's Hospital, member of Board of Consultation in Orthopaedics	1950–?
Boston Lying-In Hospital, Consultant in Orthopaedics	1952–?
Lemuel Shattuck Hospital, Senior Consultant in Orthopaedic Surgery	1954–?
Alfred I. du Pont Institute for Crippled Children, member of the Medical Advisory Board	1955–?
Nemours Foundation, member of the Medical Advisory Board	1955–?
Orthopaedic Research and Education Foundation president	1959–1961

In 1947 upon returning to MGH after World War II, Barr, succeeding Dr. Marius Smith-Petersen as chief of the orthopaedic department, was promoted to clinical professor of orthopaedic surgery at Harvard Medical School. Dean George P. Berry then named Barr as the John B. and Buckminster Brown Clinical Professor of Orthopaedic Surgery upon Frank Ober's retirement. Barr was the first to hold this professorship but not also be the chief of orthopaedics at Children's Hospital. Interestingly, in 1931 this endowed chair had become "part-time" rather than "full-time" because of inadequate funds. The medical school had added "Clinical" to the title because of the partial funding. In May 1962, the Permanent Charity Fund of Boston donated money to the university; with it was established the Edith M. Ashley Fund to support a professorship in orthopaedic surgery. This fund allowed Barr to move into his professorship on a full-time basis. After Barr's death, Dr. Thornton Brown was named acting chief until Glimcher was appointed chief of orthopaedics at Massachusetts General Hospital in 1965 and became the first to hold both of the Edith M. Ashley Professorship (see chapter 24); Dr. Sledge was awarded the John B. and Buckminster Brown Professorship in 1978 (see chapter 48). Also, in 1962 Harvard Medical School received a generous gift from the trustees of the New England Peabody Home for Crippled Children, which provided the Harriet M. Peabody Professorship in Orthopaedic Surgery; Dr. William T. Green was named the first professor of this chair (see chapter 21).

CLINICAL CONTRIBUTIONS

Dr. Barr published more than 80 articles on a variety of topics in orthopaedic surgery, mainly regarding backache and sciatica, polio, and scoliosis. He also championed orthopaedic research at MGH.

Back Pain and Sciatica

At the turn of the twentieth century, physicians understood the rarer causes of back pain but did not recognize the etiology in many less extreme cases. Uncertainty plagued its treatment:

> [Around 1900] the uncommon causes of symptoms were well known and carefully described. Tumors, tuberculosis, syphilis, gout were recognized as etiologic agents, but there was little knowledge of the common causes such as disk lesions, mechanical instability, and spondylolisthesis. Treatment fifty years ago was empiric—fantastically so—leaches, cupping, purging, and acupuncture were commonly used for sciatica, which was thought to be a primary neuritis.
>
> (Mayer 1950)

Mayer (1950) also points out that, because of "pioneering work" by many of Boston's orthopaedic surgeons—including Joel Goldthwait (chapter 33), Charles F. Painter (chapter 45), Robert Osgood (chapter 19), C. Hermann Bucholz (chapter 40), and Loring T. Swaim (chapter 46)—"this vast limbo known as 'lumbago' [was transformed] into…anatomically based differential diagnoses." Research by Goldthwait, Russell A. Hibbs, and Vittorio Putti, particularly relating to the facet joints of the lumbosacral spine, suggested "mechanical strain and arthritis" as potential causes of low-back pain and sciatic, whereas "other investigators laid stress on the role of the sacro-iliac joints" (Mayer 1950). Still, even at mid-twentieth century, "there was little agreement on the location of the exact structures involved or on proper methods of treatment" (Mayer 1950). Backache and sciatica were in the 1950s—and still are today—major problems confronted by patients. "As a rule, it [sciatica] is an obstinate affection, lasting for months, or even, with slight remissions, for years. Relapses are not uncommon, and the disease may be relieved in one nerve only to appear in the other. In the severer forms, the patient is bedridden, and such cases prove among the most distressing and trying which the physician is called upon to treat" (Osler quoted in Mayer 1950).

W. Jason Mixter, the head of the Department of Neurosurgery at MGH at the time of Barr's arrival in 1929, focused the service's work on neurologic pain, reflex sympathetic dystrophy (now called complex regional pain syndrome), sciatica, and tumors of the spine. Barr and Mixter found a common interest in low back pain. Barr had spent months unsuccessfully trying to treat conservatively

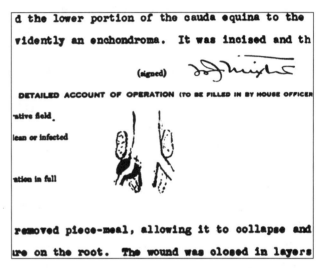

Operative report by William J. Mixter with his drawing of the small mass he found encroaching on the left S1 nerve root.
Massachusetts General Hospital, Archives and Special Collections.

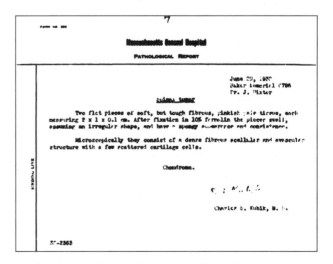

Dr. Charles Kubik's pathology report. Original diagnosis: chondroma; later revised to herniated nucleus pulposis.
Massachusetts General Hospital, Archives and Special Collections.

a 25-year-old man with intractable lumbar pain with sciatica. Barr eventually consulted with Mixter on the hunch that the man had a tumor on the spinal cord. Laminectomy allowed Mixter to identify a small mass compressing the S1 nerve root.

Barr did not believe that the excised tissue could represent a tumor, as the patient's symptoms had occurred abruptly after a traumatic injury. Indeed, pathology showed that the mass comprised cartilage rather than tumor cells. He obtained tissue samples from the "spinal enchondromas" Mixter had removed during previous procedures, and he evaluated them against normal tissue from vertebral discs that had been obtained during autopsies. The pathologist Dr. Charles Kubik also reviewed the specimens and verified that the "tumor" tissue and the normal tissue did not differ. Mixter and Barr's study of tumor specimens and normal tissue, along with details learned from reading a publication by G. Schmorl, a German researcher on disc anatomy and disc herniations, led them to deduce that ruptured herniated discs compressed nerve roots and generated radiculitis in the legs.

Throughout the rest of 1932, Mixter removed vertebral discs from three more patients because of nerve pain. One of those received a diagnosis of "ruptured intervertebral disc"—but that diagnosis came only after the procedure. Much of the medical community outside MGH questioned Mixter and Barr's approach, but, just as 1933 began, Philip Wilson, another orthopaedic surgeon at MGH (chapter 40), performed the same procedure on a patient. However, in that case there was a *preoperative* diagnosis of "herniated intervertebral disc"—providing initial support for Mixter and Barr's approach.

> "Life is short and the art long, the occasion instant, experiment perilous, decision difficult."
> —Hippocrates
> Quoted by Barr in his AAOS presidential address, this translated version is inscribed on a Harvard Medical School building

On September 30, 1933, Mixter and Barr presented their now classical paper, "Rupture of the Intervertebral Disc with Involvement of the Spinal Canal," to the New England Surgical Society at its annual meeting in Boston. In 1934, they published it with a summary of the results of surgical treatment in 19 cases—both lumbar and cervical lesions. In their introduction, they reviewed the contributions of other surgeons such as Goldthwait and Walter Dandy, who "have been reporting cases of spinal cord pressure from intervertebral disc lesions" (Mixter and Barr 1934). For Mixter and Barr (1934), however, Schmorl's work was "the most complete, painstaking and authoritative that has ever been done in this condition [but is] purely pathological" and must be "correlate[d] with clinical findings." They then described their own brief path to understanding the herniated disc syndrome:

> Our interest in this group of cases was stimulated particularly by a case seen by us two years ago in which the main symptoms were referable to root pain and in which the tumor was situated in the intervertebral foramen without cord or cauda equina compression...
>
> Investigation of the cases of spinal cord tumor treated at the Massachusetts General Hospital and in our private practice has shown a surprisingly large number...classified as chondromata, to be in truth not tumors of cartilage,

NEW ENGLAND SURGICAL SOCIETY
RUPTURE OF THE INTERVERTEBRAL DISC WITH INVOLVEMENT OF THE SPINAL CANAL*
BY WILLIAM JASON MIXTER, M.D.,† AND JOSEPH S. BARR, M.D.†
N. E. J. OF M.
AUG. 2, 1934

Mixter's and Barr's classic article on ruptures of the intervertebral disc. *New England Journal of Medicine* 1934; 211: 210.

but prolapses of the nucleus pulposus or fracture of the annulus…Nineteen of our cases are rupture of the disc and six are true cartilaginous tumor or unclassified…Diagnosis has been made difficult and operation has been delayed…on account of the indefinite nature of the symptoms and signs and their similarity to those found in various conditions such as back strain, arthritis, sacro-iliac disease, etc. (Mixter and Barr 1934)

Mixter and Barr (1934) made six conclusions based on their study of these 19 cases of ruptured intervertebral disc in both the lumbar and cervical spines:

- Herniation of the nucleus pulposus into the spinal canal, or as we prefer to call it, rupture of the intervertebral disc, is a not uncommon cause of symptoms.
- This lesion frequently has been mistaken for cartilaginous neoplasm arising from the intervertebral disc.
- In reality rupture of the disc is more common than neoplasm; in our series in the ratio of three to one.
- This lesion should be borne in mind in the study of certain orthopedic conditions, particularly in those cases which do not respond to appropriate treatment.
- A presumptive diagnosis may be made in many instances and that operation whether for this or for supposed spinal cord tumor should always be planned with the possibility of finding this lesion.
- The treatment of this disease is surgical and that the results obtained are very satisfactory if compression has not been too prolonged.

In a discussion of their paper Barr noted that Mixter performed the surgery on almost all of their 19 patients, whereas his own interest lay in their "orthopaedic aspects." With the help of Dr. Benjamin Castleman, a resident pathologist at MGH, Barr:

compared the histology of the material removed at operation from eighteen cases with the histology of intervertebral disc and…found that seven…represent purely annulus tissues, four cases nucleus pulposus only and seven contained elements of both…In ten of the nineteen cases the lesion was either between the fourth and fifth lumbar vertebrae or the fifth lumbar and the sacrum. Every one of these cases… clinically resembled lumbosacral or sacro-iliac strain, and several of them were treated under this diagnosis for a considerable period of time. (Mixter and Barr 1934)

Although some were initially skeptical of Mixter and Barr's conclusions, their article "led to a revolutionary change…regarding the origin of low back pain. Whereas before it had been ascribed to 'arthritis' of the lumbosacral junction or 'sacro-iliac' strain, it can be said without contradiction that Barr and Mixter established conclusively that lower back pain with sciatica is in a large majority of cases due to injury of the intervertebral disc. As a result, an enormous number of patients have been relieved of their disabling condition" (Cave, n.d.). According to Brown et al. (1966), this was Barr's most important work.

Case 38.1 describes the procedure and investigation done by Mixter and Barr for their first patient with a herniated disc, to whom they referred as "case 14." In 1985, Frymoyer and Donaghy reported a 50-year follow-up of case 14 (a man with the initials "K.N."):

There is no doubt that this patient was the first one when Mixter and Barr diagnosed the lesion now known as a herniated intervertebral disc. On February 7, 1946, Mixter wrote to one of us [Donaghy], "K.N. is of particular interest as he is the first patient in whom a ruptured intervertebral disc was recognized as such and as the cause for sciatica. Therefore, he is the man who started all the damn trouble." Mixter also wrote…"I remember K.N. very well. He was operated on following a long period of hospitalization under Dr. Ober's care, during which Dr. Barr saw him frequently…When he was operated on at the Baker Memorial, a diagnosis of tumor of the low cauda equina was made and at operation a rounded swelling was found on the margin of the fifth lumbar intervertebral disc. The pathology report was enchondroma. Dr. Barr and I 'smelled a rat' in this diagnosis… [K.N.'s] pain had followed closely on a severe skiing accident…[Upon] consultation with [the] pathologist, Dr. Kubik, we found that the material examined was normal cartilage…[K.N.] was the first case that focused an attention on rupture of the intervertebral disc with sciatica [and thus] is the key case in the development of the surgery of ruptured intervertebral disc."

After the operation on K.N…he [Mixter] and Barr met in the corridor of the Old Bulfinch Building. Barr was recorded as stating: "K.N.'s symptoms had followed an injury and therefore a diagnosis of tumor was unsound"…Barr suggested that "the lesion found in K.N.'s spine might be a Schmorl's node." Barr examined the slides with Kubik and was struck by the lack of cellular material…and compared [material from a normal disc] with the specimen from…K.N. The two tissues seemed to Barr and Kubik to be identical [and thus that from K.N. was] not a neoplasm.

K.N.'s laminectomy had successfully relieved his sciatic pain.

In a 1986 letter to the editor of the *Journal of Bone and Joint Surgery*, Dr. Jonathan Cohen noted that he had talked with Barr 22 years earlier (at a 1964 faculty meeting at Harvard) about

Case 38.1. Rupture of the Intervertebral Disc with Involvement of the Spinal Canal

"A twenty-five-year-old white man was admitted to the Massachusetts General Hospital June 13, 1932 complaining of pain and stiffness in his left leg of two years' duration. A few months before the onset the patient sustained a severe ski fall, but had no immediate disability. He noticed at first only mild discomfort in his back and the posterior portion of his left thigh, but it increased gradually until he was unable to work. The pain radiated down the calf and into the heel. There was a little discomfort in the other leg. He finally consulted one of us, who treated him with adhesive strapping and corset to support his back, with a tentative diagnosis of low back strain. He spent several months in absolute recumbency on a Bradford frame without relief. On account of lack of improvement, it was decided to institute a complete neurological investigation.

"On admission he presented the clinical picture of a man suffering from an extremely acute back strain. He stood with his knees flexed, the trunk listed forward and to the right. The motions of the lumbar spine were almost abolished by muscle spasm. Straight leg raising was limited to 25° on the left and 80° on the right. Neurological examination was negative except for absent ankle jerk on the left. There was tenderness along the course of the sciatic nerve, especially in the sciatic notch.

"Lumbar puncture showed questionable partial block and a definite elevation in the total protein to 108 milligrams. Lipiodol examination was negative.

"On June 29, 1932 an exploratory laminectomy from the second lumbar to the first sacral inclusive, was done. After prolonged search a mass one centimeter in diameter was found in the intervertebral foramen pressing on the left fifth lumbar root and displacing the cauda equina to the right. It was removed piecemeal from the intervertebral disc and the wound was closed. Recovery was complete and uneventful. He had complete relief from pain immediately after the operation and has remained well since his recovery from the operation.

"Pathological examination of the specimen showed it to be composed almost wholly of dense eosin staining fibrous connective tissue characteristic of annulus fibrosus. The original report classified this specimen as a chondroma."

(William J. Mixter and Joseph S. Barr 1934)

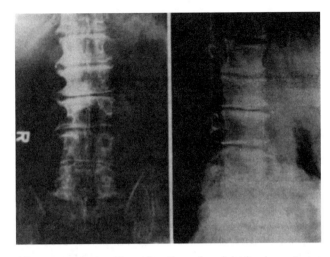

Anteroposterior and lateral radiographs of the lumbar spine of the first patient that Mixter and Barr correctly diagnosed a ruptured herniated disc as a cause of sciatica—49 years later. The patient had no back or leg pain.

J. W. Frymoyer and R.M. Donaghy, "The ruptured intervertebral disc: Follow-up report on the first case fifty years after recognition of the syndrome and its surgical significance," *Journal of Bone and Joint Surgery* 1985; 67: 1113.

Barr's "extensive consultative experience concerning impairments related to discal pathology and its surgical treatment." He reported Barr's thoughts on the matter:

> He said that he was sorry that the discovery of herniation of the disc had led to so high an incidence of "back cripples," and he thought that they were more common and more severely impaired after surgery than they would have been had no surgical treatment been pursued. This fact, in my opinion, was part of the "damn trouble." Dr. Barr also was concerned with the attribution of back pain to the so-called bulging disc, and the diagnostic and surgical measures aimed at that (arguable) observation. Part of the "damn trouble," therefore, also consisted of Barr's realizing that the pathological changes...in the intervertebral disc were diverse, and did not always allow as easy correlation between the lesion and the signs and symptoms. (Cohen 1986)

Barr continued to study intervertebral disc disorders throughout his career. Over the next 23 years, he published 18 articles on his clinical experiences. As early as 1937, he mentioned coupling spine fusion and laminectomy in patients with a disc herniation, stating, "Our experience indicates that the back is stronger," when such a combination is used (Barr 1937). In 1941, Barr and Mixter reported results regarding back pain and strength after laminectomy:

> [They] found that 60 percent of their patients deny having any back symptoms, and consider themselves as strong physically as before the onset of their disability. Thirty-two per cent complain of slight to moderate back weakness or discomfort, and 8 per cent consider themselves markedly disabled. In other words, 40 percent would probably have had to seek lighter work if their occupation entailed manual labor...There are two probable explanations for...a weak, painful back. The mechanical derangement due to the ruptured disc is obvious...Secondly, the laminectomy itself may weaken the back to a greater or lesser degree, particularly if sacrifice of an articular facet is necessary...Seventy-three per cent of the patients having fusion considered their backs of normal strength whereas only 52 per cent of those without fusion had no complaints...This series of cases is as yet too small to allow definite conclusions...but there is a place for spine fusion at the time of laminectomy in perhaps 20 to 30 per cent of the cases of protruded intervertebral discs.

Barr continued supporting the use of spine fusion in patients with low back pain, lumbar instability, or both after laminectomy. In 1947, he reported his experience at the US Naval Hospital in Bethesda, Maryland, where he worked with neurosurgeons to complete such combined operations:

> Before my arrival [the neurosurgeons] had been operating on ruptured discs, without

spine fusions...but they were not entirely satisfied with their results and they...requested the Orthopaedic Service to cooperate with them in doing a series of cases by the combined operations, the neurosurgeons...to remove the ruptured disc, the orthopaedic surgeons fusing the spine and caring for the patient postoperatively. All of the patients with ruptured discs at Bethesda during the period from August 1944 to December 1945 had this combined operation. The fusion was done according to Bosworth's technique...Almost all of the officers were returned to full duty...In my opinion, any patient in whom a facetectomy has been done, either partial or complete...should have a spine fusion done at the same time... (Barr 1947)

Investigations of the end results of various studies indicated that back pain or weakness occur after excision without fusion in up to 50% of patients. Barr listed the various methods surgeons at MGH applied when performing spinal fusion:

- Hibbs's method
- Hibbs's method combined with a bone graft from the tibia
- a bone graft from the tibia, using wiring to fixate the graft to the spinous processes
- interbody fusion
- Gibson's clothespin graft, as modified by D. Bosworth

For his part, however, Barr discontinued the use of interbody fusion after only a few attempts because it was "too dangerous."

In 1951, Barr wrote in the *Journal of Bone and Joint Surgery* that there was still no definitive consensus on whether to always use the combined operation (laminectomy with fusion), and at MGH it was performed in only select cases (~30–40%): "since our first recognition of the syndrome 19 years ago...Our staff has been aware of the potential benefits to be derived from this operation, but we have also recognized its technical difficulties."

Barr's last publication—which wasn't published until after his death—listed him as the first author and included five others as coauthors (including Maureen K. Molloy, said to have been the first female resident in the Harvard Combined Orthopaedic Residency Program [see chapter 11]). The authors mention the ongoing debate over the appropriateness of the combined operation (simple excision vs. excision and spinal fusion), noting that some at MGH endorsed it, whereas others claimed the risk and extended recovery time canceled out any advantages. The paper reviewed results from 644 private patients operated on at MGH over 10 years (from January 1947 through December 1956) for ruptured discs at the fourth and fifth lumbar spaces and for the occasional lesion at the third lumbar space. After a careful analysis of all results—including poor results and failures after the combined operation—the authors recognized that fusing the spine does not provide significantly better results. On the basis of extended hospitalization after the procedure, a longer recovery period, and the potential for severe postoperative complications, surgeons at MGH continued to reduce their use of the combined procedure. Although more than a decade earlier Barr had noted, on the basis of patient reports, that the combined procedure reduced back pain, in 1967 the authors determined that the results were similar for both simple excision and excision combined with fusion.

Scoliosis

The Research Committee of the American Orthopaedic Association, supported in part by a grant from the Alfred I. DuPont Institute, reported an "End-Result Study of the Treatment of Idiopathic Scoliosis" in 1941. Barr was a member of this committee, along with Drs. Paul C. Colonna and Lawrence Noall; Dr. A. R. Shands Jr. served as chairperson. They reviewed the end results of 425 cases from 16 clinics throughout the United States. Their conclusions were surprising, as conservative (nonoperative) care was not successful:

1. Practically none of the patients with scoliosis are cured, if correction of lateral deviation is a criterion.
2. In approximately 60 per cent of those treated by exercises the deformity increased and in 40 per cent, it remained unchanged.
3. Correction without fusion resulted in complete loss of correction after support was discontinued, in the majority of instances.
4. Correction by the turnbuckle jacket and subsequent fusion has yielded better results in this series than have other types of treatment. (Shands et al. 1941)

Treatment with the turnbuckle jacket and then fusion remained the treatment of choice at Children's Hospital from that time through the beginning of the 1970s, when internal fixation with a Harrington rod replaced it.

Polio

Barr was also interested in poliomyelitis and published 11 articles on a variety of topics including tendon transfers, leg length inequality, and stabilization of the paralyzed shoulder. He chaired the Research Committee of the AAOS, which in 1942 surveyed 20 polio clinics in the US regarding the results of stabilization in patients with a paralyzed shoulder. The committee reported that:

arthrodesis of the shoulder joint is the operation of choice in all cases of infantile paralysis with complete paralysis of the deltoid...The optimum position of fusion was...45 to 55 degrees of abduction, 15 to 25 degrees of flexion and 15 to 25 degrees of internal rotation...Postoperative fixation in plaster [lasts] from a minimum of three months to a maximum of five months...The satisfactory muscle transplantations were found only in those cases possessing fair power in the deltoid preoperatively. (Barr et al. 1942)

In 1950, Barr, then chair of the Section on Orthopedic Surgery of the American Medical Association, addressed the organization, speaking about "Poliomyelitis Hip Deformity and the Erector Spinae Transplant." With the assistance of Drs. John A. Reidy and Thomas F. Broderick, Barr had reviewed the records of 50 consecutive patients who had an erector spinae transplant through the method described by Ober in 1927 (and by Dr. E. W. H. Groves that same year). Patients were followed at MGH and in the Crippled Children's Division of Vermont's Department of Public Health, where Barr consulted for more than three decades. In his summary, Barr stated that patients with hip contractures with accompanying deformity of the lumbar spine after polio must be evaluated carefully and continually for fascial contractures, as the iliotibial band has a tendency to shorten as a child grows. Surgeons must make all efforts to prevent such contractures, but when they occur, surgery is required in order to resolve the problem. Barr recommended transplant of the erector spinae muscle with soft-tissue release.

Barr was surgeon-in-chief at the New England Peabody Home for Crippled Children for almost 15 years, a position he maintained until 1961. According to T. Brown, writing for the *Harvard University Gazette* in 1966, Barr's extensive knowledge of polio and experience caring for patients with the disease made his work there invaluable.

A SURVEY OF END RESULTS ON STABILIZATION OF THE PARALYTIC SHOULDER*†

REPORT OF THE RESEARCH COMMITTEE OF THE AMERICAN ORTHOPAEDIC ASSOCIATION

JOSEPH S. BARR, M.D., *Chairman*
JOSEPH A. FREIBERG, M.D.
PAUL C. COLONNA, M.D.
PAUL A. PEMBERTON, M.D., *Research Fellow*

THE JOURNAL OF BONE AND JOINT SURGERY   VOL. XXIV, NO. 3, JULY 1942

Dr. Barr as chair of the AOA research committee reported the results of the committee's survey on shoulder fusion. Their recommended position of a fused shoulder remains the standard today. *Journal of Bone and Joint Surgery* 1942; 24: 699.

THE SURGICAL EXPERIMENT

In 1951, Barr was elected president of the American Academy of Orthopaedic Surgeons, after having helped to establish the organization in 1934. In his presidential address at the AAOS annual meeting that year, he spoke about "The Surgical Experiment." He discussed variables that could affect surgical procedures and focused specifically on implants to be left inside the patient's body after surgery:

> We scarcely need to be reminded that every surgical operation is an experiment in which many variable factors are present, most of them not under the control of the surgeon. Because of these uncontrolled variables, the results of operative treatment are predictable only in a statistical fashion by post hoc analysis of results obtained in a significant number of similar cases. We recognize that the outcome in an individual case is not accurately predictable and that chance plays a role in determining the result...The variable factor which I particularly wish to consider today relates to the surgical materials left in the patient's body...We must use every means at our disposal to lessen the peril of the surgical experiment. In doing so, we are true to the physician's mission in life— "The multiplying of human enjoyments, and the mitigation of human suffering," [as we promise to first do no harm]. (Barr 1952)

During his speech, Barr urged the medical community to establish a multidisciplinary committee to study surgical materials. His suggestion resulted in the organization of the American Surgical Materials Association, a consortium that worked toward "the standardization and quality control of surgical implants" (Brown et al. 1966). In effect, that talk in 1951 "was largely responsible for present-day awareness of the need for adequate research in development of surgical implants to be used in the human body" (Brown et al. 1966).

In 1954, Barr, then chair of the Joint Committee for the Study of Surgical Materials, pushed the editor of the *Journal of Bone and Joint Surgery* to publish the committee's work in order to further the goal of creating the as yet unrealized American Surgical Materials Association: "For the past two years, the Joint Committee...has been hard at work. Our report should be of interest to all orthopaedic surgeons and we would be grateful if you would publish it...The proposed American Surgical Materials Association has not yet come into being. We hope that our report will serve to outline the magnitude of the problems and will be the basis for appropriate action."

The Joint Committee consisted of Drs. E. F. Cave, F. H. Mayfield, and F. L. McLaughlin, representing the American College of Surgeons; Drs. J. Grandlay, M. Gage, and R. De Forest, representing the American Medical Association; and Drs. L. Peterson, H. Smith, and Barr, representing the AAOS. Their report described those organizations' joint effort to thoroughly review the current status of manufactured materials, quality control issues, damage units, and existing organizations, e.g., the American Society for Testing and Materials and perhaps implant manufacturers, and to propose by-laws for and develop the structure of a new organization.

In 1962, the AAOS joined with the American Society for Testing and Materials (ATSM) forming the Committee F-4 on Surgical Implants to establish standards for all surgical implants. It is known today as the ATSM Committee F-4 on Medical and Surgical Materials and Devices.

ORTHOPAEDIC RESEARCH

Barr had long recognized the need for research if the orthopaedic department was going to continue to be one of the best. However, he had a difficult time starting a research program because he had no funds, no orthopaedic surgeon who was skilled in basic laboratory research, and no support for research from MGH. And then opportunity knocked: Melvin Glimcher was a senior resident with a strong basic science background and an interest in research. Barr recruited him to obtain further basic research experience at MIT and open a basic orthopaedic research laboratory in MGH. With approval of the trustees, he was given a space and permission to use the balance of money left by Goldthwait after building Ward I to furnish the lab with equipment. (For more on this, see chapters 24 and 43.) According to E. F. Cave (n.d.), Barr's "second most important accomplishment [after identifying the condition of herniated disc with Mixter and Kubik] was the establishment of the Orthopedic Research Laboratories at the Massachusetts General Hospital. This had been a dream of his for years, and it became a reality in 1960."

On September 11, 1960, Dr. Franklin C. McLean, professor emeritus (physiology) at the University of Chicago, gave the keynote address at a luncheon to celebrate the opening of the new Orthopaedic Research Laboratory, before more than 200 attendees from the orthopaedic staff, MGH, Harvard Medical School, and other medical schools and hospitals. In his address, Professor McLean began with a quote from a 1947 AAOS instructional course that highlighted the important connection between orthopaedics and basic science, noting that "your success in practice will be measured not only in terms of your ability to deal with injury and deformity, but equally in terms of your grasp of the metabolic and systemic problems that come to you." McLean lamented the long-standing lack of a relation between research and the practice of medicine, but he believed that a revolution of sorts began in the early twentieth century in bridging the two. This revolution created burgeoning connections between medical education and research—such as the opening of research departments at major educational institutions such as the University of Pennsylvania and the publication of the Flexner report—and between medical practice and research, as embodied by the opening of the Hospital of the Rockefeller Institute of Medical Research. In McLean's words, institutions were beginning to recognize the need to make hospitals both a "locus for" and an "instrument of" research. He describes numerous early examples of this—from the organization of the *American Society for the Advancement of Clinical Investigation* in 1909 (and the ongoing search for the most appropriate definition of "clinical investigation") to the creation of a clinic and labs for clinical investigation by David Edsall at MGH in 1912.

After driving home the importance of research and clinical investigation to specialty knowledge and practice, McLean went on to describe how the new Orthopaedic Research Laboratory at MGH would continue to strengthen that connection through an understanding of both basic science and the clinical practice of orthopaedics, and through collaboration with researchers at other institutions:

> The Orthopedic Research Laboratories, by deliberate policy, will engage in basic or fundamental research, in the extreme sense in which these terms are applied. This does not say that the patient is to be lost sight of; it does say that any research bearing on the musculo-skeletal system is a proper field for inquiry, to be carried out in a hospital and under hospital auspices. We may expect to see publications originating from these laboratories, reporting on research carried on by all the methods available in the physical and biological sciences. In a sense this is a return to the 1909 definition of clinical investigation, which I have quoted, as "medical research...by men actively engaged in the practice of medicine," since it is their interest in medicine that brings them together.
>
> I do not mean to imply by this that all of those who work in these laboratories will be physicians; this will by no means be true. As long ago as 1914 physicists were brought into the problem of cancer in the Collis P. Huntington Memorial Hospital for Cancer Research.

This tradition has been carried on in the Massachusetts General Hospital up to the present time; the contributions of the Massachusetts Institute of Technology in research at the M.G.H. have been many and important; there is no doubt that this collaboration will continue, as well as collaboration with the "departmental institutes of medical science" at the Harvard Medical School. We may expect every tool available to the investigator in the biological sciences to be brought to bear on the problems to be studied in these new laboratories, and we may expect to have, in a paraphrase of the words of S. J. Meltzer "a differentiation of orthopedics into a science and a practice." (McLean 1960)

The MGH orthopaedic research laboratories have remained active and continue to contribute major scientific advancements; thus fulfilling Dr. Barr's original vision.

A LASTING LEGACY

Barr received many honors during his career. He was granted an honorary membership in the British Orthopaedic Association, and he was welcomed into the American Academy of Arts and Sciences in 1944. Thirty years after graduating from the College of Wooster, in 1952, his alma mater conferred on him an honorary doctor of science degree. In 1957, he gave both the Samuel Higby Camp

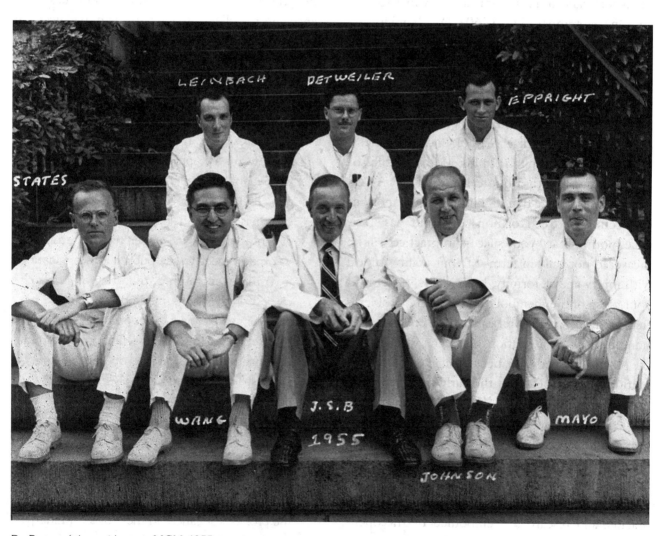

Dr. Barr and the residents at MGH, 1955. MGH HCORP Archives.

Lecture (at the University of San Francisco) and the Sir Robert Jones Lecture (to the Royal College Surgeons in London), during which he discussed "Theoretical and Practical Considerations with a Follow-up Study of Prosthetic Replacement of the Femoral Head at the Massachusetts General Hospital." In these prestigious lectures, Barr reviewed his experience using the Austin Moore prosthesis (a femoral head replacement) for hip fractures, and it became his only publication on hip fractures (in 1964). His large series of cases (>600) make his findings quite intriguing:

> Arthroplasty of the hip, using the Vitallium mold…has been in continuous use at the Massachusetts General Hospital for more than twenty years…Certain patients with hip disability are not suitable candidates…[and] in 1952 we began using the Austin Moore Vitallium prosthesis for ununited intracapsular fractures of the hip, avascular necrosis of the femoral head, and selected fresh fractures of the femoral neck…In the ten years…more than 600 patients…have been treated by this method in our hospital…The results were satisfactory or better to the surgeon in 84 per cent of the patients…Satisfactory results…in other conditions such as degenerative arthritis, post infection arthritis and congenital dysplasia or dislocation of the hip, were much less frequent…Mold arthroplasty appears to be preferable to prosthetic replacement in rheumatoid arthritis and in burned-out pyogenic infections. Reconstructive surgery for neurotrophic hip disease, in our limited experience, was unsuccessful. (Barr, Donovan, and Florence 1964)

In 1955, Dr. Barr helped found the Orthopaedic Research and Education Foundation. He was a member of its board of trustees, and he served as its president from 1959 to 1961. He also served for many years as a senior medical consultant at both the Chelsea Naval Hospital and the Boston Veterans Hospital in Jamaica Plain, Massachusetts.

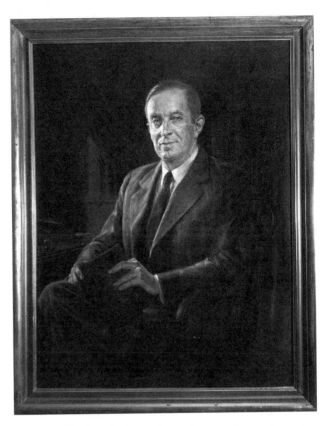

Portrait of Dr. Barr by Pietro Pezzati. Massachusetts General Hospital, Archives and Special Collections.

He had been a consultant to the Division of Handicapped Children's Services in Vermont, attending the annual summer clinics for over 30 years. Upon his retirement in 1963, the Division established the Joseph S. Barr Visiting Consultantship.

Barr was a member of the American Medical Association, American Board of Orthopaedic Surgery, Boston Orthopaedic Club, Interurban Orthopaedic Club, Harvey Cushing Society, New England Surgical Society, Boston Surgical Society, American College of Surgeons, and International Society of Orthopaedic Surgery and Traumatology.

Clement Sledge, once one of Barr's students and later his successor to the Buckminster Brown Professorship, characterized Barr as a "gentle scholar": "His gentleness and his consideration for medical students and residents was legendary… He never stopped being a student, was continually taking notes, and had an openness and an intellectual honesty that was very impressive for a young person to see" (Sledge, n.d.).

Barr had emphysema, even though he had never smoked, and it progressively worsened as he aged. Despite those physical effects, he continued his work until October 28, 1964, when he retired. He died soon after, on December 6. He was 63 years old. He was survived by his wife, Dorrice (Nash), a daughter (Mary), and a son, Joseph S. Barr Jr., who also became an orthopaedic surgeon (see chapter 40). After Barr's death, MGH established the Joseph S. Barr Memorial Fund to "strengthen resident training and...to help finance the orthopaedic operating room suite."

In 1966, Brown et al., in a bio of Barr written for the *Harvard University Gazette*, noted that: "His passing deprived him of the satisfaction of seeing his efforts bear fruit—the transition of the Orthopaedic Service at the Massachusetts General Hospital, which was largely clinically oriented, to an academic service with proper balance between clinical and research activities." Brown et al. summed up Barr's impressive career and his leadership eloquently:

> [Barr's] career as a teacher, investigator, and practitioner of orthopaedic surgery spanned thirty-six years, a time when this surgical specialty passed through its greatest period of growth and development. During these years of great progress Dr. Barr was amongst the leaders...His reputation was international, and his friends were worldwide...Joseph Barr had an inquiring mind with an unusual ability to analyze problems or situations and to reach wise decisions. He was one of the great teachers of orthopaedic surgery of our generation.

CHAPTER 39

William H. Harris
Innovator in Hip Replacement Surgery

William Hamilton Harris was born in Great Falls, Montana, on November 18, 1927. His family moved to Harrisburg, Pennsylvania, and he attended Haverford College, where he was both a Corporation Fellow and a Clementine Cope Fellow. He graduated in 1947—achieving high honors in chemistry and being elected into Phi Beta Kappa. After having also been elected into Alpha Omega Alpha and obtaining his medical degree from the University of Pennsylvania in 1951, Harris remained there as an intern and an assistant resident in surgery. He then completed a two-year military obligation as a captain in the 5005th USAF Hospital (Elmendorf) in Anchorage, Alaska.

EARLY RESEARCH AND CONTRIBUTIONS

In 1955, Dr. William Harris was accepted in the Boston Children's Hospital–Massachusetts General Hospital (MGH) Combined Program, spending his first year in research at the Boston Children's Hospital. Supported by a grant from the Orthopaedic Research and Education Foundation, he coauthored his first paper in basic science, "The Three-Dimensional Anatomy of Haversian Systems." He was an orthopaedic resident from 1956 to 1959, and, in 1959, he was chief resident in orthopaedic surgery at MGH. He continued to pursue his interest in research and specialization

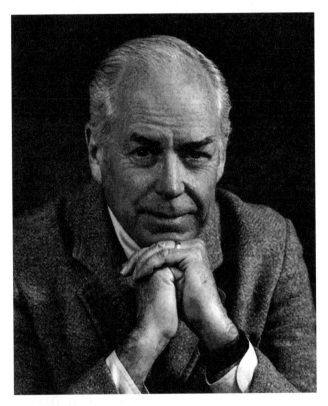

William H. Harris. Wikimedia Commons, courtesy of Louis F. Bachrach on behalf of Bachrach Studios.

Physician Snapshot

William H. Harris
BORN: 1927
DIED: —

SIGNIFICANT CONTRIBUTIONS: Compulsive developer of new techniques, equipment, and implants in hip replacement; instrumental in improving the durability of polyethylene; leader in discovering the pathophysiology of "particulate disease"

> The Three-Dimensional Anatomy of Haversian Systems*†
>
> BY JONATHAN COHEN, M.D., AND WILLIAM H. HARRIS, M.D., BOSTON, MASSACHUSETTS
>
> From the Department of Orthopaedic Surgery and the Division of Laboratories and Research,
> The Children's Medical Center, and the Harvard Medical School, Boston
>
> THE JOURNAL OF BONE AND JOINT SURGERY
> VOL. 40-A, NO. 2, APRIL 1958

A detailed understanding of the Haversian System was produced by Cohen and Harris during Harris's year in Cohen's research laboratory at Children's Hospital. *Journal of Bone and Joint Surgery* 1958; 40: 419.

in orthopaedics, and he served two fellowships: in 1959 at Oak Ridge Institute of Nuclear Studies, and from 1959 to 1960 in the Department of Morbid Anatomy of the Royal National Orthopaedic Hospital in London.

After his fellowships, Harris returned to Boston in 1960 as an assistant in orthopaedic surgery at MGH and an instructor in orthopaedic surgery at Harvard Medical School (HMS). In a personal interview, Harris described his early influence and experience:

> I came here [to MGH,] and I stayed here for two reasons: basically, the question of excellence and the question of innovation. Over long periods of time, this place has been premiere, and by that, I mean, primarily from my point of view, two specific elements. As big as this place is, it really cares. And as important as innovation is, it has never lost its belief in the optimum care of each individual. So, it's a remarkable combination. There are places in which the research element and the commitment to innovation dominate and it's hard to get a doc to go to see a patient. Conversely, there are places in which absolutely top-flight care dominates to...the exclusion or minimization of innovation. And if you go over the long-term history of this place, to me those were the two things that really count...you're surrounded by people who have the same deep belief that you do...
>
> The intensity of...total commitment to medicine [by many physicians today] is not as strong...as it was previously. That is to say, I used to say medicine owns my body 174 to 176 hours each week. Two hours I'm on the tennis court...But the rest of the time there was no such thing as on or off, or 40 hours, or somebody else is covering for me, or I can't get back. I owned the responsibility...There was an intense dedication to the craft of medicine, both the art and the science...I'll give you an example. Think about this. Smith-Petersen had some emotional ups and downs and he'd periodically get into a funk...During one of his "down" periods, Walter Bauer, the chief of medicine, scooped him up and took him to Bermuda for a week, and temporarily, partially abandoned his responsibilities as chief of medicine for a week...Unbelievable. That is commitment. It worked...
>
> Smith-Petersen worked 8 days per week. He got his idea for the cup arthroplasty on a Sunday taking a piece of glass out of the back of a Harvard student. A guy came in with a lump in his back and, in his office, on a Sunday, he took out his scalpel and cut into this lump and found at the base of it a piece of glass... and around it grew a synovial membrane!... And from that comes an observation that led to a major development [the mold arthroplasty]. Great observation and doing something with the observation...I'm speaking about the kind of compulsive dedication to the field [that] I don't see...today...It's not a 40-hour-a-week job. Smith-Petersen's a perfect example.
>
> [Regarding] the issue of innovation... There are lots of good institutions that innovate. But...if you go back over the history of this place and its commitment, there are not a whole lot that have innovated as much and very few that have innovated more...[For example]

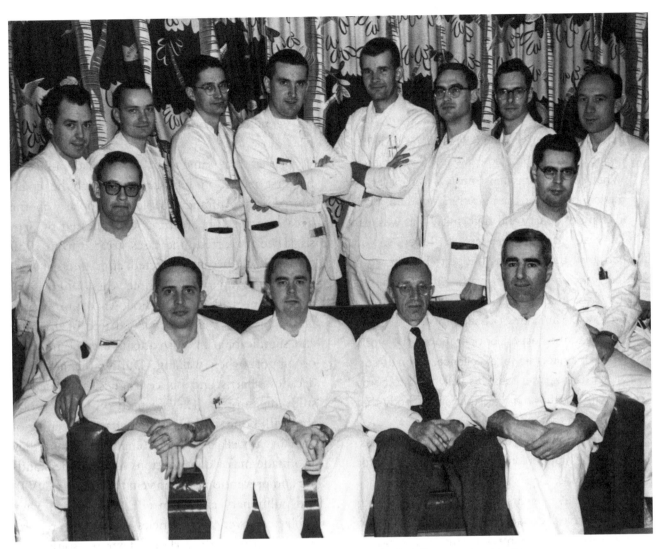

Dr. Barr with MGH residents, mid-1950s. Dr. Harris is in the back row at the far left. MGH HCORP Archives.

in the area of the hip I credit Bigelow in the mid-nineteenth century…[He made] a simple set of clinical anatomic observations on dislocation of the hip. On the other hand, those were the only tools that he had at the time and everybody…had those same tools. And in my view Smith-Petersen was the second most innovative orthopaedic surgeon in the history of the field [only Dr. Charnley was more innovative]…if you take the anterior incision…the hip nail…the cup arthroplasty…remarkably, the awesome spinal osteotomy…and the so-called Darrach operation: most of us would be happy to look back at the end of our career and tick off the just one of those five. (Harris 2009)

When Harris first started his practice, he worked from Dr. Marius Smith-Petersen's old office with Dr. Otto Aufranc, and he began to concentrate his practice on hips and knees. In his first year, he completed six cup arthroplasties. It wasn't long before he focused more and more on hip surgery.

The demands of trauma surgery are significant, and Harris began to innovate early in his career. In 1962, Harris—a member of a team of 12 surgeons—successfully, for the first time, replanted a 12-year-old boy's right arm. The team was headed by Dr. Ronald Malt, the chief resident in surgery. By 1964, Harris was promoted to Clinical Associate in Orthopaedic Surgery at HMS, and in 1965 he was an American British Canadian (ABC)

Traveling Fellow and visited Sir John Charnley in Wrightington. Total hip replacement surgery was introduced into the United States not long after this visit to Charnley. When asked about the experience in Wrightington, Harris recalled:

> [Charnley] started using polyethylene total hip replacement in 1962, so I saw it 2½ years later. What he could demonstrate was an order of magnitude better than anything we had, both in terms of quality and uniformity. This was just 2½ years after the disaster with Teflon, so you had to sit there and say I hope to hell this stuff [polyethylene] lasts longer than the Teflon, but if it does, school's out. He's got something very remarkable and now it's been proven, I think, to be, by far, the best major operation in the world if you do uniformity of excellence, if you do survival rate over decades. It's very hard to come up with another major assault on the body that has results that match this…
>
> [If Teflon were used in the United States, the total hip] couldn't have happened here for two reasons. One is the FDA. The FDA did not permit it even years later…The second thing is…Charnley conquered the Teflon disaster. Charnley's mental mechanisms were unique. That is to say, the combination of his drive, his willingness to take abject failure and turn it into success by refusing to quit, and his basic smarts were so unusual that, as I said, I put him at the top of the best of innovative people…And you had to have someone of this unique type in order to make that huge departure from conventional wisdom. (Harris 2009)

Earlier that same year, Harris had published his first paper on hip surgery, which he coauthored with Aufranc: "Mold Arthroplasty in the Treatment of Hip Fractures Complicated by Sepsis." They reported nine cases, treated from 1950 to 1963; all became infected after internal fixation. Follow-up averaged three years (range: 1–11 years). One patient died. Following cup arthroplasty, the other eight remained free of drainage and significant pain. All patients used some form of support when walking. During the next two decades, Harris and his colleagues continued to study hip surgery. They focused on issues associated with bone stock replacement and loosening of implants as well as vascular complications, and they also made major contributions to the understanding and prevention of deep vein thrombosis (DVT) and pulmonary embolism (PE) in patients. They published over 175 articles—including reports on prevention with warfarin, dextran, aspirin, and physical measures, culminating in the 1986 Otto Aufranc Award given by The Hip Society.

Classic article on the importance of anticoagulation in patients with hip fractures, by Salzman, Harris, and DeSanctis.
New England Journal of Medicine 1966; 275: 122.

Article in which Harris, Salzman and DeSanctis proved the importance of prophylactic anticoagulation in a controlled trial of patients undergoing elective hip surgery.
Journal of Bone and Joint Surgery 1967; 49: 81.

By 1966, Harris was promoted to Assistant Clinical Professor at Harvard, and, in 1967, he published "A New Lateral Approach to the Hip Joint," in which he described a new approach for cup arthroplasty of the hip contrasting with the traditional approach used at MGH and described by Smith-Petersen. In the lateral approach, Harris made a U-shaped incision with the base at the level of the posterior aspect of the greater trochanter, elevated an anterior flap of the fascia lata, the vastus and the tensor fascia lata, and osteotomized the greater trochanter with the abductor muscles attached. This approach provided a full view of the entire acetabulum, which allowed Harris to use the power tools he would later design in 1970.

LEADING INNOVATOR IN HIP SURGERY

Harris was quickly promoted to associate clinical professor at HMS by 1968, and, in 1969, he was appointed lecturer in the Department of Mechanical Engineering at the Massachusetts Institute of Technology as well as visiting orthopaedic surgeon at MGH. Aufranc had left MGH that same year, and it was Harris who continued to advance innovations in hip surgery at MGH. The two surgeons were among the few initiating the transition to the Charnley total hip replacement technique from the cup arthroplasty technique, and they each developed their own unique model and techniques. That year, Harris developed his hip rating system (later known as the Harris Hip Score) and compared it to Dr. Carroll Larson's "Iowa Hip Score"—designed in 1963—as well as to Dr. Margaret Shephard's system created in 1954. Using this comparison of the three systems in specific cases, Harris wrote that his system expanded the pain classification:

> from two categories...in the Shephard system to three...in the new scheme [making] classification of individual patients easier...Comparison of the two rating schemes shows that hips rated by the Larson system tend to fall into a more narrow range...The wider spread of rating in the new [Harris] system made the recognition of difference between hips easier and appeared to be a more accurate representation of each patient's functional state. (Harris 1969)

The editor-in-chief of *Clinical Orthopaedics and Related Research*, however, noted in a 2013 editorial that all three rating systems were prone to bias and overlooked those variables most integral to patient satisfaction. The Harris hip score was studied again in 2001 by Drs. Söderman and Malchau, and they concluded, "The current study indicates high validity and reliability of the Harris hip score. The motion domain had lower viability, but this domain contributes a maximum of only four points to a total score. The Harris Hip Score can be used for total score as it is" (Söderman and Malchau 2001).

Harris was appointed Orthopaedic Surgeon at MGH in 1971, and the following year the orthopaedic department was reorganized into specialty services after the arrival of Dr. Henry J. Mankin as the new chief of the service. Harris remained at MGH throughout his professional career and led a successful research laboratory while limiting his clinical practice to reconstructive hip surgery. Harris served as chief of the Adult Reconstructive

Traumatic Arthritis of the Hip after Dislocation and Acetabular Fractures: Treatment by Mold Arthroplasty
AN END-RESULT STUDY USING A NEW METHOD OF RESULT EVALUATION*
BY WILLIAM H. HARRIS, M.D.†, BOSTON, MASSACHUSETTS
From the Department of Orthopaedic Surgery, Massachusetts General Hospital, Boston
THE JOURNAL OF BONE AND JOINT SURGERY
VOL. 51-A, NO. 4, JUNE 1969

Article in which Harris first reported his Harris Hip Score—the accepted standard today. *Journal of Bone and Joint Surgery* 1969; 51: 737.

Unit (Hip and Implant Service) 1974–2003 and as director of the Harris Orthopaedic Biomechanics and Biomaterials Laboratory 1974–2004. In 1975, he was also promoted to Senior Lecturer at Massachusetts Institute of Technology and promoted to Clinical Professor at HMS. It was during this period that he began a 50-year program of basic and clinical research at MGH: a series of innovative advances ranging from power instrumentation, new hip implant and designs (both femoral and acetabular components), polymethylmethacrylate (bone cement) fixation, techniques in the use of bone cement, the concept of the hybrid total hip, and eventually the development of a bone ingrowth prosthesis with Dr. Jorge Galante. Harris led a very productive research program in his biomechanics laboratory, and he described his experience in a personal interview:

> There is a price to pay if you are going to also try and run a lab...it became clear that two things had to happen: First, you had to figure out how to fund it. Second, you had to control the clinical practice. Otherwise, it drowned you. You'd love that; that's all fine, but if you have in mind doing something else...and that was one of the major reasons that I went away from trauma because trauma kills you in terms of controlling your time. Arthroplasty had the advantage of being programmed and planned and probably elective. When I was doing stuff in the E.W., it would shoot the idea of being in the lab at the time...So, it was necessary to rigorously control the ingress of clinical activities. You had to have some gate on that and then you could do a number of different things, but the most disruptive one was trauma...I chose hip surgery because the dominating thing was at that time was hip surgery...the most demanding and the hardest nut to crack. (Harris 2009)

He continued his limited practice in reconstructive hip surgery, and also continued to report patient outcomes with each new development. He published more than 542 papers, 50 chapters, and five books.

In less than 10 years after total hip replacement was available in the United States, a unique and potentially game-changing complication had presented itself. Localized bone resorption began to be seen about the implants on x-rays. Charnley had reported similar changes in England, as did Dr. Willert in Germany in 1974. In 1976, Harris and colleagues reported four cases of hip pain (**Case 38.2**) and extensive bone loss that developed about the femoral component in patients 2.5–5 years after total hip replacement. Histologic specimens at revision revealed:

> sheets of macrophages, birefringent particulate matter (which was ultracellular, extracellular, or both), a few giant cells, and some bone lysis in the absence of either acute or chronic inflammatory cells...We found no clear-cut distinction between methylmethacrylate and polyethylene particles on the basis of size or shape...the wide distribution of the birefringent material...was more compatible with methylmethacrylate than with polyethylene... The cause of bone resorption is unknown.
> (Harris et. al. 1976)

Surgeons around the globe began to direct their efforts to improving the techniques and use of methylmethacrylate (bone cement) to achieve

---

Extensive Localized Bone Resorption in the Femur following Total Hip Replacement

BY WILLIAM H. HARRIS, M.D.*, ALAN L. SCHILLER, M.D.*, JEAN-MARIE SCHOLLER, M.D.*, RICHARD A. FREIBERG, M.D.†, AND RICHARD SCOTT, M.D.*, BOSTON, MASSACHUSETTS

From the Orthopaedic Research Laboratories of the Department of Orthopaedic Surgery and the Department of Pathology of the Massachusetts General Hospital, and Harvard Medical School, Boston

THE JOURNAL OF BONE AND JOINT SURGERY
VOL. 58-A, NO. 5, JULY 1976

Harris's first article on osteolysis after total hip arthroplasty.
Journal of Bone and Joint Surgery 1976; 58: 612.

Case 38.2. Extensive Localized Bone Resorption in the Femur Following Total Hip Replacement

"A man, fifty-nine years old, had a left total hip replacement for severe osteoarthritis. He was not aware of hip disease prior to the onset of symptoms at the age of forty. There was no history of infection, trauma, or other joint involvement. His total hip replacement was done through a lateral incision with osteotomy of the greater trochanter and the insertion of Simplex P bone cement which did not contain barium sulphate. At operation, the methacrylate appeared to fill the medullary canal fully and to polymerize normally. Excess bleeding did not occur. Gross and histological examination of the femoral head showed osteoarthritis without evidence of infection, inflammatory reaction, or other pathological process. One gram of streptomycin intramuscularly and one gram of oxacillin intravenously were given preoperatively, and one gram of oxacillin intravenously every four hours was continued for forty-eight hours postoperatively. The wound healed normally, and the greater trochanter united. The postoperative course was uncomplicated except for the development of thrombophlebitis, which was treated with warfarin. The patient regained excellent function, was able to carry out his daily activities without difficulty, and resumed playing tennis.

"Thirty-eight months later he noted a vague ache in the left hip and a roentgenogram showed marked localized lysis of the cancellous and cortical bone in the proximal part of the femur without evidence of loosening of the femoral component or the cement. The lytic area was near the lesser trochanter and did not involve the cortex near the tip of the prosthesis or distal to it.

"The patient was afebrile. The hip area showed no abnormality. The sedimentation rate was within normal limits, the white blood-cell count was 5700, and the differential count was normal with 1 per cent eosinophils. Serum calcium, phosphorus, alkaline phosphatase, acid phosphatase, total protein, albumin-globulin ratio, and electrophoretic pattern were within normal limits, as was the chest roentgenogram. No other evidence of infection or malignant disease was present. Patch tests for sensitivity to methylmethacrylate monomer and methylmethacrylate polymer were negative.

"Under general anesthesia, fluid was aspirated from the left hip joint and an open biopsy was performed to obtain tissue from the lytic area, which was approached through a window in the anterior cortex. The space between the cortex and the methacrylate was filled with yellow, firm, rubbery tissue and fragments of methylmethacrylate ranging in diameter from one to nine millimeters: a small amount of clear yellow serous fluid was also noted. Although the cement and femoral component appeared to be solidly fixed on first observation, closer inspection showed slight mobility when the hip was stressed either between the femoral component and the cement or between the cement and bone. Multiple samples of the fluid and tissue from the medullary canal, as well as fluid aspirated from the joint, were cultured immediately for aerobic and anaerobic organisms and for acid-fast organisms and fungi by the infectious disease consultant who was in the operating room. Smears were also made from these samples for gram-staining. However, all cultures and smears were negative, and there was no histological evidence of malignant disease or infection.

"The factors considered in planning further treatment were as follows: The lack of bone support for the mid-portion of the cement, the fragmentation of the cement, and the slight motion present suggested that fatigue failure of the femoral stem might occur. On the other hand, new cement and a new femoral component might be hazardous if the tissue reaction was an adverse response to a constituent of the joint replacement. However, if the bone lysis was caused by a tissue reaction to fragmented cement and motion, further resorption might be anticipated if the old femoral component was left in situ.

"Four months after biopsy, both components were loose and were replaced. At reoperation, multiple samples were submitted for bacteriological and histological examination, but no evidence of infection or neoplasia was present. The medullary canal of the proximal portion of the femur, including the lytic area and the area previously occupied by the intact methacrylate and femoral component, was thoroughly curetted. Two packages of methacrylate (Simplex P with barium sulphate) were used to fill the proximal part of the femoral canal and secure a long-stem femoral component. The wound healed normally: eighteen months later, the hip was functioning well and there was no evidence of further bone lysis, neoplasia, or infection."

(Harris, Schuller, Schollar, Freiberg, and Scott 1976)

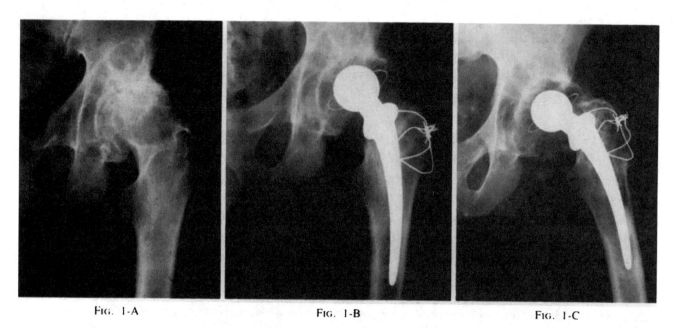

Radiographs of the hip: left: preoperative with severe osteoarthritis; middle: one week after total hip arthroplasty; right: 38 months postoperative with extensive resorption of cortical and cancellous bone about the femoral stem. W. H. Harris et al., "Extensive localized bone resorption in the femur following total hip replacement," *Journal of Bone and Joint Surgery* 1976; 58: 613.

better implant fixation in bone. Harris and his research team developed a system in the early 1980s to accomplish secure fixation with methylmethacrylate by use of distal plug in the femur, insertion of the cement from the plug proximally using a specially-designed cement gun, and then, without using the common finger packing method used at the time, pressurizing the cement by means of a specially-designed cement impactor. Similar techniques for pressurization of the cement were developed for the acetabulum. They also centrifuged the cement to eliminate any air pockets in the cement. These techniques were adopted by surgeons throughout the United States.

Osteolysis persisted after total hip replacement despite these and other advances. Failures occurred on both the femoral and acetabular sides of the prosthesis. Surgeons then turned attention to using implants without bone cement; instead, they used bone ingrowth type prostheses. Numerous designs appeared on the market. Harris and Galante joined together in the development of the Harris-Galante Prosthesis (HGP), and they reported their findings in 60 patients treated for failed cemented prostheses that were not infected: "Among those with a minimum two-year follow-up...none of the components has required revision" (Harris et. al. 1988). The bone ingrowth cementless total hip became a popular new choice of prosthesis in the late 1980s. However, even without the use of cement, osteolysis with implant failure continued to be a problem. Alternative bearings, such as ceramic components or metal on metal protheses, were designed. Research continued into the cause of osteolysis in non-cemented metal/polyethylene implants, and numerous

Harris's article recognizing osteolysis following uncemented total hip arthroplasties. *Journal of Bone and Joint Surgery* 1990; 72: 1025.)

investigations in both Europe and the United States identified another type of small particles causing the inflammatory reaction around total hip components (and total knees): polyethylene particles of wear from the acetabular component. Harris and colleagues reported the occurrence of localized osteolysis around noncemented bone-ingrowth type prostheses (HGP and porous coated anatomic prostheses):

> In the biopsy material from the three hips…that were studied in detail, there were fewer giant cells and histiocytes than are usually found in lytic areas around a cemented hip prosthesis. Small amounts of fine particulate polyethylene and metallic debris were seen in the femoral membrane from two patients…No gross metallosis was noted in the tissue…No patient had evidence of infection…It is possible that polyethylene wear debris caused the lysis… birefringent particles were seen…the focal lysis…in most [cases] was identified after three years. (Maloney et. al. 1990)

Harris and his research team continued to report outcomes of his total hip cases and new innovations related to implant design, cement techniques and basic biomechanical, and biomedical and biomaterials research. In a 1991 editorial comment before the Hip Society Proceedings, Dr. Robert Poss wrote:

> The greatest threat to long-term success of the THA [Total Hip Arthroplasty] is loss of bone stock. How can the accumulation of particular debris and the resulting osteolysis that it produces be minimized or eliminated? (Poss 1992)

At that same meeting, Harris presented his report "The First 32 Years of Total Hip Arthroplasty. One Surgeon's Perspective," in which he discussed five important warnings for cementless implants that had been overlooked up to that point in time:

1. Severe osteoporosis can occur in the proximal femur…a rare clinical problem…
2. A new condition exists characterized by bone lysis in association with cementless femoral components called "cementless [or particulate] disease."
3. Bony ingrowth does not occur from bone grafts…
4. Only small amounts of bony ingrowth are commonly found in many retrieved porous implants.
5. Revision operations have much smaller bony ingrowth than primary operations.

He noted additional warning signs for cemented implants:

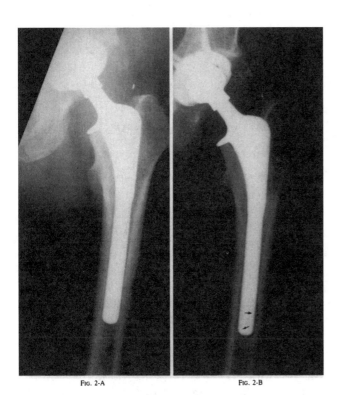

Fig. 2-A   Fig. 2-B

Radiographs of the hip: left: immediately following an uncemented total hip replacement; right: 3 years after total hip replacement with osteolysis in Zones 3, 4 and 5.

W. J. Maloney et al., "Endosteal erosion in association with stable uncemented femoral components," *Journal of Bone and Joint Surgery* 1990; 72: 1029.

1. Cement is the weak link...
2. For cemented femoral components, the failure mechanism is initiated...at the cement-metal interface...
3. Virtually every long-term 40–50% of cemented sockets [are] loose at ten years. In retrospect, the past 32 years of the practice in reconstructive hip surgery has been extraordinary [a] miraculous change from the days of cup arthroplasty to the opportunities of today in THA for helping patients with extraordinary arthritis problems. (Harris 1992)

By the mid-1990s, Harris and his team, in collaboration with AMTI (a spinoff of MIT), designed and built a hip simulator in order to determine the wear of the polyethylene acetabular component. After key modifications to replicate the actual motion of the femoral head in the acetabulum (including rotation), they were able to produce the polyethylene wear that is seen in patients after a metal/polyethylene total hip replacement. Harris and his colleagues received their second annual Otto Aufranc Award from the Hip Society in 1996 for their paper: "Skeletal Response to Well-Fixed Femoral Components Inserted with and without Cement." In this paper, they analyzed "forty-eight femora" retrieved "from 24 patients with unilateral cemented and cementless hip replacements... The maximum cortical bone loss...was at the middle section for the cemented femurs and at the midproximal and middle sections for the cementless femurs...The proximal medial cortex still represents the specific region of maximal bone loss for both types of implant fixation[, and] it seems that the less dense the bone is before hip replacement [then] the greater the extent of bone loss after... regardless of the fixation type" (Maloney et. al. 1996). That same year, using the hip simulator in his lab with Dr. Ed Merrill from MIT and Orhun Muratoglu, Harris's research team invented a new, resistant to wear, polyethylene, which was an electron-beam irradiated, melted, highly cross-linked ultra-high molecular weight polyethylene.

Shortly thereafter, in 1997, Harris was named the incumbent Alan Gerry Clinical Professor of Orthopaedic Surgery at HMS. Harris made many other major contributions to orthopaedic surgery—specifically total hip arthroplasty, and he has been recognized for his major contributions with numerous national and international prestigious awards (**Box 38.2**).

Box 38.2. Examples of Awards Granted to William H. Harris

> Harris has been granted a multitude of national and international awards for the breadth and depth of his contributions to orthopaedic surgery, but a few examples include:
>
> - The Kappa Delta Award for Outstanding Orthopaedic Research (twice)
> - The John Charnley Award from The Hip Society (four occasions)
> - The Frank Stinchfield Award from The Hip Society (three times)
> - The Otto Aufranc Award from The Hip Society (twice)
> - The Maurice Miller Award for Life-time Achievements in Orthopaedic Surgery

LEGACY

In 2000, Harris received an honorary D.Sc. degree from his alma mater, Haverford College. He was a founding member and first president of the Hip Society in 1968, and founding member and president (1993) of the International Hip Society. He is a member of various professional organizations, including the Boston Orthopaedic Club, The Interurban Orthopaedic Club, the Massachusetts Medical Society, the American

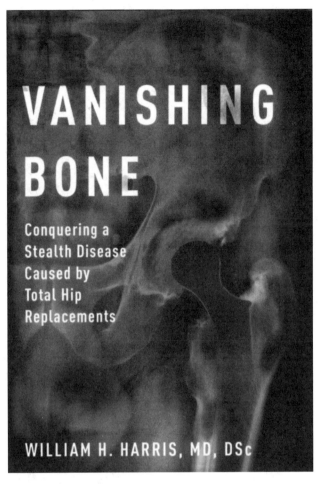

Cover of Dr. Harris's book.

Vanishing Bone: Conquering a Stealth Disease Caused by Total Hip Replacements by William H. Harris, © 2018 Oxford University Press. Reproduced with permission of the Licensor through PLSClear. X-ray photo on the cover courtesy of William H. Harris.

Medical Association, the American Academy of Orthopaedic Surgeons, the American Orthopaedic Association, SICOT, the Argentine Medical Association (Honorary Member), the Argentine Association of Orthopaedics and Traumatology, the Orthopaedic Research Society, the Society of Biomechanics, the Society of Biomaterials as well as the British, Canadian, and the Japanese orthopaedic associations.

Harris had initiated an annual course in Total Joint Replacement Surgery, held in Boston, under the Department of Continuing Education of Harvard Medical School in 1970. He remained course director for 30 years. He led a successful fellowship program in adult reconstruction and has trained many leaders in the field of arthroplasty today. As a major leader and contributor in his field he has given many invited and named lectureships around the world. He retired from orthopaedic surgery in 2004 but continued to contribute to research in the Harris Laboratory at MGH. In 2018, he published a new book *Vanishing Bone: Conquering a Stealth Disease Caused by Total Hip Replacement*, in which he tells the remarkable story of the discovery, pathophysiology, and treatment of osteolysis associated with total hip replacement.

CHAPTER 40

MGH
Other Surgeon Scholars (1900–1970)

The period between 1900 and 1970 was one of immense growth for orthopaedics at Massachusetts General Hospital (MGH). The trustees established the first outpatient orthopaedic department in 1903 as well as the Zander Room (the prototype of the modern physical therapy clinic). A new department of orthopaedic surgery (Ward I) opened in 1907, and, in 1922, orthopaedic staff were supplied with an operating room in the general surgical building. In 1940, the orthopaedic service moved from Ward I to the White Building; the physical therapy department, however, remaining in the old building. These monumental changes were led by numerous distinguished orthopaedic chiefs, including Drs. Joel E. Goldthwait (1904–1908), Elliott G. Brackett (1911–1918), Mark Rogers (Interim 1918 and 1922), Robert B. Osgood (1919–1922), Nathaniel Allison (1923–1929), Marius N. Smith-Petersen (1929–1946), Joseph S. Barr (1946–1965), Thornton Brown (Interim

Zabdiel B. Adams	228
Otto E. Aufranc	236
Joseph S. Barr Jr.	247
Robert J. Boyd	253
Thornton Brown	257
Carl H. Bucholz	264
Edwin F. Cave	270
Hugh P. Chandler	277
Thomas L. Delorme Jr.	281
Ralph K. Ghormley	288
William N. Jones	291
Robert J. Joplin	293
William L. Kermond	298
Carroll B. Larson	300
Harry C. Low	304
William R. MacAusland Jr.	308

Henry C. Marble	312
Paul L. Norton	317
Donald S. Pierce	320
Eric L. Radin	322
Eugene E. Record	329
John A. Reidy	331
Frederic W. Rhinelander Jr.	335
Sumner M. Roberts	338
William A. Rogers	343
Carter R. Rowe	350
Morten Smith Petersen	361
O. Sherwin Staples	362
George W. Van Gorder	364
Philip D. Wilson	369
Edwin T. Wyman Jr.	376

1964–1965 and 1970–1972), and Melvin S. Glimcher (1965–1970)—and later by Henry J. Mankin (1972–1996), William W. Tomford (Interim 1996–1998), and Harry E. Rubash (1998–2018).

Some surgeons are recognized for the quality of their work and their specialist contributions rather than by any particular high-ranking titles or academic pursuit. These practitioners have often proven integral to advancing the field of modern medicine. Harvard calls these clinicians "surgeon-scholars." The surgeon scholars covered in this chapter were integral to moving the needle forward at MGH between 1900 and 1970. They include:

ZABDIEL B. ADAMS

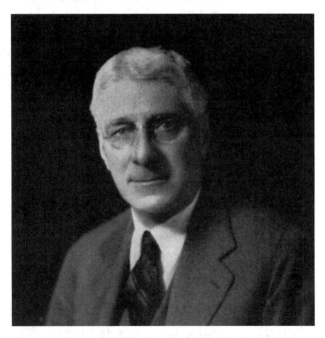

Zabdiel B. Adams. "Zabdiel Boylston Adams 1875-1940," *Journal of Bone and Joint Surgery* 1940; 22: 465.

> **Physician Snapshot**
>
> Zabdiel B. Adams
> BORN: 1875
> DIED: 1940
> SIGNIFICANT CONTRIBUTIONS: Supported Forbes's method of treatment of scoliosis; led the American Orthopaedic Association (AOA) Commission on Congenital Dislocation of Hips (1921); president of AOA in 1929

Zabdiel "Zab" Boylston Adams III was born in 1875 in Framingham, Massachusetts. He was named after his father, also Zabdiel Boylston Adams, "a physician of prominence and wide reputation" ("Zabdiel Boylston Adams" 1940); his mother was Frances (née Kidder) Adams. The young Zab "followed naturally in his [father's] footsteps," and "after three years at [the] Massachusetts Institute of Technology, he entered Harvard Medical School, graduating in 1903" ("Zabdiel Boylston Adams" 1940). His interest in orthopaedics had begun early, and he completed a surgical internship at the Boston City Hospital. "In 1907 he married Helen Foster of Brookline" ("Zabdiel Boylston Adams" 1940); they had two children.

After his internship, Adams began practicing as an orthopaedic surgeon at various Boston institutions. He began as an assistant surgeon at the Boston Children's Hospital in 1905, and as an orthopaedic surgeon at the Massachusetts General Hospital in 1906, a position he held until 1924. His time at MIT had given him the skills to hone his abilities as a surgeon: "His thorough knowledge of anatomy, combined with an unusual degree of mechanical ability and skill… furnished a sound basis for his work in orthopaedic surgery. He worked with intensity on the problems with which he was occupied and gave himself to both his hospital and private work with this spirit of devotion" ("Zabdiel Boylston Adams" 1940).

Early Orthopaedic Contribution and Military Service

Adams published about 16 articles throughout his career, including 7 on scoliosis and 5 on congenital dislocation of the hip. "At times he made special investigations and studies on the principles and methods of treatment of [these conditions], at a period when the lack of fuller knowledge rendered the care of these cases difficult" ("Zabdiel Boylston Adams. 1875–1940" 1940). Adams published his first paper in 1910, "The Treatment of Severe Scoliosis by Plaster Jackets with Windows and by Braces of a Similar Pattern." He had applied plaster jackets made while the patient was either standing (with or without the head in traction) or lying supine on a Bradford frame; the cast applied pressure to the convexity of the curve of the spine. He cut windows in the jackets to allow expansion of the chest during breathing and growth, and to care for the skin and allow shirts to be changed. He followed 10 patients at MGH and 20 patients at Children's Hospital for one year. On the basis of his similar research on five puppies, he concluded: "It is not my belief that the correction gained [by these patients] will be maintained unless an adequate brace is worn permanently" (Adams 1909).

In 1910, he published another two papers on the importance of congenital deformities of the vertebral bodies or articular processes, and a case report of sacralization of L5 as a cause of scoliosis (see **Case 40.1**).

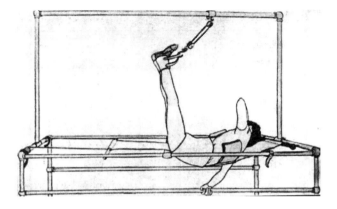

Drawing of a patient with a right dorsal scoliosis--on a frame with pelvic traction, pads in place and shoulders rotated to the right in preparation for a body cast (Forbes method).
Z. B. Adams, "Treatment of Lateral Curvature of the Spine by the Forbes Method," *American Journal of Orthopedic Surgery* 1913; s2-11: 97.)

> "Little bits of foot strain,
> Little squeaky knees,
> Make the Goldthwait sickness
> Sacro-iliac disease"
> —Source unknown, quoted in Z. B. Adams,
> "Mechanics of Back Strains," *JAMA*, 1925

At that time in the history of the treatment of scoliosis, the new technology of roentgenology prompted in-depth discussions of the deformities seen in scoliosis: lateral bending, rotation of the spine, kyphosis and lordosis, and rib deformities. A supporter of the Forbes method of treatment (versus the method of Abbott), Adams described both methods in a paper he read before the American Orthopaedic Association in May 1913: "Abbott with the spine in flexion pulls in the direction… which pull tends to rotation of the ribs towards the left, which increases the spring tension in the right rib, causing the vertebra to further rotate to the right. Forbes with the spine flexion rotates the shoulders to the right thus tending to restore the symmetry of the thoracic cross-section found at the point of greatest curvature."

In the lengthy discussion following Adams's presentation, Dr. Walter Truslow (1913) of Brooklyn stated, "The distinction lies between the question of whether one attacks the primary curve first, as Dr. Forbes enunciates, or whether the secondary curve is attached, as I think is the principle on which Dr. Abbott works." Truslow (1913) then showed a "picture [of]…the three planes in which the deformity exists." Dr. Adams (1913) responded with the goal of clarifying the difference between the two processes by providing more detail about Abbott's method: "Dr. Abbott puts his patients in flexion. That increases the mobility of the dorsal spine, as it separates the articular processes. Then he puts a circular strap around the thorax, just as Lovett used to do, and pulls down in this direction…[Now] that simply increases the rotation. You must rotate in the other direction, in order to restore the thorax to its normal form." Dr. A. H. Freiberg (1913), of Cincinnati, also commented: "It is not sufficient to pay attention to the element of torsion without attending to the element of lateral duration. It seems to me that Dr. Abbott, by attending to both, has given

Case 40.1. Scoliosis Relieved by a Procedure on a Vertebral Transverse Process

"The case is that of a Jewish girl sixteen years old, born in Russia. She entered the Out-patient Orthopedic Department, February 2, 1907, with the following history:

"Mother died of consumption. No nervous diseases in the family.

"Patient was perfectly well until present trouble started in October 1905. First complaint at that time (i.e., sixteen months before her first visit) was that right hip was growing out. Patient was then treated at another hospital for hip disease by a plaster spica and crutches, without relief.

"Treatment, including Zander exercise, hydrotherapeutic baths, plaster jackets with and without spicas, manipulations under ether and prolong recumbency, were all employed without relief, the deformity and other symptoms growing constantly worse during thirteen months of treatment. Ether manipulation always failed to correct the lumbar scoliosis.

"Eleven radiograms were taken during three months in an effort to find the cause. Those of the last lumbar vertebra showed a wide transverse process on the right which came in contact with the crest of the ilium and its epiphysis about to ossify; the unusually broad and long process had made a slight facet in the ilium.

"March 13, 1908, one year and one month after her first visit to the Out-patient Department, patient was admitted to the Orthopedic Ward.

"She complained of dull pain over the right sacroiliac articulation. Walking was not seriously interfered with but prolonged motion caused pain in leg.

"P.E. Well developed and nourished girl of seventeen years. Heart and lungs negative. Patient stands with right hip very prominent and back muscles visibly spastic upon the right side. Back presents scoliotic curve. As patient lies in bed, the right thigh is slightly rotated inward and very slightly flexed (about 10°). The right hip is drawn up making the legs appear of different length. Measurements show no shortening, however. Flexion of the right thigh is restricted to 90°; outward rotation is free; inward rotation very slightly restricted; the thigh is held adducted about 25°, and no abduction from this position allowed; extension is normal. No atrophy.

"March 19, operation. Service of Dr. Goldthwait. Ether. Usual preparations, patient lying on face with lumbar spine exposed. Vertical incision over fifth lateral process. Skin and aponeurosis of muscles split and retracted. Erector spinae muscle split by blunt dissection, down to the tip of the lateral process of fifth lumbar vertebra. Lateral process cut across with bone forceps near its middle and outer end removed with sequestrum forceps. Rough edge of stump trimmed with rongeur forceps. Bleeding was very slight. Aponeurosis of muscles closed with silk sutures. Skin with silkworm gut. Dry dressing. Sent to ward in good condition. Operation. --Excision of lateral process of fifth lumbar vertebra for abnormal development with scoliosis.

"Patient suffered considerable discomfort following operation and complained of right leg being "dead and immovable." Examination showed knee-jerks active and equal on both sides. No apparent sensory disturbance. No swelling or discoloration of that extremity. General condition good. Patient suffered slight pain in the wound.

"Patient had an uneventful convalescence. A few days after operation a plaster jacket was applied. When first allowed to walk patient shuffled the right foot and complained of hyperesthesia of the dorsum of the foot.

"She left the hospital in excellent condition on April 2, 1908, the spine having straightened considerably.

"April 14, 1908, patient could correct curvature and bend back equally to the two sides. The jacket was reapplied with straps.

"May 14, 1908, a corset brace was applied, consisting of two light steel uprights

"March 14, 1910, patient was wearing ordinary corset which gives good figure. The back caused no trouble. Photograph and radiogram at this time are given."

(Z. B. Adams 1910)

us an element of distinct advantage." In response to numerous questions, Dr. A. Mackenzie Forbes (1913) closed the discussion:

> the form of treatment suggested by me differs from that of Dr. Abbott in that...[he] attacks the secondary curve first and that I attack the primary curve fist...it is but rational to attack first the primary or organic curve allowing, as far as possible, the secondary or compensatory curves to look after themselves...Dr. Adams is the ablest exponent of the form of treatment which I have suggested...Treatment should aim at attacking the primary or organic change. True it is often difficult to say which this is, but to-day with x-rays at our disposal we ought to be able to come to some conclusion.

Adams published another three papers over a five-year period. In addition to cases he reviewed at MGH and Children's Hospital, he had access to anatomy professor Thomas Dwight's collection of spines in the Warren Museum. He summarized his thinking and his previous published research in 1915. First, he listed previous orthopaedists who studied scoliosis and various causes:

> The treatment of structural lateral curvature is now advancing...made possible by the investigations of Drs. Bradford, Lovett, Feiss and Forbes and of late the study...of Dr. Abbott of Portland. Dr. Bradford and Lovett...found there was no side bending without rotation and no rotation without side bending...In structural curvature...there are many causes...bad seating at school, faulty postures, malleability of the vertebrae, osteomalacia, rachitis, infantile paralysis, empyema, numerical variations, extra and fused ribs, lateral half of centrums missing, fused vertebrae, etc. – all have a bearing on the subject, some, but not all...are true causes... (Adams 1915)

He went on to describe asymmetrical sacralization (as seen on roentgenograms) as a rare cause of scoliosis:

> Roentgenograms of the scoliotics at Children's Hospital showed but few in which there was asymmetrical sacralization...At the Massachusetts General Hospital, in taking roentgenograms of subjects with...pains in the back, or when renal or ureteral store...is suspected, asymmetrical sacralization in all degrees is often found but there is no scoliosis. If ever a cause it is a rare cause. The Dwight Collection of spines in the Warren Museum further bears this out. Of the nineteen spines showing asymmetric sacralization but one has scoliosis and that one also shows an absence of the right neural process of the first sacral segment, which is of far greater importance...as the cause of scoliosis is concerned...Congenital defect of the articular processes were of far greater importance than asymmetric sacralization [Dr. Max Böhm]... The late Professor Thomas Dwight once said, "Anomalies of the fifth lumbar vertebra are so common that we hardly know what the normal sacrum should be." This is equally true of the sacrum... (Adams 1915)

He also commented on other involved joints, and procedures to correct such issues:

> The joints of greatest consequence...as the site of the cause of scoliosis is concerned, are those in which the surfaces between the centra have a sharp downward inclination, the lumbosacral and those between the sacral segments...The frequency of these anomalies in scoliosis is well illustrated by the clinic of the Massachusetts General Hospital. Of fifty consecutive cases in which careful roentgenoscopy has been made by Dr. Walter Dodd and Dr. Holmes, forty-four subjects showed bony defects in the sacrum or two lowest lumbar vertebrae. This study brings out the value of the flexed position.

In attempting correction, not only should the thoracic spine be flexed, but the lumbar spine should be flexed on the sacrum…

In some of these cases…operation should either precede or follow correction. In the first class it should be to replace the fifth lumbar centrum…or to remove asymmetric overgrowth of the processes, which prevent restoring the base to a position of equilibrium; and in the second class to prevent recurrence…by measures of bone graft to lock the fifth centrum to the sacrum; or on the articular processes to hold the vertebra in its place. It is evident that the lumbo-sacral region is not…the only region…found [as a cause] of congenital…scoliosis, but it is one of the most frequent sites of the cause…in girls about the age of puberty. (Adams 1915)

In closing during the discussion of his paper, Adams (1915) stated, "Asymmetrical sacralization is found in Roentgenray clinics…Out of this collection [19 spines from the Warren Museum] there was but one that showed scoliosis…[which also had] asymmetrical sacralization…It can be treated by exercises…[but] in the more severe cases, with a large transverse process on one side, surgical measures are demanded."

Early in his career Adams volunteered with the Medical Reserve Corps, and in 1917, during World War I, Adams began active service:

serving first as Captain and later as Major with Base Hospital No. 6 at Bordeaux [France]. He remained with that organization until transferred to special duty, when he was placed in command of the Special Training Battalion at Harchechamp [~225 miles slightly southeast of Paris], where he was given charge of the rehabilitation of groups of men, so that they might return to active service at the front. This was a difficult task, but he accomplished it with an efficiency that made the camp a definite success. ("Zabdiel Boylston Adams" 1940)

In April 1918, during the annual meeting of the American Orthopaedic Association, Adams reported his experience with rehabilitating soldiers in this special training battalion: "analysis of the first 373 cases admitted showed that 86% of the cases have defects that can be corrected by proper orthopedic treatment and training, while 14% have defects which require either hospital care or operative treatment or will permanently incapacitate them for combat men." After completing his service with the special training battalion, Adams went back to Base Hospital No. 6, and then moved to Base Hospital No. 114 at Beau-Desert, France. "On his return to the United States he was assigned to hospital duty, caring for the wounded soldiers, until [his] discharge from active service" ("Zabdiel Boylston Adams" 1940).

Later Orthopaedic Contributions

At this point in his career, Adams also held appointments at Harvard Medical School—as an instructor in orthopaedic surgery (beginning in 1918) and as an associate in anatomy (beginning in 1919)—until 1924. Adams's second main orthopaedic interest was congenital dislocation of the hip, and in 1920 he was appointed as a member of the American Orthopaedic Association's Commission (or Committee) on Congenital

STATISTICAL REPORT OF THE COMMISSION ON CONGENITAL DISLOCATION OF THE HIP, FOR 1921.

BY Z. B. ADAMS, M.D., BOSTON.

JBJS, 1921, Volume 3, Issue 8

Adams's report of the AOA Commission on Congenital Dislocation of the Hip—summarizing the results of different treatments used in the United States. *Journal of Orthopedic Surgery* 1921; 3: 357.

Dislocation of the Hip. Such commissions were common in the AOA during this period. They were established to examine such issues as infantile paralysis, scoliosis, ankylosing operations on the spine, and foot-stabilizing operations in infantile paralysis. With regard to congenital hip dislocation: "The Commission study of these problems was leading us to more definite ideas as to the value of methods in vogue and to standardization of the best surgical and other therapeutic procedures" ("Editorial" 1921).

The Commission on Congenital Dislocation of the Hip reviewed 713 cases of congenital hip dislocation, and Adams presented the Commission's report in 1921. **Table 40.1** lists the various reduction methods and results (categorized by children <6 and those ≥6 years old) used in these cases. After presenting the results, Adams (1921) called for analysis against other reported results that indicate few repeat reductions: "Now gentlemen, we must compare these results with those reported by M. Le Docteur Edouard Papin of Bordeaux, who reports…on 725 hips done since August 1914. They have reduced every hip with only 11 re-dislocations, and of these…nine were re-reduced. He uses the simple manual method of M. Le Professor Denucé, and puts much emphasis upon the fact that no force ever is used in the reduction."

In a publication the following year, Adams (1922) recalled this Commission report and noted that those findings, as well as "the end-results of treatment of congenital dislocation of the hip at the Massachusetts General Hospital were functionally, as well as anatomically, far from what could be desired and far from perfect." Adams also referred to Dr. Herbert P. H. Galloway's 1920 paper, in which Galloway had briefly described the introduction of open reduction to the United States, noting the initially overall poor results:

> Twenty-five years ago congenital dislocation of the hip was regarded on this continent as practically incurable…Rumors that Lorenz of

Table 40.1. Reductions Reviewed by the American Orthopaedic Association Commission on Congenital Dislocation of the Hip

Reduction	Cases (n)
Method	
Ridlon	348
Manual	155
Lorenz	150
Bradford machine	80
Hibbs table	80
Open	12
Preliminary osteotomy	11
Position after reduction	
Lorenz	188
Lange	140
Mid-position	7
Schlessinger	2
Worndorf	1
Results	
Children <6 years old	
Procedures (n = 311 in 250 hips; 11 surgeons)	
Hip reduction	198
Hip dislocation	34
Ridlon (n = 305 in 271 hips)	
Hip reduction	178
Hip dislocation	83
Children >6 years old	
Procedures (n = 70 in 60 hips; 11 surgeons)	
Hip reduction	24
Hip dislocation	29
Ridlon (n = 146 in 141 hips)	
Hip reduction	30
Hip dislocation	58
Function	
Children <6 years old	
Good	118
Fair	48
Poor	26
Questionable	3
Children ≥6 years old	
Good	1
Fair	1

Adapted from Z. B. Adams' "Statistical Report of the Commission on Congenital Dislocation of the Hip, for 1921." *Journal of Orthopedic Surgery*, 1921.

Vienna had perfected a method of bloodless reduction had crossed the Atlantic, and when this surgeon visited America and gave his reduction demonstrations the keenest interest was aroused, and our orthopaedic specialists set resolutely to work to remove the reproach of incurability...As has often happened before, zeal outran judgement...About one year after the visit of Lorenz, the late Dr. H. Augustus Wilson presented to the American Orthopaedic Association...a series of cases treated by manipulation, some...by Lorenz himself, and others by Wilson and his assistants following the Lorenz method...The average result... was not such as to arouse enthusiasm... [but] the method...[continued] to be the routine treatment...In June 1904, Dr. Henry M. Sherman of San Francisco read a remarkable paper [AOA]...opposing manipulative reduction, and following arthrotomy as the routine treatment...Disgusted with the downright failures and fictitious successes of the manipulative method, he definitely abandoned it in 1898...Dr. Sherman [stated that] "from what we have seen of the Lorenz results, scattered between Boston and San Francisco [including fractured bones, injured nerves, lacerated muscles, torn capsules and ruptured blood vessels], we cannot believe that he ever really got good anatomic results in half of all his cases...[Ridlon] claims only 10 percent...Is this enough?" (Galloway 1920)

Galloway had then discussed his own experience and advocated for open reduction for all congenitally dislocated hips:

Immediate after my return from Boston, where I had gone to see Lorenz operate, I had a female patient of three years with congenital dislocation of both hips...a true anatomical reduction was easily affected on both sides...but unfortunately subsequent experience was far less satisfactory...after hearing Dr. Sherman's paper I began to try out cautiously the open operation in selected cases...

Records show that I have opened the hip for congenital dislocation fifty times in thirty-seven patients. Seven of these operations in four patients are excluded...because they were adults in whom nothing was attempted except removal of the head...[With other exclusions] a total of thirty-eight operations in thirty-one patients [were reviewed]...Cured, 12; good results, 14; failures, 6; doubtful, 6 [insufficient follow ups]; total, 38. (Galloway 1920)

Despite previous poor results, Adams (1922) noted his interest in a reduction procedure being performed by Professor Maurice Denucé in Paris:

Having read...[Dr. Edouard Papin's] thesis, I was interested enough to go last summer to Bordeaux, in order to report to this Association my impressions of this treatment of Professor Denucé and of his end-results—anatomically and functionally...at Children's Hospital in Bordeaux...Since the outbreak of the war...he has reduced over nine hundred luxations or subluxations of the hip, with but few failures...

The reductions are all done manually by Professor Denucé's very ingenious method... not very unlike the method of Dr. John Ridlon, but it is not the same...The reduction is preceded by a manual stretching of the adductor muscles, and of this Dr. Ridlon does not approve. This stretching is done by gentle stroking of the adductors with the soft part of the palm of the operator's hand—beginning at the pelvis, and stroking downward in the longitudinal axis of the thigh, the skin having been covered with powder...[Professor Denucé] lays great stress upon the point that no violence or force is to be used.

After the adductors are stretched satisfactorily, the surgeon then attempts a gentle reduction of the hip:

The head is felt to slowly come forward and lodge in the acetabulum. As some of the doctors have suggested, it "oozes" in. At times, the shock is very slight. After the reduction, the hip is tested for stability...with fair stability...[the hip] is put up in..."ninety-ninety", that is ninety degrees of flexion and ninety degrees of abduction...the hip being reduced...[is] put in plaster. Should he fail in his first attempt to reduce the hip, he...puts the child up in traction for three weeks—drawing the head down, and then in a second attempt to reduce, he repeats the...[previous] steps...At the end of six months...the plaster is bivalved...and the parents are instructed...[in] his method of after-care...[:] exercises are given twice a day...no passive motion of the hip, but active motion...No weight-bearing is permitted on these hips until the center of ossification of the upper epiphysis of the femur is seen to have begun to increase in size markedly, and the head to shape itself, which is usually three to five months after removal of the plaster. Then walking is begun.
(Adams 1922)

The technique Adams described is very similar to one I learned from Dr. William T. Green while I was a resident at Boston Children's Hospital.

During this period, Adams may have been appointed the chief of the Orthopaedic Service at MGH (circa 1923), though I was unable to substantiate this. From 1925, he served as a consulting orthopaedic surgeon for the Lakeville State Sanatorium, "where he conducted a large and active service in the department of tuberculosis of the bones and joints" ("Zabdiel Boylston Adams" 1940). I could not locate any articles by Adams on tuberculosis, despite his long experience at the Lakeville State Sanatorium. Adams continued to research congenital dislocation of the hip, and in 1926 reported a case of a bilateral hip dislocation in a three-year-old whom he treated with Professor Denucé's technique:

The heads both entering the sockets with slight shock...Hips were held in ninety-ninety degrees position for six months...At six months the whole plaster was taken off...After [another] four months...the heads were felt plainly in front. X-ray showed the heads in front of and below the sockets...Open operation was done. The right hip had a strong transverse band in the front of the capsule (a fold of the capsule?) Which was cut through...and then the head went into the socket with ease...The left hip was also opened. Here the bands were found deep in the socket at the back, possibly a thickened cotyloid ligament folded in before the head, at the first reduction. This band being cut...[and] the head was secure in the socket.

Adams was a member of the American Orthopaedic Association, and he served as its president during 1929–30. That year, the annual meeting was held in Boston. The presidential speech he gave there was not published, but Dr. H. Winnett Orr (1937), in his history of the first 50 years of the American Orthopaedic Association, stated:

Dr. Adams in his presidential address emphasized the importance of accuracy in recording observations in orthopedic surgery and the employment of our experience to establish standard methods in treatment. It was interesting to me to observe that he called attention to the fallacy of certain claims with reference to the treatment of tuberculosis by sunlight...[As president-elect] "Zab" Adams...[had visited] Rollier in Switzerland...in the "Sun-cure clinic" at Leysin...and reported that results in tuberculosis joint patients were not particularly different from those he saw in Boston and in adult patients not even quite as good.

Adams was also a "valued and efficient member of the Board of Associate Editors of the *Journal of Bone and Joint Surgery*" ("Zabdiel Boylston

Adams" 1940). Adams held memberships in the American Medical Association, the International Orthopaedic Association, the Massachusetts Medical Society, and various local medical organizations.

An Unexpected End

Adams died at his home in Brookline in 1940. It happened suddenly; he was 66 years old. He left behind his wife, Helen, and their son, Samuel, and their daughter, Nancy.

An obituary for Adams published in the *Journal of Bone and Joint Surgery* referred to him as a "typical New Englander," a man:

> with strong, uncompromising convictions which had come down by inheritance from the rugged character of the early Puritans. He had an innate sense of justice and was intolerant of anything which suggested insincerity, and never temporized in his dealings with what he felt to be right. This made him strong in his dislikes and generous and loyal to his friends. These characteristics made themselves evident by an outspoken frankness and directness, which, although not always tactful, was the expression of his firm convictions and rather endeared him to his friends, who recognized in this trait an evidence of his integrity and honest thinking. ("Zabdiel Boylston Adams. 1875–1940" 1940)

OTTO E. AUFRANC

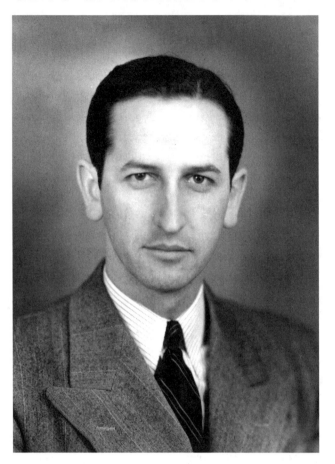

Otto E. Aufranc. Massachusetts General Hospital, Archives and Special Collections.

Physician Snapshot

Otto E. Aufranc
BORN: 1909
DIED: 1990
SIGNIFICANT CONTRIBUTIONS: Nailed the first fractured hip at Boston City Hospital; excellent anatomist and gentle surgeon; expert in cup arthroplasty of the hip; chief of the MGH Fracture Service beginning in 1957; led the establishment of the Division of Orthopaedics at the New England Baptist Hospital

Otto Elmo Aufranc was born July 19, 1909, on a farm in Callaway County, Missouri. His parents were sharecroppers and first-generation Americans—their parents were from Bern, Switzerland. Otto was one of 10 children (5 boys and 5 girls). When he was 10, his parents purchased a farm 30 miles away in Boone County. Otto worked on the farm and attended Deer Park, a small school about a quarter of a mile from the farm. He liked school, loved to read, and did well. In his senior year he won a year's tuition to college in a state-wide contest.

In 1927 he began attending the University of Missouri, only seven miles from home. He remembered, "From the first year at college and all through medical school I worked and supported myself...In my first year, after taking hygiene courses, I was paid for grading papers and doing other odd jobs. Summers I worked on the highway" (Butler and Dickson 1995). Aufranc focused on pre-law and pre-engineering courses; for him, the latter "were interesting but [the] math requirements [were] too tedious so I...took chemistry, physics, and biology courses I really liked. Medicine then became my goal" (Butler and Dickson 1995). Toward this end, Aufranc later became a night orderly at the university hospital, where he worked for two years during college. He graduated from the University of Missouri with a bachelor of arts degree in 1931 and a bachelor of science degree in 1932.

Aufranc stayed at the University of Missouri to complete their medical school program (during that time it offered only a two-year program) and continued in his work as a night orderly. While there he met Dr. Kenneth Coonse (see chapter 61), whom he later worked with after he transferred to Harvard Medical School. During the summers at Harvard Medical School, he worked as an assistant in Dr. Elliot Cutler's surgical research laboratory, where he collaborated with Dr. Coonse. After graduating from Harvard Medical School in 1934, Aufranc accepted an internship at Boston City Hospital. He completed a full general surgery residency program (during which he developed a bleeding peptic ulcer, from which he fully recovered), was chief resident on the surgical service there, and planned to receive further training in orthopaedic surgery.

Residents at Boston City Hospital received no income; rather, they were given room and board and two uniforms. Aufranc recalls donating blood each month to obtain spending money. Aufranc began his training in the role of anesthetist, in which he spent four months with little guidance: "Just a can of ether, a paper mask and go to work...So, for four months, I was the anesthetist...I never had a death" (Butler and Dickson 1995). He then spent four months as outpatient surgeon and did a four-month externship, finally taking on the role of house surgeon; many of his procedures were in trauma patients at Boston City Hospital, but he also had his own patients. He later remembered, "I learned from doctors like Frederick [sic] Cotton, Horace Binney, George Payson, Otto Hermann and my old friend Kenneth Coonse...there were a few follow-ups on patients at the B.C.H. But I had my own cases come back on Saturday or Sunday for check ups" (Butler and Dickson 1995). While at Boston City Hospital, Aufranc led the charge on a new procedure: nailing fractured hips; he was the first to perform the procedure there. In the early 1930s, 30% to 40% of patients with a fractured hip died. Aufranc recalls "read[ing] about hip nailing in a publication from the MGH by Smith-Petersen, Van Gorder and Cave. I showed it to Dr. Newton Browder who became interested...He went to Sears and Roebuck and bought a drill and some wires. The hospital got some nails from the MGH" (quoted in Butler and Dickson 1995).

Aufranc moved from Boston City to Boston Children's Hospital in 1936, when he was accepted on the orthopaedic service there. He said, "I applied and was accepted for the orthopedic service at Children's Hospital even though it was non-paying...I definitely wanted orthopedics...[but] I was told I had to take a year of pathology first" (Butler and Dickson 1995). After spending a required year in pathology at Boston Children's Hospital, Aufranc entered the Boston Children's Hospital/Massachusetts General Hospital combined residency program. He, along with Dr. Carroll Larson and Dr. Carter Rowe, were residents under Dr. Marius Smith-Petersen.

Early Orthopaedic Contributions and World War II

Smith-Petersen had previously begun performing glass cup arthroplasties during the mid-1920s. This work helped Smith-Petersen to realize that glass was not the best material—nor was wood, Bakelite, or Viscaloid. Upon the suggestion of Dr. John Cook, Smith-Petersen's dentist, he tried Vitallium. According to Aufranc, "1938 was a very special year" (Butler and Dickson 1995). That June "the first successful Vitallium mold arthroplasty [was] performed [by Smith-Petersen], replacing the unsuccessful attempts with Bakelite and Pyrex glass" (Rowe 1990). It became the standard procedure for hip arthroplasty for more than 25 years; and Smith-Petersen, Aufranc, and Larson continued to perform and study hip arthroplasty. Smith-Petersen named Aufranc as senior resident at MGH that October (a position he held until September 1939), afterward appointing him an assistant in orthopaedic surgery. Smith-Petersen also invited Aufranc to join his private practice at 266 Beacon Street in 1939. Larson joined them later, and, according to Aufranc, the three cultivated a positive working relationship and published extensively together. Aufranc and Larson learned to perform hip surgery by doing

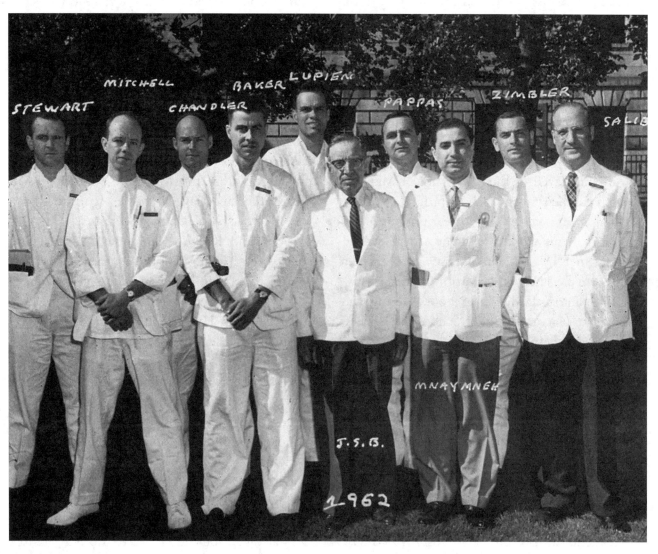

Dr. Barr with MGH residents. Philip Salib is in the front row on the far right. MGH HCORP Archives.

it, and by dissecting cadavers and evaluating hips that had undergone arthroplasty. (These hips were collected at MGH and eventually displayed in the first orthopaedics exhibit at the Museum of Science in Boston by Dr. Philip Salib.) Aufranc noted, "In my first year of private practice I was very busy, put on Staff as a Visit from the start...I supervised both of the orthopedic training programs on the ward...In addition to hip and spine surgery we did knees, shoulders, and elbows and as surgeons on the arthritis service we did all kinds of operations on hands and wrists. All this was done on what was called the 'free service'" (Butler and Dickson 1995).

> "The longer and the more philosophically we contemplate this subject, the more obvious it will appear, that the physician is but the minister and servant of nature; that in cases like those which have been engaging our consideration, we can do little more than follow in the train of disease, and endeavor to aid nature in her salutary intentions, or to remove obstacles out of her path."
> —Dr. Jacob Bigelow, presentation to the Massachusetts Medical Society, 1835

Aufranc practiced in Boston, with Smith-Petersen and at MGH, until May 1942, when he began active duty during World War II. He "served as Chief of the Orthopaedic Service in the 6th General Hospital (the Massachusetts General Hospital Unit), which saw active duty in North Africa and Italy" (Rowe 1990) (see chapter 64). Aufranc published with Smith-Petersen and Larson on various orthopaedics-related topics, beginning during his period of military service. Their first article together, "Useful Surgical Procedures for Rheumatoid Arthritis Involving Joints of the Upper Extremity," was published in 1943; this was also Aufranc's first publication. Despite the accepted practice at the time of not operating during an acute phase of rheumatoid arthritis because of a lack of success with fascia lata arthroplasty and synovectomy, Smith-Petersen, Aufranc, and Larson had success with Vitallium mold arthroplasty performed during an acute phase. They reported improved function after pain was relieved by acromioplasty (first performed in 1935), excision of the radial head, and wrist arthrodesis with excision of the distal end of the ulna. They emphasized the importance of early surgery, performed far in advance of extensive joint damage.

The three surgeons also treated patients with kyphosis, and Aufranc described their trial-and-error process and lengthy discussions to determine the location at which an osteotomy should be performed. The first osteotomy was done around 1940 and was used in patients with kyphosis secondary to Marie-Strumpell disease. Aufranc described it and the reason for the spinal osteotomy:

> We had many patients with Marie-Strumpell arthritis with a marked kyphotic deformity. Dr. Smith-Petersen had developed a method of straightening these out...under ether anesthesia, placing a blanket roll under the patient's back and gently assisting gravity in straightening the spine [and] we often gained as much as 30° of straightening. However, Dr. Larson and I saw these patients eight of nine months later when they returned with the same deformity...[We] suggested to Dr. Smith-Petersen that the spine be fused after...as much correction as possible...doing an osteotomy of the spine which had never been done before. One morning Dr. Smith-Petersen[was] very excited [and said] he knew how to do an osteotomy of the spine...but electing the level took several hours of discussion and argument. Dr. Smith-Petersen wanted to do the osteotomy at the apex of the deformity...[I] thought it should be done where there wasn't much bone...Dr. Larson thought that the best place...was the lumbosacral junction where the cord would not be injured.

In the first case…the osteotomy was [at] T10 or 11, and we got practically no correction. We then moved down to L3-4 and got a little correction. On our first try…[doing] the osteotomy at the lumbosacral junction…[we] took out a lot more bone. As the spine began to straighten, there was a sudden pop and it straightened almost completely. Our hearts were in our throats, but the patient awakened with only a sore abdomen from the shortened muscles being stretched. He developed a little ileus but no paralysis…During the next few years we did some forty cases. (Butler and Dickson 1995)

They reported their initial results in six cases in the *Journal of Bone and Joint Surgery* in 1945.

After the war, in November 1945, Aufranc returned to Boston. He received the Bronze Star that year for his service (**Box 40.1**). Upon his return, he became affiliated with the Newton-Wellesley Hospital as a staff surgeon; he had previously moved into the role of consultant there in 1940 where he remembered operating "on weekends and holidays" (Butler and Dickson 1995). He also picked up again at MGH and in practice with Smith-Petersen. He recalled that at the time "there were few beds…available in the hospital [because] the doctors who had not gone to war had been extremely busy" (Butler and Dickson 1995). He remembered:

In our early work with Dr. Smith-Petersen, Carroll Larson and I would help do a hip in the morning and one of us would go to the ward to help him do one in the afternoon. We must have done some two hundred or more rheumatoid…patients on the ward in the first few years after the war. That is when we learned how to expose the hip…Initially we would manipulate all the hips about two months postoperatively…But one month later the patients would be right back where they started…Dr. Larson and I went around daily helping the patients

Box 40.1. Aufranc Receives the Bronze Star for Meritorious Service

> Aufranc received the Bronze Star in 1945, and his son shared with me the letter Aufranc received with the award, which had been signed by Captain Karl R. Ottesen, of the Military Airlift Command, who had been adjutant of the 6th General Hospital in the Mediterranean Theater of Operations:
>
> "[To] Otto E. Aufranc, 0398072, Major, Medical Corps, 6th General Hospital for meritorious achievement in connection with military operations in North Africa and Italy from 15 May 1943 to 8 May 1945. As the only experienced orthopedic surgeon in the 6th General Hospital, Major Aufranc performed his routine duties in a highly commendable manner and personally trained, with great skill and patience, the several officers with whom he worked, with the result that a high standard of excellence was attained by his entire section. In addition Major Aufranc summarized, in a series of articles, the results obtained with various types of treatment and devised and put into service a number of simple, useful orthopedic appliances. Major Aufranc's contribution to the field of orthopedic surgery in the Mediterranean Theater was four-fold in that he proved himself an accomplished surgeon, an ingenious improviser, an able teacher, and astute observer and reporter. Entered service from Boston, Massachusetts."

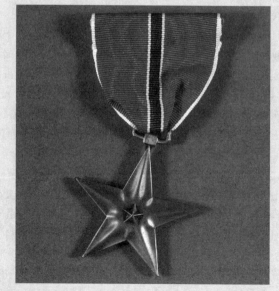

Bronze Star. Smithsonian National Air and Space Museum.

move...never forcing their hip. These patients did the best of all...[However] all patients did worse with the physical therapist...It was because of this experience that later I employed our own therapist. (Butler and Dickson 1995)

Those physicians and surgeons at MGH who had served during the war "considered forming a group practice for a number of reasons. Returning from wartime experiences in military medicine, they were faced with the uncertain prospects of rebuilding their old solo practices, they wanted to continue their wartime 'working together', and they were aware of the prerequisites and tax benefits that salaried group work might offer" (Castleman, Crockett, and Sutton 1983). Aufranc and many other staff, including Drs. Daniel S. Ellis, Marshall K. Bartlett, Daniel Holland, Edward F. Bland, Earle Chapman, Joseph S. Barr, and Stanley Wyman, "made up an informed group called the Associates[,] which later became an official staff organization, the MGH Staff Associates" (Castleman, Crockett, and Sutton 1983).

Later Orthopaedic Contributions and the MGH Fracture Service

In 1947, almost a decade after the first Vitallium cup arthroplasty, Smith-Petersen, Larson, and Aufranc published their first paper on the cup arthroplasty, "Principle of Mold Arthroplasty as Applied to the Hip." They also identified problems with the cup itself:

> The original cup was bell shaped and had a flare inside the cup that was designed to prevent it from sinking into the acetabulum. After a few years we realized that the flare was catching on the new capsule and even on the iliopsoas tendon...We also kept seeing the high spots on the femoral head and acetabulum, the so-called 'corns' which was really an area of bare bone, so we tried our best to make the cup and hip fit better...One thing I always thought and still

> believe is that the cup should fit loosely and not bind in any position...it was better to be too loose than too tight. (Butler and Dickson 1995)

Smith-Petersen, Aufranc, and Larson's article, "Principle of Mold Arthroplasty as Applied to the Hip." *Surgical Clinics of North America* 1947; 27: 1303.

The cup was not the only equipment they modified as they learned to better perform hip surgery; they also adjusted hand tools such as gouges and reamers. They also learned to treat mobility issues with daily gentle manipulation. They hired their own therapist to exercise the patients and ensure they received appropriate therapy.

Two years after their 1947 publication, Aufranc began teaching at Harvard Medical School as an instructor in orthopaedic surgery. His career progressed over the next decade, as did his work on arthroplasty. In 1954, he became a visiting orthopaedic surgeon at MGH and was named assistant chief of the MGH Fracture Service under Dr. Edwin Cave (Cave is discussed later in this chapter). Aufranc was responsible for organizing the popular postgraduate fracture courses. In 1956, Dr. Joseph Barr was chief of the Orthopaedic Service. Barr asked Aufranc to provide a brief outline of Aufranc's accomplishments in the preceding year. He responded:

1. Clinical work...follow-ups of patients with mold arthroplasty and Moore prosthesis...

2. Clinical research...post-mortem examination of shoulders with...cuff tears...plus surgical demonstration of acromioplasty on autopsy material

3. Teaching assignments...[including] those... with the Harvard Medical School and the resident staff at the MGH

4. Publications: Chapter on Arthroplasty of the Hip in Campbell's...Lectures included...[six in national meetings and post-graduate courses]...extra time has been spent on organizing chapters for the forth-coming Fracture Book...with Dr. Morten Smith-Petersen

In his response to Barr, Aufranc didn't just list his accomplishments; he also provided some suggestions that would enhance the Orthopaedic Service:

1. ....a double view box...attached to the wall of the conference room...

2. a simple set of view boxes...on the wall out in the corridor...

3. ...view box of the double type should be attached to the wall in the plaster room...

I believe each member of the staff ought to have some voluntary project that he works on throughout the term of his hospital appointment...[like] my project with the hips...Our knee arthroplasty program is a very slow turtle...because of the lack of proper cases...I believe we should be on the lookout for suitable cases for mold arthroplasty of the knee.

The following year, Aufranc was appointed assistant clinical professor at Harvard and he also succeeded Cave as chief of the Fracture Service. When he took on that position, MGH began three-day "mini-courses," an idea he had suggested previously but hadn't been approved until he was chief.

In 1957, Aufranc also published his, Smith-Petersen's, and Larson's combined experience with 1,000 cases (200 bilateral) over a 15-year period. To maintain objectivity, Aufranc had Dr. Elliot Sweet, another orthopaedic surgeon who had not been involved in the cases, examine numerous patients who had undergone arthroplasty at MGH and review all the data. Sweet's "over-all evaluation of *satisfactory* indicates the patient's condition has been improved and that the surgery was worth doing" (Aufranc 1957). These results are shown here in **Table 40.2**. Aufranc (1957) then went on to describe lessons learned:

Aufranc's review of 1,000 cases of cup arthroplasty of the hip at MGH. *Journal of Bone and Joint Surgery* 1957; 39: 237.

Table 40.2. Results from 1,000 Hip Arthroplasties over 18 Years

Overall results	Cases (n)
Excellent	45
Good	175
Satisfactory	600
Unsatisfactory*	180
Complications	
Thrombophlebitis	50
Pulmonary embolus	37
Subluxation	16
Femoral fracture	5
Dislocation	4
Death	3
Severed femoral nerve	2
Peroneal palsy	2

Adapted from data in Aufranc 1957.
*In some revisions, fibrocartilage was found over the femoral head.

The motion and friction of partial, comfortable weight-bearing are the elements that make for a durable joint. Weight-bearing must be actively protected until the full range of motion has been obtained…Another lesson learned has been the need to transplant the iliopsoas tendon to the anterior medial border of the distal portion of the capsule…to give the tendon a direct pull for function…In patients with a short femoral neck or…with no neck, as in shaft arthroplasty, it is necessary to move the greater trochanter…down the lateral portion of the shaft…[O]ther lessons…[are] unsupported by statistical evidence…[and] I list them on simple faith…The reconstruction of the hip is not complete until the hip is relatively stable through its major functional positions…The head of the femur and its acetabulum both need to be reconstructed…A full range of motion should be obtained before full strength is tried for…A long period of walking with crutches… is recommended…[sometimes] as long as two and three years after the operation…[then] adequate support…[with a cane or crutch] to prevent limping is necessary.

The following year, Aufranc began collaborating with the *Journal of the American Medical Association* to publish a "Fracture of the Month" column. The column was "patterned after the grand rounds presentations held at the MGH… [and] proved to be very time consuming. I enlisted every Resident and Fellow as they came along to help me with it. I asked Dr. William Jones to be a proof reader and Dr. William Harris to be an editor" (Butler and Dickson 1995). They published a total of 105 cases in this monthly feature. The column was suspended around 1972.

Two years after Aufranc's publication of his, Smith-Petersen's, and Larson's experience with more than 1,000 cases, Aufranc and Sweet published an accurate follow-up survey of 246 hips in 213 patients who had undergone Vitallium mold arthroplasty between 1946 and 1953. They stated seven conclusions presented in **Box 40.2**.

Box 40.2. Results of Aufranc and Sweet's Follow-up Survey Vitallium Mold Arthroplasties between 1946 and 1953

Aufranc and Sweet recorded the following results from their survey.

"Surgical hazards are not great

Disabling pain relief

    Complete: 27%

    Partial: 58%

    None: 15%

Walking

    No support: 30%

    Cane needed: 55%

    Crutches needed: 15%

Range of motion

    Unilateral hip: wide range

    Bilateral hips: limited range

Results

    Satisfactory: 82%

    Good/Excellent: 28%

No correlation with result and patients' evaluation

    Supplementary surgery required in 12%"

(Aufranc and Sweet 1959.)

FRACTURE OF THE MONTH

FRACTURE OF THE TIBIA AND FIBULA

PRESENTATION OF CASE

Otto E. Aufranc, M.D., Boston

J.A.M.A., July 30, 1960
Vol. 173, No. 13

Aufranc's first article in the JAMA "Fracture of the Month" series. *Journal of the American Medical Association* 1960; 174: 389.

Aufranc's experience culminated in the 1962 publication of his classic monograph, *Constructive Surgery of the Hip*, based on his personal experience with more than 3,000 patients (**Case 40.2**). In the preface, he recognized that not all the results were excellent, and some of the procedures were even considered failures. Aufranc notes, however, that the failures were necessary so that procedures, instruments, molds and prostheses, and management techniques could evolve. He acknowledged the contributions of his associates at the time—Dr. Morten Smith-Petersen, Dr. J. Drennan Lowell, and Dr. William H. Harris (and Drs. William Cochran and Hugh Chandler). Carroll Larson wrote the book's foreword, in which he states that Aufranc was the embodiment of Francis Peabody's teaching on patient care. Aufranc believed the goal of the surgeon to be the reduction of pain and disability through a holistic combination of skilled, discriminating surgical procedures and careful rehabilitation.

> "The Secret of the care of the patient is caring for the patient."
> —Dr. Francis Peabody
> Boston City Hospital, Lecture to Harvard students, October 21, 1925

Barr died in late 1964, just two months after retiring (see chapter 38), and MGH leadership had to choose a new surgeon to head up

Case 40.2. Cup Arthroplasty of the Hip

"This 68-year-old woman had had stiffness and some pain in both hips for years. Eventually the right hip became intolerably painful, and the pain persisted even at rest. When the patient sought orthopedic advice, she brought one anteroposterior view of the pelvis, which had been interpreted as showing bilateral osteoarthritis of the hips-mild.

"The examination revealed a stern, stoical type of New England woman who walked with obvious discomfort and limited motion in the right hip. There was a fixed flexion deformity that could be gently stretched to neutral. All motions, however, were painful. On palpation there were fullness and pain to pressure over the front of the hip and in the area of iliopsoas bursa. Active or passive stretching of the psoas aggravated this pain.

"The anteroposterior and frog leg x-ray films revealed on the right:

1. Narrowing of the joint line
2. Marginal osteophyte formation in the subcapital area in the neck with thickening of the cortex of the neck above the lesser trochanter
3. Slight flattening of the weight-bearing surface of the head"

"**Surgery:**

"At the operation [cup arthroplasty] there was excessive fluid in the joint under pressure, as well as a markedly thickened and irritated synovia and capsule, a large iliopsoas bursa, numerous barnacle-like osteophytes on the neck of the femur, and a complete loss of articular cartilage in weight-bearing areas."

"**Result:**

"Complete loss of pain and a full return of function with a greater range of motion than on the left side.

"This determined person probably would have made a success of any operation that improved the mechanical function of the hip. I am inclined to discount her claim of "complete loss of pain" as relative. Yet, she has made a will leaving her hips to our Orthopedic Department. She considers that she has been saved from the wheelchair and that even if the other hip continues to deteriorate she can tolerate surgery on that one if necessary.

"The x-ray films, if carefully studied, often cast the shadow of what may be found at surgery. Whereas a quick glance may be accurate, the interpretation may be misleading."

(Otto E. Aufranc 1962)

the Orthopaedic Service. Although asked about his interest, Aufranc declined, saying, "I felt I had reached an age [55] where I didn't feel I had enough time to do an adequate job as Chief of Service, but I agreed to stay on as Fracture Chief. I did offer suggestions as to whom I thought should be considered and some...I felt should not. For the remainder of my stay at the MGH, I supported the choice of Chief [Dr. Melvin Glimcher] even though it was not my selection" (Butler and Dickson 1995). In the late 1960s, Aufranc had achieved the peak of his academic career. Many of his honors and awards are listed in **Box 40.3**.

As the decade drew to a close, Aufranc, after 30 years at MGH, began phasing away from that hospital. At one point during the mid-1960s, he

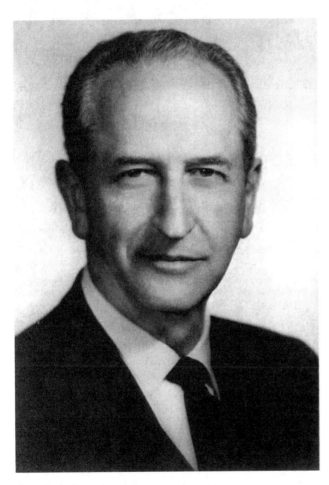

Otto E. Aufranc. C.R. Rowe, "Otto E. Aufranc, M.D. 1909–1990," *Journal of Bone and Joint Surgery* 1990; 72: 950.)

Box 40.3. Otto Aufranc's Honors and Awards

- Knight's Cross, Knight First Class, Royal Norwegian Order of St. Olav, 1948
- President, Boston Orthopaedic Club, 1962
- Vice-president, American Board of Orthopaedic Surgery, 1965; in 1967 he was elected Vice-president, American Academy of Orthopaedic Surgeons, 1967
- Citation of Merit, University of Missouri Alumni Association, 1967
- Co-founder, the Hip Society with Frank Stinchfield, 1968 (ca. 1985 the Hip Society began awarding annually the Otto Aufranc Award for innovative clinical or basic research in hip disorders)
- Samuel Higby Camp Visiting Professorship, University of California, San Francisco, Medical School, 1969
- Second Philip D. Wilson Lecture, Hospital for Special Surgery, date unknown
- Silver Dagger Award from the Pasha of Marrakech, Moscow, Russia, date unknown

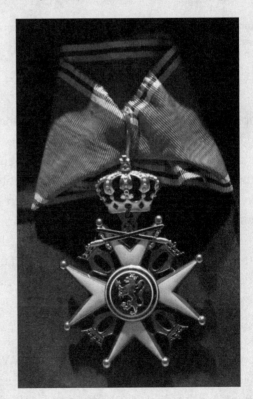

Knight's Cross, Royal Norwegian Order of St. Olav. Sandberg/Wikimedia Commons.

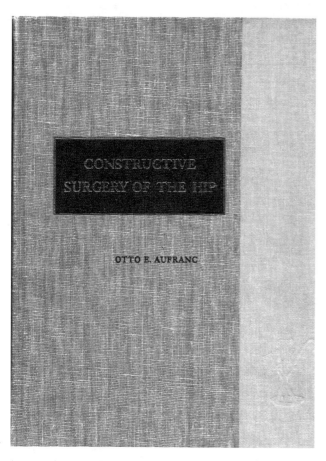

Aufranc's classic monograph, *Constructive Surgery of the Hip*. St. Louis: The C. V. Mosby Company, 1962.

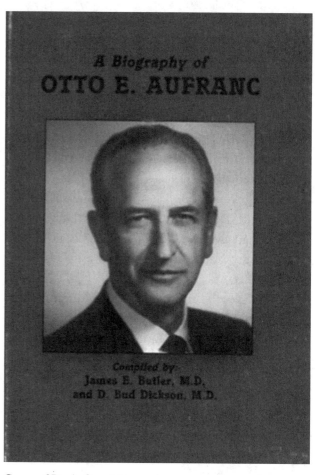

Cover of Dr. Aufranc's biography. Courtesy of James E. Butler.

had 115 patients on his service at MGH—in the Phillips House, in the Baker Memorial, and in the White Building. This represented most of the patients admitted from the Massachusetts General Orthopaedic Group and proved to be problematic in relation to not only bed availability but also operating room (OR) time. The average hospital stay for a cup arthroplasty was six weeks (three months for a bilateral case). Although he started rounds early in the morning, Aufranc was not able to see every patient on his service every day.

Aufranc had previously operated on the hip of the New England Baptist Hospital's president, Eleanor Kirkby, greatly relieving her pain. While she had been at MGH during her six-week recovery after the procedure, she realized that OR starting time was a big problem there. She convinced Aufranc to schedule a few cases at New England Baptist, guaranteeing him an on-time start in the OR. Apparently, everything ran like clockwork. This seemed to seduce Aufranc to move much of his work there; and with the help of Dr. Roderick Turner, one of Aufranc's recent fellows and chief of orthopaedics at the Lemuel Shattuck Hospital (Aufranc was a senior consultant there in 1969); he transitioned his elective reconstructive hip practice to the New England Baptist Hospital. There, Aufranc always started in the OR on time, and their staff made every effort to make the transition successful.

In his biography, Aufranc wrote about the New England Baptist Hospital, which at the time had no orthopaedic service. He recalled that Kirkby encouraged him and Turner to establish such a department and granted his request to create an orthopaedic fellowship there. He had fully transitioned to New England Baptist by 1970, where he held the position of chairman of the Division of Orthopaedic Surgery.

Legacy

Just a couple years after moving to New England Baptist, however, Aufranc developed myasthenia gravis. He retired from surgery in 1972, though he continued to teach. That year, Aufranc agreed with Dr. Henry Banks to include a rotation at New England Baptist for orthopaedic residents at Tufts University, and Aufranc was appointed as a clinical professor of orthopaedic surgery at Tufts. He continued to serve at the Baptist Hospital as a member of the board of directors and a trustee. Throughout his career, Aufranc published ~158 papers (17, plus 122 Fracture of the Month columns in *JAMA*, at MGH), 3 Orthopaedic Surgery Reviews in the *New England Journal of Medicine*, 3 books, and several book chapters.

On March 7, 1990, at age 81, Dr. Aufranc died of a massive heart attack. He was survived by his wife, Randolph (née Arnold), an artist who created many of the illustrations in his book *Constructive Surgery of the Hip*. She also painted the portrait of Smith-Petersen that used to hang at the entrance to the Smith-Petersen conference room. He was also survived by his son, Dr. St. George Tucker Aufranc (named after Randolph's brother), who followed his father as an orthopaedic surgeon at the New England Baptist Hospital.

JOSEPH S. BARR JR.

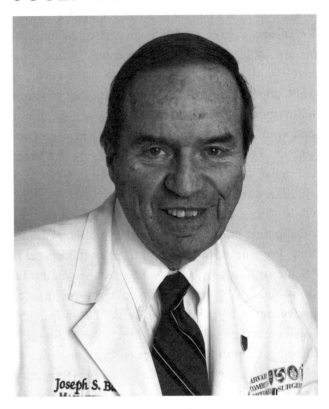

Joseph S. Barr Jr. Massachusetts General Hospital.

Physician Snapshot

Joseph S. Barr Jr.
BORN: 1934
DIED: —
SIGNIFICANT CONTRIBUTIONS: Led amputation clinic at MGH (1975–98); chief of the Division of Orthopaedic Surgery at Faulkner Hospital (1989–2006); president of the Cervical Spine Research Society

Joseph Seaton Barr Jr. was born on November 20, 1934, to Dr. Joseph S. Barr and Dorrice (née Nash) Barr. His mother was Dr. Frank Ober's secretary, and Ober was Joe Jr.'s godfather. His godmother was Nellie Smith, whom Joe called "Aunt Nellie"; she was the supervisor of the Peabody Home for Crippled Children, where Joe's father was chief of surgery.

At age six, Joe sustained a closed supracondylar fracture, which Ober reduced under ether anesthesia in his office. Joe Jr. graduated cum laude from Milton Academy in 1952 and went on to Princeton University, where he received a bachelor of arts degree in 1956. He attended medical school at Harvard Medical School, graduating in 1960. While in medical school, Joe received a $500 stipend from the dean for a summer research fellowship. On the advice of his father, he spent one summer working with Dr. Melvin Glimcher and Dr. Francis O. Schmidt at MIT. At the time, Glimcher was taking courses (advanced physical chemistry and advanced thermodynamics) at MIT while doing research on the physical chemistry of appetite and collagen in the biology laboratory. Joe worked with Schmidt every three weeks: "Schmidt [had]...planned out what he wanted to do in the lab...[every three weeks] so my job was pretty much to be recordkeeping" (Barr Jr., personal interview with the author, 2009). Joe Jr.'s father greatly influenced him to become a physician or an engineer. In addition to his laboratory experience with Schmidt and Glimcher, Joe Jr. often went with his father on rounds at the hospital on Saturday mornings.

After medical school, Barr took a surgical internship at the Peter Bent Brigham Hospital. He then spent another year in general surgery at Children's Hospital and the West Roxbury Veterans Affairs Hospital. The next two years (1962–64), he served in the US Naval Medical Corps as an assistant surgeon; he was assigned to the US Naval Station Hospital in Taipei, Taiwan. After this service he took on a residency in the Children's Hospital/Massachusetts General Hospital Orthopaedic Program (1965–68). As a resident, he spent a "couple of weeks...[in] California to take the prosthetics course and I spent a week at Rancho Los Amigos...[with] Vern Nichol...and Jacqueline Perry...They had...first use[d] the halo...in 1967 or 1968" (Barr Jr., personal interview with the author, 2009). During our interview, Barr Jr. revealed that he was impressed with his father's position and the number of famous persons (medicine, sports, etc.) he knew. As a medical student, Barr Jr. scrubbed in on one case with his father (a spine fusion), and he was amazed by how technically challenging it was. The elder Barr died before Barr Jr. started his residency, and I imagine that he wanted to continue in his father's footsteps as a spine surgeon. Barr maintained this interest in spine problems and amputations, and the rehabilitation of patients with such issues, throughout his career.

After completing the residency program, he joined the staff at Faulkner Hospital, where he remained for decades. In addition to his roles at Faulkner Hospital, Barr was appointed instructor in orthopaedic surgery at Harvard Medical School in 1969; he also served as a clinical instructor from 1969 until 1979, when he was promoted to assistant professor (part-time). He was active on the staff at the Massachusetts General Hospital; he was chief of the Amputation Clinic from 1975 to 1998, and he became very involved in teaching orthopaedic residents and medical students. He worked in rehabilitation with Dr. Donald Pierce at MGH. He was also appointed medical director of the Department of Physical and Occupational Therapy at Faulkner Hospital in 1979, a position he held until 1999; and he held the position of chief of the Division of Orthopaedic Surgery from 1989 to 2006. (During that time, in 1998, the Faulkner Hospital merged with the Brigham and Women's Hospital [BWH]. In 2006, the hospital reorganized the orthopaedic service as a department; Dr. Michael G. Wilson from the BWH was named as chairman.)

Boston Interhospital Augmentation Study (BIAS)

A team of specialists—including orthopaedic surgeons (Barr and Dr. Henry Banks), a general surgeon, a physiatrist, and a prosthetist—formed a community group in Boston called the Boston Interhospital Augmentation Study (BIAS). The group was funded by the Veterans Administration and studied whether the technique of immediate application of plaster pylon after a surgical procedure, as described by Dr. Earnest M. Burgess, would be successful among a loosely organized group of 53 surgeons and 18 hospitals. In 1973, they published two conclusions. First, the surgeon performing the surgical procedure must be a member of the team that administers the plaster pylon after the operation in order to ensure that the technique goes smoothly. Second, a preparatory prosthesis was most practical in the context of the study, as study group members could not supervise every application; a plaster cast to the mid-thigh was the next best option. In a symposium on fractures of the hip published in *Clinical Orthopaedics and Related Research* in 1973, Dr. Augusto Sarmiento, the guest editor of the issue, assembled a collection of articles, including one by Barr Jr. titled "Experiences with a Sliding Nail in Femoral Neck Fractures." Barr reported a series of 81 patients who had been treated by more than 20 surgeons (staff and residents) using a Vitallium sliding nail with a McLaughlin or Thornton side plate, and then followed for a minimum of two years. In a summary of his retrospective study, he stated, "60 were displaced fractures and 44 (73%) were successfully united at two years or more…[Disregarding] the five technical failures and…4 patients with segmental necrosis the success rate increases to…87 percent…A healed, vascular femoral head has been achieved in a large number of instances and this condition is superior to prosthetic replacement" (Barr Jr. 1973).

Active Service to Professional Organizations

Barr has been very active in professional organizations. For example, in the American Academy of Orthopaedic Surgeons, he's served on the Committee on the Spine and as chairman of both the Instructional Course Committee and the Committee on Educational Programming. He's been medical director and a trustee of the Orthopaedic Research and Education Foundation, an associate on the editorial board of the journal *Spine*, and treasurer and president of the Cervical Spine Research Society. He gave the presidential address to that society at its 1993 annual meeting in New York City.

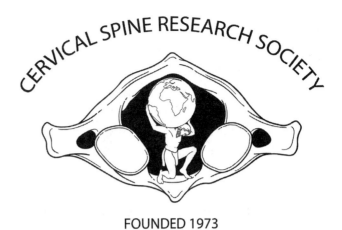

Logo, Cervical Spine Research Society. Courtesy of Cervical Spine Research Society.

After reviewing the history of the first two decades of the Cervical Spine Research Society, Barr focused his remarks on the society's next decade. Emphasizing the importance of the society to create close ties with surgeons and other stakeholders—including industry and government players, e.g., the US Food and Drug Administration (FDA), he reviewed the hotly disputed issue of pedicle screws being classified by the FDA as class III devices, thus requiring surgeons to disclose to patients that these screws are not approved devices. Barr was one of the representatives in a workshop (with Drs. Edward Hanley and Martin Krag) with the goal of helping resolve the problem. The workshop participants decided to study the use of such screws in fractures and degenerative spondylolisthesis.

Another *Clinical Orthopaedics and Related Research* symposium, this one on low-back pain published in 1977, included a lecture Barr Sr. had given at the San Diego Naval Hospital's Officers Club in 1961. Dr. William Stryker had invited Barr Sr. to give the lecture; Dr. Vernon Nickel had recorded it, and Dr. Leon Wiltse had transcribed it. Barr Jr. shared the unedited lecture for inclusion in the symposium. Much of this lecture is reprinted here in **Box 40.4**.

When he's not working, Barr enjoys sailing, especially in the ocean and in races—he's

Box 40.4. Joseph Barr Sr.'s Lecture on Low-Back Pain

"My first concepts with regards to lumbar disk lesions as causing clinical symptoms dates back to 1932. At that time I was just a little over 30 years old, had graduated from medical school, had a surgical internship, orthopedic residencies (children's and adult) and was in private practice. Those of you who are old enough to know about 1932 know that there wasn't much private practice at that time. It was scratch as scratch can. There wasn't a great deal of work and the work there was went to much older and much wiser doctors than I was at the time at that time and perhaps ever will be.

"In any case I work with Dr. Ober and those of you who know Dr. Ober know that he is a unique sort of person—blunt, independent, a down–Maine Yankee who called his shots as he saw them. He took his hat off to no man. He said he was the only Democrat in the state of Maine. He was just that sort of person.

"In any case in 1932 a young fellow came down to see Dr. Ober. I examined this fellow. [see chapter 38] His name was Kenneth Newton. He was in his 30s. I don't have any notes except my recollections because I hadn't expected to talk tonight. So, I can't verify what I have to say. You can consider these as reminisces of a campaigner if you want to and discount as much as you choose. But this is the way I remember it.

"Kenneth Newton had what we now recognize as a classical disk syndrome. He had hellish pain down his leg. He had a list in his back and he was miserable. Plain X-rays were negative. We put him in a little hospital to cool off. He stayed uncomfortable. Well, in those days we thought the cause of this syndrome was either sacroiliac strain as exemplified by Dr. Smith Peterson [sic] or perhaps lumbosacral strain. Phil Wilson was a great person to defend the sacroiliac region as the cause of low back pain and sciatic pain. We knew that spondylolisthesis caused pain in the legs sometimes. We knew that infectious arthritis did also. We knew that tumors did and then we sort of stopped and we didn't know much more about it than that.

"Anyway, Kenneth Newton did not do very well under conservative treatment so we considered manipulating his back. This was a standard form of treatment. I couldn't understand if it was strained, why it failed to be relieved by complete bedrest. It seemed to me very odd that this could be true. Any other strain of ligaments that I had ever heard of would be relieved by rest. It was also hard to understand why strain of any ligament could reduce what appeared to be typical nerve pain, deepseated [sic] and agonizing.

"So I said to Dr. Ober, 'Before we manipulate his back, isn't it possible that we are missing something?' Dr. Ober said, 'Yes, he might have a tumor. Let's get Jason Mixter to see him.' Jason Mixter was a neurosurgeon, of course, and the man in New England who knew most about the spine. Not even Harvey Cushing, I think, had opened as many backs as Mixter had, and had looked in for a variety of tumors. So Jason saw the patient and said, 'Well, it could be a tumor all right.' He had operated on a few chondromas of the spine and he advised that we do a lipiodol myelographic examination. We put in 2 cc of lipiodol to fill a big broad spinal sac and those 2 cc ran a little pencil line up and down the back. We didn't even know enough to do fluoroscopy. We just took a couple of films. These were negative as far as this was concerned. The patient was no better.

"Jason said he would be willing to explore the spine. So he did. Here I missed an excellent opportunity because I wasn't present at the exploration. I was busy doing some orthopedic examination or other and didn't see the surgery. But I was told the patient had a chondroma of the spine. I saw the operative note and in the clinical records at the M.G.H. is a very lovely pin-and-ink sketch that Mixter had made. He found the tumor by opening the dura, doing a rather radical laminectomy, removing the 2 laminae and removing the tumor through the opening in the dura. He found the first sacral nerve root under compression and removed it transdurally. The patient was much better, in fact was completely relieved of his back and leg pain.

"I wasn't so busy in those days and so on the next Sunday morning after the report had come back from pathology, 'chondroma of the spine,' I went over to the Pathology Department (Tracy Mallory was in charge), got the slides out and asked to see them. Here was this tumor but I couldn't see any cells. That seemed to me very odd. I asked Tracy about this chondroma that didn't have any cells.

He said, 'Well that is characteristic of chondromas of the spine. They don't have cells.'

"Just about that time something happened which gave us a clue. I was sent a book by Schmorl and Junghanns. I won't give the German title of it but it was a book on the spine in disease and health and, as you all know, Schmorl was a German pathologist who spent his life, especially his later years, studying spines which have been removed at autopsy. He described these little posterior protrusions which he saw which he thought were of no clinical significance.' 'Nicht wichtig' they were called. I had been asked to review this book. My German was very bad. It took me about 3 or 4 weeks of hard slogging before I could make out just what this was all about. I asked Tracy Mallory if this could be a disk protrusion because from Dr. Mixter's description this had arisen from an intervertebral disk. Tracy said he did not know. It might be. I went to the medical school and asked to see some slides of disk tissue and there were no pathological histological slides of normal intervertebral disc tissue at Harvard Medical School. This was extraordinary, but it was a fact. It was a tissue of no importance.

"So we made some disk tissue slides and compared them with this 'tumor.' Of course, it was the same sort of material. Fortunately, the Pathology Department had a very lovely index of all material they had ever examined at the M.G.H. since it was opened in 1812 or so.

"We were able to find about 20 or 30 cases of chondromas of the spine. They ranged from the cervical spine on down to the lumbar spine with 1 or 2 in the dorsal spine. And of these 'chondromas' of the spine, there were 3 or 4 of them that anybody, even a fourth year medical student, could tell were chondromas. They had cartilage cells in them. The rest of them all looked like normal disk tissue.

"So we were on the hunt then for other clinical cases with this same type of thing. Our first case in which we made the diagnosis preoperatively was a fellow by the name of John Andrade who was a Portuguese chap from down on Cape Cod.

"Phil Wilson and I operated on him. He had a severe forward and lateral list of his spine so he was cocked off to the side. Phil Wilson was sure that strain had a lot to do with this. So we took a massive tibial graft and did a fusion on him after the disk had been removed. He fused solidly but he fused with the list still present. John Andre is living today with his spine bent off to the side about 30 degrees and listed forward about 30 degrees.

"Then the struggle was on. We had a very difficult time getting the neurologists to accept the possibility that a tumor pressing on a nerve root could be present without producing objective neurologic changes. It just seemed to them incredible that such a thing could be true. If the ankle jerks were present and the knee jerks were present, the patient couldn't have this lesion. It took some doing and courage to operate on cases in which the neurologist had come out flatfootedly and said, 'there is no use in doing one of these new-fangled lipiodol injections because he has got any neurological changes. He's all right.' But we persisted and gradually we collected a number of cases.

"In 1934 Jason Mixter and I published our first paper. This paper included cases with lesions from the base of the skull down. We covered the waterfront. Cervical, dorsal and lumbar lesions are all included in his first article. But I could not get over this first case that I followed, severe sciatica with low back pain, and I finally collected 20 patients with characteristic lumbar and sciatic pain. I wrote a thesis for the AOA on this subject. It was excepted and published in about 1935 or 1936.

"But in any case I may say that these first 20 cases taught me 90% of what I have learned about disk lesions. There is a sort of pattern. Once you see see a pattern, it is there and it does not take 100 or 200 or 300 cases to see what the pattern is. It is there for anyone to see.

"In 1933 I read my first paper. This was at a Peter Bent Brigham Hospital reunion of which I was a graduate. There were 42 cases. Elliott Cutler, who has since died, was there. He was a good surgeon and a good neurosurgeon. He said it was very interesting but that he had never seen a case. He said that, if he had ever had one, he would ask me to see it. That was the last I heard from the Brigham Hospital staff.

"I won't go into the history of it. At first it was very uphill. No one believe this I think, practically at first. Yet the literature is strewn with references to it. If you start before our first paper in '34 and just collect the literature which was then in print, you would have a book shelf full of references. This has been known for many years. We didn't discover anything. We rediscovered something. Kocher was a famous Swiss surgeon, who described a case accurately in the 1800s…And there were a couple of Scottish surgeons, Middleton and Teacher who described this. Walter Dandy described it. Elsberg and Stukey described it. We didn't discover anything new. We rediscovered something that had been known. The point was that we were able to take what had been known in the pathology laboratory and what we could see clinically and had access to a group of cases which made a syndrome…It is very easy to accept now but then it was rather hard. We could scarcely believe it ourselves. It seemed too good to be true. We thought that there must be something phony about this. And every case we did, there was always a very skeptical surgeon looking over our shoulders to see this little bit of tissue that was brought out and claimed to be the cause of the trouble. The surgery wasn't nearly as skillfully done then as it is now. We didn't have the tools you have now. We didn't even have the pituitary rongeur until finally Jason Mixter found that this was the proper tool to get into the disk space with. All the technique had to be developed the way it has been recently.

"Well, that is the background and I think it is fair to say that we didn't discover disk lesions. They have been known for a long while. We certainly didn't discover what the original discoverers did, the fact that disk lesions can produce sciatic pain, because that had been known for a long time. They had been called chondromas – tumors. We had some difficulty in deciding what we would call these things, whether they would be called protrusions or ruptures or what. That led to a very long period in which there was a great deal of indecision and lack of knowledge about what the actual causes of these protrusions were. I think our Swedish confreres have pretty well proven that degenerative change is a primary cause….

"Probable degenerative change which is a weakening process plus some acute strain is the basis for most of our disk lesions. I think that it is very rare that trauma alone is the cause of disk lesions. Certainly only 30-40% of our cases give an out-and-out clearcut history of antecedent trauma which one can really relate to….

"There is a lot that hasn't been explained about disks yet…why remissions and exacerbations occur is still to me very much an unknown quantity….Why patients get spontaneous remission and exacerbations particularly in the L-4, 5 lesions is anybody's guess and I am sure we all have ideas but I don't know of anything that has been certainly proven about this.

"Then comes the matter whether you are going to stabilize the spine or whether you are not going to stabilize it…As most of you know, I have felt that in general a disk which is ruptured or protruded is no longer an intact mechanism as far as its motion is concerned. And probably that segment would be better off if it were well stabilized postoperatively….

"Some of the people here think that open surgery for disk lesions will probably be primarily thing of the past. This seems incredible but I suspect it may be true. I hope it is true. Surgery has its place. It is a tremendous thing to have a patient wake up and say, 'My leg pain is gone, I feel 100%. I am wonderful.'…I will be surprised if some of us here don't see the day when disk surgery is abolished or nearly so…If you can shrink the lesion and stabilize the spine by biochemical methods, the surgeon is going to have to fold up his tent and silently steal away. I think this could be true. Disks are 90% water…I don't know how we are going to do it but I believe it can be done and I think it will be done."

(Barr 1977)

participated in dozens. He "started sailing as a teenager…while spending a couple of summers at Tabor Academy [in Marion, Massachusetts]…For years my family has had a place in Maine on the St. George River, just on the western side of Penobscot Bay. We sailed small boats and as time went by, larger boats" (quoted in Jacquet 2008).

ROBERT J. BOYD

Physician Snapshot

Robert J. Boyd
BORN: 1930
DIED: —
SIGNIFICANT CONTRIBUTIONS: Director of the problem back clinic at MGH; influential in the formation of the Massachusetts General Hospital Physicians Organization

Little is known about Robert J. Boyd's early life and family. Details become available during his time at Harvard College, from which he graduated in 1952 with a degree in biochemistry. While there, he was active in both the Glee Club and the Harvard Band. From 1952 until 1956, he was a medical student at McGill University School of Medicine, where he was elected as a member of the Scarlet Key Society. Those who receive scarlet keys, and thereby membership in the society—known as "Keys"—are in the top 15% of their class; they are recognized because they embody several character traits, including: leadership, a commitment to excellence, commitment and determination, and have completed a project that has had beneficial effects.

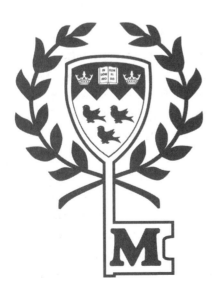

Logo McGill's Scarlet Key Society. Courtesy of the Scarlet Key Society.

After graduation, Boyd was an intern (1956–57) and general surgery resident (1959–60) at Stanford University. In the interim two years, he served as a captain in the army; he was stationed in Germany. After completing his year as a surgical resident, he remained at Stanford for another year (1960–61) as a US Public Health Service Research Fellow in surgery. In 1962 he joined the Children's Hospital/MGH orthopaedic program as an assistant resident. In addition to working at both of those hospitals, he rotated to Lynn General Hospital and the Lemuel Shattuck Hospital. After serving as chief resident at MGH—he was Dr. Joseph Barr Sr.'s last resident—Barr asked him to join the visiting staff at MGH in 1965. He remained active on the staff at MGH until his retirement in 2000—a 35-year tenure.

With a strong interest in research, Boyd cowrote more than 33 articles and coedited one book, *Trauma Management*, with Dr. Edwin F. Cave and John F. Burke; it was the last of a series of several books on fractures and trauma that began to be written by clinicians on the Fracture Service at MGH. In 1973, he published, with Burke and Dr. Theodore Colton, an article titled "A Double-Blind Clinical Trial of Prophylactic Antibiotics in Hip Surgery" in the *Journal of Bone and Joint Surgery*. Because of conflicting reports on the effectiveness of preoperative antibiotics, they had randomized 348 patients to receive either the treatment (sodium nafcillin) or a control (glucose) in a double-blind investigation:

> [T]he rate of postoperative wound infection was found to be one in 135 (0.8 percent) in…patients who received nafcillin; and seven in 145 (4.8 percent) in…control patients who received glucose as a placebo; a statistically significant difference…Our results…support the thesis that antibiotics used for prophylaxis in hip-fracture surgery are effective in reducing the rate of postoperative wound infection…if they are given before, during, and after operation…It does not seem reasonable…to pursue

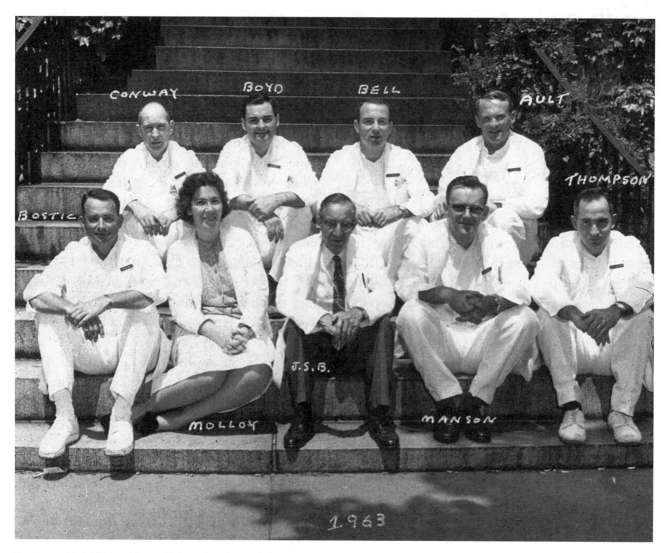

Dr. Barr with MGH residents. Robert Boyd is in the back row second from the left. MGH HCORP Archives.

investigation of the prophylactic effects of antibiotics given only after operation. (Boyd, Burke, and Cotton 1973)

Boyd limited his practice to spine and trauma. For 20 years (1980–2000), he was director of the Problem Back Clinic at MGH. During this time, Boyd also had a teaching appointment at Harvard. Six of his publications were related to the spine, reflecting this interest and expertise. In a series of six patients with pyogenic osteomyelitis of the spine, Drs. Kattapuram, Phillips, and Boyd described the superiority of computed tomography (CT) in evaluating the condition. It can indicate the size and location of the area of infection in the soft tissue in relation to the surrounding tissues and anatomic landmarks, e.g., the aorta and spine, and it can identify abscesses, which may need to be drained. CT scans over time can help to confirm that treatment is working and that the mass is indeed reducing in size.

In 1986, Boyd and Huddleston, along with Drs. Fred Mansfield and Kenneth Polivy, published their results of the use of chymopapain to treat herniated disc disease in patients with sciatica. Dr. Lyman Smith had previously published the paper "Enzymatic Dissolution of the Nucleus Pulposus in Humans" in the *Journal of the American Medical Association* in 1964. This had been preceded by another article by Smith, "Enzyme

Dissolution in the Nucleus Pulposus," published the year earlier in *Nature*. After these publications by Smith, the popularity of chymopapain increased. Boyd and Huddleston advanced their 1986 study by administering a follow-up questionnaire to 146 patients who had received chymopapain (Discase) injections to treat sciatica caused by a herniated nucleus pulposus 10–14 years earlier. The responses revealed a satisfactory result in 66%. Among the 102 patients rated as having excellent or good results, 5% required surgical discectomy. They identified a failure rate of 34%. In an editorial comment preceding the *Clinical Orthopaedics and Related Research* symposium on chemonucleolysis in which they presented their results, Dr. Eugene J. Nordby summarized the results of all 13 studies reported in the symposium. Average satisfactory results were obtained in 77%; average failure rate was 23%.

Boyd was not only a respected researcher, but also a recognized expert in spine surgery. As such he was often asked for his medical opinions by the press. For example, a study about the use of MRI of the lumbar spine in patients without back pain showed that "many people without back pain have disk bulges or protrusions but not extrusions... The discovery by MRI of bulges or protrusions in people with low back pain may frequently be coincidental" (Jenson et al. 1994). Boyd agreed that MRI was done too often for patients with back pain. Boyd told the *New York Times* that "overuse of M.R.I.'s [is due to] insecurity, threat of lawsuits, inexperience and the potential for economic gain...Surgery doesn't put new backs in and it doesn't give better long-term results...It is indicated when pain doesn't respond to conservative treatment and is clearly associated with nerve root compression...[but] only about 5% of people with back pain fall into the category" (quoted in Kolata 1994).

Boyd recalled working with Barr Sr., whose office was located in the Warren Building. He remembered that Barr:

> had stopped operating when I was his resident and he was ill enough, or so with his emphysema that he was unable to get out of his desk chair to go examine the patient [see chapter 38]. So the resident's responsibility was, and mine, to take the patient, sit there and listen to Dr. Barr interview the patient and then I would go into the examining room, examine the patient and while the patient was dressing, come back and give the findings to Dr. Barr...Then the patient would come in and Dr. Barr would advise him as to diagnosis and recommended treatment. And I must say I learned more in those six weeks... it was absolutely wonderful to see how the man synthesized information from the history. He was a wonderful interviewer and he was a brilliant and experienced and wise person...[Dr. Barr at that time] was very short of breath... and did not operate. I had information about his operating skills...[he had been] a paragon of efficiency; he had outstanding surgical skills.

(Boyd, personal interview with the author, 2009)

During our interview, Boyd also described the long hours he willingly put in during his time at MGH:

> [Dr. Barr] forgot to tell me, or he neglected to tell me, that it's [MGH] such a fascinating place to work you usually didn't get bored until 9 or 10 at night...making consults, visiting other

---

A Double-Blind Clinical Trial of Prophylactic Antibiotics in Hip Fractures

BY ROBERT J. BOYD, M.D.†, JOHN F. BURKE, M.D.‡, AND THEODORE COLTON, S.M., SC.D.§, BOSTON, MASSACHUSETTS

From the Departments of Orthopaedic Surgery and Surgery, Harvard Medical School at the Massachusetts General Hospital, and the Department of Preventive Medicine, Harvard Medical School, Boston

THE JOURNAL OF BONE AND JOINT SURGERY
VOL. 55-A, NO. 6, SEPTEMBER 1973

Boyd, et al article, "A Double-Blind Clinical Trial of Prophylactic Antibiotics in Hip Fractures." *Journal of Bone and Joint Surgery* 1973; 55: 1251.

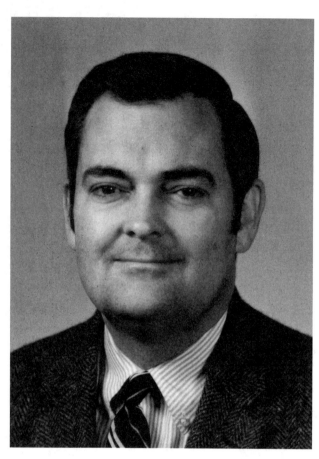

Robert J. Boyd. MGH HCORP Archives.

staff members. There were a cadre of us who would do a lot of consults in the hospital that were added on to our otherwise busy day, and we took time with patients...And so, I didn't get home...living in Weston...until 9 or 10 at night, most nights. And my Saturdays were half days, which was until 5 p.m., and Sundays as well. So, it was a way of life. But it was an absolutely wonderful, collegial place. There was no jealousy that I perceived between disciplines or within the department of orthopaedics. We all helped one another...There was a wonderful cooperative relationship between neurosurgery and orthopaedics and spine. Bob Ojemann and I did a lot of cases...but Bill Sweet...one you didn't see and relate to very much...was the chief, but he never interfered with us. (Boyd, personal interview with the author, 2009)

Boyd loved the MGH and his close personal and professional relationships with his colleagues. He worked long hours, frequently including weekends—he was totally committed to his patients and the hospital.

Boyd became very involved in hospital politics and held positions on many committees. He chaired the Staff Associates for a couple of years and was a significant leader, together with Dr. Gerald Austen and others, in the formation of the Massachusetts General Hospital Physicians Organization (later called the MGPO). Because of his success, he was placed on both the board of trustees and the general executive committee at MGH. Later, as the MGPO began to function, the Staff Association was dissolved. The hospital leadership supposedly asked Boyd—who was about to retire—to lead the MGPO, but he preferred an independent physician organization and so declined. He was eventually joined in practice by James Huddleston at Zero Emerson Place. The two worked together for a few years before Huddleston moved to Naples, Florida, where he opened a private practice. He retired from MGH and from his position as assistant clinical professor of orthopaedic surgery at HMS in 2000.

THORNTON BROWN

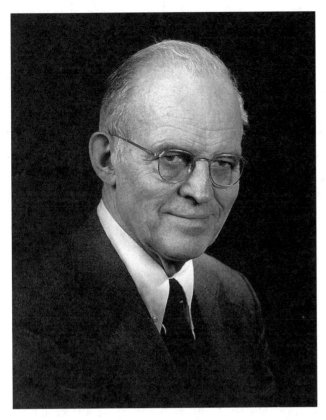

Thornton Brown. P.H.C., H.R.C. and J.C., "Thornton Brown, M.D. 1913-2000," *Journal of Bone and Joint Surgery* 2000; 82: 1675.

> **Physician Snapshot**
>
> Thornton Brown
> BORN: 1913
> DIED: 2000
> SIGNIFICANT CONTRIBUTIONS: Editor of the *Journal of Bone and Joint Surgery* for 20 years (1958–78); served as president of the American Orthopaedic Association in 1979

Thornton Brown, or "Thornie, as he was affectionately known, came from an old and distinguished New England medical family" (Curtiss, Cowell, and Cohen 2000). He was born November 24, 1913. His father was Dr. Lloyd T. Brown (see chapter 46), an associate of Dr. Joel E. Goldthwait. The elder Brown was very influential at the Robert Breck Brigham Hospital, where he served as president of the board of directors from 1932 to 1951. He also descended from John Ball and Buckminster Brown. In his book *Lest We Forget*, Dr. Carter Rowe (1996) stated that it was this illustrious background of quality in orthopaedic practice that made Thornie an excellent orthopedist and an admirable man. Despite this claim by Rowe, however, I was not able to verify that Thornton Brown was related to Dr. John Ball Brown and his son, Dr. Buckminster Brown.

Thornie "graduated from Harvard College in 1936 and from Harvard Medical School in 1940" (Curtiss, Cowell, and Cohen 2000). He served with the US Marines in the Pacific theater during World War II; he was a battalion surgeon with the Naval Medical Corps. After being discharged, he returned to Massachusetts. He married Sarah Tyler Meigs in 1944, and they lived in Milton, Massachusetts. In 1948, he "completed an orthopaedic residency in the Massachusetts General Hospital/Boston Children's Hospital program," after which he "practiced orthopaedics at the Massachusetts General Hospital" and was a consultant at Milton Hospital (Curtiss, Cowell, and Cohen 2000). When he joined the staff at MGH, the following surgeons were members of the Department of Orthopaedic Surgery: Drs. Marius Smith-Petersen (chapter 37), Joseph Barr Sr. (chapter 38), Edwin Cave, William A. Rogers, George Van Gorder, Sumner Roberts, Paul Norton, and Otto Aufranc (each described within this chapter).

Research on Back Pain

Brown became interested in back pain early in his career at MGH. Over a four-year period, he cowrote three papers: one on psychological factors in back pain, another on the development and use of a back brace, and the third on the mechanical properties of the lumbar disc. In the first paper, "Psychological Factors in Low-Back Pain," published in the *New England Journal of Medicine* in 1954, Brown, Barr Sr., and others described their evaluations of 36 patients; each evaluation comprised "an orthopaedic work-up…[including an]

Brown et al.'s first paper on low back pain. *New England Journal of Medicine* 1954; 251: 123.

x-ray study of the lumbar spine, and...myelography...[and a] psychiatric investigation [that] consisted of two or more psychiatric interviews... [The psychiatric] opinion indicated whether... the patient had psychological factors significantly complicating his condition." They went on to describe six:

> striking characteristics [that] appeared repeatedly in a number of patients:
>
> The first consisted of a history...that was vague because of confused chronology and material that seemed nothing to do with the injury and symptoms.
>
> The second was an expression of either open or veiled resentment toward and criticism of the doctors and allied personnel because of alleged mismanagement and neglect.
>
> The third comprised dramatic descriptions of the symptoms and the patient's reaction...
>
> The fourth was difficulty in localization and description of pain and other symptoms...
>
> The fifth consisted of failure of the usual forms of treatment to give significant relief from pain.
>
> The sixth included accompanying neurotic symptoms. (Brown et al. 1954)

They concluded that the number of symptoms correlated with the extent to which psychological elements contributed to the patient's condition: "In a patient showing four or more of the characteristics...psychological factors are an important part of the illness; in a patient with two or fewer characteristics, psychological factors are not important" (Brown et al. 1954).

Brown wrote his second paper, "The Immobilizing Efficiency of Back Braces; Their Effect on the Posture and Motion of the Lumbosacral Spine," with Paul Norton; it was published in 1957 in the *Journal of Bone and Joint Surgery*. I discuss it in the section describing Paul Norton later in this chapter. The final paper cowritten by Brown (with Robert Hansen and Alvin Yorra) was titled "Some Mechanical Tests on the Lumbosacral Spine with Particular Reference to The Intervertebral Discs." It exemplifies Brown's interest in basic research regarding the etiology and treatment of low-back pain and his collaboration with scientists at the Massachusetts Institute of Technology. After reviewing the literature about intervertebral discs as a cause of low-back pain, the authors stated: "This preliminary report concerns a program of tests of the mechanical strength and elastic properties of the intervertebral discs" in the lumbar spines of cadavers (Brown, Hansen, and Yorra 1957).

They enumerated four conclusions that they believed justified additional investigation of their tests:

1. Under axial compressive stress, failure of the disc complex invariably took place in the cartilaginous plate...Failures of the end-plate may play a role in the causation of pain in some back injuries when the roentgenograms show no abnormality...

2. Failure of the annulus fibrosus occurred only as the result of extremely rapid cyclic binding compared with mild axial compression. However no protrusion of disc material was produced in this short period but rather a linear horizontal tear through all but the most peripheral fibers which still remained intact.

3. ...The anulus invariably bulged on the concave side, apparently as a result of compression between the opposing vertebral surfaces...

4. Under axial compressive loads the volume losses of the intervertebral discs before failure...were [1.0 to 2.5 cm^3]. (Brown, Hansen, and Yorra 1957)

In 1983, Brown contributed a chapter titled "Orthopedic Surgery" for the book, *The Massachusetts General Hospital, 1955 to 1980*, edited by Benjamin Castleman, David C. Crockett, and Silvia Barry Sutton. In it he described various issues hampering research in low-back pain at MGH:

with Paul Norton and Thornton Brown as the orthopedic surgeons involved, several projects were begun in collaboration with the department of structural engineering at MIT, the American Mutual Liability Insurance Co., and the MGH Psychiatric Service. However, an ongoing investigation of the low back syndrome failed to materialize primarily because of the lack of innovative talent. The problem clearly was to find an orthopedist investigator with the ability and motivation to start a research program of such outstanding promise that it would attract the large-scale financial help needed to build and support the work of orthopedic research laboratory at the MGH. (Brown 1983)

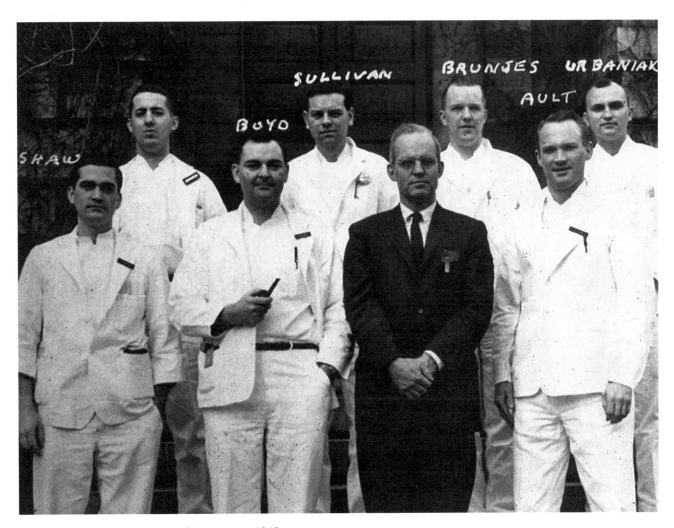

Dr. Brown (interim chief) with MGH residents, 1965. MGH HCORP Archives.

Such financial and staff roadblocks were not the only problems: Brown's personal involvement in low-back-pain–related research ended because, in 1958, he was selected to follow Dr. William A. Rogers as the editor of the *Journal of Bone and Joint Surgery* (*JBJS*). He had been an assistant to Rogers for several years during Rogers's editorship.

Dedication to the *Journal of Bone and Joint Surgery*

After his appointment as editor of *JBJS*, Brown maintained only a small clinical practice and no longer operated. As a resident in the late 1960s, I don't remember ever seeing Brown's name on the daily surgical schedule. Brown believed that the position of editor required full-time engagement, and he did not limit the hours he worked.

Brown "served as Editor until his retirement in 1978…[At the time] *The Journal* (which had been joined by its British counterpart in 1947) was the sole major orthopaedic journal. With the rapidly increasing number of orthopaedic subspecialties, however, it was only a matter of time before many of them would wish to have their own journals" (Curtiss, Cowell, and Cohen 2000). Throughout Brown's 20-year tenure as editor, he and the journal's editorial team tried to counter the pressure for more orthopaedic journals, more flexible editorial standards, and more prompt publication of accepted manuscripts through "efforts to shorten the time from submission of manuscript to publication, [which they

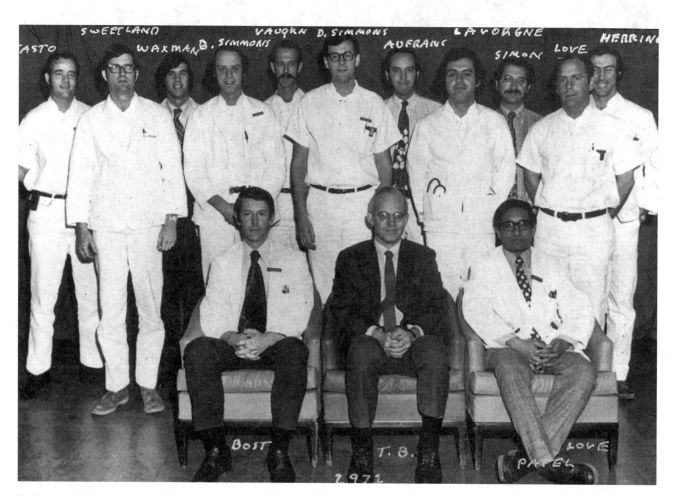

Dr. Brown (interim chief) with MGH residents, 1971. MGH HCORP Archives.

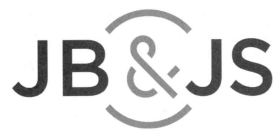

Logo, Journal of Bone and Joint Surgery (JBJS).
Courtesy of *Journal of Bone and Joint Surgery*/Wolters Kluwer.

achieved] by streamlining editorial procedure, increasing the number of issues published yearly to eight[,] and publishing *Orthopaedic Transactions*" (Curtiss, Cowell, and Cohen 2000). (*Orthopaedic Transactions* was published in 1977 and included abstracts of papers presented at annual meetings of various orthopaedic societies.) Brown also increased the standards required for publication in that journal, "partly because of Dr. Brown's requirements but chiefly because of… [his] expertise in editing. He rewrote many manuscripts word by word to make them of most use to the readers" (Cowell 2000). Brown's efforts only delayed the inevitable, however, and "new journals were published, one of the first being the *Journal of Hand Surgery*, first published in 1976" (Curtiss, Cowell, and Cohen 2000).

While Brown was editor, *JBJS* collaborated with the National Library of Medicine (NLM) to publish the *Annual Bibliography of Orthopaedic Surgery*. In 1976, *JBJS* took over this publication from the association, which had published the first edition in 1969. *JBJS* and the NLM published the *Annual Bibliography* "through 1996, when the National Library of Medicine discontinued providing camera-ready copy to The Journal because of the availability of such information online" (Cowell 2000). In addition to the *Annual Bibliography*, *JBJS* also put out six versions of the *Five-Year Cumulated Bibliography of Orthopaedic Surgery* between 1970 and 1995.

Publishing in *JBJS* in 2003, Cohen and Heckman described "the Brown era" of the journal's history as having "one important characteristic that was not obvious in the accounts of previous eras: [A] prime effort to be the journal of record":

> It is apparent that, in addition to a greatly increased number of articles in 1973 compared with 1963…from 144 to 200 articles, despite no increase in the number of issues (eight) or the number of pages (about 1800). The number of articles on the extremities increased by a factor of five; articles on the hip and on injection quadrupled; fracture articles tripled; and articles on the spine and on tumors more than doubled. Obviously, the pages per article had to decrease…[W]e must emphasize how he [Brown] elevated the standard of reporting. Many authors were in prolonged correspondence with him; they clarified, condensed…and in a word, perfected them…No previous Editor contributed so much to the establishment of JBJS as the outstanding, internationally recognized organ of orthopaedic surgery. (Cohen and Heckman 2003)

Dr. Mark Coventry, in "The American Orthopaedic Association and the Written Word"—his presidential address at the 1977 American Orthopaedic Association annual meeting—wrote about Brown's "philosophy regarding his style of editing":

> He believes that the rules he endeavors to follow have developed over the years in an effort to ensure clarity for all readers…[He] thinks that scientific articles should be clear rather than obscure and novel…He believes that the interests of both authors and readers are involved and that the two are not always reconcilable. [Brown said:] "Our fervent desire is no more than to publish the best articles we can in the clearest, most concise, and most reasonable fashion possible, just as rapidly as we can…During the first half of the 20th century an orthopaedic surgeon could with some assurance assume that if he read the Journal

completely he would keep up to date, at least with respect to the major clinical and research advances in his specialty."

Coventry (1977) also noted, however, that despite Brown's efforts, *JBJS* was no longer the only source for such information: "A list of journals...in the *Year Book of Orthopedics and Traumatic Surgery* includes fifty-five journals."

Through "patient negotiation" on Brown's part: "In 1978, The Journal became the official organ of publication of the Orthopaedic Research Society and the Canadian Orthopaedic Research Society" (Curtis Jr. 1979). Brown had "ensur[ed] that research articles relevant to the practice of orthopaedics would continue to be published in The Journal rather than being dispersed in purely research publications. This effort has been greatly helped by the addition...of a Deputy Editor for Research and a Board of Consulting Editors for Research" (Curtis Jr. 1979).

American Orthopaedic Association Presidency

In 1979, shortly after his tenure as *JBJS* editor ended, Brown was elected president of the American Orthopaedic Association in recognition of his contributions to the profession of orthopaedic surgery. In his presidential address that year he recalled the glorious past of the AOA but highlighted the association's failure to take full advantage of its resources:

> The Association must consider what it should do to advance orthopaedic surgery, what it can do that will be 'better' and not just more... Nearly fifty years ago, when the Association decided not to enlarge, many assumed that as the senior organization it would function much as the Senate does in the federal government, while the newly organized Academy would be the House of Representatives...However, the growth of the Academy and the emergence of the other organizations make a senatorial role for the Association rather unrealistic. Similarly, the...Annual Meetings...in the secluded surroundings of a resort hotel...[is] the setting... reminiscent of a "retreat" or "think tank"...the stage for creative thought. But is the Association taking full advantage of these features? The answer, I fear, is not an unqualified "yes."

He went on with suggestions for how the AOA should move forward in the years ahead:

> I suggest that the Association develop procedures to identify and analyze problems. The goal would be to bring the expertise of the membership and invited experts...to focus on current problems and thereby to stimulate, augment, or supplement the deliberations and actions of other organizations in the community of orthopaedic Societies...Like any catalyst, however, it [the AOA] did not change as the reactions it produced progressed. Instead it remained small, relinquishing to other, larger organizations the activities that require substantial financing and manpower resources. Although this turn of events has limited the Association's options, I envision a need that the AOA can fulfill uniquely. If indeed the emphasis is likely to be more on improving what we have and less on increasing it, then a major goal must

---

The American Orthopaedic Association — Its Role in a Troubled World*

BY THORNTON BROWN, M.D.†, BOSTON, MASSACHUSETTS

THE JOURNAL OF BONE AND JOINT SURGERY
VOL. 61-A, NO. 7, OCTOBER 1979

Dr. Brown's AOA presidential address. *Journal of Bone and Joint Surgery* 1979; 61: 1112.

be perfection in all orthopaedic activities...If our organization played this role to the full...the AOA would have reason to be as proud of its efforts during the last decades of the twentieth century as it is of its role at the beginning. Such pride would indeed be justified if the Association's wise counsel, watchful eye, and insistence on perfection helped to ensure that the best possible orthopaedic care was available to all at reasonable cost and that orthopaedics was not shackled by excessive government regulation. (Brown 1979)

After Retirement

Brown retired from MGH and Milton Hospital in 1993 and continued to live in Milton another 7 years. His hobbies consisted of organic farming, splitting wood, hiking, and sailing. His wife, Sarah, died in 1998, and Brown followed her two years later, on July 4, 2000. He was 86 years old. At the time he was living at the Orchard Cove Retirement Community in Canton, Massachusetts. Sarah and Thornie left behind a son and three daughters.

A surgeon publishing as "D. L. H." in *JBJS* in 2001, wrote a tribute to Brown, including a personal reminiscence:

> I first met him [Brown] in 1966 when I went to Boston for a year and an orthopaedic fellowship at Harvard and Massachusetts General Hospital...Dr. Brown invited me to the Journal Office, then based in the Countway Medical Library...I was...surprised by the man, who seemed very relaxed and informal, quite unlike the stiff, severe, senior figure whom I had expected to meet. He provided me with much help and advice on publishing research findings during the rest of my year...I shall remember him for the kindness and interest which he showed to a young British trainee in what was then a very foreign land.

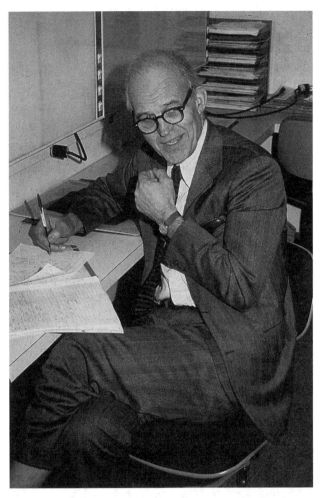

Dr. Brown completing chart documentation after seeing a patient on rounds. MGH HCORP Archives.

CARL H. BUCHOLZ

> **Physician Snapshot**
>
> Carl H. Bucholz
> BORN: 1874
> DIED: Unknown
> SIGNIFICANT CONTRIBUTIONS: Ran the Medico-Mechanical and Hydrotherapeutic Departments at MGH from 1906 to 1914; published *Therapeutic Exercise and Massage* in 1917

I was unable to find much information about Carl Hermann Bucholz except that he graduated from the University of Leipzig in 1901. He was a member of the Deutsche Gelsellshaft fur Chirurgie (the German Society for Surgery) and Deutsche Gelsellshaft für Orthopädische Chirurgie (the German Society for Orthopaedic Surgery), and he specialized in orthopaedic surgery. Throughout his career, he published two books on therapeutic exercise, so-called mechanotherapy, and massage, as well as 15 articles on the same subjects.

Although I was unable to uncover the circumstances of his transition from Germany to Boston, it is likely that leadership at MGH (probably Joel Goldthwait) recruited Bucholz (and Max Böhm before him) in the early 1900s to establish a program using the Zander equipment there. Bucholz was likely familiar with it from his time at university. In the late 1800s, European physicians such as the Swede Gustav Zander, with their mechanical and scientific approach to orthopaedic conditions, had designed complex equipment to assist patients while exercising their upper and lower extremities and spine. Such equipment obviously predates and may be considered a prototype for modern gym exercise equipment. As the new century began, German physicians embraced Zander's system, and use of the equipment spread worldwide. The Zander Room was created at MGH "in

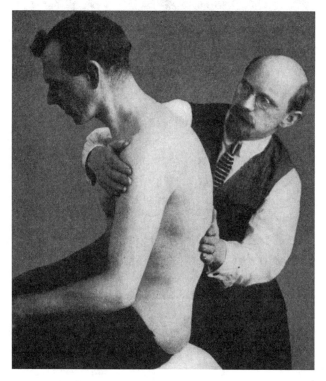

Photo of Carl Hermann Bucholz.
A Manual of Therapeutic Exercise and Massage Designed for the Use of Physicians, Students and Masseurs by C. Hermann Bucholz. Philadelphia and New York: Lea & Febiger, 1917. Harold B. Lee Library, Brigham Young University/Internet Archive.

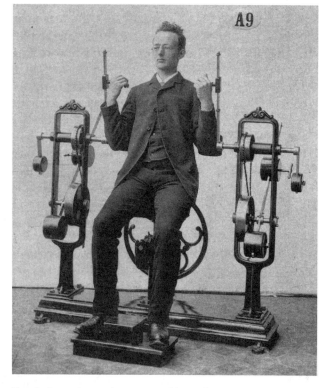

Zander's mechano-therapy machines: A.
Dr. G. Zander's medico-mechanische Gymnastik by Dr. Alfred Levertin. Königl. Buchdruckerei: P. A. Norstedt & Söner, 1892. Smithsonian Libraries and Archives/Internet Archive.

1903[, when] the seats had been removed from the large 1867 Operating Theatre [in the basement of the outpatient department] and from the space thus obtained, a corridor to the Gay Ward petitioned off. The remaining floor space and a gallery formed by the roof of this corridor was used to house the fifty-four machines invented by Dr. Zander and, with one exception, all imported from Stockholm" (Washburn 1959). By 1907, hydrotherapy and heat and massage, with the apparatus for electro-therapy, were added to the mechano-therapy machines. Their intended purpose was "to perform all the motions of the body and so exercise all the muscles. The patient was strapped to the apparatus, the motor started, and willy-nilly the joints and muscles were exercised. While very ingenious and producing good results in many cases, the machines failed to be satisfactory because they operated without any volition on the part of the patient or the development of any will to recover on his part" (Faxon 1959) (see **Case 40.3**).

We know that at Harvard Medical School, Bucholz was initially listed as an assistant in orthopaedics and physical therapy. In 1908, he was listed as assistant to the orthopaedic surgeon to outpatients (then Dr. Robert Osgood) and surgeon-in-charge in the Medico-Mechanical Department at MGH. Bucholz had replaced Dr. Max Böhm, another German trained in physiotherapy, who in 1904 had become the first surgeon in charge of that newly formed department in what was then

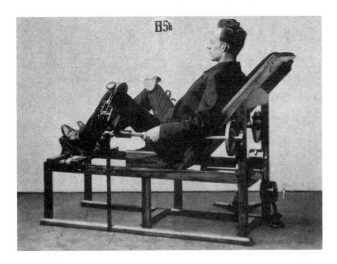

Zander's mechano-therapy machines: B.
Dr. G. Zander's medico-mechanische Gymnastik by Dr. Alfred Levertin. Königl. Buchdruckerei: P. A. Norstedt & Söner, 1892. Smithsonian Libraries and Archives/Internet Archive.

Case 40.3. Treatment of Paralysis with Exercise

"Infantile Paralysis. J. W. P., male, sixteen years of age, had partial paralysis of his trunk, pelvis, and both legs, since November 1909. The cause was probably a transverse myelitis, but differential diagnosis of anterior poliomyelitis was considered in the Nerve Department. A short period of total paralysis was followed by gradual improvement, which has continued up to the present time.

"In January 1911, when first seen in the Medico-Mechanical Department, the patient showed the following symptoms. He walked with very marked lack of support, very much like patients with double congenital hip dislocation. In standing on one leg he was not able to balance the body in a normal manner, but showed a marked Trendelenburg's symptom. The forward bending of the body was possible, but the patient could not hold himself without help in that position and had great difficulty in raising up his body again. He could hardly bend his body sideways. The movements of the legs were all possible, but very weak and unsteady. Both feet were markedly pronated and flattened.

"Under a nine week's exercise treatment and massage the patient has been markedly improved, as he says himself. His gait is much better. He can balance his body fairly normally when standing on one leg. He raises up his body after stooping forward rather easily and can hold himself in a stooping position without assistance. The sideward movements of the trunk are nearly normal. His legs are moved much easier and are rather steady. He has procured plates for his deformed foot, which correct them somewhat.

"The patient is still under treatment. With this marked improvement which has shown in two months, the prognosis of a good final outcome seems very favorable."

(C. Hermann Bucholz 1912)

called the Zander Room. (At that time, Dr. Joel Goldthwait was chief of the Orthopaedic Service; he advocated conservative treatment with exercise and massage for many painful orthopaedic conditions. Goldthwait resigned in 1908 [see chapter 33.]) Five years after leaving MGH, Dr. Böhm published a book, *Massage. Its Principles and Technique*. It was edited by Dr. Charles Painter, then Professor of Orthopaedic Surgery at Tufts. An excerpt from it appears in **Box 40.5**, underscoring how underappreciated physical therapy was in the United States at the beginning of the twentieth century. When Bucholz took over for Böhm in the Medico-Mechanical Department in 1908 at MGH, visiting surgeons there included Drs. Charles Scudder and Elliott Brackett, Dr. Ernest Codman was an assistant visiting surgeon. Dr. Walter J. Dodd was the skiagrapher. Physicians in the orthopaedic outpatient department included Osgood, the orthopaedic surgeon to outpatients; Drs. William R. MacAusland, Mark H. Rogers, and Zabdiel B. Adams, who were assistant orthopaedic surgeons to the outpatients; and, in addition to Bucholz, Carl C. Crane, Warren F. Gay, Frederick J. Goodridge, Henry L. Langnecker, and Harvey F. Newhall as assistant orthopaedic surgeons to outpatients. While at MGH, Bucholz's office was located at 139 Beacon Street; he lived at 427 Cambridge Street in Allston.

By 1914 Bucholz had been surgeon-in-charge of the Medico-Mechanical Department for six years. In that year, Bucholz published in the *Journal of the American Medical Association* his experience with the department. **Table 40.3** shows the numbers and types of cases treated during his

Box 40.5. Status of Physical Therapy in the United States in 1910

> In the "Introduction" to Dr. Böhm's *Massage. Its Principles and Technique*, Dr. Painter wrote:
>
> "In Germany physical therapeutics in all its forms is employed far more widely than it is here. The beneficial effect of massage is much more fully appreciated than with us…
>
> "In some of our larger cities there are few hospitals where fairly complete physical therapeutic facilities are to be had, but in very few of them is the value of these facilities appreciated…
>
> "The profession at large, however, are not securing for their patients the benefit that they might, because they do not know enough of the advantages inherent in the various therapeutic measures to think of making use of them…What is needed…is a more widely diffused and personal knowledge on such matters, and it is with the hope that the technique of one of the most important of these physical therapeutic measures… clearly demonstrated in this little book of Böhm's, may be brought within the reach of a great number of the medical profession."
>
> (Böhm 1913)

Table 40.3. Cases Treated in the Medico-Mechanical Department at MGH, 1908–1914

	No. of cases treated (N = 4,904)
Fractures	1,258
Dislocations	128
Stiff joints	354
Arthroplasties	9
Contractures	118
Contusions and sprains	166
Subdeltoid bursitis	331
Myositis	12
Arthritis	788
Back problems	681
Foot problems	265
Nerve diseases	547
Internal diseases	
Circulatory system	33
Respiratory system	16
Digestive system	38
Other	60
Miscellaneous	100

Adapted from Bucholz 1914.

tenure (1908–14). For Bucholz (1914), "The steady growth of the number of new patients shows how the department has become more and more an important factor of the hospital; particularly the surgical and medical departments [who] use it." Bucholz's detailed description of the workings of the department is provided in **Box 40.6**.

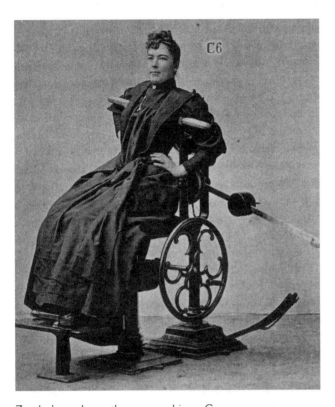

Zander's mechano-therapy machines: C.
Dr. G. Zander's medico-mechanische Gymnastik by Dr. Alfred Levertin. Königl. Buchdruckerei: P. A. Norstedt & Söner, 1892. Smithsonian Libraries and Archives/Internet Archive.

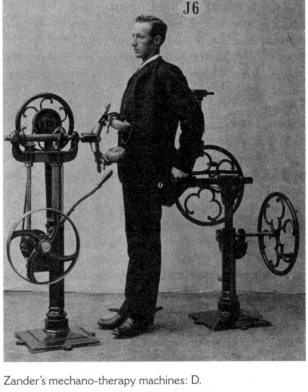

Zander's mechano-therapy machines: D.
Dr. G. Zander's medico-mechanische Gymnastik by Dr. Alfred Levertin. Königl. Buchdruckerei: P. A. Norstedt & Söner, 1892. Smithsonian Libraries and Archives/Internet Archive.

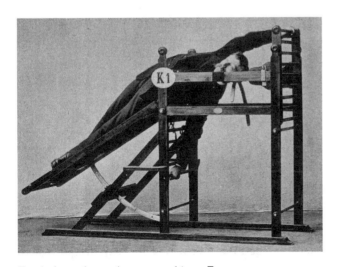

Zander's mechano-therapy machines: E.
Dr. G. Zander's medico-mechanische Gymnastik by Dr. Alfred Levertin. Königl. Buchdruckerei: P. A. Norstedt & Söner, 1892. Smithsonian Libraries and Archives/Internet Archive.

SIX YEARS' EXPERIENCES AT THE MEDICOMECHANICAL DEPARTMENT OF THE MASSACHUSETTS GENERAL HOSPITAL*

C. HERMANN BUCHOLZ, M.D.
BOSTON

JOUR. A. M. A.
NOV. 14. 1914

VOLUME LXIII
NUMBER 20

Dr. Bucholz's review of cases treated with Zander's equipment at MGH, 1908–1914. *Journal of the American Medical Association* 1914; 63: 1733.

Box 40.6. Workings of the Medico-Mechanical Department at MGH

"The medicomechanical department consists of a large room with the Zander Apparatus, a balcony for the special corrective work, two small rooms for massage and manual exercise as well as baking, and an office for examination and manual treatment...Machines are a good compensation for the exercise in many ways, but...[not] a full substitute, nor are they, in my opinion, indispensable in obtaining the local effect. Most of our surgical and orthopedic patients have to begin their treatment with the manual methods of passive and active, assistive and resistive exercise, and become ready for apparatus treatment only when they have gathered sufficient strength to control the apparatus...On many days sixty, eighty and even up to 100 patients are to be treated in from three to four hours. The average time of one treatment being considered twenty minutes. The apparatus does not necessarily require a trained attendant, though of course an intelligent and expert supervision is desirable....

"For the general effect on the circulatory, respiratory, digestive and nervous systems and on the general metabolism the apparatus is of great value and have a decided preference over the manual treatment...In close connection with the medicomechanical department is a hydrotherapeutic department in my charge...many patients get both...on the same day or on alternating days. Of Bier's methods only the baking is used to a large extent...The various methods of electrical treatment which represent another branch of physical therapeutics are distributed among the Roentgen-ray and nerve departments...The Zander room is a subsidiary department in that outpatients have to belong primarily to one of the regular clinics and are sent to the Zander room for treatment. Thus, the medical man, the surgeon, the orthopedist or the nerve man makes the indication as to the treatment in the medicomechanical or hydrotherapeutic department. He also may suggest the form of treatment which he considers best...But it must be insisted that the director of such a department has absolutely free hand to decide as to the form and amount of treatment, as well as to refuse treatment if he considers it not a suitable case...

"At present the surgeon in charge of the medicomechanical department is holding a position as orthopedic surgeon to the outpatient, while his assistant holds a place at the same department. This personal union of the orthopedic department and the department for physical therapeutics is in my opinion of greatest value...to the orthopedic cases, but also for the whole hospital, and becomes more and more so with the growing field of orthopedic work. The value of this union is acknowledged by the university in the appointment of the surgeon in charge as assistant in orthopedics and physical therapeutics at Harvard Graduate School of Medicine. We meet the same union in many German university clinics and hospitals...

"Such a department must have the intelligent and wilful support of the whole hospital and all physicians must feel that it is not an institution for the worst type of cases... [In the discussion Dr. Bucholz stated] In our orthopedic department, where about fifteen or twenty physicians are working, there are a lot of young men...when asked what they would do they could not tell. I tell them they ought to be ashamed to call themselves orthopedic doctors and not know anything about this treatment."

(Reprinted with permission from Bucholz 1914.)

The year 1914 also brought with it World War I, and "Bucholz, being a German, [eventually] had to depart, and the Zander Room was turned into a ward for naval wounded. Wartime retrenchment also forced the closing of the Out-Patient Department [Zander Room], [and the] hydrotherapy room, and physiotherapy reverted to the simplest forms of treatment. The Zander Room never reopened" (Faxon 1959). The medico-mechanical department remained closed after the war, and Bucholz returned to Germany in 1920. At that time, he had been an assistant visiting orthopaedic surgeon, along with Z. B. Adams and Mark H. Rogers; Osgood was chief of the Orthopaedic Service. Drs. Lloyd T. Brown, Andrew P. Cornwall, Murray S. Danforth, Louis A. O. Goddu,

Dr. Bucholz's book, *Therapeutic Exercise and Massage*.
Philadelphia and New York: Lea & Febiger, 1917. Harold B. Lee Library, Brigham Young University/Internet Archive.

Harry C. Low, Marius N. Smith-Petersen, Loring T. Swaim, and Philip D. Wilson were orthopaedic surgeons to outpatients, and Drs. L. P. Felch and W. J. LaMarche were their assistants.

As the 1920s progressed, "physical and occupational therapy apparently came on hard times. In 1929 [Marius] Smith-Petersen noted that 'the outstanding need of the department is the reestablishment of a Physiotherapy Department'" (Brown 1983). Over the next decade, however, "little was done until…[October 1, 1939,] when Arthur L. Watkins, who had recently completed his neurologic residency at the MGH, was appointed chief of the Physical Therapy Department[,] which was established on the second floor of the Domestic Building" (Brown 1983). After the floor was remodeled the new facility was equipped with some apparatus remaining in the Out-Patient Department and some new equipment. Occupational therapy, which operated as a separate entity, was located in an adjoining room, and "in 1945 physical and occupational therapy were combined under Watkins as the Department of Physical Medicine" (Brown 1983). We do not know what became of Bucholz after he returned to Germany, but the legacy of his leadership lived on as the department continued to evolve and grow.

EDWIN F. CAVE

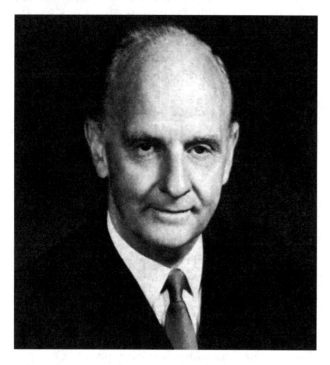

Edwin F. Cave. O.S.S., "Edwin French Cave, MD 1896-1976," *Journal of Bone and Joint Surgery* 1977; 59: 840.

Physician Snapshot

Edwin F. Cave
BORN: 1896
DIED: 1976
SIGNIFICANT CONTRIBUTIONS: Chief of the MGH Fracture Service, 1947–1957; president of the American Board of Orthopaedic Surgery (1958), the American Orthopaedic Association (1961), the American Association for the Surgery of Trauma (1967), and the Orthopaedic Research and Education Foundation (1968)

Edwin "Eddy" French Cave was born in 1896 and raised in Mexico, Missouri. His father was a physician, which perhaps started Eddy on the path he would take. He obtained an undergraduate degree from the University of Missouri (probably around 1920) and then matriculated at Harvard Medical School. While there, he became an elected member of the Boylston Medical Society, an honorary undergraduate society. After graduating from Harvard in 1924, he was appointed as a surgical house officer at MGH, a role in which he spent two years. He then completed an orthopaedic residency in the Children's Hospital/MGH combined program; Drs. Robert Osgood and Nathaniel Allison were his supervisors. After his residency, Cave joined Marius Smith-Petersen's practice and the staff at MGH; around that time, in 1929, Smith-Petersen was named chief of the Orthopaedic Service there. Other notable surgeons were on the visiting staff around the time Cave began, including Joseph S. Barr (began in 1929); William A. Rogers (1924); Armin Klein, who was also chief of orthopaedics at the Beth Israel Hospital (1920); Sumner Roberts (1929); George Van Gorder, who had recently returned from teaching at Peking Union Medical College in Beijing, China (1929).

Cave published five articles during his first 13 years at MGH. His first was the now-classic article "Intracapsular Fractures of the Neck of the Femur," which he cowrote with Smith-Petersen and George Van Gorder in 1931 (see chapter 37). At that time, Cave was just 35 years old. Cave noted that the steel used to create the triflanged nail he had helped Smith-Petersen develop in the mid-1920s was of poor quality and eventually eroded. In 1935, Cave published an article describing anterior and/or also a posterior capsulotomy through an anterior flap on either the medial or lateral side of the knee and thereby enter the joint without damaging the medial or lateral collateral ligaments. This allowed improved exposure to excise cysts or a meniscus. The following year Cave, with Sumner Roberts, published an article on measuring and recording joint function: "When the Fracture Clinic at the Massachusetts General Hospital began end-result studies, the need for a standard system of measurement of joint function became apparent...Individual methods...vary considerably and, when grouped together, may be confusing...This system [use of a goniometer or protractor to measure motion/angles] has been made as simple as possible...It is the result of ten year's trial, plus helpful suggestions received from twenty-five members of the

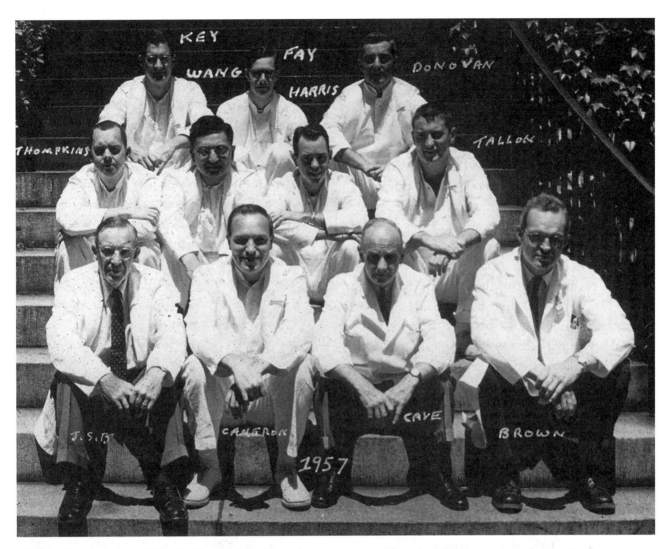

MGH staff and residents, 1957. Dr. Cave is seated in the front row, second from the right. MGH HCORP Archives.

Fracture Committee of the American College of Surgeons to whom this method was submitted for comment" (Cave and Roberts 1936).

That same year—six years into his tenure at MGH—Cave married Louise "Weezie" Fessenden. They settled in Brookline and eventually had two daughters. In 1937, just a year after their marriage, Cave opened his own private practice. Dr. O. Sherwin Staples joined him as an associate two years later. Staples joined the army in 1942, and because of this theirs "was [only] a brief professional association, but [it] led to a lasting and warm friendship" (Staples ["O.S.S."] 1977).

As the US became enmeshed in World War II, Cave began active duty as a major in the Army Medical Corps in 1942. He was "assigned to the Harvard Unit (5th General Hospital). After division of the Harvard Unit, he went to Queensland, Australia, as Chief of the Orthopaedic Service, 105th General Hospital [see chapter 64]. Later, Lieutenant Colonel Cave was Chief of the Surgical Service. When the unit moved to Biak Island, Dutch East Indies, Colonel Cave was its Commanding Officer. His final military position was Chief of the Surgical Service at Camp Edwards on Cape Cod, Massachusetts, from 1945 until his discharge on February 13, 1946" (Staples ["O.S.S."] 1977).

After his military service Cave returned to Boston, where he resumed his private practice. Dr. Carter R. Rowe joined him shortly after; this was "the start of a professional association and close friendship which continued all his [Cave's] life" (Staples ["O.S.S."] 1977). Also, at that time Gerhard Küntscher, during a visit to the US, demonstrated the application of the clover leaf rod and described challenges with its use. Cave was selected among various orthopaedic surgeons to assess an updated version of that rod: the intramedullary Kuntscher femoral rod (the German army had used it with great success during the war). "Thereafter Eddy's career was one of increasing pre-eminence on local [and] national...scenes" (Staples ["O.S.S."] 1977).

Cave became chief of the Fracture Service at MGH in 1947, a position he held for a decade (see chapter 31). Until that time, fracture cases at MGH were admitted to the surgical services or the orthopaedic service, but when Cave took over as chief—the first orthopaedic surgeon to do so—all fracture cases were admitted to the orthopaedic department. "All inpatient care was provided in the orthopaedic wards, while ambulatory treatment of fractures in the Emergency Room fell, in large part, to surgical residents on their orthopedic rotation" (Castleman, Crockett, and Sutton 1983). In addition to his role as chief, Cave was an assistant clinical professor of orthopaedic surgery at Harvard Medical School (beginning in 1953) and a consulting visiting orthopaedic surgeon at MGH (beginning in 1957); he remained in both those positions until 1969. By that time, "he had a large and very active practice" (Staples ["O.S.S."] 1977). (See **Case 40.4**.)

Cave also focused some of his research on torn ligaments in the knee, and not many orthopaedists had yet studied this topic. Dr. Don O'Donoghue traveled to Boston in the mid-1950s to discuss with Cave what O'Donoghue called the "terrible triad"—an injury to three parts of the knee simultaneously (the medial collateral ligament, the anterior cruciate ligament, and the medial meniscus). Cave suggested that O'Donoghue keep on with his research on the knee and pushed him to write up his findings.

Case 40.4. Achilles Tendon Injury

"A.B. (No. 803701, March 4, 1954), a forty-eight-year-old woman entered the hospital with the complaint of pain and weakness in the right leg. Four hours prior to entry, while attempting to push off on her right foot for a forehand drive in tennis, she had a sudden onset of pain and giving way of the right lower extremity. Pain was localized to the posterior aspect of the right ankle joint. She was unable to walk afterward and was taken to the hospital where examination revealed moderate swelling of the right ankle and the lower leg with definite tenderness over the Achilles tendon and a palpable defect at the junction of the tendon and muscular portion of the Achilles tendon. Forced plantar flexion was impossible. Passive dorsiflexion produced pain. X-rays revealed no bone injury. The next day at operation the tendon was found completely ruptured at the junction with the muscle; the plantaris tendon was intact. Repair was carried out with mattress sutures of fascia which was reinforced with silk. The wound was closed with cotton in the superficial fascia and with silk in the skin. A long leg cast was applied with the knee flexed 45 degrees. At the end of eleven days the long leg cast was replaced by a short one and this was worn for an additional thirty-six days. The patient was in a walking cast twenty-eight days after her operation. This was removed six weeks from the time of operation. Since that time, she has been walking about, wearing ordinary shoes and doing mild exercises to strengthen her calf muscle. At the end of four months the patient was walking on her toes without difficulty and had ½ inch atrophy of the calf. She had not yet returned to playing tennis but was driving a car and walking normally."

(Lawrence, Cave, and O'Connor 1955)

An Interest in Teaching

As his career progressed, Cave developed an interest in education of up-and-coming physicians, and although "he was active in teaching at the student, resident, and postgraduate levels...His interest in resident education was manifest in many ways"

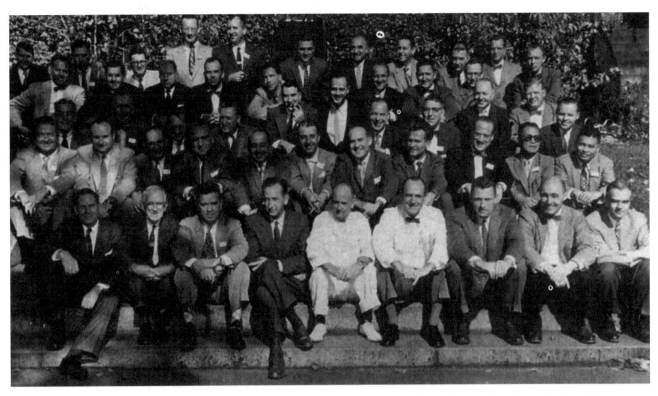

Fracture course attendees, late 1950s. Seated in the front row, right to left, second from the end: Dren Lowell, Tom Delorme, Carter Rowe, Eddy Cave, and Otto Aufranc. MGH HCORP Archives.

(Staples ["O.S.S."] 1977). One main effort was the "Fracture Courses" held at MGH; these had been suspended during World War II, but Cave reinvigorated them, and they "reached their zenith during his time [as chief of the Fracture Service]" (Staples ["O.S.S."] 1977). He also made efforts through a more traditional educational route: textbooks. "Through his energy and determination the old text, *Management of Fractures and Dislocations* edited by Philip D. Wilson and published in 1938, was reincarnated under the title, *Fractures and Other Injuries*, published in 1958" (Staples ["O.S.S."] 1977).

Cave reincarnated *Fractures and Other Injuries* at the behest of postgraduate students who had attended the MGH Fracture Courses. Cave enlisted 39 contributors—mainly orthopaedists, general surgeons, and internists on staff at MGH—to write the updated text. Cave dedicated the book to the Harvard faculty and the practitioners in the MGH Fracture Clinic—"past, present and future"—who "loyally" embody the "Spirit of Teaching" (Cave 1958). "His influence was the major motivating force that led to the publication of the second edition of the book, [renamed] *Trauma Management*, in 1974. He was honorary editor of this volume, which was dedicated to him" (Staples ["O.S.S."] 1977).

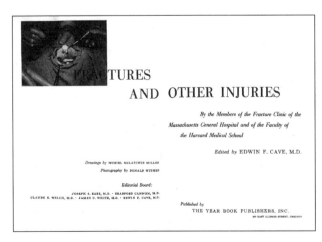

Cave's book, *Fractures and Other Injuries*. Chicago: The Year Book Publishers, 1958.

His dedication to resident education reached its peak with the creation of the Louise and Edwin F. Cave Traveling Fellowship, established through MGH in 1972 "to finance the travel of recent graduates of the Orthopaedic Residency Program... [and] endowed with funds donated by Dr. Cave, his patients, and his family" (Staples ["O.S.S."] 1977). Recipients had to agree to return to service on staff at MGH and implement the new knowledge they had acquired (see chapter 11).

Efforts on the National Scene

Cave gave the presidential address at the 1961 American Orthopaedic Association meeting in Yosemite, California. It was titled "Trauma and the Orthopaedic Surgeon," and he began by stating, "The name of our branch of surgery certainly does not describe it adequately, nor does it indicate that trauma has any place at all in our specialty..." (Cave 1961). He then described the development of orthopaedic surgery, particularly with regard to the effects of World Wars I and II:

> [I]n 1894 Phelps observed: "It is my earnest conclusion that within a very few years fractures and dislocations will be treated by the orthopaedic surgeons"...Actually...orthopaedic surgery was reborn and expanded during and after World War I, largely because trauma to the extremities became a part of orthopaedic surgery for the first time...Outstanding in the development of the traumatic side of orthopaedic surgery in World War I were Goldthwait, Osgood, Allison, Leo Mayer and Gallie; also Porter and Mackenzie Forbes...In 1919, Galloway wrote: "The war has done more to bring orthopaedic surgery into its true inheritance than would have been accomplished by any other agencies in many years"...[However] relatively few orthopaedic clinics throughout our country had the privilege of caring for fractures and other trauma after the war of 1914–18; at best, they shared the management of extremity trauma with the general surgeons....
>
> World War II changed all this. The sections of orthopaedic surgery in military hospitals often represented the largest divisions on the surgical services...Wounds of the extremities made up to 70 per cent of the case load of evacuation hospitals...[A survey regarding trauma management was recently sent to] eighty-three directors of orthopaedic training centers. A 100 percent response was obtained...Eighty-one... stated that fractures are largely in the hands of the orthopaedic surgeons. Thirteen indicated that general surgeons are treating fractures in their clinics...A significant observation was that [in] children's orthopaedics...there was a relative increase in fractures and other trauma... (Cave 1961)

Trauma and the Orthopaedic Surgeon*
BY EDWIN F. CAVE, M.D., BOSTON, MASSACHUSETTS
THE JOURNAL OF BONE AND JOINT SURGERY
VOL. 43-A, NO. 4, JUNE 1961

Dr. Cave's AOA presidential address, 1961. *Journal of Bone and Joint Surgery* 1961; 43-A: 582.

"Man was not made to sit a-trance,
And press, and press, and press his pants;
But, rather, with an open mind,
To circulate among his kind.

"And so, my son, avoid the snare
Which lurks within a cushioned chair;
To run like hell, it has been found,
Both feet must be on the ground."

—Theodore F. McManus
"Cave Sedem," published in *The Book of Fireside Poems*, ed. William Bowlin, 1937, and quoted by Cave in his AOA Presidential Address

Cave (1961) went on to predict the importance of trauma in the field of orthopaedic surgery:

> Next to obstetrics and gynecology we represent the largest single specialty group in surgery. The proposal to establish a Board of Trauma was correctly opposed in 1957...The American Orthopaedic Association has taken the lead in advancing orthopaedic surgery throughout its seventy-four years...[but] we have not put forth our best effort toward the injured patient...We can no longer simply sit as consultants...Realizing that three-fourths of all trauma is to the skeletal system, I believe frankly that we...are not responding sufficiently to our opportunity and responsibility in the management of trauma...the future of orthopaedic surgery will lie to a great extent in the field of trauma.

Cave also gave three endowed lectures: the first Scudder Oration of Trauma for the American College of Surgeons and the 7th Murray S. Danforth Oration of Rhode Island Hospital in 1963, and the Sir Robert Jones Lecture at the Hospital for Joint Diseases in 1965. In the latter two lectures, Cave chose specific orthopaedic topics: "Healing of Fractures and Nonunion of Bone" for his Danforth Oration, and knee derangements and trauma to the elbow for his Sir Robert Jones Lecture, which was titled "Twins (Extra Ordinary): The Knee and the Elbow." Cave spoke more broadly in his Scudder Oration, however; it was titled "Trauma, Specialization and the College." Cave recognized that specialization is part and parcel of the medical field, and he voiced his concerns at the time about a movement by some surgeons (including previous Scudder orators) to develop a new specialty—namely, trauma surgery. Such surgeons would treat both skeletal injuries and injuries to other anatomy and soft tissue, such as the head, extremities, and torso. However, Cave cited trauma statistics that indicated that among 800 patients admitted for trauma-induced injuries, fractures comprised more than three-fourths of the injuries, whereas injuries to the head (4%), soft tissue (7%), and the maxillofacial area (12%) were substantially fewer. Despite this potential for further specialization, Cave encouraged collaboration among surgeons—whether specialists or generalists—in order to push the field of surgery to new heights in the US.

Cave's national celebrity grew in 1964. In June of that year, Senator Edward Kennedy had fractured his spine in a plane crash and had been confined to a Stryker frame at the New England Baptist Hospital for almost five months. In November, Cave was one of four doctors to examine Kennedy and radiographs of his spine to determine when he could get out of the Stryker frame; the other three physicians were Dr. Frank Stinchfield from the New York Presbyterian Hospital; Dr. George Hammond, an orthopaedic surgeon at the New England Baptist Hospital; and Dr. Herbert D. Adams, director of the Lahey Clinic and chief of surgery at the New England Baptist Hospital. Cave "held many important offices and received many honors" (Staples ["O.S.S."] 1977); these are listed in **Box 40.7**. Throughout his career Cave published ~33 articles and edited or coedited 2 books.

Box 40.7. Edwin Cave's Professional Honors

- American Board of Orthopaedic Surgery: member, 1956 to 1964; president, 1958; on the Advisory Council, 1964 to 1969
- American College of Surgeons: second vice president, 1957; member of the Graduate Training Committee; member, Committee on Surgical Education in Medical Schools
- American Academy of Orthopaedic Surgeons: chairman, Committee on Fractures and Traumatic Surgery
- American Orthopaedic Association: 74th president, 1960–61

(Staples ["O.S.S."] 1977.)

A Second Act

Later in life, Cave enjoyed many activities outside his work: he "enjoyed the outdoors, riding and jumping his horse in the early mornings and at other free times, and working in his garden. In the winter he was an enthusiastic 'curler', participating in many competitions between the Country Club and other clubs in the United States and Canada" (Staples ["O.S.S."] 1977). However, Cave's professional success was interrupted by personal heartbreak: "In 1966 [his] happy life was shattered by the sudden passing of Weezie [Cave's wife]. Despite this devastating loss, Eddy carried on his practice and other activities as before" (Staples ["O.S.S."] 1977).

He continued his high-level work, and just after Weezie's death he was president of two national organizations: the American Association for the Surgery of Trauma (1967) and the Orthopaedic Research and Education Foundation (1968). His presidential address to the American Association for the Surgery of Trauma was titled "Trauma: Past and Present." In it, Cave traced the history of trauma from *Homer's Iliad* and advances made throughout history, including both world wars. In his concluding comments he recalled the contention and dispute upon the establishment of the association in 1939, but he then recognized the subsequent proliferation and the interdependence of surgical specialties.

> "Now I must stop before someone says
> That he who thinks in inches and talks
> by the yard should be kicked by the foot"
> —Edwin F. Cave
> AAST Presidential Address, published in the *Journal of Trauma*, 1968

Four years after Weezie's death, Cave—then 74 years old—married Joan Tozzer Lincoln. Soon after, however, Cave had a stroke. His friend and colleague O. Sherwin Staples (1977) noted, "Anyone else with a right hemiplegia and…handicap in speech and mobility might well have given up and become a recluse, but Eddy…[was] almost always cheerful." Cave also continued to practice as best he could: he "continued to visit his office daily after a session of physical therapy…On occasion he came to Orthopaedic Rounds at the Massachusetts General Hospital and attended the annual meetings of the American Orthopaedic Association and the Interurban Club" (Staples ["O.S.S."] 1977).

Cave spent just six years with Joan. In December 1976, just before the new year, Cave, at age 80, died at home in Chestnut Hill, Massachusetts. Upon his death: "Orthopaedic surgery lost one of its outstanding leaders, and many persons over the world lost a kindly and loyal friend…He was an unusually gifted man" (Staples ["O.S.S."] 1977).

HUGH P. CHANDLER

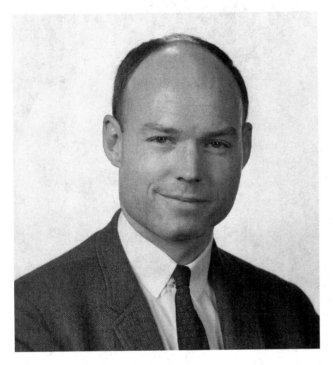

Hugh P. Chandler.—Massachusetts General Hospital, Archives and Special Collections.

Physician Snapshot

Hugh P. Chandler
BORN: 1931
DIED: 2014
SIGNIFICANT CONTRIBUTIONS: Introduced the direct lateral approach to the hip in the Harvard program; created the "vastus slide" modification to the direct lateral approach

Hugh Pollard Chandler was born in Boston in 1931, the son of Dr. Paul Chandler, the chief of ophthalmology at the Massachusetts Eye and Ear Infirmary. It was his father who encouraged Hugh to go into orthopaedics. Hugh graduated from both Harvard College and Harvard Medical School. He began his orthopaedic residency in the MGH/Children's Hospital Combined Program in 1960; at the time Dr. Joseph Barr was the chief at MGH and Dr. William Green was chief at Boston Children's Hospital. After finishing that residency, Chandler completed a fellowship at Great Ormond Street in England in 1965, followed by an Aufranc Fellowship in arthroplasty with Dr. Otto Aufranc (1965–67). (Aufranc is described earlier in this chapter.) In the dedication of the first *Harvard Orthopaedic Journal*, the resident editors wrote that Chandler:

> credits [Dr. Otto Aufranc] for many of the surgical principles he has taught to the next generation of Harvard Surgeons. These principles include isolating and sealing the skin to prevent contamination, use of sharp dissection rather than electrocautery, frequent irrigation of tissues and use of wound towels and the use of hand held retractors rather than self-retaining devices to avoid tissue necrosis. In addition, Dr. Chandler closes all wounds in multiple layers, achieving anatomic reapproximation of all tissue planes…His rates of dislocation and infection after primary total joint arthroplasty are exceedingly low. ("Dedication" 1999)

After that fellowship, Chandler joined the staff of MGH, where he remained throughout his entire career in practice.

Direct Lateral Approach to the Hip

Chandler preferred the direct lateral approach for most primary total hip procedures and simple revisions. Others had described this approach, but Chandler introduced it in the Harvard program. He and Sigurd Bervin explained the approach in a 1999 article published in the *Harvard Orthopaedic Journal*:

> The muscle fibers of the gluteus medius are separated…at the anterior border of the greater trochanter…[leaving] the abductor portion of the medius in continuity with the greater trochanter…The split in the gluteus medius is limited to less than five centimeters from the tip of the greater trochanter…to protect the superior gluteal nerve…[T]he gluteus minimus is split…

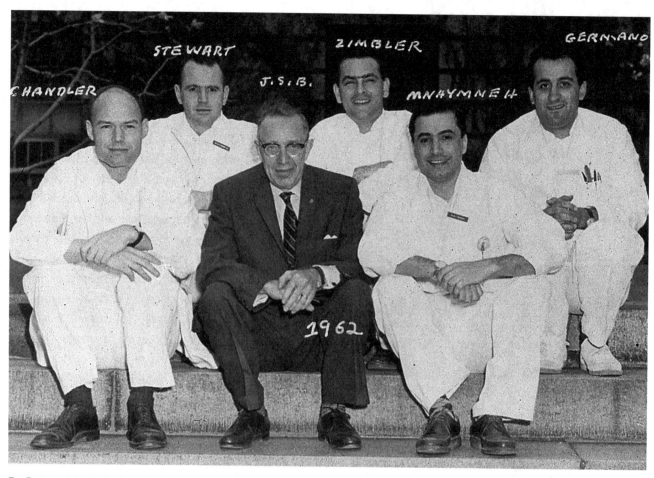

Dr. Barr with MGH residents, 1962. Chandler is seated in the front row at the far left. MGH HCORP Archives.

with the underlying capsule...The quadriceps are left in continuity with the abductors... [and] the anterior fascia of the vastus lateralis is split...six centimeters...distal to the greater trochanter...An anterior cuff of soft tissue is developed including the gluteus medius, gluteus minimus, anterior capsule, vastus medialis, and vastus intermedius...[allowing] the hip [to be] dislocated anteriorly.

Chandler also modified the direct lateral approach in what he called the vastus slide. With this modification the proximal cuff of the medius, minimus, and anterior capsule is identical to that used with the direct lateral approach, but at the distal portion of the greater trochanter Chandler incised the quadriceps fascia posteriorly, extending the incision down the shaft of the femur. This allowed him to reflect the quadriceps muscle anteriorly. With this approach he obtained excellent exposure of the acetabulum and of the entire shaft of the femur.

Chandler cowrote several articles and coedited one book, *Bone Stock Deficiency in Total Hip*

> **The Direct Lateral Approach to the Hip**
>
> Sigurd Berven, MD • Hugh Chandler, MD
> Massachusetts General Hospital

Article by Berven and Chandler containing Chandler's description of his direct lateral approach to the hip. *Harvard Orthopaedic Journal* 1999; 1.

Replacement, published in 1989. The authors aimed to describe their use of bone grafts while performing a total hip replacement. In particular, they used such grafts to reconstruct pelvic and femoral bone deficiencies (see **Case 40.5**).

Recognition

In 2003, the Arthritis Foundation recognized Chandler with its Dr. Marian Ropes Award. Dr. Henry Mankin (2003), in his presentation of the award, stated:

> Hugh did everything...and did everything not just well but spectacularly well. He was a wonderful surgeon and is perhaps one of the best hip surgeons this institution has ever known. He pioneered in such areas as acetabular arthroplasty, allograft support for the femoral shaft, lateral incision as an approach to the arthritic hip, the trochanteric slide for exposure and many, many more. He spent hours in the operating room with each patient, being absolutely sure that the procedure was done correctly...He holds the best record ever for lack of complications such as infection and dislocation. It should be evident that his patients adored him for his commitment and talent... Hugh was a mentor...a superb one. He was awarded the best Harvard teaching award

Case 40.5. Pelvic Osteolysis Associated with Acetabular Replacement

> "A thirty-two-year-old woman had bilateral osteoarthrosis of the hip secondary to dysplasia of the acetabulum. Total hip replacement without cement was done bilaterally, with a six-month interval between the procedures: the patient did well postoperatively. After recovery, her activity level was high and included cross-country skiing, bicycling, and hiking as far as five miles (eight kilometers) a day.
>
> "When the patient returned for a routine follow-up examination, seven years after the initial procedure, the only symptom was a grinding noise coming from the hips. The Harris hip score was 100 points bilaterally. Radiographic evaluation demonstrated massive osteolysis of the pelvis and the proximal parts of the femora. The components were radiographically stable. Both femoral heads were eccentric within the acetabular components; this eccentricity was indicative of polyethylene wear.
>
> "The patient was managed with revision of both hips. Thick granular tissue, darkly stained from metallic debris, was noted on the proximal part of the left femur. Some bone was located anteriorly and medially over the porous surface of the femoral component, but the remaining porous surface was visible after curettage of the granuloma from the proximal part of the femur. The acetabular liner was completely worn through, and the femoral head was articulating with the metal shell. The acetabular component was loose and easily extracted. The extensive tissue behind the acetabular implant was stained from metallic debris and there was considerable loss of bone, measuring at least 1.5 inches (3.8 centimeters) in diameter. The revision acetabular component was inserted without cement and was fixed with screws after the large defect had been packed with morselized pieces of allograft bone. The femur was reconstructed with a modular femoral component.
>
> "The findings on the right side were similar. Extensive staining of tissue from metallic debris was noted both in the proximal part of the femur and in the acetabulum. The acetabular liner was completely worn through, and the metal of the femoral head was articulating with the metal of the acetabular shell. The acetabular defect on the right side was larger than that on the left side, and the medial wall was destroyed, exposing the underlying pelvic muscles. A combination of allograft and iliac-crest autogenous graft was used to fill the acetabular defect. The new acetabular component was fixed without cement but, again, screws were used. The femoral component was stable and left in place. After the lesion of the proximal part of the femur was curetted, the defect was packed with bone graft."
>
> (Maloney, Peters, Engh, and Chandler 1993)

three times in the 80s, was revered by the residents who loved working with him and learning from him.

In an article in the *Harvard Orthopaedic Journal* the resident editors referred to Chandler as a "compassionate physician, [who listens] to patients and examin[es] them with great care" ("Dedication" 1999). He had "a passion for complex reconstructive problems in total joint arthroplasty" and "for teaching residents with patience and respect" ("Dedication" 1999).

A Passion Outside Surgery

If surgery and teaching were Chandler's passions within the field of medicine, outside of his work he had a passion "for living life with tremendous energy and infectious enthusiasm" ("Dedication" 1999). His love was sailing competitively with his wife, Betsy McCombs. For more than 30 years they raced locally and in major races such as the Block Island race, the Buzzard's Bay Regatta, the Marblehead to Halifax Ocean Race, the Marion to Bermuda race, and the Key West race, to name a few. Their first boat was called *REEB* (*beer* spelled backward). After owning a series of about six boats they eventually sailed the *Scheherazade*, a Farr 395 yacht.

> "You can yell at me, but you can't yell at anyone else. Having a non-yelling boat is crucial."
> —Motto of Hugh Chandler, captain of the *Scheherazade*, a Farr 395 yacht (Laitos 2013)

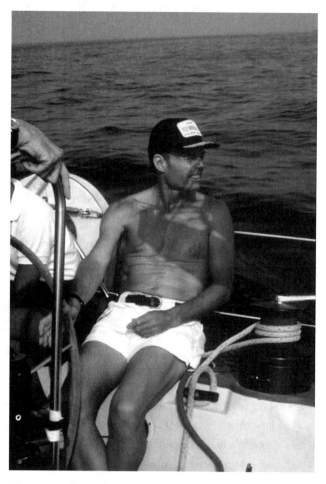

Chandler at the helm in Boston Harbor. MGH HCORP Archives.

In 1998 Chandler, aged 67, experienced a stroke, which left him with a right partial hemiplegia and an almost complete expressive aphasia. He retired from his surgical practice, but despite his disabilities he continued to sail and compete in races in the Boston area: he captained the boat; Betsy navigated. In 2012, they sailed the *Scheherazade* to victory in class 2 during the PHRF New England race. They also won the West Marine Performance Trophy in the spinnaker class.

Chandler died on October 9, 2014, at age 84.

THOMAS L. DELORME JR.

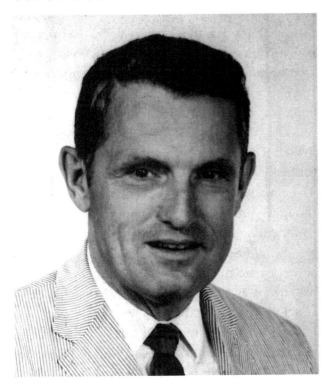

Thomas L. DeLorme Jr. "Dr. DeLorme Re-elected Head of Hospital Staff," *Quincy Patriot Ledger*, January 15, 1976. © *The Patriot Ledger* – USA TODAY NETWORK.

Physician Snapshot

Thomas L. DeLorme Jr.
BORN: 1917
DIED: 2003
SIGNIFICANT CONTRIBUTIONS: Introduced and developed progressive resistance exercises as the best way to regain muscle power after injury; created the DeLorme Table, which is still used today; led the creation of the White 9 Rehabilitation Unit at MGH

Thomas Lanier DeLorme Jr. was born in Birmingham, Alabama, on July 17, 1917. While in high school, he contracted rheumatic fever and was placed on bed rest for four months. His physicians declared that the disease had "weakened [his] heart" and his ability to perform strenuous activity thereafter would be limited. DeLorme, however, "was determined to prove the medicos wrong" (quoted in Todd, Shirley, and Todd 2014). This early experience would shape the course of his life and work. While bedridden and recovering from the fever, he began reading health magazines and other works about medicine and decided he would become a doctor. He recorded that "immediately upon leaving my sick bed I started a comeback campaign" (quoted in Todd, Shirley, and Todd 2014). A few years later, he was weight training (he created his own set of weights), exercising (strenuously, against the advice of his physician), and weightlifting competitively (in the clean and jerk he hit a personal best of 250 lb.) By 1939, when he was 22, he noted he "reached a mark of lifting 503 pounds of deadweight from the floor which exceeds the Birmingham Y.M.C.A. record by 43 pounds...I hope to win the Southern A.A.U. Championships...and possibly go on to compete in the International Olympic Games" (quoted in Todd, Shirley, and Todd 2014).

That year—after having studied at Howard University—DeLorme was accepted to the medical school at the University of Alabama. He worked to pay his way through school, and he continued his weightlifting regimen; he demonstrated lifting techniques during university football games and had achieved the 500-lb. deadlift; "at just over six feet in height, he tipped the scales at 185 pounds" (Todd et al. 2014). A Tuscaloosa, Alabama, newspaper called him "Bama Hercules." He had "became so well-known for his strength that he was invited to give a lifting demonstration at halftime during one of the University of Alabama football games. In front of the crowded stands, he lifted the front end of a truck off the ground" (Todd et al. 2014). He spent only one year at the University of Alabama, transferring to New York University Medical School in 1940. His studies and later efforts in the war did not distract from his personal relationships, and in 1941 he married Eleanor Person.

Because of World War II, DeLorme's NYU class graduated 2 months early, in April 1943. Upon graduation, DeLorme was awarded the Valentine Mott Award. Mott was a well-known surgeon and one of the founders of NYU medical school. The award was granted to an "individual who has shown exceptional support for the clinical, research and education missions of the Medical Center" (nyulangone.org). While the war continued, DeLorme completed a brief internship in New York and then, on New Year's Day 1944, joined the US Army Medical Corps as a lieutenant. A month later he went to Chicago, where he served in the Orthopaedic Section at the Ruth M. Gardiner General Hospital.

A New Method to Regain Muscle Power after Injury

The orthopaedic need at Gardiner Hospital—and at other veterans' hospitals—was overwhelming, and patients could spend as long as nine months in recovery, mainly on bed rest and doing little resistance exercise, which did not help them regain strength. Soon after beginning his service there, DeLorme recognized an "urgent need": quicker rehabilitation. This would enable patients to recover more quickly and thus make beds available faster for others. Because of his own experiences with muscle strength—both losing it through injury/disease and regaining it through exercise—DeLorme understood that resistance training would be needed if patients were to become stronger faster.

While at Gardiner, DeLorme became acquainted with Sergeant Thaddeus Kawalek, who was in a special unit that would soon head to Europe to help with recovery efforts. Kawalek was rehabilitating after surgery to treat a noncombat knee injury. During their discussions, DeLorme confided to Kawalek that he thought weight training was needed, rather than the conventional program of rest and endurance-type exercises. Kawalek was intrigued by DeLorme's ideas and invited DeLorme to create a resistance exercise program to help him regain strength in his knee. The excellent results proved that DeLorme's thoughts on resistance training during recovery had merit and could help patients do so faster.

Walter Easley, a sergeant who had ruptured the anterior cruciate and medial collateral ligaments in his knee, was another one of those patients experiencing a long period of recovery at Gardiner. He had been there more than six months, and his physicians said his prognosis for full recovery was poor and he would probably always have to wear a knee brace. Easley's quadriceps had atrophied, and he experienced extremity edema and pain. Upon Easley's invitation, DeLorme took up the challenge of his rehabilitation through weight training—high repetitions and maximum weight. As before, DeLorme's regimen worked wonders: the atrophy, swelling, and pain disappeared and Easley no longer had to wear a knee brace.

To most at Gardiner, Kawalek's and Easley's results were extraordinary. Patients began to flock to DeLorme requesting that he use what he called "heavy-resistance exercises" to help them achieve such an amazing recovery as well. (**Case 40.6** highlights just one of these many patients who DeLorme's method helped.) DeLorme's commanding officer, Colonel John Hall, approved of his efforts, and so he began a clinical trial to evaluate this new approach to rehabilitation.

On the basis of this initial study at Gardiner, DeLorme published his first paper, "Restoration of Muscle Power by Heavy-Resistance Exercises," in the *Journal of Bone and Joint Surgery* in 1945. He emphasized the difference between his method for regenerating muscle strength and that widely

---

RESTORATION OF MUSCLE POWER BY HEAVY-RESISTANCE EXERCISES

BY CAPTAIN THOMAS L. DELORME
Medical Corps, Army of the United States

From the Orthopaedic Section, Gardiner General Hospital, Chicago, Illinois

THE JOURNAL OF BONE AND JOINT SURGERY
VOL. XXVII, NO. 4, OCTOBER 1945

DeLorme's research that led to him being chosen for the Gold Key Award by the American Congress of Rehabilitation Medicine, 1964. *Journal of Bone and Joint Surgery* 1945; 27: 645.

Case 40.6. Using Resistance Exercises to Restore Muscle Power

> "A soldier sustained a complete dislocation of the knee when he fell from a four-foot platform. Two weeks after injury, a meniscectomy was performed, and the patient returned to duty, but was unable to continue because of pain on weight-bearing. Five months after the initial injury, another arthrotomy was done, a partial tear of the anterior cruciate ligament being sutured and a fascial flap placed at the site of the tibial collateral ligament. Instability persisted, and, eleven months after the initial injury, a third operation was done, at which time a fascial reconstruction of the tibial collateral and anterior cruciate ligaments was undertaken. Again the instability persisted, and the patient was fitted with a Jones knee cage. Three and one-half months after the last operation, the patient undertook the heavy-resistance exercises. At this time there was atrophy of the thigh of two and one-half inches, flexion of 58 degrees, maximum power of two and one-half pounds, and moderate swelling of the knee joint. In fifty-two days of exercise, the patient made the following gains: a power increase of sixty-two and a quarter pounds in the quadriceps, an increase of two inches in circumference, and a gain of 42 degrees in range of motion. By the end of the third week of exercise, he had discarded the knee cage. Pain and swelling rapidly disappeared. The patient was discharged from the Army because of his knee injury, took a job as a truck driver, and his knee has remained asymptomatic."
>
> (Thomas L. DeLorme 1945)

used at the time. His was "founded on the principle of heavy-resistance and low repetition exercises, whereas the generally accepted principle is low resistance and high-repetition exercises—such as stationary-bicycle riding, lifting light sandbags or other weights through ropes and pulleys, stair climbing, et cetera—which develop endurance rather than power" (DeLorme 1945). He clinically evaluated 300 cases and described the resistance program he had generally applied:

> [W]e firmly believe that even extremely atrophied muscles should exert their maximum effort at regular intervals…The patient is seated on a table with his knees flexed at an angle of 90 degrees, and the boot is strapped on the foot…Resistance is offered in the form of iron plates, graded…to twenty-five pounds each…attached to an iron boot…Fifteen is the maximum number of repetitions ever performed in a series…[whereas] ten or twelve is the number generally performed…The amount of weight lifted by the patient…[starts out] with the weight of the boot (five pounds), and increasing by small amounts . . .[, t]he patient lifts each weight ten repetitions…Once each week the patient makes an attempt to increase this…ten-repetition maximum, and when this amount is determined, no heavier weight is used during the ensuing week…[S]eventy to 100 repetitions must be performed in each workout. (DeLorme 1945)

DeLorme (1945) made eight conclusions, based on his work with those soldiers:

1. Low-repetition, high-resistance exercises produce power.

2. High-repetition, low-resistance exercises produce endurance.

3. Each of these two types of exercise is incapable of producing results obtained by the other.

4. Weakened, atrophied muscles should not be subjected to endurance-building exercises, until the muscle power has been restored to normal by power-building exercises.

5. Restoration of muscle power with return of motion in a limb has been neglected in the past. It is, in most instances, preferable to have a limited range of motion with good power than a normal range of motion with inadequate power.

6. Games and group exercises, as practiced in reconditioning programs, are unsatisfactory for producing focal muscle development.

7. In order to obtain rapid hypertrophy in weakened, atrophied muscle, the muscle should be subjected to strenuous exercise and, at regular intervals, to the point of maximum exertion.

8. In cases of meniscectomies and unstable knees, quadriceps power should be obtained by the use of strenuous, non-weight-bearing exercises. Weight-bearing exercises can produce pain, thickening, and fluid in knees, which do not have adequate muscle support.

Upon his promotion to captain in 1945, DeLorme convinced his superior offers to allocate extensive resources for physical therapy. He himself built most of the equipment housed in the new facility. One such piece was the "DeLorme table" (later the "Elgin table"), which allowed users to progress through various exercises by adjusting positioning and using pulleys; it is still in use today in various forms. DeLorme's work gained a wider audience upon a visit to Gardiner Hospital by agents from the US surgeon general's office in mid-1945. After learning about DeLorme's methods and the results he achieved, the surgeon general issued an Army-wide order: the heavy-resistance program must be applied to all orthopaedic patients.

DeLorme's commanding officer, Colonel Hall, described the efforts of his fellow officer:

> After many months of trying work, Captain DeLorme developed the section to maximum operating efficiency…It is the opinion of the staff…and of the many visiting consultants that Captain DeLorme has placed in the hands of the Orthopaedic Surgeon a new and valuable agent in promoting full recovery and restoration of

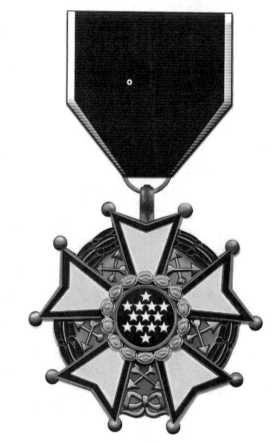

Legion of Merit medal. Wikimedia Commons.

> function…Captain DeLorme's interest and his untiring effort in applying his ideas and in developing his program have proven to be of great benefit to the Army Reconstruction program, in lessening the period of convalescence and in permitting many cases to return to duty more quickly, and others to receive maximum hospital benefits over and above those previously expected. (quoted in Todd, Shirley, and Todd 2014)

Upon Hall's recommendation, DeLorme was awarded the Legion of Merit for his work.

The Work Continues after Military Service

While working at Gardiner, DeLorme had studied the (successful) effects of his heavy-resistance exercises on 30 patients with polio. Those results were noticed by Dr. Arthur Watkins, who was leading the new Department of Physical Medicine at MGH. Watkins invited DeLorme to come to Boston to work with him to continue that earlier research. DeLorme took Watkins up on his offer, and upon his discharge from the army in late 1945, he left Chicago for Boston, where he joined MIT as the Baruch Fellow in Physical Medicine. In addition, he was accepted into a residency through the program at MGH/Children's Hospital and the West Roxbury Veterans Hospital. Although he initially studied surgery and neurology, DeLorme eventually specialized in orthopaedic surgery. He handled a large practice through MGH (both a private practice and as a member of the medical staff at MGH).

DeLorme and Watkins's research together resulted in various publications. In 1948, the two published "Technics of Progressive Resistance Exercise," in which they stated that the term *heavy resistance exercises* was misleading—for them, it implied a focus only on the amount of weight. They suggested instead the phrase *progressive resistance exercises*. In enumerating their reasons for choosing the latter as new terminology, they emphasized the application of the principles of counterbalance, loading, and repetition, as well as the use of specially designed equipment.

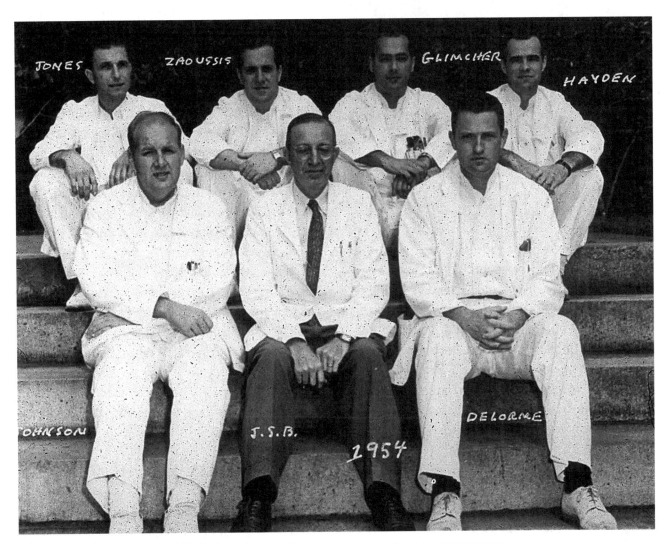

Dr. Barr with MGH residents, 1954. DeLorme is seated in the front row on the right. MGH HCORP Archives.

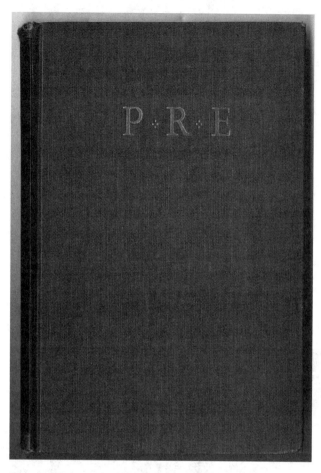

Cover of Delorme and Watkins's book, P R E (Progressive Resistance Exercise). Ottley Coulter Collection/H. J. Lutcher Stark Center for Physical Culture and Sport.

That same year they, with Robert Schwab, also published "The Response of the Quadriceps Femoris to Progressive Resistance Exercises in Poliomyelitic Patients" in the *Journal of Bone and Joint Surgery*. In 1951, DeLorme and Watkins published their book, *Progressive Resistance Exercise: Technique and Medical Application*. Their goal was for the book to serve as a "reference manual" for those medical professionals using progressive resistance exercise with their patients. Dr. Joseph Barr wrote in the foreword that DeLorme and Watkin's system of progressive resistance exercises had moved the field from an art to a science. In addition to these publications, DeLorme wrote or cowrote another ~12 articles and coedited one other book over the course of his career.

Expanding Orthopaedics at MGH

DeLorme was instrumental in expanding orthopaedics at MGH. He recognized that throughout the hospital "patients with musculoskeletal problems... especially paraplegics and quadriplegics...were not receiving optimal care" (Castleman, Crockett, and Sutton 1983). To remedy this problem, beginning in 1954 DeLorme encouraged physicians and surgeons on "the Orthopaedic Service...to play a more active role in the rehabilitation of patients in the hospital...With [Dr. Joseph] Barr's backing, DeLorme began to admit these patients to White 8 on the Orthopaedic Service and to build up a staff" (Castleman, Crockett, and Sutton 1983), working closely with the various services involved with therapists provided by the Department of Physical Medicine. Just a year later, however, a polio epidemic required a change of focus for all orthopaedists at MGH, and "the White 8 rehabilitation unit was allowed to wither...White 9 was set up as a respiratory center, and DeLorme...a junior member of the visiting staff, was primarily responsible for the orthopaedic care of these patients, many of whom were severely disabled" (Faxon 1959). As the patients with polio recovered and the epidemic waned, the team at MGH revisited the idea of a rehabilitation unit, and DeLorme, again with Barr's support, began this task. DeLorme, as the new unit's director, obtained funding from the Pope Foundation (from which he had previously received funding for his research). He brought together a team of professionals, including "Leonard Cronkite...[as] internist-in-charge [and] William Kermond of the Orthopaedic Service was assistant director" (Faxon 1959). The unit's 44 beds were never empty, and "residents from Orthopaedics now had as one of their rotations time on White 9" (Faxon 1959).

Professional Life after MGH

In 1958, just a couple of years after setting up White 9 as the new rehabilitation unit at MGH, DeLorme resigned as its director to take a position

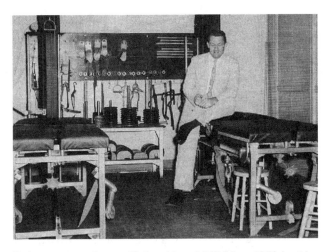

DeLorme seated on an Elgin table at MGH (late 1950s) with some of his favorite original equipment. Courtesy of the York Barbell Company.

as medical director of the research laboratory at the Liberty Mutual Insurance Company. Through his work at Liberty Mutual and his private practice he cultivated an interest in amputations. With Drs. W. Gerald Austen and Robert S. Shaw he began researching blood perfusion in amputated limbs. Dr. Melvin Glimcher, then director of the MGH Orthopaedic Research Laboratories, called their work "unbelievable." Later, while still at Liberty Mutual, DeLorme also helped develop the "Boston Arm," along with Glimcher and other scientists from MIT.

Author Recollections

I saw DeLorme's dedication to his work firsthand during my residency during the late 1960s. He was scheduled to give one of the evening lectures at MGH, but we didn't expect to see him because he was in the hospital as a patient, recovering from recent spinal surgery—he would have multiple surgeries throughout the rest of his life. To our surprise, however, he showed up in a hospital gown, with an IV attached to his arm and pulling the IV stand along with him. He was undeterred and presented his lecture to us residents. We were very impressed.

DeLorme became president of the medical staff at Milton Hospital in 1975 while continuing as research director at Liberty Mutual. He was also a clinical professor at Harvard Medical School at the time and had a busy orthopaedic practice focused on spine surgery at both MGH and Milton Hospital. DeLorme, his wife Eleanor, who taught at Wellesley College (her area of expertise was France during the Napoleonic era), and their three sons lived in Milton.

He retired around 1990. He was plagued by back pain for the rest of his life. He died on June 14, 2003, at age 86. At the memorial service, Glimcher spoke highly of DeLorme's work:

> Patients who could not walk developed enough muscles to stand and walk and kept increasing their ability to get around, take care of themselves, feed themselves, [to] use their hands and feet, to write, to paint, to use tools and so forth...Eventually an entire system of equipment and exercises and the proper way to deal with this was developed, which became a worldwide standard, referred to simply as Progressive Resistance Exercises...it was the application of his technique that he returned millions of patients back to their family and friends. (Glimcher 2003)

DeLorme had worked a "miracle" for his patients, helping them to regain strength and reclaim their lives.

RALPH K. GHORMLEY

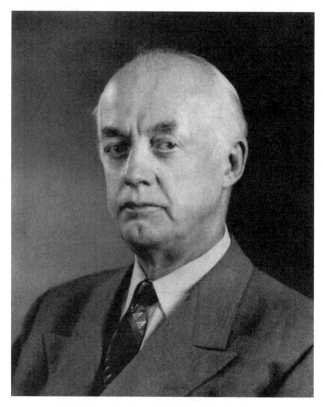

Ralph K. Ghormley. R.W.J., Jr. and J.S.S., "Ralph K. Ghormley 1893-1959," *Journal of Bone and Joint Surgery* 1959; 41: 1364.

Physician Snapshot

Ralph K. Ghormley
BORN: 1893
DIED: 1959
SIGNIFICANT CONTRIBUTIONS: Expert in tuberculosis; coined the term, "facet syndrome"; served as head of the Section of Orthopaedic Surgery at the Mayo Clinic (1938); president of the American Orthopaedic Association (1948–49); president of the American Board of Orthopaedic Surgery (1951 and 1952)

Ralph Kalb Ghormley was born in early 1893 in Portland, Oregon. He stayed on the West Coast for his undergraduate education; he attended Whitworth College, in Spokane, Washington, from which he graduated in 1914. He headed east for medical school, obtaining an MD degree from Johns Hopkins University in 1918. This was during World War I, and thus he could be said to have "graduated in medicine virtually under fire as a member of the volunteer group of medical students from Johns Hopkins who served and studied at the Johns Hopkins Base Hospital Unit in France in 1917–1918" (RWJ Jr., MC, and JSS 1959). He began his service as a private in the US Army Medical Corps; by the time of his discharge he had been promoted to captain.

After the war, Ghormley completed a year-long internship (1921–22) at New York Hospital. He then returned to Johns Hopkins for a year of training in orthopaedic surgery. In 1924, he moved to Boston, where he joined Dr. Robert Lovett's practice and became an assistant orthopaedic surgeon at Massachusetts General Hospital. That year, he also became a member of the Massachusetts Medical Society and was appointed assistant in orthopaedic surgery at Harvard Medical School; he later became an instructor in orthopaedic surgery there. After Lovett's death, Ghormley stayed in the practice with Drs. Frank Ober, Albert Brewster, and Nathaniel Allison. While in Boston, "he was [also] a resident physician at the [Peabody] home and spent many hours with the children in their outdoor recreations…[he was] a great favorite with the children" (Loughlin 1924). As he embarked on his career, so too did he embark on the adventure of marriage: he tied the knot with Jean McDougall in 1924.

Ghormley published and presented extensively during the mid- to late 1920s, and much of that research was on tuberculosis. At a Cabot Case Conference at MGH in 1925, he presented findings of his examinations of frozen sections of a foot amputated at the ankle in a patient with tuberculosis. The following year he reviewed cases of joint disease treated over a two-year period at MGH and presented his results as a thesis for membership in the American Orthopaedic Association. That paper was published in the *Journal of Bone and Joint Surgery* in 1926. In his summary he stated that in his case series:

> an effort has been carried through to reach a final positive diagnosis [and t]he predominating

> **JOINT DISEASE***
> A CLINICAL-PATHOLOGICAL STUDY
> BY RALPH K. GHORMLEY, M.D., BOSTON
> Orthopaedic Department of the Massachusetts General Hospital
> JBJS, 1926, Volume 8, Issue 4

Ghormley's AOA thesis in which he reported a 66% accuracy in diagnosing joint tuberculosis with current laboratory tests—proving a "need to further improve our present methods of diagnosis." *Journal of Bone and Joint Surgery* 1926; 8: 858.

disease of the series is tuberculosis…[This] diagnosis…is of prime importance…[and of] available aids in diagnosis, the tuberculin test deserves first mention, a negative reaction being strongly against tuberculosis. The x-ray in the early cases is of little help and in complicated cases is of little or no value…The history and physical examination are of great aid, and in a fair proportion of cases give information sufficient to give a correct diagnosis.

(Ghormley 1926)

Two years later, Ghormley cowrote, with John Bradley, a paper on tuberculosis of the spine in children. They studied radiographs of the spine taken over time in 70 patients at the New England Peabody Home for Crippled Children as well as specimens from the Warren Museum. Ghormley and Bradley (1928) made six conclusions:

1. Calcification in a lesion does not necessarily mean satisfactory healing.
2. Clearing or reestablishment of bony detail is a much better indication of healing.
3. Bony fusion or bony block is a favorable sign.
4. Decrease in the size of an abscess is a favorable sign, while increase…is decidedly an unfavorable sign.
5. Paravertebral abscesses accompanying dorsal Pott's disease are dangerous in that they cause a much wider destruction than the original lesion…
6. It is suggested that early eradication of such abscesses might be attempted, but the danger of establishing a permanent sinus is serious.

Ghormley remained in Boston for seven years. During his last three years there, he served as secretary of the Boston Orthopedic Club. At the Club's May 1929 meeting, he and Nathaniel Allison presented a paper on joint changes seen in arthritis and tuberculosis. He was becoming an expert on joint tuberculosis.

Ghormley left Boston in September 1929 to join the staff at the Mayo Clinic in Rochester, Minnesota. He continued to work with Allison, who also left MGH soon after Ghormley to become professor of surgery and chief of the division of orthopedic surgery at the University of Chicago. In 1931, they published *Diagnosis in Joint Disease: A Clinical and Pathological Study of Arthritis*.

After eight years at the Mayo Clinic, Ghormley was promoted to professor of orthopaedic surgery. He became head of the clinic's section of orthopaedic surgery in 1938. Ghormley's early experience at MGH and his later work at the Mayo Clinic helped him to become "a superb clinician, a skillful and fearless operator, [and] a teacher to both the local students and staff and also to the many professional visitors" (RWJ Jr., MC and JSS 1959). His many and varied interests, "including clinical and experimental research, is shown in his many professional contributions" (RWJ Jr., MC and JSS 1959). In all he is named on almost 300 publications. "As a constructive idealist he labored incessantly to raise the standard of training and practice in orthopaedic surgery" (RWJ Jr., MC and JSS 1959), and he held major leadership positions in orthopaedics, including on the American Board of Orthopaedic Surgery; he was its president in 1951 and 1952. He also was a member of numerous

> **DIAGNOSIS IN JOINT DISEASE**
>
> *A Clinical and Pathological Study of Arthritis*
>
> BY
>
> NATHANIEL ALLISON, M.D., F.A.C.S.,
> PROFESSOR OF SURGERY, IN CHARGE OF DIVISION OF ORTHOPEDIC SURGERY, UNIVERSITY OF CHICAGO; FORMERLY PROFESSOR OF ORTHOPEDIC SURGERY, HARVARD MEDICAL SCHOOL AND CHIEF OF ORTHOPEDIC SERVICE, MASSACHUSETTS GENERAL HOSPITAL.
>
> AND
>
> RALPH K. GHORMLEY, M.D.,
> ASSOCIATE IN ORTHOPEDIC SURGERY, MAYO CLINIC; ASSISTANT PROFESSOR OF ORTHOPEDIC SURGERY, MAYO FOUNDATION, ROCHESTER, MINNESOTA. FORMERLY INSTRUCTOR IN ORTHOPEDIC SURGERY, HARVARD MEDICAL SCHOOL AND VISITING SURGEON, MASSACHUSETTS GENERAL HOSPITAL.
>
> From the Orthopedic Service of the Massachusetts General Hospital and the Harvard Medical School (1924-1930). Assisted by the DeLemar Mobile Research Fund.
>
> NEW YORK
> WILLIAM WOOD AND COMPANY
> MDCCCCXXXI

Allison and Ghormley's book, *Diagnosis in Joint Disease: A Clinical and Pathological Study of Arthritis.* New York: William Wood and Company, 1931.

Box 40.8. Ralph Ghormley's Many Professional Roles

Memberships
- Children's Bureau of the US Department of Labor
- American Medical Association
- American Surgical Society
- Clinical Society of Orthopaedic Surgery (president, 1941)
- International Society of Orthopaedic Surgery and Traumatology
- The Robert Jones Club

Fellow
- American College of Surgeons

committees of the American Academy of Orthopaedic Surgeons and the American Orthopaedic Association. He was both secretary (1933–40) and president (1948–49) of the latter. His professional service was seemingly unending; more of his professional roles are listed in **Box 40.8**. I have purposely emphasized only Ghormley's activities and contributions before and during his career at MGH and Harvard Medical School. It's clear that during his time at the Mayo Clinic, he went on to make even more significant contributions, but I mention them only briefly here.

He served as an orthopaedic consultant for the US Department of Veterans Affairs. He also chaired the American Medical Association's Committee on Postgraduate Training in Orthopaedic Surgery; he was followed in that role by A. R. Shands Jr., who established a registry for orthopaedic residencies at the Alfred I. DuPont Institute in Wilmington, Delaware. Ghormley was also a member of the first Residency Review Committee in Orthopaedic Surgery for the AMA. The committee's first meeting was held October 23, 1953. Two years later, it reinspected 118 residency programs and approved 13 new programs.

Ghormley's career came to an end as the 1950s headed inexorably toward the new decade. In 1957, he "was honored by his former fellows...and colleagues in the Mayo Clinic by the establishment of the Ralph K. Ghormley Traveling Scholarship, designed to enable the recipients to visit leading centers in orthopaedic surgery in this country and abroad" (RWJ Jr., MC and JSS 1959). Ghormley retired in 1958. Edwin Cave (1961), one of Ghormley's colleagues, expressed gratitude to his teachers Nathaniel Allison, Marius Smith-Petersen, and "Ralph Ghormley, whom I revered all of my professional life...whose contributions to our special branch of surgery will live forever, and who taught me so much."

Ghormley died of a heart attack at age 66, just one year after retiring, in Carmel, California. He was survived by his wife, Jean, and their two children.

WILLIAM N. JONES

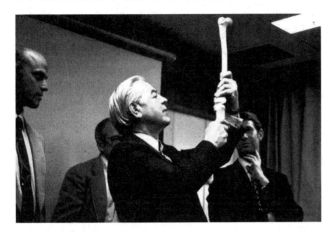

William N. Jones demonstrating the knee joint at an MGH conference. MGH HCORP Archives.

Physician Snapshot

William N. Jones
BORN: 1916
DIED: 1991
SIGNIFICANT CONTRIBUTIONS: Frequent coauthor of *JAMA*'s Fracture of the Month series; developed Smith-Petersen's mold arthroplasty of the knee (MGH distal femoral prosthesis)

I was unable to find much information about William N. Jones other than the briefest outline of his life. Jones was born and raised in Anderson, Indiana. He completed his undergraduate education at the University of Chicago in 1936 and received his MD degree from the same school in 1940. During World War II, Jones served as a major in the US Army Medical Corps with the Johns Hopkins University Medical Unit. He was married to Arlene (née MacFarlane); they lived in Hamilton, Massachusetts, and had no children.

Jones was an assistant orthopaedic surgeon at MGH, had a private practice, and was an instructor at Harvard Medical School. From 1961 until 1970 Jones cowrote with Dr. Otto Aufranc and others ~100 articles in the "Fracture of the Month" series published in the *Journal of the American Medical Association* (described in the section about Aufranc earlier in this chapter). In 1969,

Case 40.7. Mold Arthroplasty of the Knee

> "Originally, a flat cup-like mold was designed with slight bulges for the femoral condyles and with fins or keels in the intercondylar position projecting from both the superior and inferior surfaces. In October 1942, using this mold, arthroplasty of the left knee was carried out through an anterior U-shaped incision. The operation was 2 hours and 55 minutes long. A tourniquet was in place for 1 hour and a transfusion of 500 cc blood was administered during a late stage of the operation. The early postsurgical result was a very limited range of motion without pain.
>
> "A similar operation was done in December 1942 on the patient's right knee. Again, only very limited motion resulted and unfortunately the knee joint was persistently painful. The mold was removed 14 months after operation with reankylosis occurring readily at 20° flexion.
>
> "The patient felt that even the 20° range of motion in the left knee helped her in walking, and hoping to gain a wider range of motion, she underwent a revision of the knee joint in February 1944. At the second operation a new mold without projecting fins and with a higher rising shield over the anterior portion of the femoral joint surface was used. The patient's condition was improved, and at follow-up examination in 1960 she had a range of painless motion from 15° flexion to 60° flexion with a 10° active extension lag. She was unable to get out of an ordinary chair or go up or down stairs unassisted but was up and about on crutches during most of the day."
>
> (William N. Jones 1969)

Jones published the only article that he wrote alone, "Mold Arthroplasty of the Knee Joint." In it, he described his experience with Dr. Marius Smith-Petersen at MGH (see **Case 40.7**). In the article's brief introduction, Jones notes, "Except perhaps for some periods during World War II, the 5 years that I worked with Dr. Smith-Petersen were the most exciting and interesting of my experience; although largely an assistant, I remember the time as always pleasant. His qualities as a physician, his conviction of the benefits of surgery, and his skill in demonstrating them were very impressive" (Jones 1969).

Smith-Peterson had been performing mold arthroplasties on patients' hips since the early 1940s, and at that time he "hoped that the principle of interposition of a free moving mold [Vitallium] could be adapted successfully for the knee" (Jones 1969). Although those early efforts helped patients achieve better motion, it was usually limited, and they often dealt with instability and eventual declines in function. Smith-Petersen was disappointed in such results, and "he requested, somewhat casually, that I [Jones] design a new mold that would work more successfully" (Jones

Box 40.9. Continuing Evolution of the Vitallium Mold for Use in Knee Arthroplasty

In the late 1940s and early 1950s Jones worked, at Marius Smith-Petersen's request, to develop a mold that would allow extensive range of motion, improve stability, and retain the patient's initial improved function over the long-term:

"I felt that in order to achieve a wide range of motion in the knee it would be necessary to reconstitute the complex femoral joint surface rather than the simpler tibial joint surface, keeping the condylar length, or height, in flexion. A little foundry was set up in the office laboratory and a small variety of metal molds was made and tried in a series of plaster and elastic knee models...all were surface molds... unattached. None worked well.

"After several discussions, Dr. Smith-Petersen decided that it had to have a stem...The mold was...hollow with 2-mm thick walls to 'conserve stock,' to allow knee fusion if arthroplasty failed...The lateral walls were made low to allow preservation of the collateral ligaments. Initially a 4½ inch Smith-Petersen nail was used as a medullary stem...mounted well forward on the mold [at 15 valgus]" (Jones 1969).

Smith-Petersen and Dr. Otto Aufranc favored the new mold design in Vitallium, and Smith-Petersen performed the first knee arthroplasty with the newly designed prosthesis in 1952:

"A tourniquet was not used; 1500 cc blood were given during the operation of a little over 3 hours' duration... After the first operation Dr. Smith-Petersen had several suggestions for alternatives of the mold...No mold has broken...Dr. Aufranc has more recently contributed a longer (7½") stem that is heavier, blunter and tapered...but does limit the varus-valgus variability in mold placement... Dr. Morten Smith-Petersen [Marius Smith-Petersen's son]...accomplished what his father tried to do more than 10 years earlier, i.e., having the manufacturer cut down the inner walls of the condyles of the mold...to allow preservation of the cruciate ligaments..." (Jones 1969).

In May 1953, a patient in whose left knee Smith-Petersen had previously inserted a free mold returned for an arthroplasty on the right knee, using the new mold:

"The boy's knee had long been ankylosed and it was a year before a gain of motion to a maximum of 85° was attained. Extension never was quite complete...[although] function remained very good and the patient's life continued to be active, involving farming and tractor driving" (Jones 1969).

Smith-Petersen became ill then and could not perform the procedure (he died soon after, in June 1953). It was probably Jones who performed the procedure in Smith-Petersen's place.

Despite the loss of their friend and colleague, Jones and Aufranc, with Smith-Petersen's son, Morten (also an orthopaedic surgeon), continued the work. The positive results in that patient helped to keep alive interest in the new mold, and the mold arthroplasty procedure itself— particularly considering the poor results in earlier cases. Jones (1969) summarized the results of subsequent mold arthroplasties they performed into the later 1960s:

"In 1958, Dr. Aufranc and I, and in 1967, Dr. Aufranc, Dr. William Kermond and I reported stabilities concerning this procedure [unpublished data]...Mold Arthroplasties were performed in 83 knees of 65 patients. Seventy-five percent had severe rheumatoid arthritis...21 had completely ankylosed knees...Molds were removed because of infection; 12 of the 14...from rheumatoid knees...The results...at 6 to 12 months will remain the same for at least 5 years [average range of motion 66°]...[I]t was believed that an attempt to preserve motion was justified since...if failed, fusion could be done easily."

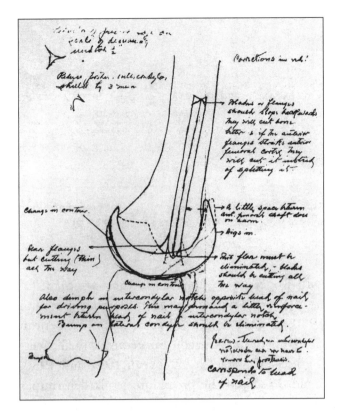

Dr. Smith-Petersen's sketch of the MGH femoral stem prosthesis—with alterations suggested after the first clinical use of a prototype. *Clinical Orthopaedics and Related Research* 1969; 66: 85.

1969). Thus, Jones began to help Smith-Petersen advance the molds used in knee arthroplasty, keeping in mind Smith-Petersen's preferences to avoid, when possible, both replacing bone with synthetic materials and using a Judet hip prosthesis, which Smith-Petersen believed was not durable and thus would not stay fixed in place. Jones documented "the development of the last mold, which, unfortunately, he [Smith-Petersen] was able to use only once [in 1952] and without success. He expected that it would allow reconstruction of many badly damaged knees and to a considerable extent this has been realized [it was commercially available for some time]." **Box 40.9** includes further details describing the continuing evolution of this mold over the subsequent 15 years.

Not much is known about Jones's work in the latter part of his career. We know that he retired in 1983, after 35 years at MGH. He died eight years later at age 75.

ROBERT J. JOPLIN

Physician Snapshot

Robert J. Joplin
BORN: 1902
DIED: 1983
SIGNIFICANT CONTRIBUTIONS: Developed the sling procedure to correct splay foot and hallux valgus; first president of the American Orthopaedic Foot Society (1969)

Robert J. Joplin was born in 1902 in Texas. After graduating with a bachelor's degree from the University of Texas in 1923, he went to Boston to attend Harvard Medical School. He received his MD degree from Harvard in 1929. After internships at Children's Hospital and MGH, Joplin limited his practice to orthopaedic surgery, mainly at MGH. In 1933 he followed Dr. William T. Green as a resident in orthopaedic surgery at Children's Hospital. In 1936, Joplin was an assistant orthopaedic surgeon at Children's Hospital and Robert Breck Brigham Hospital, and an assistant in orthopaedic surgery at Harvard Medical School.

In 1936, he published the paper "Convalescent Care in Chronic Arthritis" (his first) with Dr. John G. Kuhns, Chief of Staff at the Robert Breck

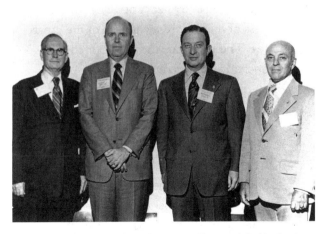

First four presidents of the American Foot and Ankle Society. Left to right: Robert J. Joplin, Robert Samilson, Nathaniel Gould, and Nicholas Giannestras. Photo used with permission from the American Orthopaedic Foot & Ankle Society.

Brigham Hospital. They surveyed 661 convalescent patients and concluded that three factors were important in these patients' care: close supervision, good treatment started early, and early diagnosis and treatment of any complications. While at MGH, Joplin wrote or cowrote five articles on the foot and the textbook *Slipped Capital Femoral Epiphysis*, which he wrote with Drs. Armin Klein (chapter 53), John Reidy (mentioned later in this chapter), and Joseph Hanelin.

Sling Procedure for the Foot

Despite this work in arthritis and slipped capital femoral epiphyses, Joplin's main interest and focus was foot surgery, especially his "sling" procedure (see **Box 40.10**). In 1947, he published his first article on the foot, written with Dr. William A. Rogers, titled "Hallux Valgus, Weak Foot and the Keller Operation: An End-Result Study." The data in that article:

> revealed that the Keller operation, employed for the most part...hardly gave satisfactory results...The following unsatisfactory results were found repeatedly:
>
> 1. The...push-off mechanism either appeared weaker after operation...or was unchanged in 89 per cent...due to weakness of the flexor mechanism of the great toe. The tendency to splay-foot either was unchanged or increased...
>
> 2. Ninety-one per cent...failed to show improvement in the structure of the foot...
>
> 3. ...[Ninety] per cent of the patients were employed in sedentary occupations...
>
> 4. Varus of the first metatarsal was unchanged in 90 per cent...[whereas] in 9 per cent it had increased. (Joplin 1950)

Although he had performed the first sling procedure in October 1947—the month his article

Joplin's article in which he describes his sling procedure for splay feet. *Journal of Bone and Joint Surgery* 1950; 32: 779.

with Rogers was published in the *Surgical Clinics of North America*—he didn't introduce it until 1950, in a paper he read at that year's American Academy of Orthopaedic Surgeons Annual Meeting in New York City. Between 1947 and 1950, Joplin had used the procedure to fix deformities in 131 feet. He noted that his aim had been to create a procedure that would provide better results than could be achieved with the Keller operation. To do so, he used amputated limbs to evaluate "experimental corrective procedures" that used the adductor hallucis (first reported by McBride in 1928). Joplin described the procedure in detail:

> To enable...[the adductor hallucis] to function effectively, it seemed physiologically sound to attach it to some structure on the medial rather than on the lateral aspect of the first metatarsal...Consequently...a drill hole is made through the shaft [of the first metatarsal] to permit the attachment of the adductor hallucis tendon to the capsule on the tibial side...To prevent the adductor hallucis...from suddenly overstretching, some reliable method was needed to overcome...[t]he splay or spreading forces...The logical structure seemed to be the long extensor tendon of the fifth toe... [The tendon is] divided as far proximally as possible...The distal portion of this tendon [is then] anchored securely to the neck of the fifth

metatarsal, while the little toe was held in neutral position…The tendon of the abductor digiti quinti…[is] then brought upward and sutured to the extensor of the fifth toe, distal to the tenodesis… (Joplin 1950)

As a next step, the fifth toe extensor tendon is passed, with the use of a tendon passer, across the foot beneath the necks of the lateral four metatarsals. It is brought over the dorsum of the first metatarsal neck, in a latter modification; in the original technique, it is brought through a hole made in the first metatarsal where the adductor tendon is passed medially. Then, with a gauze wrapped tightly around the forefoot, the extensor tendon and the adductor tendon are sutured tightly, in a complex fashion, incorporating the medial capsule of the first metatarsal phalangeal joint and the short abductor muscle/tendon unit. Residents were responsible for the name of the procedure, "the first of which was done in October 1947. It "was referred to by the house officers as the 'sling procedure'" (Joplin 1950), and the name stuck for a number of years.

In the discussion of Joplin's paper, Dr. Earl D. McBride (1950) commented that "we do need a procedure for correcting the laxity of the broadened, ungainly splay foot." Although McBride felt it would be too extensive for use in removing large bunions and that challenges arise when drilling near and fracturing the first metatarsal, he thought that "The tendon operation which he [Joplin] describes should be an excellent procedure for splay foot" (McBride 1950).

Joplin continued to use and develop the sling procedure. In 1964, he reported his experience with the operation in 615 feet. He advocated use of the sling procedure in teenage patients and adults—even older adults "in their seventies, provided the soft tissues are healthy and the circulation good" (Joplin 1964). Although complications had occurred, they "were not severe. The most common complication was mild to severe stiffness of all the toe joints…Calluses always disappeared

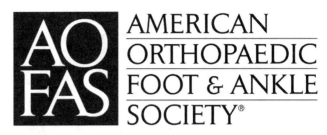

Logo American Orthopaedic Foot and Ankle Society. The society changed their name from the American Orthopaedic Foot Society in 1983. Used with permission from the American Orthopaedic Foot & Ankle Society.

during convalescence…Medial subluxation of the sesamoid with hallux varus occurred in eight feet…There have been no wound infections since the first report…Loss of correction of the splay foot deformity occurred in six patients" He also delineated the indications for the procedure, which at the time included "splay foot, metatarsus primus varus, and hallux valgus sufficient to cause difficulty fitting shoes or pain when standing or walking" (Joplin 1964).

Joplin was one of the founders of the American Orthopaedic Foot Society, and at a 1972 symposium of that organization, chaired by Dr. James E. Bateman, Joplin reported a 22-year follow-up of the sling procedure he had performed on a 12-year-old boy in June 1948. Joplin believed this to be the longest reported follow-up in a child. On the basis of the results over that extensive follow-up, Joplin (1972) concluded that:

deformity of the bony structures can be altered while growth exists if correction is obtained by the sling procedure…Comparison of a series of preoperative and postoperative roentgenograms reveals the immediate changes obtained by surgery; improvement continues until the epiphysis is closed and even beyond…and [such improvement] has not been shown to occur after this operation on an adult's foot. The changes reveal what may be called a "growing child syndrome" following [the] sling procedure.

Box 40.10. Sling Procedure to Correct Splay Foot and Hallux Valgus

"A curvilinear incision, two inches long, is made over the dorsum of the big-toe joint, damage to the extensor-tendon sheath being carefully avoided. The incision is terminated proximally when the tendon of the abductor hallucis has been exposed. The medial aspect of the capsule is then opened with a linear incision, about one and one-half inches long, which is extended from the proximal phalanx across the joint, through the bursa, and over the exostosis, to the middle of the neck of the first metatarsal. The dorsal and plantar edges or flaps of this capsule are separated by sharp dissection from the exostosis, which is subsequently excised with a thin, sharp osteotome.

"Attention is then directed to the space between the head of the first and second metatarsals. Dissection is carried down through the overlying sheath to expose the adductor hallucis tendon. When this sheath has been retracted, the adductor hallucis (oblique and transverse portions) and the flexor hallucis brevis muscles are exposed; together, their tendons are found inserted into the lateral lip of the proximal phalanx. The insertion of the adductor hallucis is carefully removed, as much tendon length as possible being taken. This detached tendon is then grasped with an Allis forceps and lifted upward, while sharp dissection is used to separate it from the capsule, the lateral sesamoid, and the lateral head of the flexor hallucis brevis. This dissection should be meticulously performed. A strong tendon, about one-half to three-quarters of an inch long and from one-eighth to three-sixteenths of an inch wide, may be obtained. With the relaxation of the lateral capsule of the joint facilitated by the removal of the adductor hallucis, the hallux valgus can be corrected easily.

"The flexor hallucis brevis is permitted to remain attached to the lateral sesamoid bone, which becomes restored to its anatomical position beneath the head of the first metatarsal. The surgeon should be warned here against a possible danger. If all the tendons (adductors and flexor brevis) should be transplanted and no restraining or stabilizing structure allowed to remain on the lateral aspect of the proximal phalanx, the great toe may assume a position of marked varus. The long extensor tendon likewise may shift to the tibial side of the joint and thus create a persistent bowstring effect, contributing further toward maintaining an overcorrected position or varus deformity.

"A five-millimeter twist drill is used to make an opening transversely (parallel with the sole of the foot) through the neck of the first metatarsal. The exact location of this opening is determined by holding the tendon of the adductor hallucis up and out of the wound under slight tension. The drill hole is placed at the point where the tendon crosses the neck of the first metatarsal.

"Attention is then directed to the opposite side of the foot. A short curved incision is made over the fifth metatarsophalangeal joint. Dissection is carried down to the capsule, which is incised between the tendons of the abductor digiti quinti and the extensor longus.

"The proximal position of the long extensor tendon of the fifth toe is demonstrated by tension placed on its distal portion.

"A small transverse incision is then made within the natural skin fold at the designated point, just anterior to the ankle. Dissection is carried down to the anterior ligament, which is incised transversely for a short distance, to expose the bundle of extensor tendons. The fifth tendon can be recognized when gentle traction again is applied distally. The foot is then strongly flexed to facilitate removal of as much of the tendon as possible. The severed distal end, when grasped with curved Kelly forceps, may be easily passed down the common tendon sheath, if the curve of the forceps is kept upward to conform to the contour of the foot and ankle.

"This procedure usually frees the tendon mesentery and enables the operator to draw the tendon through the distal wound without incising the skin through its course.

"The exostosis over the distal, lateral aspect of the fifth metatarsal is exposed and excised with a rongeur. Great care is taken to avoid unnecessary exposure of the joint or trauma to the articular cartilage. A towel clip is used to make an opening in the cancellous bone, just proximal to the head of the fifth metatarsal. Through this small hole a silk suture is passed to fix the extensor tendon to the raw bone surface, the fifth toe being held in neutral position. The abductor digiti quinti tendon is brought anteriorly and sutured to the long extensor tendon of the fifth toe, over the base of the proximal phalanx, to prevent permanent toe flexion should the transplanted tendon later become stretched. The capsule is carefully replaced.

"A small tendon passer is then inserted between the retracted abductor digiti quinti tendon and the shaft of the fifth metatarsal; it is passed across the sole of the foot, just beneath the necks of the lateral four metatarsals, care being taken to keep within the plane of the transverse head of the adductor hallucis and parallel with its fibers. The towel clip is removed from the edges of the first incision to permit the tendon passer to deliver the extensor tendon across and out, between the first and second metatarsals, where it is left temporarily.

"The two ends of a fairly strong (size 2–0) silk suture, firmly attached to the freed tendon of the adductor hallucis, are brought through the previously made drill hole; one end is passed through the dorsal flap of the capsule, the other through the plantar flap. The extensor tendon is likewise passed through the same opening, carried slightly distally, and inserted through the plantar capsule.

"A gauze sponge is placed around the fore part of the foot. While its two ends are drawn firmly together to squeeze the metatarsals together and thus correct the splay-foot deformity, a large Kocher clamp fastens the end of the sponge to maintain this position while the tendons are being fastened firmly. To accomplish this fixation, the extensor tendon, which had just previously been passed through the plantar flap of the capsule, slightly distal to the drill hole, is directed proximally around a slip of the abductor hallucis tendon, up through the dorsal flap, and back toward the proximal phalanx. It is held there under moderate tension while silk sutures, previously placed through the dorsal and plantar flaps of the capsule, are passed through the fifth tendon graft and tied. The amount of capsule on the medial side of the great-toe joint which is allowed to remain following the reefing procedure may affect the degree of motion of the great toe. For example, placing the tendon graft too near the phalanx necessarily restricts movement.

"Furthermore, the transplanted adductor tendon should not be pulled at an acute angle, for rubbing against the edges of the drill hole may cause chafing or division. The tendon graft should pass straight through the drill hole into the capsule at such an angle that free motion of the great-toe joint is permitted. The range of motion of the great toe should be observed before the wound is closed.

"The tendon graft thus serves three purposes: (1) It approximates the metatarsals, thus correcting the splay-foot and primus varus; (2) it corrects the hallux valgus by abducting the great toe; and (3) it advances the attachment of the abductor hallucis tendon to a position nearer the phalanx by taking a reef in the medial side of the capsule. Thus it repairs the capsule while correcting the deformity.

"The gross over-all deformities of the foot are thus corrected, while the function and the configuration are restored to a more nearly normal state.

AFTER-CARE

"Following closure of the skin incision and application of dry sterile dressings, plaster-of-Paris shoes, extending from the toes to above the malleoli, are applied, as well as rubber heels, to permit weight-bearing. After four or five days, the patient is allowed to start walking with the aid of crutches. The amount of walking is kept to a minimum as long as standing produces swelling of the toes. The patient is encouraged to keep his feet elevated at all other times and to do toe-curling exercises...

"After three or four weeks the plaster shoes are removed and the patient is permitted to wear leather shoes as soon as they can be fitted. Compression bandages should be worn to prevent swelling, if walking in loose bedroom slippers is allowed. Physical therapy, in the form of heat and massage with active exercises, is helpful. Standing on tiptoes is discouraged until after six weeks. The patient may expect to resume his usual activities from eight to ten weeks after operation."

—Robert J. Joplin, 1950

Legacy

Joplin was the first president of the American Orthopaedic Foot Society. His 1969 presidential address was titled "The Proper Digital Nerve, Vitallium Stem Arthroplasty, and Some Thoughts about Foot Surgery in General." In his introduction, he shared his excitement about future opportunities in the field of foot surgery: "Today a rare opportunity awaits the young orthopaedic surgeon who is interested in foot problems, because in this special field, which remains almost unexplored, he has a chance to exert his ingenuity as in no other branch of surgery that I know of today" (Joplin 1971). The body of his speech cited brief case reports related to the topics listed in the title of his address.

Joplin was on the board of consultation at MGH, where he had risen to the role of visiting orthopaedic surgeon. At the end of his career, he was an attending in orthopaedic surgery at the Boston Veterans Administration Hospital and an instructor in orthopaedic surgery at Harvard Medical School. He was a member of numerous organizations including the Massachusetts Medical Society and the American Academy of Orthopaedic Surgeons. His office was at Zero Emerson Place in the city; he lived in Chestnut Hill.

I found very little information about the last 10 years of Joplin's life. He died on May 8, 1983, at age 81, in Kennett Square, Pennsylvania. He was survived by his wife and their four children (two sons and two daughters).

WILLIAM L. KERMOND

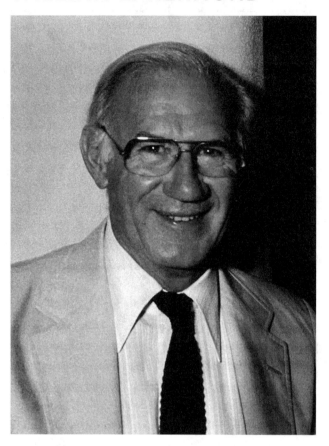

William L. Kermond. Courtesy of Ellen Fador.

Physician Snapshot

William L. Kermond
BORN: 1928
DIED: 2012
SIGNIFICANT CONTRIBUTIONS: Private practitioner interested in rehabilitation; volunteer with Por Cristo, providing orthopaedic care to children in Ecuador

Dr. William L. Kermond was raised and educated in Victoria, Australia, where he attended Newman College at the University of Melbourne. I was unable to find much information about him; however, some details are available regarding his university education, training, and practice. After graduating from Newman, he traveled to London to continue his education at the Royal College of Surgeons. At some point he emigrated to the United States, and he practiced and taught in

Boston: as an orthopaedic surgeon at Winchester Hospital, an assistant in orthopaedic surgery at Massachusetts General Hospital, and an instructor in orthopaedic surgery at Harvard Medical School.

In addition to his role as assistant in orthopaedic surgery at MGH, Kermond was also assistant director of the hospital's White 9 Rehabilitation Unit under Dr. Thomas DeLorme for a brief period. In his history of orthopaedics at MGH during the twentieth century, Carter Rowe indicates that Kermond was promoted to chief of the unit when DeLorme resigned as its director in 1958. Thornton Brown, however, in his chapter on orthopedic surgery in the 1983 book *The Massachusetts General Hospital, 1955–1980*, wrote that DeLorme "was succeeded first by Irving Ackerman and later Robert Jones, an assistant in Medicine who held the position of coordinator of rehabilitation until 1965 when he accepted an appointment elsewhere." Kermond practiced mainly at Winchester Hospital, along with Dr. Frank Bates (chapter 23) and R. Wendell Pierce. He oversaw the Orthopedic Back Center in Winchester, a clinic that provided care to people experiencing back pain.

Kermond cowrote two papers while at MGH. In the first, titled "Disease-Simulation Technics in Rehabilitation Teaching," published in 1964; he, Dr. Robert H. Jones, and an orthopaedic research fellow, Dr. John H. Bowker, described their efforts to modify normal function by attaching to participants (third-year medical students) devices that simulated hemiplegia, a knee disarticulation, or rheumatoid arthritis of the hand. Their objective was to develop "a state of empathy in which the fuller appreciation of a disability, including the patient's emotional reaction to it, leads to its knowledgeable analysis and correction. The 'patient' feels very real frustration on being unable to manage self-care…conditions are imposed that are similar to those facing a patient as he becomes the 'student' requiring instruction in substitution patterns or in the use of prosthetic devices" (Bowker, Kermond, and Jones 1964). In the second paper, "Determination of Leg Length Discrepancy. A comparison of Weight-Bearing and Supine Imaging"; cowritten with providers from the MGH departments of orthopaedic surgery, radiology, and physical therapy; the authors showed that estimations of leg-length discrepancy significantly differed between physical examinations and radiographic investigations. When determining leg-length discrepancy, they considered radiography to be superior to a physical exam.

During his career, Kermond volunteered with Por Cristo, a federation of health care providers who travel to Ecuador to train physicians in orthopaedics and provide such care to patients (mainly children). He also played golf and tennis, flew planes, and enjoyed sailing. He died on February 18, 2012; his wife Evelyn (née Conway) and their five children (three sons and two daughters) survived him.

CARROLL B. LARSON

Physician Snapshot

Carroll B. Larson
BORN: 1909
DIED: 1978
SIGNIFICANT CONTRIBUTIONS: Chaired the Department of Orthopaedics at the University of Iowa for 23 years; coedited numerous revisions of the popular reference *Calderwood's Orthopedic Nursing*; president of the American Academy of Orthopaedic Surgeons

Carroll Bernard Larson was born on September 10, 1909, in Council Bluffs in Western Iowa, across the Missouri River from Omaha, Nebraska. His parents, Charles Bernard and Ida Caroline, owned a hardware store. In high school, Carroll excelled academically and in track and field (pole vaulting). He attended the University of Iowa, and while there he was active in the Phi Beta Pi medical fraternity and the US Army ROTC program; he was elected the outstanding cadet in the ROTC honor fraternity (Pershing Rifles). He graduated in 1931 with a bachelor of science degree, and he remained at the University of Iowa during medical school, receiving an MD degree in 1933.

Early Training and Practice

After graduating, Larson accepted a three-year surgical internship and residency at Santa Clara County Hospital in San Jose, California. (About four decades after Larson's tenure there, the hospital became affiliated with Stanford University.) In his early days in San Jose, he met Nadine West Townsend, whom he married in 1934. Shortly after their marriage, however, and after just two years in the surgical program at Santa Clara County Hospital, Larson had to return to the Midwest for one year to fulfill ROTC obligations in Duluth, Minnesota, and while there he worked part-time with physicians in Indianola and Ida Grove. Upon completing his ROTC commitment in 1937, Larson and Nadine moved to

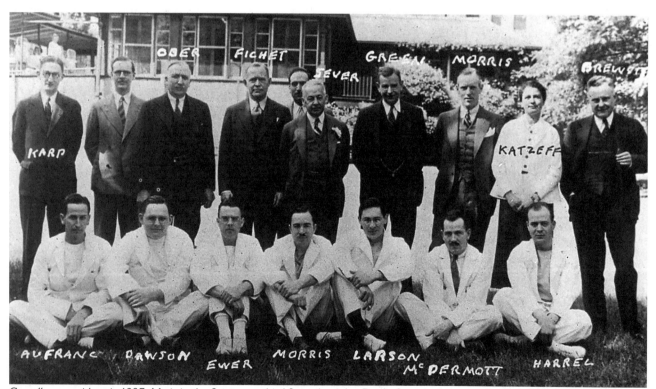

Carroll as a resident in 1937. He is in the front row, third from the right. Dr. Aufranc is sitting on the far left of the first row.
MGH HCORP Archives.

Boston so he could spend two years training in the Children's Hospital/MGH Combined Orthopaedic Residency Program. Larson successfully completed his orthopaedic residency in 1939, and Dr. Marius Smith-Petersen asked Larson to join him and Dr. Otto Aufranc in private practice (see the section about Aufranc earlier in this chapter) as an assistant in orthopaedics.

Soon after the US joined World War II, Aufranc was sent overseas (see chapter 64). Larson remained in Boston to help Smith-Petersen and to teach: he supervised the graduate and undergraduate teaching of orthopaedic surgery at MGH and was responsible for creating and presenting a continuing course on trauma for physicians in the military medical corps (see **Case 40.8**).

The King Report

Around the time World War II ended, leadership at MGH recognized that social changes would require the hospital to adapt and plan for the future, and in 1945 the hospital's general executive committee created the Committee on Staff Reorganization and Office Building—colloquially referred to as the "King Committee" after its chairman, Donald S. King. The other committee members were Leland S. McKittrick, Allan M. Butler, Langdon Parsons, and Larson. The King Committee "presented a report in the next year on hospital organization which profoundly influenced the future of the hospital" (Faxon 1959). With regard to staff organization, the committee made five recommendations:

1. The professional staff of the Massachusetts General Hospital should, as in the past, consist of full- and part-time doctors.
2. The part-time staff should be limited to those who would contribute to the development of the Hospital by teaching or by clinical laboratory investigation. [This was to eliminate "dead wood" and assured a working staff.]
3. Facilities, that is, an office building, should be provided which would make it easier for the members of the active professional staff to work together in private practice as well as in hospital activities....
4. Some form of staff organization should be developed around the men in the proposed office building which would give office patients the same benefits of group care as are now enjoyed by patients in the Baker Memorial... [This recommendation resulted in the formation of the Massachusetts General Hospital Staff Associates.]

Case 40.8. Primary Closure with Local Treatment of Septic Wounds in Osteomyelitis

> "A student of nineteen had multiple foci of osteomyelitis, occurring over a period of seven years. In July 1944, acute symptoms from a new focus, in the mid-shaft of the right femur, developed. Operation included saucerization, and insertion of two vitallium cannulae, with wound closure. Free pus was encountered in the medullary canal. The postoperative course was smooth. The patient was particularly appreciative of the absence of painful dressings, because of his previous experience with them.
>
> "Systemic penicillin, 100,000 units in twenty-four hours, was administered for ten days after operation, and for a week after the removal of the cannulae. Local penicillin was injected every four hours: ten cubic centimeters, 250 units per cubic centimeter. This was continued up to the time of the removal of the cannulae.
>
> "The cannulae were removed on the twenty-sixth post-operative day under pentothal anaesthesia, and the defects were closed. A small rubber catheter was left in place, and penicillin was continued locally for ten more days.
>
> "The wound was entirely healed six weeks after the original operation. Roentgenograms at that time showed satisfactory progress of bone repair.
>
> "Only ten months have elapsed since operation, but so far there has been no local recurrence of sepsis."
>
> (Smith-Peterson, Larsen, and Cochrane 1945)

5. Such an office building and clinic would be feasible only if the staff were provided with more private beds… (Faxon 1959)

"The 'King Report' had been debated at length for two years, by the General Executive Committee, by the Staff in meetings and in the dining room and corridors" (Faxon 1959). In the report, the King Committee:

recommended that all active members of the Staff should function actively in at least one of the following directions: (1) care of ward patients, (2) teaching, (3) research. This made it necessary for the Chief of each service to decide how many physicians he needed on his staff in the various grades and to prepare a roster. The pending reorganization of the surgical services and the possibility of an office building made this difficult. Another problem was the status of Pathology, Radiology and Anesthesiology which came to be designated as 'supporting departments.' The staffs of these departments were all on full-time salaries. What should be their relationship to private patients and to 'third-party' patients as regarding professional fees? The matter of professional fees for patients in the General Hospital paid by third parties…was settled by having the Hospital collect these in the name of the attending physician, placing them in a fund, to be disposed of according to the direction of the staff involved, with Trustee approval…Physical changes at the Hospital were many in 1948 [none seemed to involve orthopaedics.]…Storrow House in Lincoln, for convalescent patients…was opened on August 8. (Faxon 1959)

Contributions to Orthopaedic Research and Nursing Education

In 1946, the year the King Report was presented, Larson was promoted to assistant orthopaedic surgeon at MGH. All told Larson spent ~10 years on the staff at the MGH and in private practice. He cowrote four articles with Smith-Petersen, Aufranc, and Dr. Williams Cochran. Larson's main interests were the spine and arthritis, the latter particularly in relation to hip arthroplasty (see chapter 37 and the section about Aufranc earlier in this chapter). He collaborated with Dr. Joseph Barr, Dr. William Mixter, and others in neurology, pathology, and radiology to perform early studies of herniated discs. Larson was also interested in nursing education, and he held a position as a lecturer at the School of Nursing at MGH, which had opened in 1873.

During this period, in 1948, Larson also traveled to Oslo, Norway, to assist Smith-Petersen during the back operation he performed on Princess Martha. While there Larson assisted Smith-Petersen in performing cup arthroplasties on numerous patients as well. That same year, the government of Norway bestowed on him the honor of Royal Commander of the Order of St. Olaf for his work with Smith-Peterson in that country, and he was also selected as one of the American Orthopaedic Association's first group of ABC traveling fellows.

In 1950, Larson resigned from the MGH and was elected to the board of consultants. He had decided to leave Boston and MGH for Iowa, as

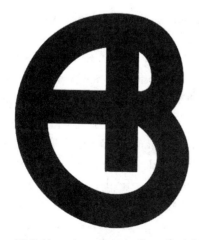

Logo of the ABC (American, British, Canadian) fellowship.
Courtesy of the American Orthopaedic Association.

he had been chosen to chair the Department of Orthopaedics at the University of Iowa, succeeding Dr. Arthur Steindler; he also became a professor in that department. While at Iowa, Larson continued his work around nursing education: he collaborated with Marjorie Gould to revise the second edition of Robert Funsten and Carmelita Calderwood's *Orthopedic Nursing*, which had by then been reprinted three times. Larson and Gould's work resulted in 1953 in the third edition of the newly titled *Calderwood's Orthopedic Nursing*, which was subsequently republished in at least seven editions. The book was "presented primarily to furnish a background of medical information and principles of care of the orthopaedic patient for nursing students...appropriate emphasis is placed on the role of the nurse on the health care team" (Gassman 1962).

Legacy

Larson had influential roles in many organizations in the field of orthopaedics; some of these are listed in **Box 40.11**. He remained in the position of chairman of the orthopaedic department at the University Iowa until 1973, when he retired after 23 years at the helm. Larson died on October 3, 1978, after a prolonged illness. After his death, his University of Iowa colleagues Dr. Reginald Cooper and Dr. Michael Bonfiglio (1979) described Larson as:

> a quiet man with a sense of personal dignity needed in the approach to problems not lending themselves to easy solutions. He listened; he constructively counseled without intrusion of his own concepts on those who sought his counsel or assistance. Perhaps this is the greatest gift that a man can give to his patients, his friends, his students, and his family – to present help in a manner which is acceptable to them. This he could do without rancor, without dominating, and without demeaning an idea no matter how frivolous it might have been. He gave assistance willingly and worried lest the recipient feel beholden to him. (Cooper and Bonfiglio 1979)

They described a man who aimed to give only his best to his patients, his colleagues, and his profession.

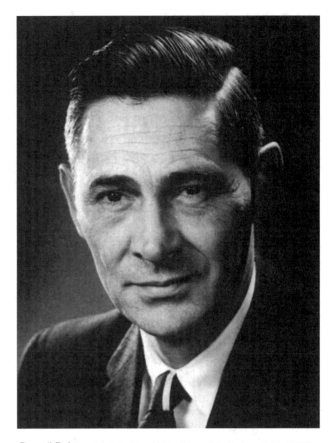

Carroll B. Larson. R.R.C. and M.B., "Carroll B. Larson 1909-1978," *Journal of Bone and Joint Surgery* 1979; 61: 151.

Box 40.11. Carroll Larson's Professional Roles

- Treasurer and president, American Academy of Orthopaedic Surgeons (1966)
- Charter member, Orthopaedic Research Society (1954)
- Associate editor, *New England Journal of Medicine*
- Editorial Board member and trustee, *Journal of Bone and Joint Surgery* (1968–74)
- Advisory Medical Board member (1957–66), Executive Medical Advisor (1966–68), and Director of Medical Affairs (1968–76), Shriners Hospitals

HARRY C. LOW

Physician Snapshot

Harry C. Low
BORN: 1871
DIED: 1943
SIGNIFICANT CONTRIBUTIONS: Spent 10 years as surgeon-in-charge of the Infantile Paralysis Clinic at MGH; first chairman of the Committee on Occupational Therapy

Harry Chamberlin Low was born in 1871 and raised in Salem, Massachusetts. He stayed in his home state to receive his education: he graduated from Harvard College in 1893 and Harvard Medical School in 1897. He interned at Children's Hospital in 1898 and then spent three years (two of which he spent in pathology) at Boston City Hospital. As the twentieth-century began, he left Boston for London and Vienna, where he spent a year studying medicine. He moved on to Italy, but after five months there he returned to Boston, having decided to practice orthopaedic surgery. Soon after his return, on June 18, 1902, he married Mabel C. Chapman. He set up an office at 409 Marlboro Street. For the next approximate six years, in addition to his private practice, Low worked as an assistant pathologist at Children's Hospital (see **Case 40.9**) while also possibly holding a similar position at Boston City Hospital.

In 1909, he was an assistant in orthopaedics at the Massachusetts General Hospital; after two years in that role he was promoted to assistant orthopaedic surgeon to outpatients. In 1915, while practicing at MGH as an orthopaedic surgeon, Low published his only orthopaedic-related article, titled "A Study of the Scope and Efficiency of a Large Orthopedic Clinic." In it he described the beginnings of the orthopaedic outpatient clinic at MGH—which at the time had not yet been operating for a decade—the cases and populations its physicians treat, and the types of diagnoses they identify. An excerpt from this article is provided in **Box 40.12**.

A STUDY OF THE SCOPE AND EFFICIENCY OF A LARGE ORTHOPEDIC CLINIC.

BY HARRY C. LOW, M. D.

JBJS, 1915, Volume s2-12, Issue 3

Low's review of the early experiences in the first orthopaedic clinic at MGH. *Journal of Bone and Joint Surgery* 1915; s2-12: 396.

This 1915 article was one of just eight Low published throughout his career. Two years after that publication, he became an orthopaedic surgeon to outpatients and was continuously on the service every other day.

In 1919, the MGH board of trustees appointed Low as chairman of the new Committee on Occupational Therapy. In December 1920, Low described how the committee enhanced "the value of Occupational Therapy in the wards of the Hospital":

> [T]he Committee secured the services of several Reconstruction Aides who had been in War Service. These volunteers, with students from the School of Occupational Therapy, and the Tide-Over League, have carried on the work for more than a year. At first the work was done in the medical, surgical, and the orthopaedic wards. In the wards of an acute hospital, like the Massachusetts General Hospital, occupational therapy has consisted mainly of keeping up the morale of the patients, thereby shortening the period of convalescence. In a few instances, by special request of the doctors, work has been undertaken with patients to facilitate the restoration or function in fracture and joint disability.
>
> The number of patients under our treatment during the year (274) is much less than

Case 40.9. Acetonuria Associated with Death after Anesthesia

"M.J.B. a girl, aged eight years, of Fitchburg, entered the Children's Hospital on October 6, 1903. She had an extensive infantile paralysis involving most of the muscles of both lower extremities which came on five years before, and necessitated the use of crutches in walking.

"On several occasions during the preceding year, the child had several very acute attacks of severe and persistent vomiting, accompanied by marked prostration and rapid pulse, and the physician in attendance stated that the condition of the child at the time of these attacks, very closely resembled that described to him as existing on the first day of the fatal one. The attacks were severe enough to cause considerable alarm as to their outcome.

"The child seemed rather delicate, but was well nourished, and physical examination showed nothing abnormal aside from the infantile paralysis already mentioned. The urine was acid, with specific gravity of 1,020, free from albumin and sugar. The pulse was 100; the temperature was 100.

"Four days after entrance the child was etherized, and three tendons were transplanted. The loss of blood was insignificant, though the operation and the application of the plaster bandages kept the child under ether about an hour and a half. The child took ether rather badly, being rather blue, and having a rapid pulse, but at no time during or immediately after the operation, was there ground for anxiety in regard to the condition.

"During the recovery from ether the child vomited as usual, and then seemed comfortable, and in good condition till twelve hours later. She then suddenly began to vomit persistently. The vomitus was at first watery and light green in color, but later dark. The pulse became very rapid, jumping to about 190, the temperature rose to 106. The vomiting lasted for about thirty hours. The child, who had been restless, gradually sunk into a delirious stupor, and died forty-two hours after the operation, thirty hours after the vomiting began.

"In this case no test was made of the urine for acetone or diacetic acid. It was clearly recalled afterward, however, that the peculiar odor of the breath was very strong. Stimulation had no effect.

"Autopsy, Oct. 12. Dr. H. A. Christian.

"Body of a well-developed, well-nourished female child…

"Spinal cord shows, particularly in the lower lumbar region, an atrophy of the anterior horn on one side. The blood vessels lie on the surface of the cord, are much congested. No other lesion found.

"Anatomical diagnosis. —Chronic poliomyelitis, anterior.

"Cultures.—One culture spleen – bacillus of colon group. Two culture liver – very slight growth of same.

"None of three show any staphylococci or streptococci.

"Histology. – Spinal Cord: The anterior horn of one side shows marked atrophy with almost complete disappearance of the anterior nerve cells.

"Anterior mediastinum: The loose tissues of the anterior mediastinum show an acute inflammatory process of slight degree, evinced by the presence of polynuclear leucocytes in the tissue, adjacent to the gas cysts described in the gross. Sections of this tissue stained by Gram-Weigert method show no micro-organisms. Sections of liver, spleen, kidneys and lungs are negative. From these sections it is evident that to the marked process in the cord there is added some slight acute inflammatory process in the anterior mediastinum."

(Brackett, Stone, and Low 1904)

it would have been had we been able to carry on the work continuously with a full force of workers. The large number of pupil volunteers that we have had was due to the experience and supervision they received, under our able head aides, Miss Hurd, Miss Hayward, and Miss Wigglesworth.

The curative value of the occupational side of this work has been very evident, and in some cases the physiotherapeutic side has been brought out also. This latter will be more important as the co-operation between the surgeon and this department in the treatment of handicapped patients is developed. There is a field for the work in all the wards of the Hospital, and it has recently been started by two volunteers in the Skin Ward, where the problem of infectious disease of the hands has to be met. Also, a worker is devoting five days in the week to a new development of this occupational

Box 40.12. Early Experiences in the Orthopaedic Outpatient Clinic at MGH

In 1915 Low published an article detailing the efforts of providers caring for patients through the orthopaedic outpatient clinic at MGH:

"The orthopedic outpatient clinic of the Massachusetts General Hospital...[was] started at that time as a new department taking many of its cases from the medical clinics it received from 10 to 12 patients three days in the week. It soon became a daily clinic...at first the distinctions made as to which were orthopaedic cases were very limited; including only spinal deformities, flat-foot and rickets. During the last three or four years we have seen the numbers doubled until it now ranks as one of the largest of the outpatient clinics and out of 400 to 500 cases treated daily the orthopedic clinic receives an average of 50 to 60. Last year there were treated in the orthopedic department over 14,000 cases of which 2100 were new patients.

"The data for this study of 500 consecutive cases...was made by one of the social service workers in order that we might find out what we were doing. A previous survey of 247 consecutive new cases had shown many surprising things. In this clinic from thirty to ninety patients daily the outpatient surgeon or the assistant outpatient surgeon sees and directs the treatment of all new cases, following and advising any changes in the treatment of old cases. There are also on service daily three assistants to the surgeon, various graduate volunteers, students, house officer, nurses, orderlies, etc....all the morning hours of some five to eight doctors are occupied...

"You will notice that the clinic is not largely a neighborhood one as only 21 percent are from the city. The large Boston City Hospital, the Carney, and the Children's Hospitals are almost purely for the citizens of Boston. At the Massachusetts General Hospital, the clinic is increased by many patients from all throughout Massachusetts and the three Northern New England states, so that the variety of unusual and interesting cases is great. We must appreciate that the patients are using several dollars for carfare and time taken off from work and coming to us for an opinion that must be well considered and a treatment that should be well judged.

"The birthplace is much in accordance with our population; The Russian Jew being more numerous on account of the immediate neighborhood of the hospital...It will be observed that the clinic is chiefly an adult one...[with] three high points...ten to fifteen, twenty to twenty-five and thirty to fifty years. The first increase is in youth with its postural and scoliotic changes; the second at the time of life when the slightly weak or inefficient man succumbs to the stress and strain of the ordeal of work-a-day life... we see the back and foot strains in poorly developed or congenitally defective individuals. From 30 to 50 the curve rises again to reach its maximum in the period of life most afflicted with arthritic troubles – infections, toxic, hypertrophic, etc....

"From our chart we would judge that four to five visits will suffice for the cure of most cases in the clinic...many of the cases of back and foot strain, slight arthritic troubles, etc., are easily cured. A large number of cases purely orthopaedic as tuberculous arthritis have made from ten to thirty visits and you will realize that thirty visits coming

work in the Children's Ward following the ideas of Montessori.

The need of occupational therapy in a large active hospital may be found to be as great as it is recognized to be in the chronic institutions where it has had its greatest development. Up to now this has not been thought to be true, but the change that is wrought by occupational therapy in the mental attitude and physical well-being of the patients and its effect on the ward as a whole has been noticed by both our doctors and the nurses, so that the demand for this work is rapidly increasing. It is hoped that the department can soon be established on a more permanent basis, with a paid Head Aide in charge and a regular allowance for materials and equipment granted. ("Editorial 'Selections from the Annual Report of the Orthopaedics Department'" 1920)

Beginning in 1921, Low spent a decade as the surgeon in charge of poliomyelitis at MGH. His

> every two months represent a treatment covering several years. We notice that forty-four cases (less than 10 percent) made only one visit...
>
> "In the earlier survey of 247 cases there were over 20 per cent who visited only once...In the diagnosis group you will notice the large number of cases having trouble with the feet...Next in number are the nontubercular arthritic cases. However, adding the cases of postural and other back strains associated with sacroiliac, lumbar, and sciatic pain and symptoms (30 plus 34) and also a fair proportion of sixty-nine 'Miscellaneous other than Orthopedic' cases which were diagnosed as visceroptosis, etc. (38), we have 102 cases of one class. In recent years the corrective measures of orthopedic surgery...and the advance made by the orthopedist in the study of back and leg pains has done much to increase the scope of this specialty.
>
> "With most of the other clinics our relations were simply those of consultant. From the genitourinary and the dental clinics their gonorrheal and pyogenic causes of arthritis we received by 8 of the 500 cases. Possibly the cases coming for treatment there are so well cared for that they suffer no arthritic symptoms...we referred to those departments fourteen and nineteen patients we found needed special treatment for the cause of their arthritis. We realize that more than this 4 per cent of our orthopedic cases need dental treatment. This lack of cooperation between the different clinics is to be regretted. It is further shown as we only sent twenty-three cases to the Children's and twenty-nine to the throat departments. Tuberculosis still bears a fair proportion, but that of rickets, infantile paralysis, fractures and dislocations is small. The tuberculous diagnosis chart shows the well-known proportion of the afflictions of the various joints...
>
> "Thanks to the efficiency of the admitting physician and the wide variety of cases that are now recognized as primarily orthopedic there were over 60 per cent of the cases that came directly to our clinic...By the reference of old patients we received from the medical service eighty-seven cases, from the surgical sixty-nine cases...We are sending more cases to the medical (150) than anywhere else...our relative use of the Zander and hydrotherapy and the need of social service help is over 14 per cent of the cases...
>
> "Our means of diagnosis...in 247 cases, 118 X-rays were made, 7 Wassermann tests, 3 tuberculin and 2 gonorrheal...of the 42 nontubercular arthritic cases, X-rays were taken in 14-general physical examinations, recorded in only 5, Wassermann and gonorrheal tests in one. Of the tuberculous cases, 18 in number, 4 had general physical examinations, none had tuberculin...The diagnosis may often be well made from clinical symptoms and the number of X-rays shows the dependence we put on them...
>
> "We have to thank the social service department for helping us in many ways in carrying out the treatment which has been advised...We still feel the great need of more thorough study of the treatment of patients in the hospital clinic and that by such studies much can be gained."
>
> (Low 1915)

efforts in the hospital's Infantile Paralysis Clinic were described in 1920 as "unusually devoted" ("Editorial 'Selections from the Annual Report of the Orthopaedics Department'" 1920). Because of Low's work at the New England Home for Little Wanderers (he likely treated orphans with polio who were housed there) and the Children's Sunlight Hospital at Scituate—Low was president of that hospital's repair shop—these institutions were used regularly to house patients with polio who were being treated at MGH, and their families.

Low retired from active service at MGH in 1931. In 1935 he sustained a stroke but continued to work in public health until 1937, when he had a second stroke. His wife cared for him in their summer home in Hanover, Massachusetts. He died September 13, 1943. Dr. Robert Osgood (1943) recalled that Low was a "hidden servant... who quietly, unselfishly and successfully planned his life and went about doing only good."

WILLIAM R. MACAUSLAND JR.

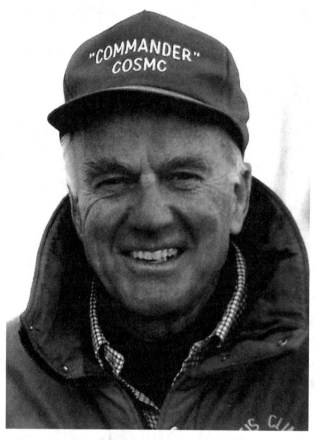

William R. MacAusland Jr.
J.S.B., Jr. et al., "William Russell MacAusland, Jr., MD 1922–2004," *Journal of Bone and Joint Surgery* 2004; 86: 2582.

Physician Snapshot

William R. MacAusland Jr.
BORN: 1922
DIED: 2004
SIGNIFICANT CONTRIBUTIONS: Served as the 48th president of the AAOS in 1980; proposed the establishment of an AAOS Learning Center; helped found the Carlos Otis Stratton Mountain Clinic in Vermont; instrumental in establishing the emergency medical technician specialty

William Russell ("Mac") MacAusland Jr. was born in Boston on December 9, 1922. His family had "a rich orthopaedic heritage, as both his father, William R. Sr., and his uncle, Andrew R., were practicing orthopaedic surgeons in the Boston area" (Barr Jr. et al. 2004). His mother was Dorothy (née Brayton) MacAusland. MacAusland Sr. had graduated from Harvard Medical School in 1903 and after an internship in Worcester was an assistant to Dr. E. G. Brackett for a short period. He then went into private practice; published numerous papers on arthroplasty; especially of the hip, knee, and elbow; and eventually became chief of orthopaedics at Carney Hospital and a clinical professor of orthopaedic surgery at Tufts University.

The younger William attended school at Milton Academy and Harvard College. He followed in his father's footsteps to Harvard Medical School, where he received a medical degree in 1947. Upon his graduation he married Frances Prescott Baker, and the two moved to Rochester, New York, where MacAusland began his surgical training at the University of Rochester Medical Center followed by a residency in orthopaedic surgery at the New York Orthopaedic Hospital. He "became lifelong friends" with John Gartland while there and was residency partners with him (Barr Jr. et al. 2004). After finishing his residency MacAusland entered the US Air Force as a captain and spent two years at Maxwell-Gunter Air Force Base in Alabama.

Early Career

After completing his military obligation, he returned to Boston, where he joined the practice of his father and uncle. MacAusland's "boundless energy enabled him to work in several hospitals in Boston and its environs" (Barr Jr. et al. 2004). He also held academic positions at Harvard and Tufts Universities. MacAusland "loved to be 'on service' and work with the residents" (Barr Jr. et al. 2004). He unhesitatingly took on "the most difficult cases to prove to the residents that fractures should be treated by orthopaedists. If called to the emergency room in the middle of the night, Bill was quickly there to help and to teach. He never shied away from the toughest case or complication" (Barr Jr. et al. 2004).

He published several papers early in his career. He cowrote three papers with John Gartland on the use and effects of hyaluronidase; these were published in 1952, 1953, and 1954. Between 1953 and 1956 he cowrote another five papers, each on a different topic related to his experiences at Maxwell Air Force Base—a bone flaking device, a radiographic table for use during hip procedures, a penicillin-streptomycin bone bank, local infiltration anesthesia in knee surgeries, and boat-nail fixation in cancellous bone.

MacAusland and Eaton's article reporting successful treatment with retaining intramedullary rod fixation in infected femur fractures. *Journal of Bone and Joint Surgery* 1963; 45: 1643.

Author Recollections

One case I worked on with MacAusland during my time as chief resident on White 6 at MGH in 1970 epitomizes his ebullient attitude. One night, two intoxicated young men were pushing their car in the North End when they were struck from behind by another car. The results were catastrophic: in both men, both knees were dislocated with open fractures, with nerve and vessel injuries. They arrived at the emergency department at MGH sometime after midnight. I called MacAusland, the visiting physician on service, and he arrived in the operating room about the same time our team of residents did. Without hesitation he started to operate in one room with resident assistants; I was operating in another room. We had stabilized all four knees before rounds the next morning. None required amputation.

Pinnacle of a Career

MacAusland was busy during the latter half of the twentieth century: "One resident commented that bill 'wore his shoes backwards' to get out of the operating room faster and onto his next task!" (Barr Jr. et al. 2004). He became a fellow of the AAOS in 1956 and served on many of the association's committees. In 1961 he received an ABC traveling fellowship with the AOA, and three years later he became a member of that association. MacAusland continued to publish throughout his career, and more than half of the 15 articles he wrote were about trauma.

While teaching residents, MacAusland often referred to two papers he published on trauma in the early 1960s. The first, published in 1962, described the "Treatment of Olecranon Fractures. Indications for Excision of the Olecranon Fragment and Repair of the Triceps Tendon." In it, he and his colleagues described 132 olecranon fractures treated at MGH over a decade: the olecranon had been removed in 28, though only 18 were followed up. They suggested excising the olecranon (with triceps insertion repair) when the fractures are so extensive that normal anatomical positioning cannot be achieved, or when internal fixation is inadequate or results in nonunion. They purposely underscored that olecranon excision does not affect the stability or range of motion of the elbow joint.

In the second article, "The Management of Sepsis Following Intramedullary Fixation for Fractures of the Femur," published in 1963, MacAusland and Dr. Richard G. Eaton reviewed 14 patients treated at MGH between 1950 and 1962 (see **Case 40.10**). They found "no conclusive evidence as to the value of one antibiotic over another or the effect of dosage or duration of antibiotic therapy," and with "adequate

Case 40:10. Sepsis after Intramedullary Fixation of a Femoral Fracture

> "M. W., a housewife, forty-three years old, had a closed comminuted fracture of the upper third of the right femur treated promptly at another hospital by Küntscher-rod fixation. Wound infection developed at the fracture site seven days after operation, and incision and drainage were immediately carried out. Ten months after operation the wound was still draining. The Küntscher rod was removed and a hip spica was applied.
>
> "Twenty-two months after fracture, when the patient was admitted to the Massachusetts General Hospital, the extremity was immobilized in a spica cast, the wound was draining, and there was non-union with shortening, rotation, and marked angulation. Two sequestrectomies were performed and the limb was maintained in balanced suspension. Two months after the second sequestrectomy, the wound was completely dry and without tenderness, but there was shortening of ten centimeters with angulation. The pseudarthrosis was excised, and a Küntscher rod was introduced after correcting the deformity caused by 90 degrees of anterior angulation and 120 degrees of internal rotation. After operation, infection recurred but responded to incision and drainage and subsequent sequestrectomy.
>
> "Four months after rod fixation, moderately advanced callus formation was present medially and drainage was decreasing. Nine months after operation, union was solid and there was only scant drainage.
>
> "Contact was made with the patient by telephone more than two years after insertion of the second Küntscher rod because she had moved. She said that the wound had continued to drain for more than three years, but had now been dry for ten months. Motion in her knee was restricted and she used a cane when walking outdoors."
>
> (MacAusland Jr. and Eaton 1963)

surgical drainage with maintenance of rigid internal fixation," both infections and fractures healed (MacAusland Jr. and Eaton 1963). They also made a case for strict internal fixation:

> Unless internal fixation is maintained, non-union, angulation, and shortening are certain to occur, and drainage will persist. Once union is established, the infected soft tissues and bone are stabilized and healing is promoted… If drainage continues after consolidation of the fracture, removal of the internal fixation is generally advisable…Sepsis is usually eradicated after removal of the rod and, if necessary, sequestrectomy…A plea is made for the maintenance of rigid internal fixation, even in the face of seemingly disastrous infection, in order to achieve union of the fracture." (MacAusland Jr. and Eaton 1963)

Two years later, MacAusland published the book *Orthopaedics: A Concise Guide to Clinical Practices*, which he cowrote with Dr. Richard Mayo. That same year, he traveled to Nigeria for six weeks with Orthopaedics Overseas, then a new organization with the goal of teaching orthopaedics to physicians in developing countries. In 1968, he went to Mexico City as a physician for the US Olympic Team. Back at home, MacAusland was practicing with Dr. Edwin Wyman at an office on Beacon Street. They began consulting for Harvard Health Services and with "the Shriners Burns Institute at Massachusetts General Hospital, and developed innovative methods for burn surgeons to use when immobilizing patients for skin grafting" (Barr Jr. et al. 2004).

In the late 1960s, MacAusland worked extensively to expand education and training for emergency responders and with the AAOS Committee on Injuries to create the book *Emergency Care and Transportation of the Sick and Injured*, better known as the "orange book," in 1971. He also "helped to develop and teach many courses for emergency personnel" through the American College of Surgeons (Barr Jr. et al. 2004). He had a hand in developing a specialty for emergency medical technicians. MacAusland was well-known for these endeavors: "If one was out to dinner with

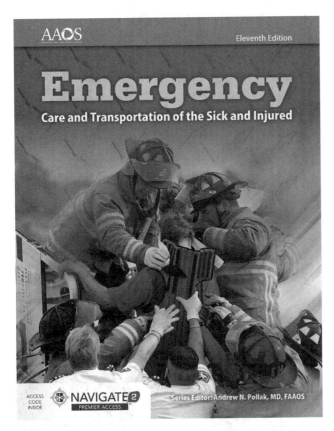

Cover of the AAOS Emergency Care and Transportation of the Sick and Injured ("orange book").
Reproduced with permission from © American Academy of Orthopaedic Surgeons, and image © Glen E. Ellman.

Bill, it was not uncommon to see a police officer or a firefighter come by the table and say, 'Dr. Mac, how are you?'" (Barr Jr. et al. 2004).

MacAusland was an avid skier—I recall his fondness for the sport. We both belonged to the Rocky Mountain Trauma Society and regularly attended its yearly meeting at the Snowmass Ski Resort at the height of the ski season. In 1971, MacAusland parlayed his love for skiing into his professional work by helping to open the Carlos Otis Stratton Mountain Clinic, in Stratton Mountain, Vermont. The clinic cared for patients with skiing injuries and "became a model for others throughout the skiing world" (Barr Jr. et al. 2004). From its opening, and for more than 30 years (until he retired in 2003), MacAusland, his family, and orthopaedic residents spent time at the clinic during winters, and Harvard offered a month-long rotation there for medical students. Staff at the clinic "fondly referred to [Bill] as 'The Commander'" (Barr Jr. et al. 2004).

MacAusland eventually became treasurer of the AAOS and then second vice-president in 1977. MacAusland was first vice-president of the Academy in 1980—the year he was subsequently elected president—and gave an address titled "Crossroads for Orthopaedics" at the annual meeting in Atlanta. After reading all of the Academy's previous presidential addresses, MacAusland (1980) began his own by stating, "in no other document or source material can you get the real flavor of the past, the visions of our predecessors, the growth, the problems, the strength and excitement of our Academy," which he described as, "an organization that believes in the development and preservation of excellent patient care through education and research." He then suggested some of his hopes and desires, such as making available a junior membership status for surgeons who are well into their residencies and would eventually be candidate members of the AAOS. He went on to suggest, "the Academy should be restructured to permit it to be more responsive to…questions" about economics, social conditions, legislation, regulations, and regionalization of major surgical procedures and to "become more sensitive to the needs of our patients and the issues surrounding health care" (MacAusland Jr. 1980). To do so, he proposed that the Academy's own Committee on Manpower needs to continue its study…to

MacAusland's AAOS presidential address, "Crossroads for Orthopaedics." *Journal of Bone and Joint Surgery* 1980; 62: 674.

develop accurate and useful data...[on] the effectiveness and availability of orthopaedic care for the community in the future...There is, however, an immediate and very serious crossroad facing the Academy...How do we establish proof of continuing competence of a practicing orthopaedic surgeon...? The American Board of Orthopaedic Surgery can test orthopaedic cognitive knowledge and that only. It should be the Academy's position to develop a mechanism attesting to the competence of the orthopaedic surgeon to continue to practice...Let us never forget first and foremost we are doctors of medicine, that our primary responsibility is to our patients...We must share in the pain, suffering, and worries of our patients and their families" (MacAusland Jr. 1980).

In his leadership roles with the AAOS, "One of his most important initiatives was to propose that the Academy build a fixed educational facility" (Barr Jr. et al. 2004). In his 1980 vice-presidential address, MacAusland asked: "How can the Academy better serve the needs of its membership and the orthopaedic community in the field of education? One answer...is a permanent educational facility...a building or group of buildings containing the entire educational package of the Academy." The AAOS took that suggestion to heart, and although "It took a number of years...eventually the Learning Center in Rosemont, Illinois came to fruition" (Barr Jr. et al. 2004).

After Dr. William MacAusland's retirement in 2003, he volunteered at the West Roxbury VA hospital. He had pursued a plethora of interests throughout much of his life and was an avid sports fisherman and beekeeper who also enjoyed tennis and golf. He developed a terminal illness soon after retiring, and the next year he died at age 81 at his home in Dedham. He was survived by his wife, Frances, and their children (four sons and two daughters).

HENRY C. MARBLE

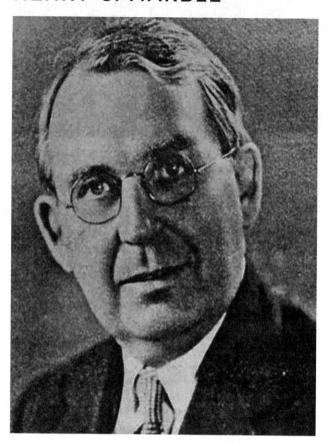

Henry C. Marble. Courtesy of the American Association for the Surgery of Trauma.

Physician Snapshot

Henry C. Marble
BORN: 1885
DIED: 1965
SIGNIFICANT CONTRIBUTIONS: One of the three physicians to perform the first blood transfusion at MGH in 1912; generous and dedicated teacher; established the Hand Clinic at MGH in 1925; served as chief of the MGH Fracture Service from 1929 to 1940; helped to found the American Association for the Surgery of Trauma, and served as its president in 1942 and 1943; one of the founders of the American Society for Surgery of the Hand

---

Henry Chase Marble was born in 1885 and raised in Worcester, Massachusetts. He received his undergraduate education at Clark University, graduating in 1906. He then went on to Harvard

Medical School, obtaining an MD degree in 1910. He spent the next two years as a surgical intern on the West Surgical Service at MGH. After completing that internship, he remained on the staff at MGH. His faculty appointment at Harvard Medical School was assistant in surgery.

Work with Blood Transfusion

Marble was part of a groundbreaking effort immediately upon beginning his career at MGH. In 1912, while still an intern, he helped Drs. C. A. Porter and Adams Leland perform:

> The first blood transfusion at MGH...to prepare an anemic woman patient for operation. The donor's radial artery and a vein in the patient's arm were exposed simultaneously, and one end of a double curved Elsberg cannula inserted in the artery, the other end in the vein. No reaction took place...after forty-five minutes, no change being noted in the patient, a second vein was tried. Still no change. Next a basilic vein was used, and after fifteen minutes the patient's cheeks became red and she felt warm, but the donor felt faint. The transfusion was considered successful. (Faxon 1959)

In 1901, "[Karl] Landsteiner had announced his discovery of blood groups," and in 1909 William L. Moss "had published his studies on iso-agglutinins and isohemolysis" (Faxon 1959). At that time, however, "no practical method of typing and crossmatching blood had come into general practice" (Faxon 1959). In his 1959 history of MGH from 1935 to 1955, Dr. Nathaniel Faxon (1959). shared Marble's personal memories of the transfusion technique he and his colleagues used without the benefit of knowing the patient's blood type:

> There was no blood typing. That the transfusion of blood from one person to another could cause reactions was recognized and guarded against by giving the first 20 cc. very slowly and watching for the symptoms of reaction. If the patient showed a flushed face, chills, swollen tongue, and pain in the kidney region, the transfusion was stopped. Caution and judgment resulted in few severe reactions. If the artery to vein method was used one could only guess at the amount of blood transfused. With other methods the delay necessary to test for reaction often resulted in the clotting of blood in the flask, tube or syringe, and the loss of the whole lot.

Early Orthopaedic Contribution

This early work with blood transfusions seems to be the extent of his efforts outside the field of orthopaedics (although he also published single papers about recurrent hernias, gall stones, and surgical disorders in patients with psychoses). About four years after he joined the staff at MGH, he was appointed assistant surgeon in the outpatient department, a position he held until 1925. However, one year later, Marble joined the US Army Medical Corps and served in France at Base Hospital No. 6 during World War I (see chapter 63). In July 1917, he joined other physicians from MGH at the base hospital, where he was initially the adjutant and registrar. A year later, he "was named Chief of the Orthopedic Department and continued in that capacity until the hospital was relieved of duty on February 1, 1919" (Ballantine Jr., n.d.).

Upon the return of the Base Hospital No. 6 orthopaedists to MGH after the war, they reinstated the Fracture Service there. Its chief was Dr. Daniel F. Jones (who followed Dr. Charles Scudder) a general surgeon; Dr. Robert Osgood was the first representative from the MGH Department of Orthopaedics. "Marble, then in his late 30s, was one of the 'younger surgeons' assigned to the Fracture Service" (Ballantine Jr., n.d.). His wartime experience and his work on the MGH Fracture Service sparked his "sustained interest in the problems of fractures" (Ballantine Jr. n.d.). In 1921, Marble took on two other posts in addition to those he held at MGH: he became the director of the Boston Clinic of the American Mutual Liability Insurance Company, and he was appointed as a consultant to the Bedford Veterans Administration Hospital.

The MGH Fracture Service had much success, which "led Dr. Marble to believe that there should be a special service devoted to injuries to the hand. Thus in 1925, the Hand Clinic came into being [at MGH] directly as a result of his efforts" (Ballantine Jr., n.d.). This was probably the first such clinic in the US. Its goal was "not only to acquire experience, knowledge, and to improve the care of hand injuries and infections, but most particularly to impart such knowledge that was available to the House Staff" (Hamlin Jr. 1966). The service created and maintained "a most elaborate system of records," and "[m]any advances in treatment, both operative and non-operative, have originated in this clinic. Its reputation has spread throughout the country, and it has been widely copied" (Washburn 1959). That same year, he was promoted to surgeon in the outpatient department at MGH, a position he held for 10 years.

Later Orthopaedic Contributions and Publications

Four years after opening the Hand Clinic, "Marble was made Chief of the Fracture Clinic, a position that he held for many years [until 1940]" (Ballantine Jr., n.d.). During his tenure as chief of the Fracture Service, he shared responsibilities with three other orthopaedic surgeons: Dr. Nathaniel Allison (1929–30), Dr. Philip D. Wilson (1930–34), and Dr. George Van Gorder (1934–40). Marble also was active on the Committee on Fractures of the American College of Surgeons, to which he was appointed in 1933. During this period, Marble was also appointed assisting visiting surgeon at MGH in 1935, and he also served as chief of the surgical staff at Chelsea Memorial Hospital and a visiting surgeon at Faulkner Hospital. "He did a great deal [to] keep the level of care high at the V.A. between the two wars" (Hamlin Jr. 1966).

While a member of the Committee on Fractures, he advocated for more fracture cases to be admitted to MGH so that surgeons and staff could receive appropriate training—that is, they needed a volume of cases sufficient for trainees to "have an opportunity to see at least one of each type of common fracture" (Washburn 1959). Marble would take surgical interns and residents to a nearby mortuary to "dissect hands and other anatomical areas. In this way he probably taught more anatomy to the MGH House Staff than everyone else put together. And it would be a rare House Officer of that period who does not look back upon those occasions with a great deal of appreciation and affection for 'Uncle Henry'" (Hamlin Jr. 1966)—as the residents always called him. Dr. H. Thomas Ballentine recalled such a "kidnap" and trip to the morgue. He first met Marble in 1938:

> when as a young house officer, I was seized upon unexpectedly by this robust, rotund, busy, always-in-a-hurry surgeon who was in his early fifties. A muscular arm was thrown around my shoulders and I was invited (in a tone of voice that brooked no refusal) to the city morgue which in those days was almost adjacent to the Massachusetts General Hospital. The cause of this kidnap lay in the fact that Dr. Marble had just heard that there was an unclaimed body in the morgue and permission had been given to him by his friend the medical examiner to carry out an anatomical dissection. We spent three hours meticulously dissecting the knee joint and its surrounding musculature. My only previous encounter with anatomical dissections had been as a first year student and I was fascinated by this opportunity to see things as 'they really were!' (Ballantine Jr., n.d.)

He loved teaching younger surgeons: "No one liked to teach more, and fewer could teach better.

Every operation was a teaching exercise and 'Uncle Henry's' voice—which had considerable carrying power, could frequently be heard in the corridors of the operating floor" (Ballantine Jr., n.d.). Marble was known for his willingness to teach and his patience with surgeons-in-training: "[N]o matter how much he had to do on any particular day an opportunity to teach younger men, to pass on his knowledge and his wisdom, was never put off… [He] was as generous with his time at the operating table as he was in the dissecting room and was as kind to them as any surgeon that they encountered" (Ballantine Jr., n.d.).

During this time, Marble also published on a variety of topics. He wrote a chapter on fractures and dislocations of the phalanges and metacarpals for Philip D. Wilson's textbook *Fractures* published in 1938. That same year, toward the end of his tenure with the Fracture Service at MGH, he helped to found the American Association for the Surgery of Trauma. Marble was succeeded in 1940 by Dr. Arthur W. Allen, a general surgeon, as chief of the Fracture Service and Dr. Marius Smith-Petersen, who acted as orthopaedic co-chief (until 1947). When Marble stepped down from the Fracture Service, he also wrote "Emergency Treatment of Fractures," published as a Report on Medical Progress in the *New England Journal of Medicine*; it covered both the upper and the lower extremities. He also cowrote one of only three articles he produced on the hand: "Tuberculous Tenosynovitis" in the *New England Journal of Medicine*. He published "Purposeful Splinting Following Injuries to the Hand" in *JAMA* the following year.

Marble was appointed visiting surgeon at MGH in 1941, a position he held until 1945. His work with the AAST also continued, and he held the post of president in 1942 and 1943, during World War II. His first year as president, the association held its annual meeting in Boston. His presidential address was titled "Our Surgeons in the Present War." He discussed what he saw as the focus of surgeons on their practices at the expense of teaching. Cognizant of the war in which the nation was embroiled at that time, he elaborated on the need for young surgeons to be appropriately trained to provide the best care to injured soldiers, though he noted that injuries sustained in war and injuries at home are similar, that only the location varies. For Marble, soldiers who know they will be cared for well and have a good chance for recovery will be more effective in their

Logo, American Association for the Surgery of Trauma.
Courtesy of the American Association for the Surgery of Trauma.

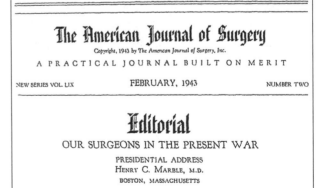

Marble's presidential address to the AAST, 1943.
The American Journal of Surgery 1943; 59: 159.

jobs. The continuing war deterred the association from having an annual meeting during Marble's second year as president.

In 1945 and 1949, "he published papers concerned with the nation-wide results of intervertebral disc surgery in industrial accident cases" (Ballantine Jr., n.d.). Over the next two years he published five additional articles (four of which were cowritten with Dr. Joseph Barr) on industrial surgery and low back disability. He was also one of the 35 founders of the American Society for Surgery of the Hand, which had held its first meeting in Chicago in 1946. Four years later—after almost 30 years of affiliation—he became the American Mutual Liability Insurance Company's surgical advisor. "In this…post he was able to pursue actively his interest in work-related injuries [having served as chairman of the Committee on State and National Legislation]. His concern over the problem of bringing the best of surgical care to the injured workmen was far reaching." (Ballantine Jr., n.d.).

In 1951, he was an associate editor, with supervising editor Frederic Bancroft, on the second edition of the book *Surgical Treatment of the Motor-Skeletal System*. Two years later, he published his third and final article on the hand "Nerve Grafts into Hands" in the *American Journal of Surgery*. In 1955, he was appointed honorary surgeon at MGH at 70 years of age, a position he held for 10 years. The following year, he was honored by his alma mater, Clark University, with an Honorary Doctor of Science Degree. The citation read: "A nationally known specialist in hand surgery. A Sunday painter, world traveler, and drama critic of no mean ability" (Jacobson 1965).

He continued to publish, and his work culminated in his book *The Hand: A Manual and Atlas for the General Surgeon*, published in 1960 and eventually translated into various languages, including Polish (in 1964). In the preface, Marble emphasizes the importance of the immediate treatment after injury in the ability of the hand to regain function. Marble's goal was to help the physicians and surgeons who provide this emergent care. For Ballantine Jr. (n.d.), "It is in the use of this word 'help' that we find another of the essential qualities of this remarkable individual: help to his patients, help to his colleagues, help for his pupils."

> "When the physician bears the patient's pain, then will medicine our fainting hope sustain"
> —Memorial to the first doctor in Jamaica, Spanishtown Cathedral, author unknown

Legacy

Dr. Marble was a board-certified general surgeon, a member of the American Medical Association, the Boston Surgical Society, and the Harvard Club (Boston). He ran his private practice out of an office on Charles Street. He lived with his wife at 15 Crystal Street in Newton Centre. He died suddenly in retirement at age 80, while on a trip in Willimantic, Connecticut, on July 15, 1965. He left behind his wife Alice (née Ingram), two sons, and a daughter.

PAUL L. NORTON

> **Physician Snapshot**
>
> Paul L. Norton
> BORN: 1903
> DIED: 1986
> SIGNIFICANT CONTRIBUTIONS: Developed (with Thornton Brown) the Norton-Brown spinal brace; expert in the fascia lata transfer to erector spinae muscles

Paul L. Norton was born in 1903, raised in East Boston (Orient Heights), and educated in the city. He was a student at Boston Latin School and East Boston High School, from which he graduated in 1921. He went on to attend Harvard College. During his freshman year (1922), a tank of liquid oxygen exploded in the Cryogenic Engineering Research Laboratory in the basement of the Jefferson Physical Laboratory, killing two students and injuring six others. Paul was one of those injured: he sustained a fracture of his left leg. He had been in a physics class one floor above, watching a demonstration of an efficiency motor generator. This accident may have influenced his choice to pursue a career in orthopaedic surgery. He graduated from Harvard College in 1925 and then was accepted into Harvard Medical School. He received an MD degree in 1930.

Early Training and Career

Norton stayed in Boston to begin his training. He completed a surgical internship at Carney Hospital and an orthopaedic residency at MGH/Boston Children's Hospital. He became a senior resident in orthopaedic surgery at MGH in 1934–35. After he completed his training, Norton practiced in both Boston and Concord, Massachusetts; he lived in Lincoln, Massachusetts, where he was a member of the town's board of health and finance committee. He joined the staff at MGH as a visiting orthopaedic surgeon and at Harvard Medical School as an instructor in orthopaedic surgery in 1935 (he held both positions until 1966). The following year, Norton began as an orthopaedic consultant at the state's Crippled Children's Service; he mainly provided services at the clinics in Hyannis and Brockton. He was also chief of the orthopaedic staff at Lakeville Hospital about that time. He was considered an expert in surgical procedures for polio, specifically fascia lata transfer to erector spinae muscles.

Norton published two papers early in his career at MGH (among seven total publications during his career). The first, "An Adoption of the Balkan Frame for Developing Motion and Abduction of the Hip," he cowrote with Fred Ilfeld and published in the *Journal of Bone and Joint Surgery* in 1938. Norton and Illfield (1938) described a "traction-suspension apparatus… [that] was evolved primarily to meet the need of early mobilization of the hip following surgery, particularly acetabuloplasties and arthroplasties. In these particular operations, early motion in flexion and abduction is [an] essential result… ordinary traction-suspension…allows adequate flexion of the hip…[but] not enough abduction." He also worked with Dr. Marius Smith-Petersen to develop an adjustable reamer for use on the femoral head; this reamer was intended to replace Smith-Petersen's original six reamers that had been "made over a period of years at considerable expense" (Norton 1940). At the end of the 1930s Norton began working with Emerson Hospital in Concord, and in 1939 he also became a member of the American Academy of Orthopaedic Surgery.

Later Orthopaedic Contributions

Norton's most significant research contribution was his collaborative work with Dr. Thornton Brown; the brace maker Karl W. Buschenfeldt; Robert L. Hansen, PhD, and Y. C. Loh of the Department of Civil Engineering at MIT; and Eugene Murphy, PhD, chief of prosthetics and sensory aids for the US Veterans Administration, that culminated in the concept of the Norton-Brown spinal brace. They began in the early

1950s by examining spinal bracing—the goals of brace use and the dynamics between the back and the brace. Using photographs, they studied the mechanics of forward and side bending and how various braces would work during and be affected by bending.

They began by taking radiographs of their four volunteers (three medical students and an engineering student) wearing the braces. They soon realized, however, that the requirement for images at numerous amounts of bend in every brace they were testing—including Arnold-Abbott, Jewett, Williams, Goldthwait, Chair-back, Taylor, and plaster jackets—would be excessive. To avoid this requirement and still be able to measure angular change at each level of the lumbar spine, they used instead Kirschner wires, which they inserted (under local anesthesia in the four student volunteers) into the lumbar spine and the posterior iliac wing. They also used electric gauges, rather than pneumatic ones, to obtain accurate measurements of the forces with bending (between 20 and 80 lbs.) of each brace on the spine.

Norton and Brown reported their research and introduced their new Norton-Brown brace at the 1955 annual meeting of the American Orthopaedic Surgeons in Los Angeles. They published their findings with the new orthotic in 1957. Despite "inadequate" data and numerous technical issues with spine immobilization, they introduced their brace. In this new apparatus they had:

> replac[ed] the paraspinal uprights with lateral uprights which extended downward to the greater trochanter and by applying force to the lumbosacral region by means of a single crossbar, two goals are achieved. First, the force is kept localized over bony prominences so that prompt and...uncomfortable pressure accompanies forward bending or slumping in the sitting position. Second, a low point of attachment for the lower straps of the abdominal pad gives good counterpressure at the lower end of the brace without impending sitting in the erect position. Incidentally, side bending is quite effectively blocked by the lateral uprights. The performance of this brace has been superior in restricting flexion of the lower lumbar interspaces in the sitting position. During standing and forward bending its effect has been variable...In its brief clinical trial, the performance of the experimental brace has been encouraging ...It is our impression that in the treatment of low-back pain a careful study of the history will often reveal whether flexion or extension seems to be the more comfortable position. This being the case, prescription of a suitable back support should not be purely empirical. (Norton and Brown 1957)

The Immobilizing Efficiency of Back Braces*†
THEIR EFFECT ON THE POSTURE AND MOTION OF THE LUMBOSACRAL SPINE
BY PAUL L. NORTON, M.D., AND THORNTON BROWN, M.D., BOSTON, MASSACHUSETTS
From the Orthopaedic Service, Massachusetts General Hospital, Boston
THE JOURNAL OF BONE AND JOINT SURGERY
VOL. 39-A, NO. 1, JANUARY 1957

Norton and Brown's article in which they described their new spinal brace for low back pain. *Journal of Bone and Joint Surgery* 1957; 38: 111.

> "The best [back] brace would be a leather strap with a tack stuck in it. The thought was that the tack would cause the patient to brace himself. After about four years of investigation we came to that conclusion."
>
> —Paul L. Norton
> "Research and Development of the Norton-Brown Spinal Brace." *Orthopedic & Prosthetic Appliance Journal* [Orthotics and Prosthetics], 1966

Norton and his colleagues conducted other experiments with their patient-volunteers; these lasted almost four-and-a-half years. Norton commented on their findings, particularly that when patients bent forward while wearing a long brace, they could achieve more lumbosacral motion than they did when wearing no brace. He also pointed out the more extensive spinal flexion with slouching in a chair than when purposely bending over as far as possible. This relaxation is important for retaining the effects of spinal fusion. Dr. Vernon Nickel, a surgeon-colleague of Norton who performed spinal surgery, said, "You know, that explains what we have been doing...for several years, stopped all our patients from sitting, following spinal fusion. We either made them stand up or lie down, and this explains why" (quoted in Norton 1966).

In 1960, he and Dr. Edward Nalebuff reviewed the treatment of young patients with congenital dislocation of the hip who began walking early, i.e., at age one to three years, at the Lakeville State Sanatorium. They had previously applied frog leg positioning between 1949 and 1958 to 22 hips and abduction/internal rotation, combined with a rotational osteotomy, to 9 hips. The frog leg position maintained reduction in just 8 of those 22 hips. Abduction and internal rotation, however, achieved "satisfactory results" in many of the hips.

Norton continued to study spinal deformity through the 1960s. He cowrote two papers on paraplegia in children and adolescents based on his work at MGH (**Case 40.11**). In the paper published in 1965, the authors reviewed a series of 104 patients with paraplegia. They found that "lordosis was by far the most common [spinal deformity]...Harrington instrumentation and spine fusion including the sacrum was found to be the most effective means of controlling spine and pelvic deformity...[but] has been used in too few patients and for too short a period of time for definite conclusions" (Kilfoyle, Foley, and Norton 1965).

As the 1960s progressed, Norton continued his long affiliations with various hospitals

Case 40.11. Spine and Pelvic Deformities in Youth with Paraplegia

> "F.R., A sixteen-year-old boy who had myelomeningocele and flaccid paralysis below the eleventh thoracic segment from birth, had walked with braces and crutches for only brief periods prior to admission to the Massachusetts Hospital School. After admission he walked with crutches, a pelvic band, and long braces. However, there developed a severe high-level lordosis and a severe left scoliosis which extended from the tenth thoracic to the first sacral vertebra and ultimately measured 81 degrees (Ferguson method). As deformity progressed his balance became worse and he was finally able to move about only in a wheel chair. He was considered many times for forced correction and fusion, but his general condition ruled out a procedure of this magnitude. His spine at the time of writing had become quite fixed and there was no hope of correcting the deformity."
>
> (Kilfoyle, Foley, and Norton 1956)

and institutions. Although in 1962 he ended his term as chief of staff at the Massachusetts Hospital School in Canton, a position he had held since 1946, he remained as an orthopaedic consultant there. He also continued at the school as chairman of the board of trustees (he had been appointed chair in 1958). In 1963, he began a four-year term as the first president of the New England Orthopedic Society. He was named chairman of surgical service at Emerson Hospital in 1965, and, in 1971, he became the head of the hospital's Department of Physical Therapy; he remained in each role for two years. In 1972, after 25 years, he ended his tenure as a consultant at Emerson. He had served as president of the Middlesex Central District Medical Society and held memberships in the American Orthopaedic Association and the American Medical Association.

In 1969, Norton published his last paper, "Intertrochanter Fractures," in which he summarized his experience treating such fractures, which he labeled as either stable (with the calcar and lesser trochanter still attached to the shaft) or unstable (comminuted with an avulsed lesser trochanter). For internal fixation, he used a cannulated Smith-Petersen nail with a McLaughlin side plate or a fixed angle Jewett nail-plate; both were popular at the time. Interestingly, he reported no data, stating, "This report, written as part of the Smith-Petersen Commemoration by one of 'his boys', has no statistics since 'Smith-Pete' hated statistics" (Norton 1969).

Legacy

In 1976, upon the end of Norton's run as chairman of the Massachusetts Hospital School's board of trustees, the hospital's leadership named a medical library after him. He probably officially retired around that time as well. He received recognition in 1983 for his 50 years in various roles at MGH. He experienced a prolonged illness and died at his home in Concord on October 4, 1986, at age 83. His wife Margaret and their five children mourned his death.

DONALD S. PIERCE

> **Physician Snapshot**
>
> Donald S. Pierce
> BORN: 1930
> DIED: —
>
> SIGNIFICANT CONTRIBUTIONS: Expert in management of spinal cord injuries; chief orthopaedic rehabilitation unit on White 9; coauthor of *The Total Care of Spinal Cord Injuries* and *The Halo Vest: Its Application and Use*; advocate for the use of the EMG as a diagnostic tool

Donald Shelton Pierce was born in 1930. He was a graduate of Harvard Medical School (HMS), and his main interest was spinal cord injuries. Little information is available about him, but after discussions with Dr. Joseph Barr Jr., my own recollections, and an article coauthored by Dr. Pierce while at Case Western University Medical School in 1964, I believe we can establish that he most likely had come to MGH from Case Western University. After joining the staff at MGH, he remained there for about 40 years.

He probably was recruited by Dr. Melvin Glimcher, because Dr. Pierce was chief in the orthopaedic rehabilitation unit on White 9 when I rotated at MGH (1968 and 1970). He had held this position for about 15 years when Dr. Henry Mankin arrived at MGH. Pierce, as chief of rehabilitation, had collaborated with the orthopaedic staff on management of amputees, spinal cord injuries, and neuromuscular diseases, in which he advocated the use of the electromyogram as a diagnostic tool. He was also an associate orthopaedic surgeon at MGH and a clinical associate in orthopaedic surgery at HMS.

Pierce published three books, several chapters, and gave an AAOS Instructional Course, "The Halo Orthosis in the Treatment of Cervical Spine Injury." His first book, *Amputees and Their Prostheses*, was coauthored with Dr. Mohinder A. Mital in 1971. The following year, Pierce stepped down as chief of the orthopaedic rehabilitation unit when Mankin replaced him with Dr. Robert

Leffert. Pierce's other two books were related to spinal cord injuries. In 1977, he coauthored *The Total Care of Spinal Cord Injuries* with Dr. Vernon H. Nickel, writing:

> The purpose of this book is to set forth the most advanced principles in surgical and medical management of the patient with an acute spinal injury...through the complete management of such patients until they are rehabilitated to a normal, healthy, active life in the community.

He also authored chapters in the book on the acute treatment of spinal cord injuries, and, with Dr. John D. Constable (a plastic surgeon at MGH), a chapter on management of pressure sores.

In the book, *The Total Care of Spinal Cord Injuries*, the authors described three treatment tools bearing Pierce's name: The first, the Pierce Collar, is a "firm felt [cervical] collar reinforced with steel stays" that can be used in the early treatment of patients suspected of having a cervical spine injury. The second, the Pierce Fusion, a modification of Dr. William A. Rogers's fusion in which:

> a wire is passed through the base of the spinous process of the lowest vertebra to be fused. It is then crossed in the spinous process of each of the other vertebra in the fusion area, tightened at each level...and twisted after passage through the base of the upper most spinous process in the area to be fused. Additional wires are passed through the same holes at the top and bottom of the fusion, passed through holes in the strut grafts, and crisscrossed and twisted over the grafts to hold them on the sides of the spinous processes and laminae after placing bone on the decorticated laminae around the strut graft.

The third, the Pierce Graft, was a method of notching the opposing cervical vertebral bodies, across the gap made by removal of a vertebral body, that allowed for stable locking of a fibular graft.

The last book, *The Halo Vest: Its Application and Use*, was coauthored with Dr. Joseph S. Barr Jr., and published in 1978 by the American Academy of Orthopaedic Surgeons. Pierce was president of the Cervical Spine Research Society in 1984. **Case 40.12** is an example of one of his later cases.

Case 40.12. Familial Bilateral Carpal Tunnel Syndrome

> "A 13-year-old boy...the brother of the patient described in case 1, had a history of idiopathic thrombocytopenic purpura at age 10 and presented with five months of hand numbness bilaterally, worse on the left. Examination was normal except for bilateral Tinel and Phalen signs, both more prominent on the left. Cervical spine, shoulder, and chest x-rays were normal. His symptoms resolved after bilateral carpal tunnel release. At surgery, the transverse carpal ligament was thick, and there was unusual bilateral thickening of the flexor retinaculum bilaterally. Pathologic examination of an excised specimen revealed normal connective tissue: a stain for amyloid was negative."
> (Leifer, Cros, Halperin, Gallico, Pierce, and Shahani 1992)

After retiring in 2015, he and his wife Janet returned to their home in Castine, Maine, on Penobscot Bay. They made a restricted grant to the department of orthopaedics at MGH.

ERIC L. RADIN

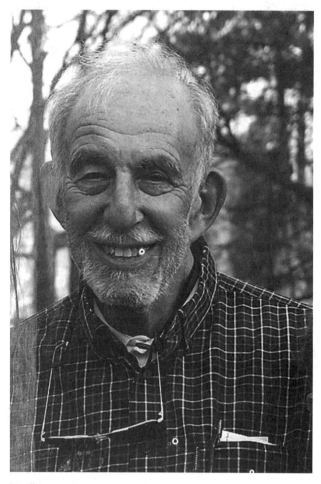

Eric L. Radin. Courtesy of Melissa Radin Goldstone.

Physician Snapshot

Eric L. Radin
BORN: 1934
DIED: 2020
SIGNIFICANT CONTRIBUTIONS: Established investigator in both joint lubrication and the biomechanics of bone; received the Kappa Delta Award (with Igor L. Paul and Robert M. Rose) for their research on joint lubrication; proponent that alterations in bone mechanical properties may be the primary etiology of osteoarthritis; chaired the Department of Orthopaedic Surgery at West Virginia University Medical School (1979–89); directed the Bone and Joint Center and chaired the Department of Orthopaedic Surgery at Henry Ford Hospital (1989–95)

Eric Leon Radin was born on September 14, 1934, and raised in Brooklyn, New York. He received an undergraduate bachelor of arts degree in experimental psychology from Amherst College in 1956. In 1960, he received an MD degree from Harvard Medical School. After a year-long surgical internship at UCLA Medical Center, he spent one year as an assistant resident in surgery at the Medical College of Virginia. From 1962 to 1966, he was a resident in the Boston Children's Hospital/Massachusetts General Hospital combined orthopaedic residency program (**Case 40.13** describes a patient Radin treated during his time at Boston Children's Hospital).

Harvard Medical School: A Focus on Basic Research

Radin's main focus was basic research, and he had three primary areas of interest: fractures, joint lubrication, and the biomechanical factors involved in osteoarthritis. Radin cowrote two clinical papers on fractures with Dr. Edward J. Riseborough; clinicians often referred to them after their publication. In the first, "Fractures of the Radial Head," published in the *Journal of Bone and Joint Surgery* in 1966 while Radin was still a resident, Riseborough and Radin examined 100 patients two years or longer after their injury. At the time, "the controversy surrounding the treatment of radial head fractures [was] based… on the failure to separate undisplaced, displaced, comminuted, complicated and pediatric fractures" (Riseborough and Radin 1966). They evaluated range of motion and early active motion in 88 isolated fractures in adult patients and found that:

> early motion may displace otherwise undisplaced fractures…if more than one-third of the radial head is displaced, limitation of motion will probably result…The range of motion depends on the anatomical result….Inferior radio-ulnar subluxation does occur, but is…of little significance…[and] can be ignored…We would treat undisplaced fractures involving less than one-third of the radial head with active motion as

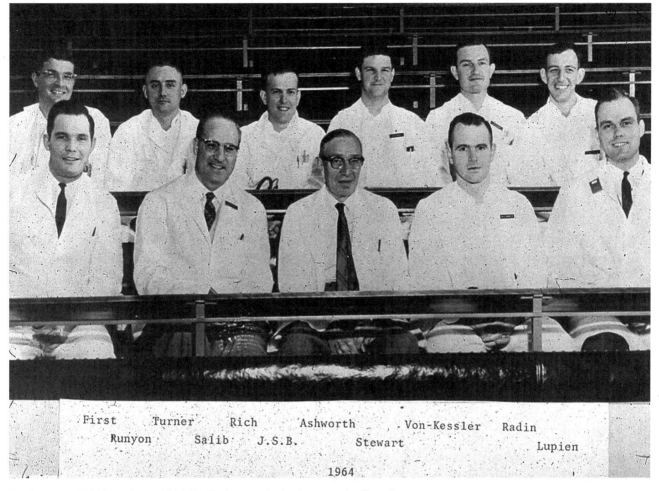

Dr. Barr with MGH residents, 1964. Dr. Radin is in the back row at the far right. MGH HCORP Archives.

soon as the patient is comfortable...Displaced fractures involving less than two-thirds of the radial head should...be treated by early active motion...Displaced fractures involving more than two-thirds...should...be treated by early total excision, as should all comminuted fractures. (Radin and Riseborough 1966)

Shortly thereafter, Radin completed his two-year military obligation (1966–68), serving as the assistant chief of the orthopaedic section at the US Air Force Hospital at Andrews Air Force Base. Simultaneously he was a special postdoctoral fellow in experimental pathology at the National Institute of Arthritis and Metabolic Diseases in Bethesda, Maryland. After completing his military service, Radin was appointed as a research fellow in the Department of Orthopaedic Surgery at MGH—this was in 1968–70, during the last two years of Dr. Melvin Glimcher's tenure as chairman. Radin held a joint appointment as a fellow at MIT.

Radin published his second paper on fractures with Riseborough in 1969, "Intercondylar T Fractures of the Humerus in the Adult." They described a reexamination of 29 of 52 patients who had been treated for such fractures at MGH over a 12-year period (1951–63) and had been followed up for at least two years. With the goal of comparing the results of various treatments, they:

defined four major types of fracture according to the amount of comminution and the degree of displacement of the fragments. We could find

Case 40.13. Neuritis in a Patient with Infectious Mononucleosis

> "A twenty-year-old white man, a business administration student, was admitted to Children's Hospital Medical Center, Boston, Massachusetts, on August 20, 1963, with a chief complaint of weakness of the right shoulder of two and one-half week's duration.
>
> "The patient had been well until six weeks prior to admission when he contracted infectious mononucleosis, characterized by fever 101.6 degrees Fahrenheit, sore throat, malaise, and fatigue. He was treated by his local physician for a week with rest in bed. His heterophil titer, when he was first seen by his physician, was 1:64 and ten days later was 1:6000.
>
> "Two and one-half weeks after the onset of his illness, the patient noted the gradual onset of sharp pain in the right shoulder, the lateral aspect of the arm, and the front of the elbow. The pain was intermittent, worse at night, aggravated by motion of the right upper extremity, and not relieved by aspirin. He was treated with an analgesic and a muscle relaxant with temporary relief during this period.
>
> "When the patient came to our Orthopedic Out-patient Department three and one-half weeks after onset of his mononucleosis, his complaint was persistent pain. At that time, there was tenderness at the right deltoid insertion and the right deltoid was weak. This was first interpreted as tendinitis which was treated with phenylbutazone.
>
> "One week later the pain had completely disappeared, but no active contraction of the right deltoid could be obtained. On the right side the triceps was rated fair plus; the biceps, good; and the external rotators of his shoulder, poor plus. Hypesthesia was detected over the apex of the right shoulder. Ten days later he was admitted to the hospital for evaluation.
>
> "In the past, the patient had had a fracture of the distal end of the humerus. A slight deformity of his right elbow remained. The review of systems was non-contributory.
>
> "Physical examination revealed a well-developed, husky, man in no distress with temperature 98.6 degrees Fahrenheit, blood pressure 100/80, and pulse seventy- two. There were no abnormal findings on general physical examination except in the right upper extremity. No adenopathy, no hepatic enlargement, and no throat redness were detected. He stood with his right shoulder slightly low and did not swing his right arm when he walked. There was a full range of motion of his right shoulder.

no classification in the literature that was satisfactory…The treatment of…[these fractures] in adults should be determined on the basis of the amount of rotatory deformity and comminution. Severely comminuted fractures do not lend themselves to open reduction and are best treated with skeletal traction…In minimally displaced fractures, good results can be obtained by immobilization in a plaster cast…Fractures with a significant rotatory deformity…are more likely to have a good result when skeletal traction is used…Open reduction and adequate internal fixation are not easy…[and] is very rarely indicated. (Riseborough and Radin 1969)

Radin's interest in lubrication began during his time as a guest investigator with the Section on Rheumatic Diseases in the Laboratory for Experimental Pathology at the National Institute of Arthritis and Metabolic Diseases (part of the National Institutes of Health). His work on fractures and lubrication overlapped, and again in 1969 Radin—this time with Frank C. Linn, a research engineer at the National Institutes of Health—published in *JBJS* an article titled "Lubrication of Animal Joints. III. The Effect of Certain Chemical Alterations of the Cartilage and Lubricant." Using dogs as subjects, they calculated in vitro the coefficient of friction in the ankle. Enzymatic treatment of bovine synovial mucin substantially affected the value of the coefficient. From this they concluded that a protein moiety in mucin and hyaluronate act in concert to give mucin the qualities of a lubricant. In some cases, human synovial joints provided similar or better lubrication that the bovine mucin. In a "Current

> "Muscle examination revealed on the right a poor-minus deltoid, good-to-normal trapezius and serratus anterior, good rhomboids, poor external rotators and latissimus dorsi, poor-plus sternal portion of the pectoralis major, normal clavicular portion of this muscle, good-to-good-plus biceps, and good-to-normal triceps. All other muscles were normal in strength.
>
> "Laboratory data included a hematocrit of forty-five, a white blood cell count of 6,200, and a normal urinalysis. Spinal fluid analysis revealed: total protein 35 milligrams, sugar and chloride normal, and 3 white blood cells and 1 red blood cell per high-power field. There was no growth on culture.
>
> "The patient was seen by a neurological consultant who felt that the findings were consistent with a neuritis of the fifth cervical root. A myelogram suggested if there were any signs of progression. During the next five days of hospitalization, the patient showed no change in his muscle power. He was put on exercises to maintain the range of motion of his shoulder as well as active assisted range-of-motion exercises, and was discharged to be followed in the outpatient department.
>
> "His sensory defect cleared within four months, but twenty-two months after discharge he still had no return of deltoid power. However, he had regained good-to-normal strength in all his other previously weakened muscles. Apparently, by stabilizing his humeral head in the glenoid with his triceps, infraspinatus, and subscapularis muscles, he was able to abduct his arm to 160 degrees with an obviously hypertrophied supraspinatus. At 90 degrees of abduction he had good-plus abductor strength. He denied any functional limitation.
>
> "Electrical stimulation of his deltoid with alternating current gave no response. With direct current, the posterior part of the deltoid contracted well in the anterior part, fairly well. There was no response when the axillary nerve was stimulated. Electromyographic examination revealed no fibrillation potentials. On maximum attempted contraction, there were some muscle potentials, but both their amplitude and duration were reduced from normal with a reduction in the interference pattern as well. On the basis of these tests, it is believed that further recovery of the deltoid function may be expected."
>
> (Eric L. Radin 1967)

Comment" in the same issue, Radin summarized the current concepts of joint lubrication and his and Linn's research. He noted that synovial mucin contains a protein portion, which is essential to joint lubrication by binding with the catilagenous surface—but other factors are also important, particularly the compressibility of cartilage, which allows interstitial fluid to flow into and out of cartilage.

During this period in his career, he became established at institutions throughout the area. He was appointed as a lecturer in the Department of Mechanical Engineering at MIT, a position he held for a decade (1969–79). He was also promoted from instructor to assistant professor of orthopaedic surgery at Harvard Medical School in 1970. With Glimcher's move from MGH to Boston Children's Hospital that year, Radin joined the acting staff at Children's as an associate; and he also began as an associate in orthopaedic surgery at Beth Israel Hospital.

CURRENT COMMENT

Synovial Fluid as a Lubricant

By Eric L. Radin

Arthritis & Rheumatology

October 1968
Volume 11, Issue 5

Radin's first article on joint lubrication. *Arthritis and Rheumatology* 1968; 11: 693.

> **A Comparison of the Dynamic Force Transmitting Properties of Subchondral Bone and Articular Cartilage**
>
> BY ERIC L. RADIN, M.D.*, IGOR L. PAUL, SC.D.†, AND MARTIN LOWY, F.R.C.S.‡,
> BOSTON, MASSACHUSETTS
>
> THE JOURNAL OF BONE AND JOINT SURGERY
> VOL. 52-A, NO. 3, APRIL 1970

Radin et al.'s early publication on the importance of subchondral bone in joints in the development of osteoarthritis. *Journal of Bone and Joint Surgery* 1970; 52: 444.

> **A Consolidated Concept of Joint Lubrication***
>
> BY ERIC L. RADIN, M.D.†, BOSTON, MASSACHUSETTS, AND
> IGOR L. PAUL, SC.D.‡, CAMBRIDGE, MASSACHUSETTS
>
> THE JOURNAL OF BONE AND JOINT SURGERY
> VOL. 54-A, NO. 3, APRIL 1972

Radin and Paul's article, "A Consolidated Concept of Joint Lubrication." *Journal of Bone and Joint Surgery* 1972; 54: 607.

As the 1970s proceeded, Radin continued to study lubrication but began to focus most of his research on biomechanics, mechanical factors in the pathogenesis of osteoarthritis, mechanical properties of trabecular bone, the importance of subchondral bone, and other mechanical issues of bones, cartilage, and joints. He published more than 30 articles on such topics during the decade of the 1970s—his last 10 years in Boston. In one of his earliest studies (1970) on the importance of subchondral bone with impact loading of joints, Radin, Paul, and Dr. Martin Lowy studied compression forces of bovine articular cartilage and subchondral bone in the laboratories of MGH and MIT. Considering that "cancellous bone is approximately ten times stiffer than articular cartilage...subchondral bone in vivo is considerably thicker," they found that:

> Under physiologic loads and...rates, a film of synovial fluid on the cartilage added nothing to the ability of articular plugs to alternate peak dynamic force; however, at very low load rates cartilage plugs coated with synovial fluid were...stiffer then specimens coated with veronate buffer. It is highly likely...that alternations in the quality of the subchondral bone could have a profound effect of the subchondral bone-articular cartilage system to withstand dynamic forces. (Radin, Paul, and Lowy 1970)

Two years later, Drs. Simon, Radin, and Paul established that loss of articular cartilage proteoglycan followed stiffening of the subchondral cancellous bone.

Radin would also go on to publish more than 12 articles on lubrication—three in *Nature*—before he left Harvard. He and his coauthors wrote about the roles of mucin, hyaluronic acid, the synovial membrane, and lubrication in total joints. In 1972, with Dr. Igor L. Paul from MIT, Radin published "A Consolidated Concept of Joint Lubrication" which described the two mechanisms of lubrication in animal joints: one in soft tissue, which "involv[es] the sliding of synovial membrane on itself or on other tissues, and a cartilage on cartilage system." Because soft tissues resist motion to a greater extent during stretching and friction than does cartilage in friction with other cartilage, they suggested that the former may be the main cause of joint stiffness:

> Lubrication of the soft-tissue system depends on molecules of hyaluronate in the synovial fluid which stick to the synovium in a layer and keep moving surfaces apart. Cartilage-on-cartilage lubrication, by contrast, is dependent

> ### Quantitative Studies of Human Subchondral Cancellous Bone
>
> ITS RELATIONSHIP TO THE STATE OF ITS OVERLYING CARTILAGE*
>
> BY JAMES W. PUGH, PH.D.†, ERIC L. RADIN, M.D.‡,
> BOSTON, MASSACHUSETTS,
> AND ROBERT M. ROSE, SC.D.§, CAMBRIDGE, MASSACHUSETTS
>
> THE JOURNAL OF BONE AND JOINT SURGERY
> VOL. 56-A, NO. 2, MARCH 1974

Radin et al.'s article on the effects of changes in the properties of subchondral bone on articular cartilage. *Journal of Bone and Joint Surgery* 1974; 56: 313.

on hyaluronic acid. A hyaluronic-free glycoprotein fraction which has been isolated from synovial fluid confers...a lubricating advantage equal to that of whole synovial fluid. Removal of this fraction from synovial fluid deprives the fluid of any lubricating advantage over buffer. The action of this glycoprotein on cartilage is a boundary phenomenon similar to that of hyaluronate on synovium. In addition to the boundary effect, cartilage surfaces are kept apart by a fluid squeeze film made up of joint fluid and interstitial fluid which weeps from the articular cartilage itself. The squeeze-film effect is probably potentiated by the undulations of the surface and the elasticity of the cartilage, which may lower fictional resistance by elastohydrodynamic effects. (Radin and Paul 1972)

One year after that publication, Radin and Paul, along with Robert M. Rose (also at MIT), received the Kappa Delta Award from the American Academy of Orthopaedic Surgeons for their research titled "Studies on Joint Lubrication." That same year, he became an associate professor at Harvard Medical School, and in 1974 he joined the active staff at Mt. Auburn Hospital; he remained in both roles until 1979. He had a clinical practice in orthopaedic surgery in these hospitals, with a focus on foot and ankle problems and trauma.

Radin continued to pursue his research on biomechanics in 1974, and—in a publication with J. Pugh and R. Rose—they were the first to accurately report that subchondral bone stiffening was "associated with early loss of mucopolysaccharide from articular cartilage...and that the stiffening disappeared as the cartilage changes became more advanced" (Pugh, Radin, and Rose 1974). In that study of 15 cadaver femurs with no evidence of osteoarthritis, "changes in the spatial arrangement of the trabeculae (rather than the gross density of the bone) are shown to correlate with the observed increase in subchondral bone stiffening associated with loss of cartilage mucopolysaccharide." (Pugh, Radin, and Rose 1974). That year Radin, Paul, and Rose also suggested that the subchondral bone in a joint has an important role in the etiology of osteoarthritis. Four years later, Radin and his colleagues reported their research on repetitive impulsive loading in New Zealand rabbits. They found that bone stiffening happens quite early as cartilage incurs damage:

> To stimulate the forces from hopping, the right foot...was subjected to 1½ the animal's body weight 40 times a minute for 20-40 minutes per day...Under these conditions subchondral bone stiffening occurred and was associated with the earliest metabolic changes of cartilage damage. When bone stiffening returned to normal the effect in the cartilage...diminished. The results suggested that subchondral bone stiffening accompanies the earliest metabolic changes in osteoarthritic chondrocytes and suggests that trabecular microfracture may occur early in this sequence of events. (Radin et al. 1978)

Later Orthopaedic Contributions

During his 11-year tenure at Harvard Medical School, he published approximately 80 papers;

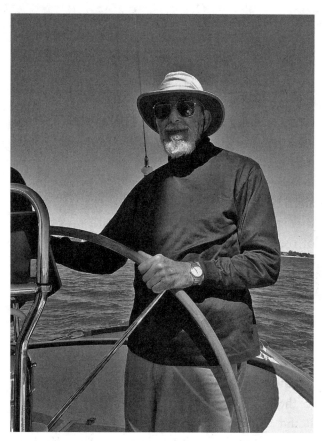

Radin at the helm of his boat in Buzzards Bay. Courtesy of Melissa Radin Goldstone.

multiple book chapters; and one book, *Practical Biomechanics for the Orthopedic Surgeon* (cowritten with Sheldon Simon, Robert Rose, and Igor Paul in 1979). However, in 1979, Radin was recruited to be a professor and chairman of the Department of Orthopaedic Surgery at West Virginia University School of Medicine. He accepted and left Boston for Morgantown. Though his tenure at MGH and Harvard ended here, his research in biomechanics continued, mainly focusing on mechanical factors as an underlying etiology for osteoarthritis. (He preferred the term *osteoarthrosis* to *osteoarthritis* because for Radin "-itis" implied inflammation, and he believed that the condition was caused by increased stiffness of the bone rather than the effects of inflammatory cytokines in the joints.) He remained at WVU for 10 years.

In 1989, he was recruited to be the director of the Bone and Joint Center and chairman of the Department of Orthopaedic Surgery at Henry Ford Hospital in Detroit, Michigan. He also became director of the residency training program there. In 1990, he was made a clinical professor of orthopaedic surgery at the University of Michigan. In 1991, he received the Breech Family Endowed Chair of Bone and Joint Medicine at Henry Ford Hospital. In 1995, he became chairman emeritus and director emeritus, and continued his professorship and his position as residency director. In all, Radin remained at Henry Ford Hospital for 10 years.

In 1999, two decades after leaving Boston, he returned to take a position as adjunct professor of orthopaedic surgery at Tufts University School of Medicine. Over his career he had published more than 200 papers and book chapters and two books on biomechanics. He retired around 2004, which freed up time for him to now focus full time on sailing, his favorite hobby, in Marion, Massachusetts. In the mid-2010s, Radin developed Alzheimer's disease and had to move into the Stone Senior Living facility in Newton. He died of coronavirus disease on April 26, 2020, during the COVID-19 pandemic. His first wife, Tova Radin, had predeceased him; their three daughters, Melissa Goldstone, Jessica Peters, and Alison Kibler, as well as his ex-wife Crete Boord Radin, survived him.

EUGENE E. RECORD

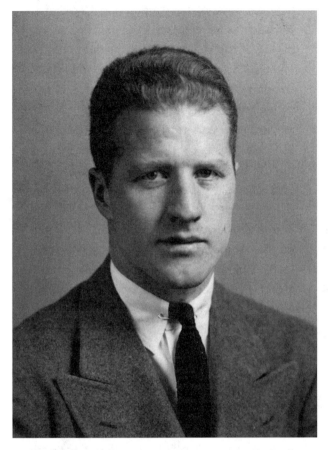

Eugene E. Record. Massachusetts General Hospital, Archives and Special Collections.

> **Physician Snapshot**
>
> Eugene E. Record
> BORN: ca. 1910
> DIED: 2004
> SIGNIFICANT CONTRIBUTIONS: Published, with Dr. Richard Warren, the book *Lower Extremity Amputations for Arterial Insufficiency* (1967); chief of orthopaedic and prosthetic appliance team at the Boston VA Hospital

Eugene E. Record—often called "Red" because of his intense red hair—was born about 1910 and grew up in the Boston area, excelling in track and field events at Brookline High School. His father worked for an oil company. Apparently, while Eugene was growing up, his family struggled with the large medical expenses resulting from his older brother contacting poliomyelitis. Eugene attended Harvard College on a scholarship beginning in 1930, and he helped pay his way by working as a tutor for the children of the influential Gannet and Aldrich families, with whom he became very close: each summer the families took him to Europe, and one had him fitted for a tuxedo in Fleet Street, London. (The families always dressed for dinner, the women in gowns and the men in tuxedos. This early exposure to formality stayed with him, and he was always in a jacket and tie—even while mowing the grass.) His work paid off and he graduated with the class of 1934.

Record left Boston briefly to attend McGill University Medical School in Montreal; he graduated in 1937. He then returned home to receive training in the Boston Children's Hospital/Massachusetts General Hospital Orthopaedic Residency Program; he was appointed chief resident at Boston Children's Hospital on September 1, 1941, succeeding Dr. Charles Sturdevant. Five months later, Record was called to active duty with the US Army Reserve and ordered to Fort Devens, where he was placed in charge of a venereal disease ward. Many years later he recalled, "It was there [at Fort Devens] that I learned to be philosophical about matters beyond one's control" (quoted in Long 2004).

After World War II, Record entered private practice and joined the staff of MGH as an assistant orthopaedic surgeon. He also practiced at the New England Peabody Home for Crippled Children as an assistant in orthopaedic surgery and at the Boston VA Hospital, where he was chief of the orthopaedic and prosthetic appliance team. I was unable to find much information about him, but I recall catching glimpses of him while I was a resident in the late 1960s. He was a tall man, quiet and distinguished. At that time, Record had an occasional patient in the hospital but never seemed to operate. According to his son, Eugene E. Record Jr., the elder Record always considered a surgical procedure as a last resort; he'd tell patients, "Let's see if we can get you better without operating" (quoted in Long 2004).

Record published five papers; he was a coauthor on three of them in the "Orthopaedic Progress" series in the *New England Journal of Medicine*. Two others were about arthrodesis of the ankle (see **Case 40.14**). In one of these, written with Joseph Barr in 1953, they highly recommended ankle fusion for fracture malunions: "Our experience with ankle fusion for painful malunion has been so favorable that we have no hesitation in recommending it as the treatment of choice in such cases...[as well as] in certain irreparable nerve lesions, in joint infections and in poliomyelitis" (Barr and Record 1953).

Case 40.14. Ankle Arthrodesis

> "[The patient], a 60-year-old woman, sustained a trimalleolar fracture in 1949; attempts at closed reduction were unsuccessful. Open operation was done, and severe postoperative sepsis occurred. When the patient was first seen about 1 year after operation, a draining sinus was present posterior to the ankle joint, the foot was extremely painful, and partial weight bearing was possible only with the aid of crutches. X-ray examination revealed a large area of decreased density in the distal tibia, which represented an active focus of infection. At operation the sinus tract was excised, and all dead bone and granulation tissue were removed, as was the cartilage of the ankle joint. No graft was used. The denuded bony surfaces united, the sinus closed promptly, solid fusion has been obtained, and the patient has an excellent functional result."
>
> (Joseph S. Barr and Eugene E. Record 1953)

Although he published about fractures, his main subspecialty interest within orthopaedics was amputation, especially in older adults. In 1963 Record presented an AAOS Instructional Course, "Surgical Amputation in the Geriatric Patient" in which he stated that:

Stump bandaging...has not been used for geriatric patients at the Amputation Clinic of the Massachusetts General Hospital. Proper bandaging of the stump to control edema requires great skill...and...[can be] hazardous to the circulation of the stump of the geriatric patient. A well-fitted elastic stump sock is [used] ... Advanced age is no contra-indication to the use of a prosthesis... [but] is contra-indicated for the above-the-knee amputee in the presence of senility...[an] inability to use the opposite extremity or the upper extremities, [and] extreme obesity...The temporary limb used at the Amputation Clinic at the Massachusetts General Hospital has a conventional foot; a drop-lock knee joint...a laced leather ischial leather weight-bearing thigh corset...a metal hip joint; and a pelvic band.

Record also published a book, *Lower Extremity Amputations for Arterial Insufficiency*, in 1967. He cowrote the text with Dr. Richard Warren, a general surgeon (see chapter 4).

Record was described as a dignified, caring, and compassionate man. Dr. Carter Rowe, in his history of orthopaedics at MGH during the twentieth century, remembered Record as a staunch ally of those working on the Orthopaedic Service and as an orthopaedist whose unflagging work helped so many patients in the amputation clinic. One published anecdote mentioned Record's efforts to stay in shape: he always took the stairs and would often have residents and colleagues lagging behind him. He died at his home in Marblehead, Massachusetts, on September 26, 2004. He was 94 years old. His four children and his wife, Emily, survived him.

JOHN A. REIDY

> **Physician Snapshot**
>
> John A. Reidy
> BORN: 1910
> DIED: 1987
> SIGNIFICANT CONTRIBUTIONS: Coauthor of *Slipped Capital Femoral Epiphysis*; chief of orthopaedic surgery at Newton-Wellesley Hospital (1954–74)

John A. Reidy was born in Albuquerque in 1910, when the city was a territory of New Mexico. His parents were John A. Reidy and Neil White Reidy. Little is known about him. but I did discover some information on his early education. He graduated from the University of New Mexico, where he was a letterman (sport unknown) and a member of the Sigma Chi Fraternity. He then attended Harvard Medical School, graduating in 1934; he served as class president.

Reidy began working (most likely as an intern) at Boston City Hospital in 1934. I was unable to find any information about his internship or residency training. He was eventually on staff at Massachusetts General Hospital and Faulkner Hospital, and he was chief of orthopaedic surgery at Newton-Wellesley Hospital from 1954 to 1974. He also served as a consultant orthopaedic surgeon at the Massachusetts Eye and Ear Infirmary and Hale Hospital in Haverhill.

Research Interests

Reidy published 12 articles on orthopaedic surgery. His main focus was initially polio, as in the articles he cowrote with Dr. Joseph Barr; later, he mostly wrote with Dr. Armin Klein about slipped capital femoral epiphysis.

His first publication, written with Barr, James Lingley, and Edward Gall, described research on the effects of irradiation on epiphyseal growth in dogs. This followed on Barr, Lingley, and E. Gail's previous publication on the effect of irradiation on epiphyseal growth in young albino rats, which had "show[n] that it was possible to impede growth in long bones by exposing the epiphyseal cartilages to…irradiation…To verify the results…and to expand the scope of the animal investigations, it seemed advisable to do a similar study on dogs…because of their possible therapeutic application to man" (Reidy et al. 1947).

Reidy et al. (1947) administered roentgen (800–1200 r) to particular joints in 6-week-old dogs, and they listed five results:

1. The epiphyseal cartilage was profoundly affected, and retardation of growth occurred.

2. The articular cartilage of the treated joints showed frank microscopic evidence of degenerative changes…

3. There was no evidence of significant abnormality in the adjacent cortical or cancellous bone…[or] soft tissues.

4. Mild bowing of the treated fore limb [*sic*] occurred in eight of twelve animals. No such deformity occurred in the hind limbs.

5. …There was evidence of stimulation of growth at the untreated epiphysis of the treated long bone.

On the basis of these findings, they concluded that "The clinical use of roentgen irradiation in growing epiphyses to control longitudinal growth inequalities in children must be considered experimental, and fraught with some potential dangers" (Reidy et al. 1947).

Reidy cowrote four papers on poliomyelitis with Barr and others, beginning in 1949 with "Prediction of Unequal Growth of the Lower Extremities in Anterior Poliomyelitis." Their study population included "166 adults in whom poliomyelitis [had] developed before the age of eleven" (Stinchfield, Reidy, and Barr 1949). Although they found "no specific relationship between the age [at] onset and the amount of discrepancy in limb length," they did identify "a definite relationship between the relative muscle strength in the two extremities and the discrepancy in leg length. These data may be utilized clinically in predicting the amount of shortening that will occur in a patient having poliomyelitis before the age of eleven" (Stinchfield, Reidy, and Barr 1949).

Dr. William T. Green (1949) was critical of the work in his discussion of the paper: "They have been forced to use groups of patients which are too few in number for statistical deduction… [and] a constant coefficient [of growth inhibition] has not occurred in their cases or in ours… There are many factors involved which cannot be dismissed…" Green noted, however, that the evidence they presented may indicate that the use of staples, as suggested by Blount, "seems to be a very good method to correct certain deformities, if used properly…[but that l]onger observation of more cases will be necessary before we can determine how dependently growth will resume after removal of the staples" (Green 1949). He agreed with the authors that "in patients under eleven years of age, the shortening at maturity corresponds with the degree of paralysis, or that it was independent of the age at onset" (Green 1949).

Reidy published again with Barr and Allan Stinchfield in 1950 regarding the use of sympathetic ganglionectomy to treat leg length discrepancy. On the basis of their results, they believed that:

> As a rule, limb length inequality of 2 centimeters or more is clinically significant and the use of a corrective lift on the shoe is required. Of the twenty-three sympathectomy cases, seventeen had a final inequality of 2 centimeters or more. Eighteen of the control group had a final inequality of 2 centimeters or more…[L]umbar sympathetic ganglionectomy can be used…but is probably best supplemented or supplanted by other methods, if the discrepancy is of any magnitude. (Barr, Stinchfield, and Reidy 1950)

Case 40.15 summarizes the case of one patient they treated in that series.

Case 40.15. Ganglionectomy in a Patient with Polio

"Summary of Case 17901 (P.B.):

"1931 Year of birth.

"1933 Patient contracted poliomyelitis, treated by local doctor.

"Patient referred to Massachusetts General Hospital. Left lower extremity flail: right, fair to good. Total muscle score: left 14, right 66.

"1937 Erector spinae transplant, left.

"1939 Arthrodesis of foot and posterior transplant, right.

"1941 Lumbar sympathetic ganglionectomy, left.

"1947 Walks with crutches and long leg brace on left lower extremity when out of doors. Crutches not used indoors.

"In this case…the skin temperatures indicated a persistent partial vasomotor denervation of the left lower extremity, six years after lumbar symptomatic ganglionectomy…not present in every case.

"Discrepancy at operation: 2.5 cm.

"Predicted final discrepancy without operation: 2.9 cm.

"Final discrepancy: –0.7 cm."

(Barr, Stinchfield, and Reidy 1950)

Two years later, along with Barr and Thomas F. Broderick, Reidy published two articles on lower-extremity tendon transplantations in patients with poliomyelitis. In part 1, "Tendon Transplantations about the Foot and Ankle," the authors described the results from 100 patients who underwent tendon transplantation—most often the peroneal tendons—in addition to stabilization of the bones in the foot. They noted, "Transplantations to reinforce power in dorsiflexion were done more frequently and…were more successful than were the posterior transplantations…to improve plantar flexion," and that "Approximately one third of the transplantations were rated as *failures*, one third as *fair*, and one third as *good* to *excellent*" (Reidy, Broderick, and Barr 1952; emphasis in the original). These results pointed them toward five main results:

1. The presence of good muscle power before operation favorably influenced the end result.
2. Operations done before the age of eleven were likely to be unsuccessful, and re-operation was necessary in 60 per cent of these cases.
3. ...[I]n the presence of good muscle power...triple arthrodesis without tendon transplant produces an excellent functional result...
4. There is some evidence that arthrodesis of the interphalangeal joints of the toes may be sufficient to correct..."cock-up" toes... without transplanting tendons to the metatarsal necks.
5. In general, the combined operation of arthrodesis and tendon transplantation should be reserved for feet with marked muscle imbalance. (Reidy, Broderick, and Barr 1952)

One of their main takeaways from this study was "that no two cases of poliomyelitis are identical" (Reidy, Broderick, and Barr 1952).

In the companion article (part 2) to the one just described, titled "Tendon Transplantations at the Knee," Broderick, Reidy, and Barr (1952)

TENDON TRANSPLANTATIONS IN THE LOWER EXTREMITY
A REVIEW OF END RESULTS IN POLIOMYELITIS *
I. TENDON TRANSPLANTATIONS ABOUT THE FOOT AND ANKLE
BY JOHN A. REIDY, M.D., THOMAS F. BRODERICK, JR., M.D., AND
JOSEPH S. BARR, M.D., BOSTON, MASSACHUSETTS

TENDON TRANSPLANTATIONS IN THE LOWER EXTREMITY
A REVIEW OF END RESULTS IN POLIOMYELITIS *
II. TENDON TRANSPLANTATIONS AT THE KNEE
BY THOMAS F. BRODERICK, JR., M.D., JOHN A. REIDY, M.D., AND JOSEPH S. BARR, M.D.
BOSTON, MASSACHUSETTS

THE JOURNAL OF BONE AND JOINT SURGERY
VOL. 34-A, NO. 4, OCTOBER 1952

Reidy et al's articles on tendon transfers in the lower extremities in poliomyelitis. *Journal of Bone and Joint Surgery* 1952; 34: 900, 914.

provided a very brief history of tendon transplantation: "Early tendon transplantations were confined to the foot following Nicoladoni's original operation in 1881. The knee offered the next logical site for experimentation and Goldthwait in 1897 reported on successful sartorius transplants to strengthen weak quadriceps muscles. Subsequently all the thigh muscles, individually or in combination, have been so employed." They then described the end results of 39 tendon transplantations at the knee in 38 patients over 25 years (beginning in 1922). The patients had received a mean follow-up of ~9 years and 2.5 months. They stated, "The subjective results...were in general good, but on objective grounds the results were disappointing. Knee-extension power following tendon transplantation was rated fair or better in only 30 per cent... Seven of twelve patients using braces were able to discard their braces" (Broderick, Reidy, and Barr 1952). Regarding function, they noted the:

> tendency to assume that the most important factor is quadriceps or extensor power. Our study suggests that other factors are of equal importance. Good hip, posterior thigh, and calf musculature will permit excellent function, even when the quadriceps is paralyzed...Tendon transplantation at the knee in some instances impairs function by the production of hypertension deformities, dislocation of the patella, or lateral instability...[I]ll-advised tendon transplantation at the knee in some instances is a subtractive operation. (Broderick, Reidy, and Barr 1952)

Reidy began publishing about slipped capital femoral epiphyses in 1949. Collaborating with Drs. Armin Klein and Robert Joplin, and later Joseph Hanelin, he cowrote multiple articles on the topic, as well as a book, *Slipped Capital Femoral Epiphysis* (see chapter 53). In addition to the articles discussed in Armin Klein's biography in chapter 53, Reidy cowrote in 1953 the paper, "Management of the Contralateral Hip in Slipped Capital Femoral Epiphysis." The research presented therein was "based on sixty-eight patients with eighty-one slipped capital femoral epiphyses treated at the Massachusetts General Hospital from 1933 to 1949...[where] about four patients appear every year at the Out-Patient Department for treatment of their slipped epiphysis" (Klein et al. 1953). Of those 68 patients, who included "five times as many boys as girls," "[t]wenty-five or 41 per cent...had bilateral slipping" (Klein et al. 1953). They described the use of roentgenology in treating these patients:

> The most constant roentgenographic indications of contralateral involvement were a widened epiphyseal plate and slipping which sometimes was of such slight extent that it could be detected only on comparison with roentgenogians [sic] of "normal" subjects of like maturation and sex...Our experience...would seem to indicate that...only one out of eight patients in whom contralateral slipping develops will require...open reduction and nailing. The majority...can be treated adequately by the simple operation of nailing *in situ*...If children...can be checked...roentgenographically every two to three months...it should not be necessary to nail contralateral hips with slipping until they become symptomatic...If...not...[then] nailing *in situ* to prevent further symptomatic slipping might well be considered. (Klein et al. 1953)

It seems that 10 years later, Reidy was also studying fractures. In 1963, he published with Dr. George W. Van Gorder an article on displaced fractures of the proximal radial epiphysis. They had reviewed patients with such fractures who had been treated at either MGH (n = 18) or Newton-Wellesley Hospital (n = 12) over the years 1924 through 1960. Those patients had been young—between 6 and 13 years old—when the injury occurred, and they were followed up for a mean of 6 years. In the summary, the authors noted, "Displacement of the proximal radial epiphysis is a rare injury...the result of a fall backward or to the side on the outstretched hand with the forearm in supination" (Reidy and Van Gorder 1963). Among the cases they reviewed:

> Eighty per cent [of patients] had displacement of 60 degrees or more...The treatment should be closed reduction if possible but if this fails, as was frequently the case...open reduction without internal fixation should be performed...[T]he children under ten years of age had a higher percentage of good and excellent results than did those in the older age group. Bone spurs on the proximal end of the radius, ulna, or both bones were noted in six of...eight children who were twelve years or older...and who were treated by open reduction. [They] tended to have greater restriction of rotation at follow-up examination. Flexion or extension was rarely limited; rotation was limited in 75 per cent of the cases. Pronation [was] the motion most frequently involved...Eighteen of the twenty-nine patients who had an end-result evaluation had normal or near normal elbow motion with minimum deformity. (Reidy and Van Gorder 1963)

Later Years

Reidy lived in Dover, Massachusetts, and was a summer resident 50 miles away in Wareham, at the northern tip of Buzzards Bay. He was an active member of the Brookline Country Club, the Dedham Country and Polo Club, the Longwood Cricket Club, and the St. Botolph Club of Boston. I was unable, however, to determine his membership status in various professional organizations. At his 25th Harvard Medical School class reunion, he presented his class's gift of $25,000 to Dean George Packer Berry. At the time, it was the largest 25-year class gift Harvard Medical School had ever received.

At age 77, Reidy died in his home after a short illness, leaving his wife Alice (née Sherburne), one son, and two daughters. (A third daughter had died before him.)

FREDERIC W. RHINELANDER JR.

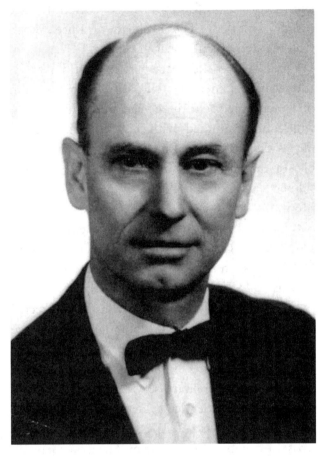

Frederic W. Rhinelander Jr. T.R.S., "Frederic W. Rhinelander, MD 1906-1990," *Journal of Bone and Joint Surgery* 1993; 75: 792.

Physician Snapshot

Frederic W. Rhinelander Jr.
BORN: 1906
DIED: 1990
SIGNIFICANT CONTRIBUTIONS: Extensively involved in research that revolutionized the treatment of burn management; authority on the blood supply to bone; chief of the Orthopaedic Service at Letterman Army Hospital (1946–47); received Legion of Merit Award for his work on bone grafting during World War II

Frederic William Rhinelander Jr. "was born on May 25, 1906, in Middletown, Connecticut. His father, Philip Mercer Rhinelander, an Episcopal minister, later became Bishop of Pennsylvania" (T.R.S. 1993). At age nine, Fred began at St. Albans School in Washington, DC, where he studied Latin, Greek, and the biological sciences. He then received his undergraduate education at Harvard University, from which he graduated cum laude with a bachelor's of arts degree in biochemistry in 1928. He continued his extensive education: he "studied English literature for one year at Oxford University in England...He received a B.A. in physiology from...Oxford University School of Medicine in 1932...followed by an M.A. from Oxford and by an M.D. from Harvard University Medical School in 1934" (T.R.S. 1993). After medical school his training advanced. He spent a year "as a graduate assistant in pathology and bacteriology at Peter Bent Brigham Hospital...The next year, he was a research assistant in the Department of Pathology at [Harvard Medical School] and served on the Arthritis Service of [MGH]. He then served a year as a surgical house officer [on the East Surgical Service in 1937] at Massachusetts General Hospital" (T.R.S. 1993). In 1938, Rhinelander began an orthopaedic residency at MGH and Children's Hospital.

In 1939, while completing the first year of his residency, he cowrote a paper titled "Exchange of Substances in Aqueous Solution Between Joints and the Vascular System." Drs. G. A. Bennett and Walter Bauer were his coauthors. (Bauer was visiting physician and physiologist at the time. He would later become the Jackson Professor of Clinical Medicine at Harvard Medical School. Bauer founded the Robert W. Lovett Memorial Unit for the Study of Crippling Diseases at MGH and served as the Unit's director from 1929 to 1958.) This paper was Rhinelander's first basic science research publication in orthopaedics and illustrates his early interest in basic science research. Rhinelander spent the second and third years of his residency (1939–41) in Philadelphia at the Shriners Hospital for Children and Temple University Hospital. Upon completing his residency, he went back to Boston, where he became an assistant in orthopaedic surgery at both MGH and Harvard Medical School., where he taught until 1947.

> THE PROBLEM OF BURN SHOCK COMPLICATED BY
> PULMONARY DAMAGE*
>
> OLIVER COPE, M.D., AND FREDERIC W. RHINELANDER, M.D.
>
> FROM THE DEPARTMENT OF SURGERY OF THE HARVARD MEDICAL SCHOOL AND THE SURGICAL SERVICES AT THE
> MASSACHUSETTS GENERAL HOSPITAL, BOSTON, MASS.
>
> Annals of Surgery
> June, 1943
> Volume 117
> Number 6

Cope and Rhinelander's classic article that revolutionized the treatment of burns. *Annals of Surgery* 1942; 117: 915.

During this period, Rhinelander "was actively involved in the treatment of burns and contaminated wounds" (T.R.S. 1993). As the 1940s commenced, Rhinelander, along with Drs. Oliver Cope, Bradford Cannon, and Francis Moore, began to study the physiology and treatment of burns…They discarded the use of tannic acid and triple dyes in favor of petrolatum sterile dressings and pressure bandages. They showed the importance of fluid balance and derived a surface area formula for the administration of fluids to anticipate and prevent shock in severely burned patients. Cannon demonstrated the advantage of immediate excision of burned areas and grafting whenever possible" (Faxon 1959). Through this work they identified the most important aspects of burn care: "management of the wound from the first protective dressing to the final healing, proper therapy in anticipation of shock, the control of infection, the maintenance of good nutrition, and help with the psychological adjustment to injury" (Faxon 1959). Their research "revolutionized the handling of burned patients" (Faxon 1959). In 1942, "soon after they had reached these conclusions," a devastating fire at the Cocoanut Grove nightclub—in which 492 people died and hundreds of others were injured—"gave them a chance to try them out as a practical way of treating large numbers of casualties. The result was good, and this form of treatment was immediately adopted by the National Research Council and recommended to be used as the standard treatment in the armed forces" and in civilian hospitals (Faxon 1959). The following year, Rhinelander cowrote the first of two papers on burns with Oliver Cope, who would later become a professor of surgery at MGH. That paper was titled "The Problem of Burn Shock Complicated by Pulmonary Damage."

In 1944, in the latter part of World War II, Rhinelander joined the US Army with the rank of captain. He spent three years in service, during which he continued with his research, including work on bone grafting, which "was responsible for the salvage of limbs of many of his fellow soldiers, and for this he received the Legion of Merit Award" (T.R.S. 1993). He also published two other orthopaedic papers during this time: "Adjustable Casts in the Treatment of Joint Deformities" in the *Journal of Bone and Joint Surgery* in 1945, written with Dr. Marian W. Ropes (who in 1958 followed Bauer as the director of the Robert W. Lovett Memorial Unit for the Study of Crippling Disease), and "Surgical Reconstruction of Arthritis" in *Surgery* in 1946. During "his last year of military service, he was Chief of the Orthopaedic Service at Letterman Army Hospital in San Francisco" (T.R.S. 1993). As chief, he wrote a "report for the Army Surgeon General, on the use of bone grafts from the iliac crest to fill large defects in long bones; [it] was included in the 1970 Medical Department of the United States Army publication *Surgery in World War II*" (T.R.S. 1993).

Upon his discharge from the service in 1947, he held the rank of major. In September of that year, he resigned from his position as assistant in orthopaedic surgery at MGH and Harvard Medical School. He moved to San Rafael, California, and began a private practice. His affiliation with the armed forces continued despite his not being on active duty, and, in 1947, he began consulting for Letterman Army Hospital (until 1948). That year, he also became an attending physician at the University of California Hospital in San Francisco. During this time, he continued working with Cope; they published together a second article on burns in 1949. Beginning in 1951 he spent four

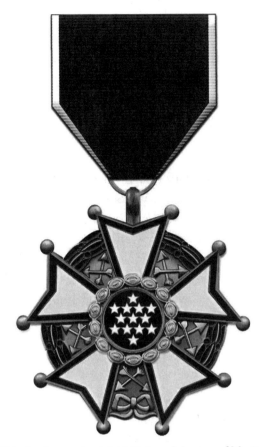

Dr. Rhinelander received the US Army's Legion of Merit for his research and use of bone grafts in injured soldiers. Wikimedia Commons.

years consulting at the hospitals on the Travis and Hamilton Air Force Bases in California.

He left his private practice and the University of California in 1955 to move to Cleveland, Ohio, where he had taken a position as an associate professor of orthopaedic surgery at the Case Western Reserve University School of Medicine, "an affiliation that was to last for twenty years" (TRS 1993). He experienced a disappointing setback during the move to Ohio: "the material for his report, on 500 cases of iliac-crest bone grafts that he had followed for five years, was lost. He had very much wanted to have this experience published" (T.R.S. 1993).

Ten years after joining the staff at Case Western Reserve University, Rhinelander became a professor of orthopaedic surgery. While there, Rhinelander produced many original research studies involving bone healing and the micro-circulation of bone as well as studies on fractures and the treatment of arthritis. Over his career, he published approximately 30 articles on these major topics, and an important chapter, "Circulation of Bone" in Geoffrey Bourne's book, *The Biochemistry and Physiology of Bone*.

He received various awards during his last few years at Case Western, and soon after leaving (**Box 40.13**). He became a professor emeritus in 1972. But his career did not end there: "Fred retired from practice in Cleveland in 1975 and moved to Little Rock, Arkansas, to become Distinguished Professor of Orthopaedic Surgery at the University of Arkansas College of Medicine" (T.R.S. 1993). He also spent three years (1975–77) as the director of orthopaedic research, after which he "was appointed Orthopaedic Research Professor Emeritus" (T.R.S. 1993).

Box 40.13. Rhinelander's Honors and Awards

- Annual Award of the Association for Osteosynthesis/Association for the Study of Internal Fixation (1971)
- Kappa Delta Award from the Kappa Delta Foundation and the Orthopaedic Research and Education Foundation (1974)
- Clemson Award in Basic Science from the Society of Biomaterials (1975)
- John Charnley Award from the Hip Society (1979)
- Alfred Rives Shands Jr. Lecture through the Orthopaedic Research Society (1979)

Rhinelander and his wife Julie, whom he had met while he had been in the army (they had married sometime during World War II), returned to California in 1979. The lived in San Clemente and spent much of their leisure time sailing. Rhinelander died 11 years later, on November 4, 1990. Julie and their seven children (three daughters and four sons) survived him.

SUMNER M. ROBERTS

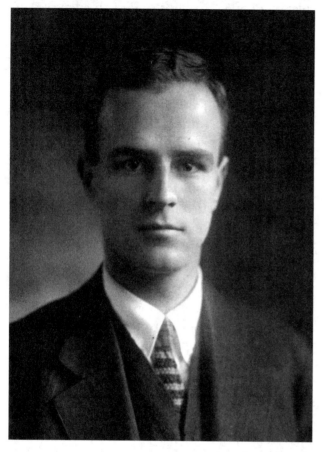

Sumner M. Roberts. Sumner Mead Roberts, 1921. (Senior Photograph) HUD 321.871 Folder 5. Harvard University Archives.

> **Physician Snapshot**
>
> Sumner M. Roberts
> BORN: 1898
> DIED: 1939
> SIGNIFICANT CONTRIBUTIONS: Described the "Pseudo Fracture of the Tibia" (a stress fracture); active member of the fracture service; brilliant surgeon and great teacher; president of the Boston Orthopaedic Club; amateur ornithologist

Sumner Mead Roberts was born to Odin Roberts, a well-known lawyer, and Ada (Mead) Roberts on January 25, 1898. After moving from Dedham, Massachusetts, to Chestnut Hill at age 10, he attended Country Day School in Newton, where he showed early leadership skills on student council and participated in multiple sports including football, baseball, and track. He attended Mesa School in Phoenix, Arizona, in 1916, before attending Harvard College. At Harvard, he continued to participate in sports and was a member of the football and baseball teams. His studies were interrupted by his naval service during World War I:

> As a preliminary training he shipped as a member of the crew on a South American cargo boat, and on his return entered the Naval Reserves Corps and [after school at Charlestown] was commissioned Ensign in the United States Navy [but he never went to sea]. He was honorably discharged soon after the Armistice and resumed his academic studies at Harvard. ("Sumner Mead Roberts, A.B., M.D., F.A.C.S. 1898–1939" 1940).

Two years before graduation, he spent the summer of 1919 in Hawaii, serving as an assistant to Professor Thomas A. Jagger with Charles Thorndike. He completed elective courses in zoology and biology, studying the crater of the volcano at Kilauea. After receiving his AB degree from Harvard in 1921, he immediately began his studies at Harvard Medical School, graduating in 1925. Next, he completed "two years of surgical internships under Dr. Eugene H. Pool at the New York Hospital, and two more years of special training in orthopaedic surgery in the postgraduate course conducted by the Harvard Medical School, the Boston Children's Hospital, and the Massachusetts General Hospital" ("Sumner Mead Roberts, A.B., M.D., F.A.C.S. 1898–1939" 1940).

He was admired by his colleagues as a "quiet, strong, able orthopaedic surgeon" ("Sumner Mead Roberts, A.B., M.D., F.A.C.S. 1898–1939" 1940).

Roberts began his private practice with Dr. Philip D. Wilson, Dr. Francis. C. Hall, and Dr. Robert B. Osgood at 372 Marlborough Street. He was also an assistant in orthopaedic surgery at Harvard Medical School, assistant visiting orthopaedic surgeon at the Massachusetts General Hospital, and orthopaedic consultant at the Massachusetts Eye and Ear Infirmary and the Robert Breck Brigham Hospital. "The treatment of fractures and the rehabilitation of the severely crippled arthritic patients were problems which particularly interested him" (Barr 1939). During this early period in his career, he also married Elizabeth Converse, who was the daughter of "the distinguished musician and composer, Frederick S. Converse" on December 27, 1927 ("Sumner Mead Roberts, A.B., M.D., F.A.C.S. 1898–1939" 1940). They lived at 74 Oak Hill Street, Newton and would have three children together.

In 1930, he was listed as Instructor in Orthopaedic Surgery at Harvard Medical School. He also held various hospital appointments throughout his career:

> He was consultant in Orthopaedic Surgery to the Huntington Memorial [Hospital] a member of the staffs of the Faulkner Hospital and the Dedham Clinic [and] a very active member of the [MGH] 'Fracture Service.' It was at the Massachusetts General Hospital that the bulk of his public orthopaedic practice was conducted. Here the light shone brightest on his unusual abilities as a brilliant surgeon and a great teacher of undergraduate and postgraduate students. ("Sumner Mead Roberts, A.B., M.D., F.A.C.S. 1898–1939" 1940)

During his 12 years in practice, Dr. Roberts published eight papers (five of which were on trauma) and the chapter "Fractures of the Upper End of the Humerus" in Wilson's Textbook *Fractures and dislocations*; he was also a coauthor on approximately 32 "Progress Reports in Orthopaedic Surgery" published in the *Archives of Surgery* from 1932 to 1939. In his first publication, he reviewed 10 years of records (1923–1932) of patients on the fracture service of MGH, and he concluded the records indicated a trend toward treating fractures of the proximal humerus with fixation and early active motion rather than with prolonged immobilization in an apparatus. At this time, there was a difference of opinion about how to treat fractures at the shoulder. Some argued for immobilization and rest; Roberts supported early active motion for stable fractures and after open reduction of unstable fractures, and he reported good results in these patients. During the period of his study, there were 96 cases of fractures of the proximal humerus. He used the MGH method of evaluating the outcomes of patients after recovering from a fracture; that is, he used the categories anatomic, economic, and functional. Each category was evaluated on a scale of 0–4, with 4 being excellent. (This was an early attempt at using outcomes at MGH and was used for a number of years. See chapter 32 for additional discussion of this method.) He concluded:

1. Classification on anatomic lines is sometimes inconvenient and difficult…

2. Fracture of the greater tuberosity is not common without associated injury… Fixation in abduction is usually sufficient treatment.

3. In fracture dislocations the most common fracture is that of the greater tuberosity… when the dislocation is reduced, the fractured fragment returns to position. Dislocations with separation of the head are difficult problems…Removal of the head should be avoided if possible.

4. In epiphyseal separation, exact reposition is necessary. Open reduction is…often indicated…

5. Transverse fractures of the surgical neck occur in young people and are prone to displacement. Good reposition…often requiring open operation…

6. Comminuted fractures occur in elderly people…Simple fixation suffices, and early motion is desirable.

This paper generated lots of discussion with both some agreements, but also some disagreements with his recommendations; these major figures included Dr. Henry C. Marble, Dr. H. Winnet Orr, Dr. James W. Sever and Dr. Henry W. Meyerding.

In 1937 Roberts published two articles on "Fractures and Dislocations of the Cervical Spine;" Part I on fractures and Part II on dislocations, complications, and operative treatment with numerous individual brief case reports. **Case 40.16** highlights an example of one of the many cases Roberts reviewed. He observed:

> Fractures and dislocations of the cervical spine should be reduced at once…Fractures are more serious than dislocations and are more liable to be fatal or to be accompanied by irreparable cord or nerve damage…Dislocations are very rarely fatal. Their reduction is not dangerous.

Case 40.16. Congenital Absence of the Odontoid Process

"On September 4, 1931, a young man, twenty years of age, came to the emergency ward of the Massachusetts General Hospital complaining of pain in his neck. The onset of symptoms had been sudden and had occurred the day previous when he had been "bridging" in a gymnasium. This meant that, lying on the gymnasium mat face upper-most, he had lifted his body off the mat by arching his back until his weight was supported only by his feet and his hyperextended head. In this position he was slowly moving his feet so that they described a circle with his head as a pivot. He suddenly felt something snap in his neck at the base of his skull and collapsed on the mat with severe pain in his neck. There was no loss of consciousness and no impairment of sensation or function in his extremities. He went home alone, but came to the hospital the next day because the pain in his neck still persisted, though to a lesser degree.

"Physical examination showed a well developed and muscular young man who held his head turned about twenty degrees to the right of the mid-line and tipped very slightly to the left. There was moderate tenderness on pressure over the spinous process of the axis and slight tenderness laterally on both sides at the same level. Visual examination of the posterior nasopharynx revealed no abnormality. All neck motions were slightly painful and were limited by muscle spasm. He could not rotate his chin to the left of the mid-line. Other motions were correspondingly restricted. Passive motion of the occiput on the atlas was nearly normal, but all other passive motions were limited by muscle spasm. A diagnosis of a forward dislocation of the left articular facet of the atlas on the axis was made.

"The roentgenographic examination confirmed the clinical diagnosis, except that the dislocation was backward on the right, instead of forward on the left, and also revealed the reason for it. The patient had no odontoid process. The odontoid had apparently failed to develop. The spot where the base of the odontoid normally would be appeared as a smooth ridge with a slight sulcus on either side at the inner margins of the articular processes.

"The patient was put to bed on a Bradford frame and five points of head traction were applied. Roentgenograms taken three days later showed the dislocation to be reduced. A molded leather collar was made and fitted and he was discharged from the hospital one month after entry. The question that arose at the time of discharge was: Was this boy constantly in danger of another dislocation, a dislocation which might readily be fatal? The answer was probably in the affirmative. Any trivial injury, such as a sudden unguarded movement, might dislocate an unstable neck of this sort. This danger was explained to the patient and a stabilizing operation advised. Operation was refused, however.

"This man was seen again one year later, during which time no untoward accident had occurred. He had not played football, but had played basketball regularly. His neck was symptom-free and all motions were normal. The danger he was running was once more explained to him and operation advised, but he again refused."

(Sumner Mead Roberts 1933)

> FRACTURES AND DISLOCATIONS OF THE CERVICAL SPINE
> PART I. FRACTURES *
> BY SUMNER M. ROBERTS, M.D., BOSTON, MASSACHUSETTS
>
> FRACTURES AND DISLOCATIONS OF THE CERVICAL SPINE
> PART II. DISLOCATIONS, COMPLICATIONS, AND OPERATIVE TREATMENT
> BY SUMNER M. ROBERTS, M.D., F.A.C.S., BOSTON, MASSACHUSETTS
> THE JOURNAL OF BONE AND JOINT SURGERY
> VOL. XIX, NO. 1, JANUARY 1937

Roberts' two articles on fractures and dislocations of the cervical spine. *Journal of Bone and Joint Surgery* 1937; 19: 199, 477.

They will not recur if properly treated…Fixation after reduction of either fracture…or dislocation must be complete and of long duration…Early complications cannot be avoided. Proper treatment begun early will less their permanent effects…Late complications are usually due to lack of early treatment and to inadequate fixation…Operation is rarely indicated except to relieve late cord symptoms. (Roberts 1937)

That same year, he published the paper "Arthroplasty of the Elbow" with Dr. Robert Joplin. They wrote that:

A majority of cases were patients with chronic rheumatoid arthritis at the Robert Brigham Hospital. All but one [a patient of Dr. Kuhn's] were operated upon in collaboration with Dr. Philip Wilson to whom entire credit is due for the establishment of the operative technique that has been used…23 arthroplasties…have been followed for periods ranging from 16 months to 11 years. Sixteen of the patients had elbows that were completely ankylosed…The operative technique used…is as follows:…the incision starts on the posterolateral aspect of the lower arm…follows down the outer border of the triceps tendon…carried down to the bones…exposed subperiosteally…[which] necessarily separates the triceps from its attachment to the olecronon…The radial head is excised…The bones should…be separated along the lines of the former joint…The periosteum…stripped…so that the entire articular surfaces of humerus and ulna, with about 2 inches of their adjacent shafts, are entirely free from soft structures…The lower end of the humerus is remodeled with rasp and osteotome… to form a single condyle …The ulna is similarly treated so as to form a long, shallow articulation…A strip of fascia…about 6 by 3 inches, is then taken from the outer aspect of the thigh. One end…is placed over the remodeled humerus, gliding surface outermost…The other end is placed over the reconstructed ulna. (Roberts and Joplin 1937).

They went on to conclude:

1. Arthroplasty of the elbow is a successful operation resulting in a useful, permanent amount of flexion [average gain in motion was 100°]…

2. Full motion…is not desirable…too great a range of motion is accompanied by instability…

3. Rotation of the forearm is more difficult to restore…The radial head and usually a portion of the lower end of the ulna should be resected.

4. Arthroplasty gives the patient a mobile elbow…useful for simple tasks…not…suitable for hard labor. (Roberts and Joplin 1937).

He published his last article with Dr. E. C. Vogt; together they discussed what was most likely a stress fracture and "a hitherto undescribed lesion of the lower leg, which they named "Pseudo Fracture of the Tibia" ("Sumner Mead Roberts, A.B., M.D., F.A.C.S. 1898–1939" 1940). He was an active participant in numerous professional associations, including as a Fellow of the American College of Surgeons and of the American Academy

> **PSEUDOFRACTURE OF THE TIBIA** *
>
> BY SUMNER M. ROBERTS, M.D., AND EDWARD C. VOGT, M.D.,
> BOSTON, MASSACHUSETTS
>
> THE JOURNAL OF BONE AND JOINT SURGERY
> VOL. XXI, NO. 4, OCTOBER 1939

Roberts and Vogt's article, "Pseudofracture of the Tibia." They believed that the lucent lines they observed were most likely sites of nutrient vessels and not a fracture—stress fractures were not recognized at the time. They reported, however, that Ollonqvist (Finland) identified similar "fractures" in the mid-third of the tibia in army recruits 8 years earlier. Similar x-ray appearances were reported with "march foot"—called "Umbauzone" or "wear-and-tear" fractures by the Germans. The x-rays in Roberts and Vogt's article show the appearance of healing as seen in stress fractures, and included two cases that went on to complete displaced proximal tibial fractures. *Journal of Bone and Joint Surgery* 1939; 21: 891.

of Orthopaedic Surgeons; and a member of the American Medical Association, the Massachusetts Medical Society, and the American Orthopaedic Association. He also participated in the Interurban Club and served as president of the Boston Orthopaedic Club.

Not long after his final publication, Dr. Sumner Roberts was killed in a car accident at just 41 years old on November 19, 1939. After impact, his car had rolled and instantly crushed him. At the time, he was returning home (on route 132) from treating a patient for a fractured spine—ironically also the result of a car accident—in Cape Cod Hospital. Afterward:

> The swift communication of the news of his untimely death by word of mouth from friend to friend and the immediate sense of grief which fell on all testify only too well to the affection and respect which his personality had engendered. He was straightforward and sincere…His modesty and reserve prevented him from becoming a favorite of the crowds, but few physicians can number more sincere friends than he among his colleagues.
> (Barr 1939)

He had been an angler and lover of nature, including "an amateur ornithologist of merit" ("Sumner Mead Roberts, A.B., M.D., F.A.C.S. 1898-1939" 1940). He "was the embodiment of a kindly calmness which his patients often spoke of as 'priest-like': it blessed them with comfort and inspired them with confidence. His natural reserve was friendly, untinged by self-esteem. His criticism of himself was severe, of his colleagues very rare and then always just and gentle" ("Sumner Mead Roberts, A.B., M.D., F.A.C.S. 1898-1939" 1940). His friends and colleagues had "felt assured that in the near future, he would be generally recognized as one of the great exponents of the specialty of orthopaedic surgery" but his life was tragically cut short ("Sumner Mead Roberts, A.B., M.D., F.A.C.S. 1898-1939" 1940).

WILLIAM A. ROGERS

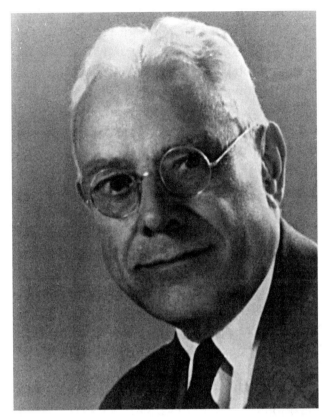

William A. Rogers. ("William Alexander Rogers, MD March 30, 1882—April 4, 1975," *Journal of Bone and Joint Surgery* 1975; 57: 438.)

Physician Snapshot

William A. Rogers
BORN: 1892
DIED: 1975

SIGNIFICANT CONTRIBUTIONS: Editor of the *Journal of Bone and Joint Surgery*—stabilized finances, started the American and British volumes, expanded the editorial board to include members of the English-speaking associations, and oversaw the independence of *JBJS* with its own board of trustees; expert in cervical spine fractures and dislocations; designed the posterior cervical spine interspinous wiring technique; avid ornithologist

William "Bill" Alexander Rogers was born in 1892 to Oscar H. Rogers, Medical Director of New York Life Insurance Company, who invented a type of sphygmomanometer, and Mrs. Rogers (I could not locate her name in the historical records), a school teacher; he was raised in Schenectady, New York. He worked first for the General Electric Company as a physicist after receiving his bachelor's degree from Union College. Afterward, he attended Cornell Medical School before graduating in 1919. He completed his orthopaedic residency at Massachusetts General Hospital (MGH). He was also the first assistant of Dr. Marius Smith-Petersen before entering a solo private practice.

Early Career

Dr. Rogers joined MGH as an assistant in orthopaedics in 1924, during a period of transition and change. Dr. Osgood had moved to Boston Children's Hospital and Dr. Allison had become chief of the Orthopaedic Department. The small operating room for orthopaedics had been recently moved from the Orthopaedic Ward's basement to a larger room in the 1900 Surgical Building. Rogers's major contribution to orthopaedic care and end results involved fractures and dislocations of the spine. In 1926, fracture cases were assigned to the Fracture Service, including fractures involving the spine without spinal cord injury. The annual report of the hospital's board of trustee's that year noted that Rogers established:

> a "follow-up" system which is of great value in ascertaining the end results of surgical treatment. Patients who have been operated upon in Ward I are asked to return to the Hospital after a period of one year. The Social Service Department co-operates in locating the patients, and on one Sunday each month the entire Orthopaedic Staff gathers in the Hospital and reviews the history, treatment and result accomplished in the patients operated upon during that month one year previous. The attendance at these 'follow-up' clinics has been most gratifying and the service is making end result records which cover over seventy

per cent of the cases that have been operated upon in the Hospital.

In 1929, Rogers was promoted to assistant orthopaedic surgeon at MGH, and in 1935 he was appointed assistant visiting orthopaedic surgeon. That same year, he presented his thesis to the American Orthopaedic Association, "Treatment of Fractures of the Vertebral Bodies Uncomplicated by Lesions of the Cord." In his thesis, he stated that fractures of the spine require early and accurate diagnosis and follow the same general principles as the treatment of large weight-bearing bones after reduction by hyperextension. He noted that the first successful reduction of these fractures was demonstrated by Arthur G. Davis in 1924 and reported in 1929, six years before he presented his thesis. Davis and Rogers were each independently using reduction maneuvers by slow and intermittent hyperextension of the spine—the keynote of reduction—on a flexible Bradford Frame or Goldthwait irons. To complete his study, Rogers reviewed 31 cases of vertebral body fractures treated between 1928 and 1932. His steps for successfully completing the reduction included:

- Obtaining lateral x-rays
- Placing the patient in a body cast when reduction is acceptable on x-ray
- Treating the patient in the body cast with bed rest for 4 months
- Using an ambulatory jacket for an additional 2 to 7 months after the patient completes the period in the body cast
- Completing the maneuver in a slow and incremental fashion

Afterward, the initial reduction restored the anatomic shape of the vertebral body, but with ambulation the deformity returned in 65% of patients. Those patients, however, remained asymptomatic. Spine fusion was indicated only when adequate reduction of a fracture-dislocation could not be obtained. He determined that:

- To ensure no injury to the spinal cord occurs, accurate early diagnosis is essential before treatment with manipulative reduction
- Reduction should not be delayed after injury and should be completed early
- The longer the time span after the injury, the more difficult the reduction becomes

Editor, *Journal of Bone and Joint Surgery*

Two years after Rogers presented his thesis, he became visiting orthopaedic surgeon at MGH, a position he held until 1952. As one of the hallmarks of his career, he was appointed editor of the *Journal of Bone and Joint Surgery* (JBJS) in April 1944. The fact that "he made such contributions to patient care and at the same time carried the mighty burden of The Journal with all its problems of the 1940's [sic] and 1950's [sic] is proof positive of his tireless energy and devotion to orthopaedics" (Brown 1975). A few years before Rogers' appointment, Dr. Elliott Brackett had died in 1942 after serving as editor for 20 years. Afterward, "Murray S. Danforth was appointed editor in January 1943. He died in June 1943 after serving only 4.5 months as editor. Charles Painter then became editor pro tem and served until" Rogers' appointment (Cowell 2000). He was:

> keenly aware that the mantle of [the biblical figure] Elijah which had fallen on his shoulders, had to be worn with becoming dignity and wisdom, he at once began a careful analysis of the Journal's affairs. The situation was complicated, the footing treacherous; he had to watch his step carefully. Actually, despite Dr. Brackett's masterful policies, Bill soon realized that...he had inherited three problems: first, an unsatisfactory relationship of the Journal to current British orthopaedic literature; second, an insecure financial policy suggesting the need for a commercial publisher; and third, the relationship

of the Journal to the American Academy of Orthopaedic Surgeons... (Mayer 1958)

For about 25 years the *JBJS* served as the British Orthopaedic Association's official publication. Nevertheless, "the number of papers submitted by the members of the British Association was disappointedly small" because *JBJS* had a very small circulation with little reach (Mayer 1958). As his first order of business, Rogers focused on methods to substantially increase the journal's circulation, and eventually:

> there crystallized in his mind the concept of a joint publication. By the spring of 1947...he submitted several alternative proposals to the officers and Editorial Committees of the [British Orthopaedic] Association and the [American Academy of Orthopaedic Surgeons], and the Board of Associate Editors of the Journal. At the same time a similar meeting occurred in England. As a result, a conference was arranged between representatives of the British Orthopaedic Association and the Editorial Committees of the American Orthopaedic Association and the American Academy of Orthopaedic Surgeons...on May 27, 1947. Sir Reginald Watson-Jones acted as leader of the British group, Dr. Rogers of the American. Thanks largely to the admirable spirit of friendliness engendered by those two great personalities, a plan of co-publication was evolved... approved in June by each of the three organizations. (Mayer 1958)

For the new joint endeavor, they determined they would publish quarterly issues in both the United States and in Great Britain. They also offered multiple options for purchase, including a single subscription to both, a single subscription to the American ("A") journal or a single subscription to the British ("B") journal. He simultaneously offered editorial board positions to the members of the Canadian, Australian, New Zealand, and South African Orthopaedic Associations. He realized the importance of "ownership" of *JBJS* by these English-speaking countries if he was going to persuade their members to purchase the journal.

This was all no small accomplishment for Rogers, but other difficulties quickly developed. Rogers directed both the journal's finances in addition to its content, and previously the journal had received donations between 1922 and 1929. After 1929, the American Orthopaedic Association members:

> had [each] contributed $15 to a Journal Fund in addition to [their] yearly subscription of $5...Members of the [American Academy of Orthopaedic Surgeons], however, had not been asked to make...such donations. Each member paid the usual $5 fee for his subscriptions, thus giving to the journal in the year 1945 about $5,500, whereas the actual cost of publishing Academy articles amounted to $15,000. (Mayer 1958)

Early in his role, Rogers was therefore presented with what seemed an unsurmountable problem; the deficit was several thousand dollars in 1948. In June of that year, the Treasurer of the American Orthopaedic Association "voiced the opinion that the 'Editor of the Journal should not be called upon to carry the financial load and that the time had come to place the responsibility of the publication of the Journal in the hands of a commercial publisher'" (Mayer 1958). Thereafter, the Executive Committee of the Association was authorized to "appoint a body...of both the Academy and the Association to explore with a major publishing house the possibility of negotiating a satisfactory contract for publishing the Journal" (Mayer 1958).

Rogers was devastated, and he was adamantly against commercial publication. About one year later, at the business meeting of the Association, he argued that profit was "contrary to the spirit in which the Journal was conceived" (Mayer 1958). He further emphasized that:

> lowering standards would be inevitable, that control would pass from the hands of the Journal to that of the commercial publisher, that the Editor would be shorn of "all but a mere vestige of control", and that the Association would be giving away a most valuable investment into which it had poured large sums of money and an inestimable amount of energy and effort. (Mayer 1958)

He won his argument after successfully influencing the treasurer who then supported him.

His challenges had not yet come to an end, however. He still needed to surmount a deficit of $9,489.79 in April 1949, so as an immediate next step, he created the Journal Finance Committee. Although his goal had been to ameliorate the relationship between the journal and the American Academy of Orthopaedic Surgeons:

> [t]he inequity of the situation was obvious...Dr. Rogers realized that the essential cause of conflict between the Association and the Academy was the ownership of the Journal by the older generation [AOA members]. The great body of Academy members—enthusiastic young orthopaedic surgeons—were anxious to share whole heartedly in the development of the Journal and felt...entitled to participate in the publication of this, the official organ of their Academy, but how could they secure a share of the ownership. (Mayer 1958)

During this time of financial upheaval, Rogers continued to simultaneously implement innovative content changes at the journal. He established the Proceedings in 1953, which were:

> abstracts of scientific papers presented at orthopaedic meetings. At first, the proceedings covered only the Annual Meetings of the AOA and AAOS, but in later decades they included reports from more than a dozen different orthopaedic meetings around the world. (Cohen and Heckman 2003)

Under his guidance throughout the 1950s, there was also "frequent collaboration between those in the clinical arena and those in the academic disciplines," such as engineering, chemistry, and physics (Cohen and Heckman 2003).

Meanwhile, together with the Finance Committee, he began the work of a complete reorganization of the Journal's ownership. In response, "the American Orthopaedic Association magnanimously relinquished all rights to the Journal and transferred these to a new corporation, The Journal of Bone and Joint Surgery, Incorporated, controlled by a board of trustees, three representing the Association, three the Academy" (Mayer 1958). This board, comprised of six trustees, was to select a seventh member who was "to be entrusted with the editorship of the Journal" (Mayer 1958). In January 1954, after granting its approval, the Academy "contributed the sum of $40,000 to the reserve fund of the Journal, thus creating a total reserve of $83,000. Dr. Rogers's financial fears were at last laid to rest, and the conflict between the Association and the Academy solved" (Mayer 1958).

Rogers was unflagging in his work seeking worthy, original contributions for the journal, and he continued to hold the journal to the highest standards in his role as editor; "not only did he read every one of the hundreds of manuscripts submitted, but he maintained a lively correspondence with the authors" (Mayer 1958). He helped finesse each author's paper, and, at the board meetings, they determined which papers they would publish. By the late 1950s, Rogers appointed two assistant editors, Thornton Brown and Jonathan Cohen. He needed help with manuscripts in response to the continued clinical and academic collaborations, and their training in basic science" made them ideal for the role (Cohen and

Heckman 2003). In *Lest We Forget*, Dr. Carter Rowe recalled the Journal's office:

> Some of us remember the Journal's office when it was located at 8 The Fenway, its busy main room with tables stacked with manuscripts, and Miss Florence Daland (assistant editor) and John Reed (business manager) presiding over all activities. Dr. Rogers's office opened off the left end of the main room. It was a small office, indeed, for the amount of work contained therein. (Rowe 1996)

Under Rogers's leadership, the journal grew from a circulation of 3,606 in 1942 to exceeding 11,500 by 1958. He also increased the number of journal issues from four to six in 1954 and then to eight in 1959 for the American volume, while always ensuring the American and British Journals always mutually benefited. Rogers was an expert "captain at the helm" and:

> It is truly amazing how he managed to keep in touch with active workers everywhere. He had his eyes and ears in every laboratory… He was also particularly eager to improve the standards of orthopaedic education by papers dealing with fundamental scientific advances… Whereas in 1936 only 5 percent of the articles dealt with basic sciences, in 1956 the percentage had risen to 22.
>
> Those associate editors…could not but be impressed by Bill's sterling qualities as Editor: his honesty, his fairness, his thoroughness, his indefatigability, his acumen, and his supreme devotion to the advancement of orthopaedic surgery through the Journal. (Mayer 1958)

Later Orthopaedic Contributions

Dr. Rogers continued to make his own contributions to the literature, notably about spinal trauma, while serving as editor of the *Journal of Bone and Joint Surgery*. **Case 40.17** highlights an example of one of the many cases he reviewed. In addition to his previous publications on the dorsal and lumbar spine, in 1942 and 1957, Rogers wrote two significant papers on fractures and dislocations of the cervical spine, including an end-result study. In the first of these papers he described:

> refinements of technique in the case of the broken neck…essential to the safety of the spinal

Case 40.17. Cord Injury with Closed Reduction of a Lumbar Spine Fracture-Dislocation

> "The patient, a man of twenty-nine, had been thrown from an automobile. For a day after the accident, there had been little or no evidence of root pressure. Slowly spreading paralysis than developed in scattered groups in both lower extremities. On the third day he was transferred from a distant hospital to the Service of Dr. W. J. Mixter with whom the writer saw him in consultation…The diagnosis of fracture-dislocation of the first lumbar vertebra upon the second was made, and extension was attempted, using ankle traction and suspension with block and tackle.
>
> "The usual traction was supplemented by manual traction by assistants before and during the extension maneuver. Morphine-scopolamine was used…All attempts to carry the extension further failed. At the point shown in the roentgenogram, the partial paralysis quickly changed to almost complete paralysis. Open reduction under local anesthesia was done the same day by Dr. Mixter and the author. When the articular facets were exposed, they were found to be locked…In order to free and to realign them, it was necessary to flex the column (done by lowering both ends of the operating table) and then to rotate them into alignment with a periosteum elevator used as a pry…Hyperextension could then be accomplished with ease, and the reduction could be completed. The jacket was applied in this position…All neurological signs cleared up, and at the end of a year the patient was symptom-free and able to engage in full pre-injury activities."
>
> (William A. Rogers 1938)

cord...[including] skeletal traction and tidal drainage...[to which he added] open reduction and internal fixation...All [injuries] must be treated with these cardinal points peculiar to the cervical spine...1. The cord must be protected at all times; 2. Reduction must be complete, or pain and recurrence may ensue; 3. The fixation must be adequate, or recurrence will follow...

Cord injury and increase or recurrence of deformity has taken place during first aid, during transport to the hospital, during the roentgenographic study, and during preliminary preparation. It has been the author's experience that all these dangers may be obviated by the used of an adjustable Thomas collar or the Forrester type...When the cervical spine is under skeletal traction [Crutchfield tongs], correctly applied, the spinal cord is safe...If skeletal traction is not successful in effecting reduction, open reduction may be indicated. Closed manipulation has led to cord injury and death... Open reduction gives sight precision... in dangerous or doubtful cases...under skeletal traction....

In flexion injuries, once reduction has been effected...internal fixation is applied...The appropriate vertebrae are wired together, and bone grafts are placed so as to bridge the interspinal and interlaminar spaces at the completion of open reduction [Rogers's technique]... Babcock stainless-steel wire, No. 24, is satisfactory, and does not cause osteolysis. In each of the spinous processes to be fixed, a small transverse hole is made at...the junction of the process with the laminae.... The wire is looped around the superior border of the upper process, and the ends are passed through the hole in that process in opposite directions. The ends are passed distally and parallel across the interspinal space, and then in opposite directions through the hole in the process below. This is repeated until the lowest process to be fixed has been included. One end is then looped around the inferior border of this process; the wire is made snug; and the ends are fastened by twisting. A pair of osteoperiosteal grafts, one on each side, are laid transversely, bridging each interspace. The adjoining portions of the pair of grafts are forced between the parallel positions of the wire fixation. Bare chips are packed in wherever possible. There has been no failure of fusion by rigid test in the eleven cases so treated...Nine of eleven patients returned to their work in an average of five months. The range of motion in rotation varied from 45 to 140 degrees, depending on the vertebrae fused. (Rogers 1942)

Meanwhile, Rogers had continued in his position as visiting orthopaedic surgeon at MGH, and, in 1952, he was appointed to the Board of Consultation. Five years later, Rogers also published the end-results of his experience treating 77 patients with 87 fractures, dislocations or fracture-dislocations of the cervical spine over a ten-year period (1940–1950) at the Massachusetts General Hospital, including several treated at the Marine Hospital of the United States Public Health Service in Boston. He noted:

All of these patients, except fourteen, were seen at follow-up examination by the author at one to twelve years after definitive treatment...For the sixty-three patients who survived the injury, the mean follow-up period was five years. Fourteen of the seventy-seven patients died from complications resulting directly from involvement of the cord, from within a few hours after injury to seven months after the injury. (Rogers 1957)

He wrote the following conclusions:

1. For the dangerous period between the time of injury and definitive treatment, and while being moved about...the patient should be recumbent, at all times, on a firm stretcher

> **Fractures and Dislocations of the Cervical Spine**
> AN END-RESULT STUDY*
> BY WILLIAM A. ROGERS, M.D., BOSTON, MASSACHUSETTS
> THE JOURNAL OF BONE AND JOINT SURGERY
> VOL. 39-A, NO. 2, APRIL 1957

Rogers' article reporting his ten-year outcomes treating cervical spine fractures and dislocations. *Journal of Bone and Joint Surgery* 1957; 39: 341.

or bed. An adjustable traction neck brace should be worn during these times, applied in the long axis of the spine in the neutral position. 2. Skull traction is the best proved means of protecting the cord during definitive treatment…3. Skull traction will accomplish reduction and maintain it in a high proportion of injuries. It is comfortable and greatly facilitates nursing care. 4. Complete reduction is ideal; satisfactory reductions may include those in which there is less than 0.3 centimeter of decrease in the anteroposterior diameter of the vertebral canal. Open reduction was accomplished in seven patients, in six of whom skull traction had failed. 5. Internal fixation and surgical fusion provide reliable stabilization of the injured vertebrae. They appear to protect the cord against attrition in patients with a vertebral-canal diameter of less than normal. 6. The treatment of cervical-spine injuries is highly specialized; technical errors in treatment may be fatal. A trained and experienced operating team is essential. (Rogers 1957)

Dr. Carter Rowe remembered Dr. Rogers as "one of the first orthopaedists with special interests in the cervical spine" (see **Box 40.14**). Rogers was innovative in his approach and in his use of equipment to treat the condition. His apparatus was unique "with its horizontal track and pulley, [and] a patient in skull traction was able to turn from side to side without losing alignment of the cervical spine" (Rowe 1996).

Box 40.14. Mental Attitude is Essential for Recovery from a Spine Fracture

> "Anxious to spike the common notion that a man with a broken back is never any good again…Dr. Rogers… presented cases…which had convinced him that the attitude of the patient…has a great deal to do with the results…two-thirds of his broken back cases are doing the same work now they did before their accidents. They have averaged three weeks in hospital. Less than six months lay-off, and a little more than $300 compensation for the injury…Dr. Rogers classified his spinal fractures as much by their mental attitude as by their physical injuries. He contrasted the results in two cases. One was a house painter, the other a roofer. The painter was 'a grand fellow, cooperative, eager to get back to work.' He was in the hospital only a couple of weeks and we got him back on his job in 5.7 months, with $317 compensation.
>
> "The roofer 'had a sister, a nurse, who was full of the idea that a spinal injury was a terrible thing and that he'd never get over it. We had him seven months in the hospital and he ran up a compensation bill of $476 for his back and $600 more for a deafness he said he'd acquired that none of us could understand.' Dr. Rogers prescribed early exercises for broken backs, 'so you won't have to go through months of bakings and massage when the plaster jacket comes off. The patient is given to understand right away that he isn't so badly off…"
>
> (*Daily Boston Globe*, September 27, 1934, p 7)

Legacy

Dr. William Rogers had continued his tireless devotion to the field despite many personal tragedies. His son died in a plane crash in 1949, while on a training flight one year after graduating from Annapolis. Before resigning as editor from the *JBJS* in 1958, he had remarried six years earlier. But his wife Emily died quickly after they had married from a health condition. After her death, "he remained in Peacham [on their farm], but soon his health also failed, forcing him to leave his precious Vermont and to return to his native heath, as he liked to call it, in Schenectady" (Brown 1975). He died on April 4, 1975, at 83 years old and was survived by his daughter and son. According to Brown (1975), "His contributions to orthopaedic surgery, notably in the treatment of fractures and dislocations of the cervical spine, are matters of record." Mayers (1958) believed that of the many honors he received, he most valued the Honorary Fellowship in the British Orthopaedic Association, which was awarded to him in July of 1952.

Rogers was fondly remembered:

> To those who inherited some of his patients after retirement, the esteem and affection with which they regarded him were little short of awesome. Patients from all walks of life were his ardent admirers…His eventual triumph over recurrent malignant disease…[led Dr. Thornton Brown to recall] a vivid recollection on the eve of his final and last-ditch operation to eradicate his disease…[where he was] sitting in his hospital bed surrounded by papers and hard at work on Journal affairs…
>
> With all his dedication to the Journal and orthopaedics, he still had a tremendous enthusiasm for life and other interests. At the annual meetings of his travel club, the Forum, only John Royal ('Dinty') Moore could keep up with him. Their early morning bird walks (Dr. Rogers was an avid ornithologist) after festive evenings even now are exhausting to contemplate.

CARTER R. ROWE

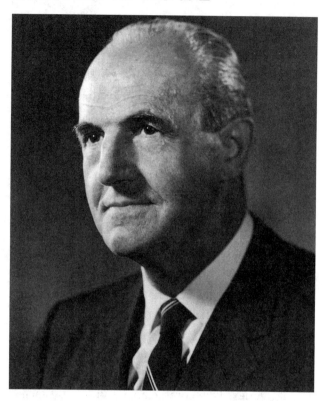

Carter R. Rowe. B.Z. and H.J.M., "Carter R. Rowe 1906–2001," *Journal of Bone and Joint Surgery* 2001; 83: 1773.

Physician Snapshot

Carter R. Rowe
BORN: 1906
DIED: 2001
SIGNIFICANT CONTRIBUTIONS: Leader in shoulder surgery; orthopaedic surgeon for the Bruins; founder of the AOSSM; founder and president ASES 1984; president AOA 1969; elected into the AOSSM Hall of Fame 2003; published *Lest We Forget*; Southern gentleman

Carter Redd Rowe was born on August 30, 1906, in Fredericksburg, Virginia. He attended both Davidson College and the University of Virginia Graduate School; he received his AB degree from the former and attended the latter for a year to study chemistry. He graduated from Harvard Medical School (HMS) with his doctorate in medicine in 1933. Dr. Rowe wrote his first article, "Cardiac Asthma," under the direction of Dr. Soma Weiss while still a student at HMS. I was, however, unable to discover whether his first medical paper was ever published. He later completed training in New York City at the Long Island College Hospital (as a medical intern for a year) and the New York Post Graduate Hospital (as a surgical intern for two years).

Early Career

In 1939, after finishing his orthopaedic residency at Massachusetts General Hospital (MGH) and Boston Children's Hospital, he returned to Fredericksburg, "where he worked for almost three years doing a bit of everything, including general surgery, obstetrics, and orthopaedics," as well as taking employment with the Medical Center there (Zarins and Mankin 2001). Not long thereafter, he joined the US Army Medical Corps during World War II. He was drafted as a captain and stationed with the Harvard Unit at the 105th General Hospital in Gatton, Australia. Toward the end of the war, he was sent to Biak Island in the Dutch East Indies and Leyte in the Philippines (see chapter 64).

During this period (1945), he also published his first orthopaedic paper, "Selection of Cases for Arthrotomy of the Knee in an Overseas General Hospital. A Two-Year Follow-Up Study," more than 10 years after he wrote his first paper at HMS. He coauthored the paper with Dr. Edwin F. Cave and Dr. Lester B. K. Yee. They reported their results of 121 knee arthrotomies over a two-year period (1942–1944). They wrote: "Of the 121 cases...sixty-five or 54 per cent. were...uncomplicated meniscus injuries...twenty-three cases or 19 per cent. were...complicated meniscus injuries... [and] thirty-three cases or 27 per cent. were operated upon for other reasons then a torn meniscus" (Cave, Rowe, and Lee 1945).

They further concluded that:

> in order to prognosticate which patients with internal derangement of the knee will return to full duty after operation, careful preoperative evaluation of the patient as a whole is essential.

Surg Clin North Am. 1947 Oct;27:1289-94

Capsular repair for recurrent dislocation of shoulder: pathological findings and operative technic

E F CAVE, C R ROWE

Cave and Rowe's first article in which they describe the Bankart procedure and their initial results in 25 cases.
Surgical Clinics of North America 1947; 27: 1289.

> This involves the sizing up of the individual from the psychological standpoint...[knowing] the mechanism of injury...a...thorough physical examination...[including examining] the opposite or normal knee...for comparison... The vast majority of patients with an uncomplicated meniscus injury can be returned to, and will remain at, full military duty...Patients whose knee disability is due...or complicated by, articular damage or instability...should not be operating upon in an overseas theatre... Exceptions...may be made in so-called 'key personnel' who ...can return to limited service..." (Cave, Rowe, and Lee 1945)

When Rowe returned from the war, he moved to Boston. Cave had offered him a position at MGH, and he accepted an appointment as staff in 1946. He also received a position at Harvard Medical School. That same year, he married Mary Moore, who he had previously courted for seven years. During these initial years at MGH, he "was also involved in the Crippled Children Service in the Commonwealth of Massachusetts, and, as a volunteer, at the Veteran's Hospital [first in Framingham and later in Jamaica Plain]" (Zarins and Mankin 2001).

The following year, Cave and Rowe published their first paper on the shoulder. While stationed together in Australia, they had learned about the Bankart procedure. They observed:

Prior to Bankart's capsular repair, Nicola's operation, consisting of transplanting the biceps tendon through the head and neck of the humerus, was the best operation. This is easily performed, and seemed to be successful in most cases. As years went by, however, there were more and more recurrences because of rupture and fraying out of the transplanted biceps tendon either at its point of exit from the tunnel in the humeral neck or at its point of entrance into the humeral head. The operation advocated by Bankart has appealed to the authors as being the most logical procedure suggested thus far. We also agree with Bankart as to the site of the lesion in the majority of cases. The lesions consistently found have been fracture and fraying of the glenoid labrum and complete separation of the capsule from the glenoid along the anterior and inferior portions...Since the lesions are consistently in one location, is reasonable to carry out the repair at this point...

In our series of twenty-five cases, three related pathologic findings were present: (1) trauma to the cartilaginous glenoid labrum; (2) trauma to the bony rim of the glenoid; (3) separation or shearing off of the capsular attachment...The most consistent finding was trauma to the cartilaginous labrum. This occurred in twenty-one of the twenty-five cases (84 per cent)...Injury to the bony rim of the glenoid was noted in 15 cases (60 per cent)...In fourteen cases (56 per cent) the joint capsule was completely torn from its attachment to the rim of the glenoid. Thirteen of these tears were in the anterior and anterior inferior portion of the glenoid, and one in the superior portion. The separation of the capsule from the glenoid rim may not be recognized easily, and it is well in each case to pass a blunt instrument along the anterior rim of the glenoid to determine the presence or absence of capsular separation...Recurrent posterior dislocations occurred in three of the twenty-five cases (12 per cent). Only one of these presented traumatic changes similar to those found in the anterior dislocations...[After the authors describe the Bankart procedure in detail they concluded:] Closure of the wound is completed with fine cotton or silk [silk later abandoned by Dr. Rowe]. After operation the arm is immobilized with a Velpeau bandage or sling and swath for ten days, and supported with a sling for an additional two weeks. Motion to the horizontal plane is allowed in six weeks and by the end of eight weeks it is expected that there will be only slight restriction in abduction and external rotation which, if permanent, is probably a good thing. (Cave, Rowe, and Lee 1945)

Leader in Shoulder Surgery

Over the next 46 years, Rowe continued to make numerous significant contributions to the field of shoulder surgery. Two-thirds of his publications on the shoulder were about instability and anterior dislocations. In 1956, he published a significant article on prognosis after a shoulder dislocation. He reviewed

admissions over the past twenty years to the Massachusetts General Hospital for shoulder dislocation...[including] patients followed by members of the staff in other hospitals...488 patients (500 shoulders)...The follow-up period

> **The Journal of Bone and Joint Surgery**
> *American Volume*
> Prognosis in Dislocations of the Shoulder *
> BY CARTER REDD ROWE, M.D., BOSTON, MASSACHUSETTS
> *From the Shoulder Clinic, the Massachusetts General Hospital, Boston*
> OCTOBER 1956
> VOL. 38-A, NO. 5

Rowe's article, "Prognosis in Dislocations of the Shoulder."
Journal of Bone and Joint Surgery 1956; 38: 957.

averaged 4.8 years...Dislocations occurred anteriorly in 98 percent and posteriorly in 2 per cent. [He summarized as follows:] In 38 per cent...the dislocation recurred. Primary shoulder dislocations were found to occur as frequently after forty-five years of age as before forty-five. The incidence of recurrent dislocation...was very high in the second decade (92 per cent), but showed marked decrease after age fifty...The age of the patient at the time of the primary...dislocation was the most significant single prognostic factor...Usually the greater the initial injury, the lower was the incidence of recurrence...Fracture of the shoulder girdle was a complication in 24 per cent...[that] of the greater tuberosity was 15 per cent... Humeral head defects were present in 38 per cent of the primary dislocations and in 57 per cent of recurrent dislocations. These were associated with an increase in the incidence of recurrence (82 per cent)...A high incidence of recurrence was noted...[when] there was no immobilization or for whom there were very short periods of immobilization, long periods of immobilization were not associated with a significant decrease in recurrence...Following primary...dislocation, 70 per cent of the dislocations which recurred did so within two years... Following operative...repair...fifty-two per cent recurred within two years...The incidence of posterior dislocation was two per cent...The incidence of bilateral dislocation was 2.4 per cent...[and] the incidence of nerve injury was 5.4 per cent...The incidence of epileptics with shoulder dislocations was 2 per cent. (Rowe 1956)

His results showed that with the Bankart operation, it did not limit external rotation and yet tended to establish that "the Bankart is the better procedure" (Carr 1956).

The following year, Rowe participated in an Academy Instructional Course Lecture on the shoulder with Drs. Aufranc and Barr, and five years later in 1962 presented his Instructional Course Lecture, "Acute and Recurrent Dislocation of the Shoulder." In his lecture he recalled his experience during the war in Australia:

World War II gave orthopaedic surgeons an opportunity to gain more experience in the surgical management of recurrent dislocations of the shoulder. Two methods emerged which were widely accepted and gave excellent results, namely, the Bankart repair and the Putti-Platt repair. Other methods used which gave a low incidence of recurrence were the Magnuson, the Hybbinette-Eden, and the Gallie-Le-Mesurier techniques. The results of all these methods...[indicate] an incidence of recurrence of less than 7 or 8 per cent. The Nicola repair did not fare well in the Army or in younger more active civilians. The experience with this procedure at the Massachusetts General Hospital showed a recurrence rate of 59 per cent. Since World War II, the Dickson procedure has been published but sufficient time has not elapsed for follow-up study. (Rowe 1962)

Dr. Rowe favored the Bankart repair, which he taught to the residents in the Harvard Combined Orthopaedic Residency Program, and he described the specific technical steps he used in his instructional course lecture. He also used, and

The Management of Fractures in Elderly Patients is Different

BY CARTER R. ROWE, M.D.*, BOSTON, MASSACHUSETTS

An Instructional Course Lecture, The American Academy of Orthopaedic Surgeons

THE JOURNAL OF BONE AND JOINT SURGERY
VOL. 47-A, NO. 5, JULY 1965

Rowe's AAOS instructional course on management of fractures in the elderly. *Journal of Bone and Joint Surgery* 1965; 47: 1043.

emphasized, the importance of cotton sutures; refusing to use silk. At this time Rowe was listed as visiting orthopaedic surgeon at the MGH and instructor of orthopaedic surgery at Harvard Medical School.

By 1963, he was recognized as a leader in the field of shoulder surgery. He published five papers that year in an edition of the Surgical Clinics of North America. He also occasionally published a paper on fractures. His classic was "The Management Of Fractures in Elderly Patients is Different," an Instructional Course in 1965. **Box 40.15** includes a description of his course.

"Over the years...Dr. Rowe gradually concentrated more and more on shoulder injuries and in the 1980s focused chiefly on shoulder problems. He had always been interested in the contribution...of Ernest A. Codman, who had written a major textbook on shoulder surgery. Carter Rowe's greatest impact was in the area of his specialty [interest]. Specifically, he developed the techniques and instruments used in the Bankart repair, a procedure that he helped to perfect and popularize. He was also a pioneer in elucidating the concepts, findings, and management of a traumatic and voluntary shoulder instability" (Zarins and Mankin 2001).

Dr. Rowe was also exceptionally active in the American Academy of Orthopaedic Surgeons (AAOS) and the American Orthopaedic Association (AOA). He "was responsible for developing and publicizing a widely used method for musculoskeletal examination and measurement" as chairman of the AAOS Committee on Joint Motion. In

---

Box 40.15. Dr. Carter Rowe's Classic Fractures in the Elderly Course

The below is a description of Dr. Rowe's classic fracture course, "The Management of Fractures in Elderly Patients is Different," in his own words:

"Several years ago, I [Dr. Rowe] inserted an Austin Moore prosthesis in a patient, eighty-four years old, for a fractured femoral neck. Postoperatively she became completely unmanageable and disoriented. Restraints were needed to keep her in bed. The patient was promptly sent home to household nursing care. Several days later, when I visited her at home, I was surprised to find her sitting up playing cards with her sister. Her disorientation had cleared up completely, she was understanding, cooperative, and apparently quite happy. I am certain that if this patient had remained in the hospital she would have died.

"With these principles in mind, I have found it very helpful to group fractures of elderly patients into four treatment categories: 1. Minimum immobilization; 2. Plaster Immobilization; 3. Traction and suspension; 4. Open surgery of some form, with or without internal fixation. Fractures requiring minimum immobilization[:] The majority of fractures of the surgical neck of the humerus...vertebral compression fractures...most fractures of the pelvis except involving the acetabulum...olecranon fractures ...impacted fractures of the femoral neck...Other fractures[:] Selected Colles', tibial-condyle, and calcaneal fractures...Fractures requiring immobilzation in a plaster cast[:] The majority of humeral shaft fractures...forearm and wrist fractures...selected tibial-condyle fractures...Fractures which may do best if treated with traction and suspension[:]...supracondylar [femur] fractures...fractures of the mid femoral shaft... intertrochanteric fractures. Fractures in which open surgery is indicated[:] Hip. Internal fixation of fractures of the femoral neck was perhaps one of the greatest advances in the treatment of fractures during the past three decades... Internal fixation of...pathological fractures of long bones... [and] traumatic fractures of long bones...Surgical resection of the fracture...olecranon...femoral head...

"Summary. 1. The primary aims in the management of fractures in the aged should be relief of pain, mobilization as soon as possible, and return to normal environment and activities within a reasonable time. 2. Discussions concerning fracture management should be based on the psychological and physical condition of the patient before injury. 3. Careful consideration must be given to the specific, and sometimes narrow, needs and functional limitations of the patient."

(Rowe 1965)

Box 40.16. Dr. Carter Rowe's Presidential Address to the American Orthopaedic Association in 1969

"Increased communications have naturally led to discussions, shared intents, and cooperative action by the combined Associations. The adoption by the six Associations...in 1964...developed by the American Academy of Orthopaedic Surgeons...[and] accepted *in toto* by the International Society of Orthopaedic Surgery and Traumatology...in October, 1969.

"A second cooperative action...in 1966, when the American Board of Orthopaedic Surgery began conversations with the British Orthopaedic Association relative to reviewing and coordinating the orthopaedic training programs...If agreement is attained by the six Associations, it is conceivable that...these decisions and standards may be considered and accepted on a broad international basis.

"During the coming ten years, our activities in the field of education should be expanded further through the medium of Exchange Fellowships...The singular success of the A.B.C. [American, British, Canadian] Exchange Program, begun in 1948, is an excellent example of what can be accomplished with careful planning and funding... There is a great need at present for coordinating our diverse orthopaedic information storage and retrieval systems...

"Among our member countries in the past ten years, there has been a rapid development of basic and clinical research programs...It is apparent that much could be gained if our Associations will establish standing committees to correlate their respective activities...In the United States in 1967, orthopaedic problems ranked seventh among the causes of patient visits to the physician and accounted for 10 per cent of...hospital admissions. With certainty that these percentages will increase...our combined Associations should give thorough study to the quality of health services and to the supply of orthopaedic manpower in our six countries.

"Rapid increase in the scientific contributions over the past ten years is...reflected in [publications]...In 1973... [The Journal of Bone and Joint Surgery] received from the American Medical Writers Association The Honor Award for Distinguished Service in Medical Journalism among Specialty Journals...For the present.. our six Associations [should] continue to coordinate our activities and compare our scientific contributions under the aegis of The Journal of Bone and Joint Surgery...

"In closing...I would encourage the American Orthopaedic Association and our member Associations to consider the establishment of appropriate standing committees on education, research and health services in each Association...meeting at specific intervals to coordinate and continue the study of problems and activities in these... areas...No reciprocal action taken by our Combined Associations would more enrich our specialty, nor foster greater friendships, than an active, growing Exchange Fellowship Program...We have recognized the need for increased communication and cooperation-- our challenge lies in expanding and strengthening these bonds."

(Rowe 1970)

1964, he had served as treasurer of the AAOS, and he was elected president of the AOA from 1969 until 1970, "presiding over that organization's Fifth Combined Meeting in Sidney, Australia in 1970" (Zarins and Mankin 2001). His presidential address was titled, "The Challenge to Orthopaedics in the English-Speaking World." His talk was a historical one. It focused first on the early development of orthopaedics in the United States and England; then on the origins and development of the American Orthopaedic Association, the Australian Orthopaedic Association, the South African Orthopaedic Association, the Canadian Orthopaedic Association, and the New Zealand Orthopaedic Assocation; followed by the growth of orthopaedic surgery in the US, Britain, and Canada; and finally he made comments on the present and future. **Box 40.16** provides an excerpt of his speech.

In 1973, with Drs. Donald Pierce and John G. Clark, he continued his research on the shoulder and reported on 26 patients who could voluntarily dislocate their shoulders (see **Case 40.18**). They wrote:

Dislocation was produced by suppression of one element of one of the muscle force-couples responsible for shoulder motion...most patients responded well to muscle-strengthening exercises...[but] patients with significant psychiatric problems did poorly after all types of surgical and non-operative treatment unless their psychiatric problem had been resolved... If surgical treatment was undertaken, a combination of procedures was necessary rather than one of the standard operations...

From this study...the following tentative conclusions were reached: 1. This syndrome begins most frequently in early childhood or adolescence. 2. The displacement of the humeral head, anteriorly, posteriorly, or inferiorly, is usually painless and is produced atraumatically by voluntary muscle action. 3. Intra-articular injury...does not occur. There is consistent absence of both the Bankart and the Hill-Sachs lesions...4. The syndrome occurs twice as frequently in males as in females. 5. Psychiatric interviews...showed that eight [of 26 patients] had definite unsolved psychiatric character problems...and eighteen did not...6. There was a significant difference in the response to treatment...Both operative and conservative treatment...[in those with unsolved psychiatric character problems]...carried a poor prognosis. In...[the other group] the prognosis was uniformly favorable, with either conservative or operative treatment. (Rowe, Pierce, and Clark 1973)

Rowe and colleagues' report on voluntary dislocation of the shoulder. *Journal of Bone and Joint Surgery* 1973; 55: 445.

Case 40.18. Voluntary Dislocation of the Shoulder

"A female oxygen therapist stated that she began dislocating her left shoulder at the age of eight and her right shoulder at age fourteen. During her initial examination she demonstrated that she could voluntarily dislocate both shoulders anteriorly, posteriorly, and inferiorly. At this time she was under the care of a psychiatrist in a nearby city with whom we maintained close contact. She repeatedly presented herself to us, requesting surgical relief of her shoulder problems which, she stated, eliminated her ability to work in the hospital or to carry out many physical activities. Her psychiatrist had identified her condition as acute schizophrenia. At one time she threatened suicide unless her shoulders were operated upon. However, with competent psychiatric help, continuing interest manifested by her physicians, and a program of shoulder exercises, the patient gradually improved, ceased dislocating her shoulders and returned to work. For the past five years she has had no shoulder complaints, has work regularly and is quite happy. Her psychiatrist identified her request for shoulder surgery as a compulsive reaction for self-mutilation."

(Rowe, Pierce, and Clark 1973)

Doctor for the Bruins

In 1976, more than 10 years after Rowe had begun to be recognized as a leader in the field of athletic injuries, he continued to concentrate his practice in shoulder surgery. His specialization occurred in sync with the establishment of the Sports Medicine Service at MGH. A sports journalist had anointed him with the moniker "Cool Hand Luke...after he had operated on one of the Bruin's players...A master surgeon... [he placed an] emphasis on surgical procedures that respected and restored anatomy. He was an advocate of early postoperative motion" (Zarins and Mankin 2001). He "was a devoted fan of the

Box 40.17. Rowe's Memories as Team Orthopaedic Surgeon for the Boston Bruins

In Lest We Forget, Rowe remembered:

"[A]n amusing incident [abduction of Phil Esposito]... During the period 1969 to 1972 when the Boston Bruins had won two Stanley Cups within three years...in a game against the New York rangers at the Boston Garden, Phil Esposito had fallen when a Ranger player...landed on his outstretched, internally rotated right leg. Those close by... could hear his knee crunch. I saw him immediately afterwards in the emergency ward at MGH. He knew his knee was badly injured, but pleaded to go home...He had never been in a hospital before...I had to impress on Phil that the ligaments of his knee were seriously torn and that his career as a hockey player depended on a strong, stable knee. In spite of his reservations he consented to being admitted and...surgery. The next day we repaired the torn ligaments...Postoperatively his right leg was immobilized in a long-leg plaster cast and suspended in a Balkan frame. When making evening rounds on the third postoperative day, I received an emergency call: 'Dr. Rowe, please call Phillips House 5. Urgent.' I called...'Dr. Rowe, I don't know what to say – Phil Esposito is not in his room, and neither is his bed!' 'I'll be right up.'

"True enough--not a sign of Phil, nor his bed, in the room. Just at this time we heard that a patient in a Balkan frame bed was being hurriedly pushed through the main corridor of the hospital and out of the North entrance. Another report quickly followed that a bed with a patient in it, and a number of escorts, was seen entering the Branding Iron Bar, across the street from the hospital. I immediately called the Branding Iron. Bobby Orr answered the telephone, 'Doc, don't worry, we are handling Phil just like a baby. He's having a beer, and we will be back in fifteen minutes.' Actually they were back in fifteen minutes with one wheel of the bed missing, but otherwise with the passenger and leg in acceptable shape...In early evening one of the players...[had posed] as a detective, called the nurses station with the request for a chart search for a possible criminal in the hospital. Phil's colleagues had time to roll Phil and his bed with its frame out to the waiting elevator, down to the main corridor, and out of the hospital. Phil said he was 'frightened to death' and covered his head with a blanket. The north door of the hospital was broken a bit getting the bed and large frame out...The Boston Globe headline the next morning, 'Patient abducted from Massachusetts General Hospital in his bed,' was followed by an article with many theories of what must have taken place...I reported it at rounds that day, simply as a 'patient complication.'"

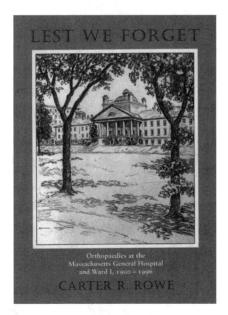

Cover of Rowe's book on the history of orthopaedics at MGH from 1900 to 1996. Courtesy of Bauhan Publishing.

Boston Bruins" ("Carter Rowe, 94; Doctor for Bruins") and the team's orthopaedic surgeon for years. He operated on many players including Phil Esposito and Bobby Orr, and John Hannah of the New England Patriots. In **Box 40.17**, Rowe recalls his experiences.

Culmination of 30 Years of Research

Three years later, in 1978, Rowe published his personal long-term results of Bankart's operation in 161 patients over a 30-year period (1946–1976). "The results...were rated excellent in 74 per cent, good in 23 per cent, and poor in 3 per cent. Ninety-eight per cent of the patients rated their result as excellent or good. Sixty-nine per cent... had a full range of motion, and only 2 percent...

redislocated...We concluded that with meticulous technique...postoperative immobilization is not necessary, early return of motion and function can be expected, and resumption of athletic activities with no limitation of shoulder motion is possible for most patients" (Rowe, Patel, and Southmayed 1978). In this paper the authors included Dr. Rowe's rating system for instability of the shoulder with which he evaluated all his patients after a Bankart repair (see **Table 40.4**.)

Table 40.4. Rating Sheet for Bankart Repair

Scoring System	Units	Excellent (100-90)	Good (89-75)	Fair (74-51)	Poor (50 or Less)
Stability					
No recurrence, subluxation of apprehension	50	No recurrences	No recurrences	No recurrences	Recurrence of dislocation
					or
Apprehension when placing arm in certain positions	30	No apprehension when placing arm in complete elevation and external rotation	Mild apprehension when placing arm in elevation and external rotation	Moderate apprehension during elevation and external rotation	Marked apprehension during elevation or extension
Subluxation (not requiring reduction)	10	No subluxations	No subluxations	No subluxations	
Recurrent dislocation	0				
Motion					
100% of normal external rotation, internal rotation, and elevation	20	100% of normal external rotation; complete elevation and internal rotation	75% of normal external rotation; complete elevation and internal rotation	50% of normal external rotation; 75% of elevation and internal rotation	No external rotation; 50% of elevation (can get hand only to face) and 50% of internal rotation
75% of normal eternal rotation, and normal elevation and internal rotation	15				
50% of normal external rotation and 75% of normal elevation and internal rotation	5				
50% of normal elevation and internal rotation; no external rotation	0				
Function					
No limitation in work or sports; little or no discomfort	30	Performs all work and sports; no limitation in overhead activities; shoulder strong in lifting, swimming, tennis, throwing; no discomfort	Mild limitation in work and sports; shoulder strong; minimum discomfort	Moderate limitation doing overhead work and heavy lifting; unable to throw, serve hard in tennis, or swim; moderate disabling pain	Marked limitation; unable to perform overhead work and lifting; cannot throw, play tennis, or swim; chronic discomfort
Mild limitation and minimum discomfort	25				
Moderate limitation and discomfort	10				
Marked limitation and pain	0				
Total units possible	100				

(Rowe, Patel, and Southmayed 1978).

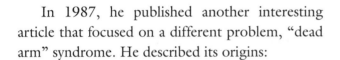

Rowe and colleagues' article on his long-term outcomes of the Bankart procedure in 161 patients. *Journal of Bone and Joint Surgery* 1978; 60: 1.

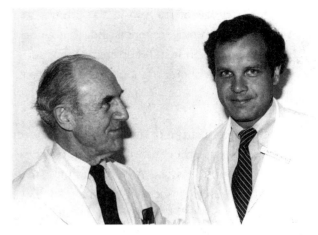

Dr. Rowe (left) with his new associate, Dr. Zarins. Courtesy of Bertram Zarins.

In 1987, he published another interesting article that focused on a different problem, "dead arm" syndrome. He described its origins:

> The author's introduction to the 'dead arm' syndrome happened in the early 1960s when a jockey sought help because he could not use a riding crop…[following] an extension injury to his arm when he fell from his horse. As he raised his arm to reach backward, he experienced a sudden pain and weakness in his shoulder, which eliminated his ability to strike the horse's flank. All studies and examinations had been negative…[from] experts across the country. His request [to Dr. Rowe]…was direct: "Doctor, I'm not paid to ride; I'm paid to win. Would you look into my shoulder? If you don't find anything, I'm no worse off. If you find something, maybe it can be fixed and I can ride again"…Before the advent of arthroscopy… the author explored his shoulder, and to his surprise, found a large Bankart lesion. It was repaired…and the jockey returned to riding and winning races again. (Rowe 1987)

He then referred to his publication in 1981, "Recurrent Transient Subluxation of the Shoulder," coauthored with Dr. Bertram Zarins, in which he concluded:

> Transient subluxation of the shoulder may cause the so-called dead-arm syndrome… characterized by sudden sharp or 'paralyzing' pain when the shoulder is moved forcibly into a position of maximum external rotation in elevation or is subjected to a direct blow. This syndrome may also occur during throwing, repetitive forceful serving in tennis, or working with the arm in a strained position above shoulder level…Two groups of patients were identified…Group I [26 patients] …[had a] sensation that subluxation was occurring when they used the arm in elevation…Group II [32 patients]… were not aware of slipping out or instability of the shoulder…
>
> A Bankart procedure was performed in thirty-two shoulders in which a Bankart lesion was found, and a modified Bankart repair (capsulorrhaphy) was done in the remaining eighteen…Results…70 per cent excellent, 24 per cent good, and 6 per cent fair. Ten shoulders were treated by non-surgical means. (Rowe and Zarins 1981)

He further noted that:

> In the active athlete, who has…experienced a forceful overextension of his elevated arm, followed by…persistent pain and weakness in

the forceful use of his arm in the position of throwing, swimming, or tennis and…has a positive apprehension test, recurrent anterior subluxation of the shoulder should be considered.
(Rowe 1987)

Anterior subluxation of the shoulder can occur in athletes who use their arm in forceful overhead activities. In some, with a previous injury (tear) to the anteroinferior glenoid labrum (Bankart lesion), such repeated activities may result in partial subluxation of the joint. With the episode of partial subluxation, the athlete may experience the "dead-arm syndrome"; i.e., sharp or "paralyzing" pain in the arm. It is usually transient but recurrent with the activity. Rowe identified the lesion early (the 1960s) and was successful in treating these patients with a Bankart repair. He and Zarins reported 94% good/excellent results.

Legacy

Dr. Carter Rowe retired at 85 after a lengthy career at MGH and Harvard Medical School. For the majority of his time on the Harvard faculty, he had been an instructor in orthopaedic surgery. Eventually Dr. Henry Mankin had supported his promotion to associate clinical professor. Rowe:

> epitomized the finest qualities of a physician and surgeon. He was truly a caring person who treated everyone with kindness, dignity and respect. He was a wonderful teacher who was admired and remembered by the residents and staff at Massachusetts General Hospital and the faculty at Harvard Medical School for the fifty years that he was associated with them.
> (Zarins and Mankin 2001)

Throughout his career, he published over 50 articles; 29 involved the shoulder, which was his favorite specialty of choice. In 1988, he had published his textbook, *The Shoulder*, a seminal work in the field.

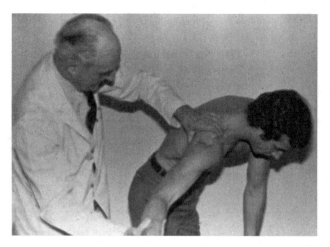

Dr. Rowe examining a patient's shoulder. Courtesy of Bertram Zarins.

Author Recollections

I fondly remember an evening with my wife, Gerry, in the home of Dr. and Mrs. Rowe for dinner. They showed us the sincere warmth of southern hospitality. Dr. Rowe was very proud of his achievement of becoming president of the American Orthopaedic Association, and he showed me his presidential medallion, while at the same time encouraging me to work hard and follow in his footsteps.

Rowe was an active member of numerous organizations, including various local, state, national, and international associations. He was an honorary member of the British and Australian Orthopaedic Associations, and he served as trustee of the Orthopaedic Research and Educational Foundation. He was also "a founding member of the American Orthopaedic Society for Sports Medicine (1972), [and] a founding member and the second President of the Shoulder and Elbow Surgeons (1984)" (Zarins and Mankin 2001).

After returning to his birthplace Fredericksburg, Rowe authored the book *Lest We Forget, Orthopaedics at the Massachusetts General Hospital and Ward I, 1900-1996*. A review assessed the book:

This book invokes memories of those who have gone before us in the field of orthopaedic surgery…Rowe…describes his life as a resident and a staff member at the Massachusetts General Hospital over the years. This is an interesting book. Perhaps it will even make the reader think about the past, an activity rarely indulged in these days, and learn for the future. (Rangaswamy 1996)

He died a few years later, at 94 years old, on June 25, 2001 in his home. He was survived by his wife, Mary, and their three sons. He was remembered fondly and held in great esteem by his colleagues:

He was extraordinary in his support for the Orthopaedic Service at Massachusetts General Hospital. Never upset or angry, Dr. Rowe was always positive in his reactions to and his relationships with people. With a charming manner and a wonderful sense of humor, he was always supportive of his students and colleagues. He selflessly helped them to deal with problems. Never petty, never parochial…[he] was a man of character with a clear vision for the future of orthopaedic surgery. (Zarins and Mankin 2001)

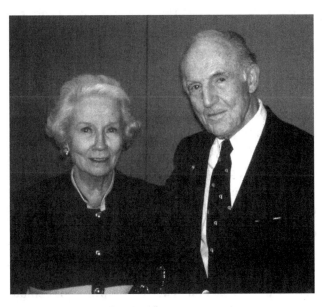

Dr. Rowe and his wife, Mary. Courtesy of Bertram Zarins.

MORTEN SMITH PETERSEN

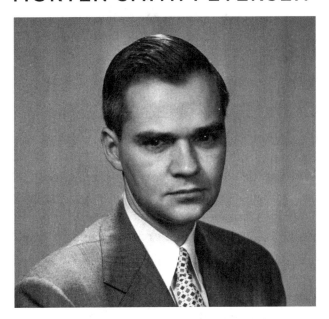

Morten Smith-Petersen. Massachusetts General Hospital, Archives and Special Collections.

Physician Snapshot

Morten Smith-Petersen
BORN: 1920
DIED: 1999
SIGNIFICANT CONTRIBUTIONS: Specialized in hip surgery; an excellent technician

Morten Smith-Petersen, the son of Dr. Marius N. Smith-Petersen (see chapter 37), was named Morten after his grandfather. He was born in ca. 1920 in Newton, Massachusetts. In 1942, he graduated from Amherst College, and in 1945 he received his MD degree from the University of Rochester Medical School in New York. He remained in the US Naval Reserves following graduation from medical school until 1953.

As a resident, I recall seeing Dr. Smith-Petersen occasionally at MGH when he was an assistant in orthopaedics in the 1960s. Dr. Joseph Barr Jr. recalled in an interview that when he was a resident he had operated with Smith-Petersen. Barr was unsure of Morten's training, but he believed it was in the MGH/Boston Children's Hospital Combined Program. He also recalled that Smith-Petersen limited his practice to hip surgery and was an excellent technician. On one occasion, Smith-Petersen, while being assisted by Dr. Barr Jr. completed a bilateral cup arthroplasty in less than two hours.

In about the middle of his career, Smith-Petersen moved his practice to the Brigham and the Baptist Hospitals. He joined the staff at the New England Baptist Hospital in 1968 and in 1973 was elected a member of the corporation. He had academic appointments at Harvard Medical School as instructor and at Tufts Medical School as assistant clinical professor. I recall one brief conversation with Smith-Petersen in which he stated that he never came to the hospital early for rounds or surgery because he never knew his dad while growing up because his dad had worked long hours. He therefore made a commitment to have breakfast with his family each morning, often taking his children to school before visiting the hospital.

I was able to find only one publication coauthored by Smith-Petersen; a letter to the editor of *Lancet* in 1974, "Sensitivity to Intrafat Heparin." The authors reported a patient reaction to bovine-derived heparin that seemed to be a local immune complex induced vasculitis, and that such a reaction, although rare, should at times be expected during hip replacement surgery. In all, they treated 18 patients with intrafat heparin prophylaxis after total hip replacement. Although no patients developed a significant venous thrombosis, 10 did develop a local hematoma and in seven of those patients the hematoma was major. Three of these seven patients subsequently had a pulmonary embolism demonstrated on lung scan after heparin therapy was discontinued. Smith-Petersen and colleagues argued the evidence was against using this method of prophylaxis for patients undergoing a total hip replacement.

Dr. Morten Smith-Petersen retired and moved to St. Petersburg, Florida. He died on Friday, July 30, 1999, at the age of 79; he was survived by his wife Evelyn (Leeming), two sons, and three daughters.

O. SHERWIN STAPLES

Physician Snapshot

O. Sherwin Staples
BORN: 1908
DIED: 2002
SIGNIFICANT CONTRIBUTIONS: Head of the orthopaedic section at Dartmouth Medical School and the Mary Hitchcock Memorial Hospital from 1946 to 1970

Oscar Sherwin Staples Jr., who preferred his name without the suffix "Jr.," was born in Boston on May 19, 1908, to Oscar S. and Nellie E. (Barnes) Staples. As a student at Harvard College, he participated in rowing, as the bow. Staples was on the 1927 Harvard crew team that lost to the teams from the University of Pennsylvania and MIT on the Charles River at Cambridge and took third place in the American Henley rowing competition. He graduated with a bachelor of arts degree in 1930 and continued on to Harvard Medical School, receiving an MD degree in 1935. After a two-year internship at Boston City Hospital (1935–37) and orthopaedic residency training in the Children's Hospital/Massachusetts General Hospital (1937–1939), he joined Dr. Edwin Cave's private practice in 1939. That year he also joined the staff at MGH as an assistant in orthopaedic surgery and at the New England Peabody Home for Crippled Children (**Case 40.19** highlights an example of a case he treated while there); he worked at both institutions until 1946. While in Boston, Staples published three articles, including one in 1941 with Cave titled "Congenital Discord Meniscus, a Cause of Internal Derangement of the Knee."

In 1942, early during World War II, he served as a captain in the army; he was posted to the 6th General Hospital with Dr. Otto Aufranc and others from MGH (see chapter 64). While in Europe (most likely in Rome), Captain Staples met Mable Hughes, a nurse anesthetist from Atlanta, Georgia, who worked at Grady Memorial Hospital and Emory University. They were married on

December 11, 1945, and at the end of that month Staples resigned his position at MGH.

The couple moved to New Hampshire so Staples could take the position of head of the orthopaedic section at Dartmouth Medical School and the Mary Hitchcock Memorial Hospital in 1946. Charles F. Carr, in his 2020 description of the history of the orthopaedic residency program at the Dartmouth Hitchcock Medical Center, designated Staples as the first orthopaedic surgeon to

Case 40.19. Osteochondritis in a Finger

> "[The patient], a girl aged two years and one month, was admitted on October 19, 1938, to The New England Peabody Home for Crippled Children with the diagnosis of tuberculosis of the spine. Five months previously, the mother had noted prominence of the lumbar spine, followed in three months by occasional pain.
>
> "The physical examination upon admission was negative, except for prominent mid-lumbar kyphosis, a cold abscess palpable in the left flank, and moderate psoas spasm on the left. Roentgenograms of the spine showed a destructive process characteristic of tuberculosis, involving the third, fourth, and fifth lumbar vertebral bodies. Roentgenograms of the chest were normal. The tuberculin test was positive in a 1 to 10,000 dilution.
>
> "The patient was treated by bed rest in a bivalved plaster jacket until February 1941, two and one-third years after admission. During the first six months that the patient was in the hospital there was a slight increase in the destructive process, as shown by roentgenographic examination, but subsequently the destructive phase stopped, and recalcification and regeneration of bone began. At the end of the first year of treatment, the patient's general condition was good.
>
> "Fifteen months after entry, the cold abscess present in the girl's left flank ruptured spontaneously. The resulting sinus healed after five months. There was no evidence of secondary infection at any time. Guinea-pig inoculation with material from the abscess was negative, but, because of the clinical course and other findings, the diagnosis of tuberculosis was maintained.
>
> "In February 1941, the patient was allowed to be ambulatory in a back brace. She was given gradually increasing periods of activity each day with no resulting ill effects.
>
> "In May 1941, two and one-half years after entry into the hospital, the patient, then four years and eight months old, complained of pain in her right index finger. As far as could be determined, there had been no previous finger symptoms or trauma of any sort. Examination revealed redness, tenderness, and swelling, confined to the region of the distal interphalangeal joint, with no evident joint effusion. The motions of the finger were normal.
>
> "Roentgenograms of the hand showed that the epiphysis of the distal phalanx of the right index finger was smaller and dense than normal. Roentgenographic study of the spine showed no evident activity of the tuberculous process. The disease appeared quiescent, with questionable spontaneous fusion of two of the vertebral bodies involved.
>
> "A splint was applied which held the affected finger in extension. The splint was removed after two weeks, when symptoms had disappeared and the hand had apparently become completely normal. No further treatment was given. There were no further symptoms or signs in the finger during the following nineteen months.
>
> "During this period the patient's general condition remained excellent.
>
> "In January 1942, a spine fusion was performed, which had been postponed previously because of the respiratory infection.
>
> "Four months after operation, the girl was again allowed to be ambulatory in a back brace, and her further hospital course was uneventful.
>
> "Roentgenographic studies of the affected finger were repeated at intervals during the nineteen months following the onset of finger symptoms. Gradual improvement was noted in repeated roentgenograms, and, after five months, the previously abnormal epiphysis was entirely normal in appearance. Final roentgenograms taken in December 1942 show no difference in the two hands."
>
> (O. Sherwin Staples 1943)

practice in the state of New Hampshire. (According to Carr, Dr. Stuart Russell came from Michigan in 1948 to become the second practicing orthopaedic surgeon there.) Three years after beginning his work at Mary Hitchcock, Staples began the process of creating an orthopaedic residency program there. He applied twice to the American Board of Orthopaedic Surgery but was unsuccessful. It wasn't until 1957 that the ABOS approved Staples's request, and he developed an orthopaedic residency training program there in earnest. Staples held his position as head of the orthopaedic section for ~27 years and residency program director for 16 years. He stepped down in 1973, turning over his administrative functions to his successor, Dr. Leland Hall. For the next eight years, he served as chief of orthopaedics at the VA Hospital in White River Junction, Vermont. In 1981, he became a consultant at the VA Hospital and retired in 1992. During his time at Dartmouth he published another 12 articles. He died on December 2, 2002, at 94 years old.

GEORGE W. VAN GORDER

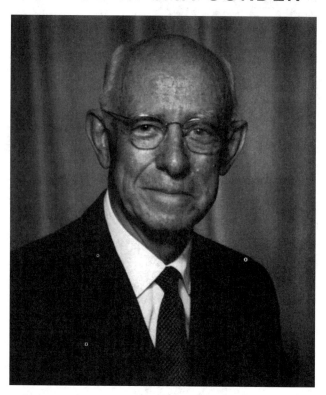

George W. Van Gorder. E.F.C., "George Wilson Van Gorder, M.D. 1888-1969," *Journal of Bone and Joint Surgery* 1970; 52: 608.

Physician Snapshot

George W. Van Gorder
BORN: 1888
DIED: 1969

SIGNIFICANT CONTRIBUTIONS: Served as co-chief of the MGH Fracture Service (1934–40); served as vice-president of the American Orthopaedic Association (1949); modified the Trumble technique for hip fusion

---

Born in 1888, George Wilson Van Gorder grew up in Pittsburgh, Pennsylvania. George had an older sister who went to China as a missionary; from a young age George wanted to follow that same path. Beginning in 1907, he attended Williams College in Williamstown, Massachusetts, where "he was an excellent student and a good athlete, being among other things captain of the hockey team" (Cave 1970). During one hockey game Van Gorder "injured his hip…and pain and limp gradually developed" (Cave 1970). Van Gorder's first diagnosis was tuberculosis, but after a few months of these symptoms Van Gorder saw Dr. Elliott G. Brackett, who at the time was the chief of orthopaedic surgery at Massachusetts General Hospital. Brackett:

> had the courage to explore the hip. He found no tuberculosis but a large spur, the result of injury, which, upon removal, gave almost complete relief of pain. George lived the remaining years of his life essentially free from disability. During his convalescence from his hip operation, exercises were prescribed and his senior by one year, M.N. Smith-Petersen, assisted George with his exercises and saw to it that the patient did them every day. (Cave 1970)

During his undergraduate years, Van Gorder spent the summer months with "Sir Wilfred Grenfell in his mission in Labrador and Newfoundland" (Cave 1970), providing medical care and various social services to the people living in rural communities there. He graduated from Williams College in 1911 and matriculated at Harvard Medical School, graduating in 1915. The Peter Bent Brigham Hospital had begun operations in 1913, while Van Gorder had been in medical school; upon graduating from Harvard he became one of the early surgical interns there.

Van Gorder joined the US Army Medical Corps with the rank of captain and began active duty on July 12, 1917, in the thick of World War I. In August he was stationed at Camp Greenleaf, Fort Oglethorpe. By September, he was transferred to Camp Meade. On October 9, 1917, he sailed to Liverpool. He was stationed at the 3rd Southern General Hospital in Oxford until June 1918; at Shepherd's Bush Orthopaedic Hospital in London from June to November 1918; and then at Base Hospital #8 in Savenay, France from November 1918 to May 1919. Van Gorder returned to the United States in May 1919 and was discharged on August 1, 1919, about two years after he had entered active duty.

Van Gorder must have continued to hold on to his early wish to follow his sister to China. After being discharged from the army, he got the opportunity to go "as associate professor of orthopaedic surgery at the Rockefeller Foundation Medical School in Peking [Peiping or Peking Union Medical College]" (Cave 1970). During his time at the Peking Union Medical College, Van Gorder published three papers in Chinese medical journals; one paper on an orthopaedic topic (the use of a plaster pylon in leg amputations); and one paper in the *Annals of Surgery*. He also met and married his wife, Helen R. Gorforth. He remained in that role in China for a decade. Upon their return to the United States in 1929, the Van Gorder family settled in Boston, where Van Gorder began private practice as an orthopaedic surgeon with Marius Smith-Petersen. He also became a member of the staff at the Lakeville State Sanatorium, the New England Deaconess Hospital, and the Newton-Wellesley Hospital. He was head of the state's Crippled Children's Clinic in Brockton, Massachusetts, and was assigned by their General Executive Committee to a specialized clinic in disorders of the peripheral circulation (recognized years ago by Dr. Charles Painter). His main affiliation, however, was with the Department of Orthopaedic Surgery at MGH, where he was initially appointed assistant orthopaedic surgeon and Harvard Medical School; at the latter he was an instructor in orthopaedic surgery. According to the 1929 report from the General Executive Committee:

> Dr. Marius N. Smith-Petersen has been promoted to the position of Chief of the Orthopaedic Department. Dr. Philip D. Wilson to the position of Orthopaedic Surgeon, Dr. Armin Klein and Dr. William A. Rogers to the position of Assistant Orthopaedic Surgeons, and Dr. Edwin F. Cave to the position of Orthopaedic Surgeon to Out-Patients. We have been fortunate indeed in adding to our staff the following men: Dr. George W. Van Gorder as Assistant

Orthopaedic Surgeon; Dr. Sumner Roberts and Dr. Joseph Barr as Assistants. (Washburn 1939)

His first publication upon returning to MGH from China was the classic paper, "Intracapsular Fractures of the Neck of the Femur; Treatment by Internal Fixation," which he cowrote with Smith-Petersen and Cave. Most of his subsequent nine papers would also deal with fractures. By 1932, he had been back in the United States for three years and had established himself in Boston. His time in China continued to influence his practice, however, and that year he published an article in the *Journal of Bone and Joint Surgery* on chronic posterior elbow dislocations that he had treated in China (see **Case 40.20**). Van Gorder became active on the fracture service at MGH, and in 1934 was named associate or co-chief of the service (Dr. Henry Marble was chief); he held that position until 1940.

Case 40.20. Surgery for an Old Elbow Dislocation

"Shang Teh Sheng, a Chinese soldier, age forty, fell from his horse three weeks before admission to the hospital, sustaining a severe injury to his right elbow, which he had held in a position of extension and supination when he attempted to break the force of his fall. Following the accident he noted that this elbow was stiff and very painful and at the same time swelling of the entire arm appeared, which subsided after a period of ten days.

"Ten days prior to admission to the hospital he had had his elbow joint manipulated repeatedly by some Army surgeons in an effort to flex the forearm, but all attempts were unsuccessful and he was still unable to use the right arm. Family history and past history were irrelevant.

"*Physical Examination*: Outside of the local surgical condition, there was nothing unusual in the general physical examination. The patient's right arm was held in a position of 175 degrees at the elbow joint with a limited range of flexion and extension of ten degrees. Pronation and supination were also markedly limited. In the cubital fossa was a mass which on palpation was considered to be the lower end of the humerus. The olecranon process of the ulna was higher than normal. There was about one-half inch of shortening of the right arm. Examination for possible nerve injury revealed anesthesia of the ulner side of the right hand with inability to abduct and adduct the fingers, and definite weakness of the ring and little fingers.

"*Diagnosis*: A clinical diagnosis of 'posterior dislocation of the right elbow with ulnar nerve injury' was made. X-ray report stated 'complete backward dislocation of the elbow joint without gross fracture, but with slight new bone production, presumably a result of periosteal stripping from the lateral epicondyle.'

"*Preoperative Notes*: An attempt at closed reduction of the dislocation was made under ether anesthesia, care being taken not to fracture the olecranon tip. The result was a failure. Following manipulation, the arm was protected and placed at rest to allow for the subsidence of swelling. Two weeks later operation was performed.

"*Operation*: Open reduction of old irreducible dislocation of the right elbow. Autogenous tendon graft from tendo achillis to triceps tendon.

"*Postoperative Course*: First dressing on the tenth day, stitches removed. Wound healed *per primum*. Cast discarded. Arm held in acute flexion by Jones sling. Gentle motion started. Postoperative x-ray report states that the bones of the joint are now in normal position.

"*Discharge Note*: Patient left the hospital one month after operation and continued physiotherapy for another month, when he was forced to return to his regiment. At this time, examination showed flexion to be perfect, rotation perfect, and extension 165 degrees. The ulnar nerve weakness showed evidence of improvement.

"*Follow-up*: One year after operation the patient was again examined. His right elbow showed almost perfect function with the exception of ten degrees' limitation of extension. The transplanted tendon was functioning very well and voluntary extension, although not quite so strong as on the normal side, was satisfactory and increasing in degree."

(Van Gorder 1932)

Van Gorder's article "Treatment of Acute Fractures of the Neck of the Femur." *Journal of the American Medical Association* 1948; 137: 1181.

Van Gorder reported his successful results using the Trumble extra-articular technique to fuse the hips in 13 patients with tuberculosis of the hip. *Journal of Bone and Joint Surgery* 1949; 31: 717.

In 1935, Van Gorder was promoted to assistant visiting orthopaedic surgeon at MGH, and, after two years, he became a visiting orthopaedic surgeon. In 1938, Dr. Wilson published the textbook *Fractures and Dislocations*; Van Gorder had contributed three chapters on fractures of different segments of the femur.

As the 1940s began, US involvement in World War II loomed. In 1942 Van Gorder and Marble participated in a series of panel discussions on fractures in a program called "War Sessions," sponsored by the American College of Surgeons. In anticipation of the war, 20% of all physicians and surgeons in the US attended these discussions at various clinics around the country to prepare for treating war injuries. Van Gorder was on the panel in New Haven, Connecticut, and Marble participated in the panel in Portland, Maine. Just nine months after the war ended, in June 1946, Van Gorder became acting chief of the Orthopaedic Service at MGH. Three years later, he became a member on the hospital's board of consultation.

In 1949, after joining the Board of Consultation at MGH and ending his position as visiting orthopaedic surgeon there, Van Gorder published his experiences with a modified version of the Trumble technique for fusing the hip. The Trumble technique was:

an ischiofemoral type of arthrodesis, advocated in 1932 by Hugh C. Trumble of Melbourne Australia. This operation is especially suitable in cases of tuberculosis of the hip...where an iliofemoral arthrodesis would not only have little chance of success, but might produce irreparable harm...[Jacques] Calvé...[predicted] that the time would come when the tuberculous hip would be fused successfully by the construction of a buttress on the adductor side of the joint...[O]ne year later, this is exactly what Trumble succeeded in accomplishing when he devised his ischiofemoral fusion operation. (Van Gorder 1949)

Van Gorder's modifications included using a one-and-one-half spica (instead of a posterior plaster shell) and using a screw to fix the tibial graft into the femur (rather than the trap-door method Trumble had used). Van Gorder preferred not to separate the posterior femoral cutaneous nerve from the sciatic nerve, and he used the same leg as a source of the tibial graft so he could leave the unaffected limb alone. On the basis of the results from 13 patients he had treated at Lakeville State Sanitarium, Van Gorder (1949) became "convinced that the Trumble type of ischiofemoral arthrodesis is the best form of extra-articular fusion of the hip joint that has been devised."

> The Central-Graft Operation for Fusion of Tuberculous Knees, Ankles, and Elbows
>
> BY GEORGE W. VAN GORDER, M.D., BOSTON, AND CHIEN-MIN CHEN, M.D., MIDDLEBORO, MASSACHUSETTS
>
> *From the Lakeville State Sanatorium, Middleboro*
>
> THE JOURNAL OF BONE AND JOINT SURGERY
> VOL. 41-A, NO. 6, SEPTEMBER 1959

Van Gorder and Chen reported their successful use of the central-graft fusion of Hatt in children with tuberculosis of the knee, ankle and elbow. *Journal of Bone and Joint Surgery* 1959; 41: 1029.

Van Gorder remained at MGH for another decade. He continued on the Board of Consultation until 1958, when he was named an honorary surgeon. He had left his private practice a year earlier. Van Gorder continued to publish through the end of his career. In 1959, he and Dr. Chien-Min Chen published another unique approach to arthrodesis. They reported on the central-graft operation, a technique devised by R. Nelson Hatt in 1940, in fusions of the knee, ankle, and elbow. Van Gorder and Chen (1959) had great success with the procedure. They noted, "One of the distinct advantages of the procedure...is that a bone graft can be driven across the central portion of a joint, thus bridging and locking its articular surfaces, although not interfering with growth of the bone. Such a procedure is especially applicable to children whose joints may require fusion, since central grafts do not arrest bone growth while they are stimulating bone union."

They also suggested replacing elbow excision with fusion through the central-graft operation, particularly in children, in whom "the operation is [especially] of supreme value because it offers a high percentage of successful joint fusions without causing cessation of bone growth...[S]olid bone fusion...was obtained in all of the fifteen children...[However] it is of extreme importance to avoid allowing the patella to become attached to the femur at the anterior epiphyseal line...[which] produced local cessation of growth with resulting marked genu recurvation and shortening" (Van Gorder and Chen 1959). In six of their patients who had "tuberculosis of the elbow, the operation was not quite so successful" (Van Gorder and Chen 1959): one graft failed, resulting in a persistent nonunion. In adults with tuberculosis of the knee, though, "the single-central-graft femur...was successful in all of the nine patients," and in nine patients (both adults and children) with "tuberculosis of the ankle...fusion was obtained in all of the patients" (Van Gorder and Chen 1959).

Van Gorder retired from MGH in 1959. Edwin Cave (1970), who had worked closely with Van Gorder, described him as "an excellent teacher and a fine surgeon" who "was especially knowledgeable about tuberculosis of bones and joints, a lot of which he had seen during his stay in China. He was [also] particularly skilled in the management of fractures." During his career, Van Gorder had been a member of various professional organizations, including the American Orthopaedic Association—he had become a member in 1934 and was its vice president in 1949—the American Academy of Orthopaedic Surgeons, the American College of Surgeons, and the American Medical Association.

One of Van Gorder's longtime friends, who had known him since their schooldays together, described Van Gorder: "I find it very difficult to express in words the magnitude of George's personality in either his work or social life, but we who knew him well, as I did, loved him for all he was and all that he accomplished" (quoted in Cave 1970). Edwin Cave (1970) called him "the most kindly of men" who "truly had the spirit of a missionary in almost everything he did." In the mid-1960s Van Gorder moved into Mount San Antonio Gardens, a retirement community in Pomona, California. He died there on January 20, 1969.

PHILIP D. WILSON SR.

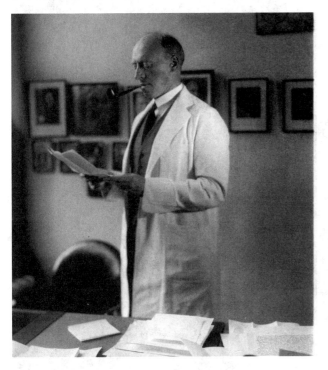

Philip D. Wilson Sr. Courtesy of The David B. Levine, MD Archives and Special Collections, Hospital for Special Surgery.

> **Physician Snapshot**
>
> Philip D. Wilson Sr.
> BORN: 1886
> DIED: 1969
> SIGNIFICANT CONTRIBUTIONS: Consultant in charge of amputations United States Armed Expeditionary Forces (AEF); co-chief (with Henry Marble) of the MGH Fracture Service; third president of the American Academy of Orthopaedic Surgeons (1934); surgeon-in-chief at the Hospital for the Ruptured and Crippled

Philip Duncan Wilson was born April 3, 1886. His father was "Dr. Edward Wilson, a much-respected family physician who also held the Chair of Obstetrics in the Starling Medical School" in Columbus, Ohio (H. P. 1969). After completing high school in Columbus, Philip matriculated at Harvard College and graduated in 1909 with a bachelor of arts degree. He remained in Boston, attending Harvard Medical School, where "he began to show his considerable talents" (H. P. 1969). He was class president and in 1912 received his MD degree cum laude. He moved directly into a two-year surgical internship at Massachusetts General Hospital. During that internship, in 1913, Wilson met and worked alongside Harry Platt, who at the time was an assistant in orthopaedics at MGH under Brackett. In his book *An American Appreciation*, Wilson (1966) recalled that Platt "was particularly impressed by the freedom given to the juniors to express their opinions about case problems, and the frank and open discussions that were conducted on ward rounds. He also enjoyed the meetings of the Orthopaedic Journal Club," which were held in Brackett's home. Journal clubs in faculty homes are something many residents miss out on today. Wilson (1966) also noted that Platt—and thus of course Wilson himself—had become "acquainted with the Boston pioneers in orthopaedic surgery, including Bradford, Goldthwait, Osgood, Lovett, Sever and others." Platt returned to the UK in 1914, just as World War I began. He would eventually be knighted and become president of both the Royal College of Surgeons of England and the British Orthopaedic Association.

Wilson himself left MGH in 1914 with plans to return to Ohio and begin practicing in orthopaedic surgery. World War I was immanent, however, and as the US became involved, Wilson "was invited to join the Harvard Unit then assembling [in Boston] under Harvey Cushing" (H. P. 1969); Dr. Robert Osgood was the unit's senior orthopaedic surgeon (see chapter 63). Both Cushing, in his *A Surgeon's Journal*, and Osgood, in the diary he kept during the war (which was never published), described the unit's "early experiences in France in 1915 at Neuilly where it was housed in the Lycée Pasteur" (H. P. 1969). One biographer of Wilson said, "The months in Neuilly at the American Ambulance were to be a turning point for Philip Wilson; perhaps the one influence above all the others which shaped his life—for working at the hospital was a Red Cross nursing aid, Miss Germaine Parfouru-Porel" (H. P. 1969), whom Wilson met. Germaine was "the daughter

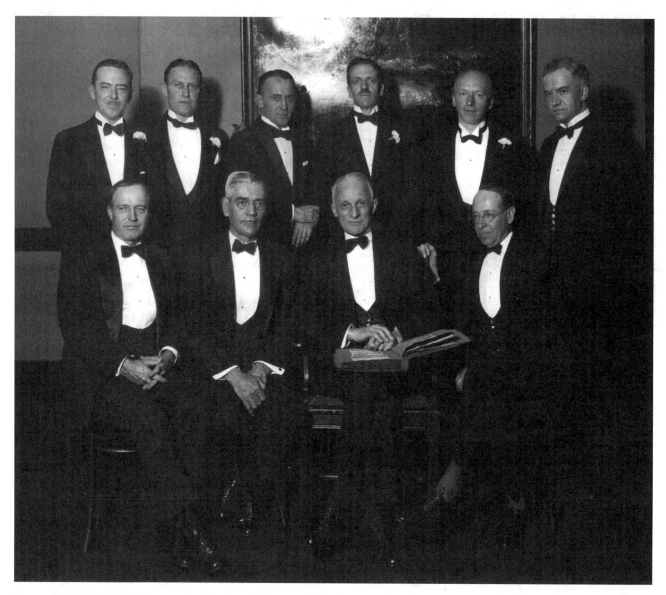

Harvard Unit, WWI. Dr. Harvey Cushing is seated, second from the right (Dr. Robert B. Osgood). Standing in the back at the far right is Dr. Smith-Petersen, and next to him is Dr. Philip D. Wilson Sr. P. D. Wilson, "Robert Bayley Osgood 1873–1956," *Journal of Bone and Joint Surgery* 1957; 39: 728.

of Madame Réjane, the great French actress…she had enjoyed meeting important personages…traveled widely, was bilingual, having been educated by English governesses, and was deeply interested in the theatre, in music and in literature" (H. P. 1969). Wilson's first tour of duty was short, and he returned to the US after only three months in Neuilly, but he returned to France in 1916. He reunited with Germaine then, and they married on July 6 of that year. After another brief trip to the US, the couple was "soon back in France with Philip now a Major in the United States Army Medical Corps. In this capacity he served from July 1917 to August 1919…as Consultant in Charge of amputations to the whole of the American Expeditionary Forces" (H. P. 1969). When the war ended and the troops demobilized, the couple returned to the US to stay, first to Columbus, and then to Boston, where Wilson became a visiting orthopaedic surgeon at MGH under Dr. Elliott G. Brackett. He also joined the staff at the Robert Brigham Hospital, "where in the next few years he perfected two important operative procedures in the surgery of arthritis[:] posterior capsuloplasty in flexion contracture of the knee and arthroplasty of the elbow joint" (H. P. 1969). Two years later, he took a position as a clinical instructor at Harvard Medical School.

Wilson became recognized as an expert in amputation during and after World War I. In 1918, while in France, he had published a chapter titled "Principles of Design and Construction of Artificial Legs" in the compilation *Publications of the Red Cross Institute for Crippled and Disabled Men*. He also focused on other areas of interest, including fractures. Shortly after Wilson returned to MGH, the hospital's fracture clinic began to function as an independent unit, with both general surgeons and orthopaedic surgeons participating in the management of fractures (see **Case 40.21**). Dr. Charles Scudder resigned as chief of the service in 1920, and Dr. Daniel F. Jones took over (see chapter 31); Dr. Nathaniel Allison was Jones's co-chief. About five years into Jones's leadership, Wilson and Dr. William A. Cochrane published their book, *Fractures and Dislocations; Immediate Management, After-care, and Convalescent Treatment with Special Reference to the Conservation and Restoration of Function*. This was the second of what would be five books on fractures published from the Fracture Service (see the section on Edwin Cave earlier in this chapter). (Scudder had published the first in 1901. Dr. Frederic Cotton, from Boston City Hospital, had published a similar book, *Dislocations and Joint Fractures*, 15 years before Wilson and Cochrane's title came out.) While they were writing the manuscript, Cochrane, a Scottish orthopaedic surgeon who had come to MGH to work with Joel Goldthwait, returned to Scotland to "resum[e] work at the Edinburgh Royal Infirmary, happily without interruption of his duties as joint author" (Wilson and Cochrane 1925).

Jones wrote the foreword to *Fractures and Dislocations*. In it, he supported Wilson and Cochrane: "It would, I believe, express the feeling of the staff of the Fracture Service of the Massachusetts General Hospital to state that they are entirely in accord with the views of the authors as expressed in this work. It is not possible, however, that all members of a large service should agree upon all minor details even though they have come to a remarkable unanimity of opinion on all the important facts. This divergence of opinions would, I believe, be quite unimportant" (Jones 1925).

In the preface the authors commented on the terrific advances that had occurred over the preceding 10 years in how fractures and dislocations had been treated: "The greater perfection of the Roentgen ray...established a new standard by which results must be judged...A new goal has thereby been set, that of complete functional

Drs. Wilson and Cochrane, *Fractures and Dislocations*. The second book published from members of the MGH fracture service. Philadelphia and London: J. B. Lippincott and Company, 1925.

Case 40.21. Open Reduction for Displacement of the Proximal Femoral Epiphysis

> "[The patient,] a boy, aged 17, admitted, Dec 1, 1921, had first felt pain in the left hip six months before, when high jumping. The pain was only momentary, and he was able to continue his athletic activities. Two weeks before admission, he had to run to catch a street car, and had boarded it when it was moving. In doing this, he wrenched the hip and immediately felt severe pain, which persisted, although it decreased in severity. He was able to walk, although he was lame. The day before, he had slipped and fallen, doubling the left leg under him. He felt a snap in the left hip and there was great pain; he was unable to rise and had to be carried home.
>
> "The patient was tall and slender. The left leg was externally rotated, and all movements of the hip were painful. The trochanter was prominent and lay above Nélaton's line. There was a shortening of one-half inch. The roentgenogram showed the characteristic deformity.
>
> "December 3, under ether anesthesia, closed reduction was attempted, following the Whitman procedure, and a long plaster-of-Paris spica was applied. Roentgenograms taken through the plaster showed an unsatisfactory position. Open reduction was performed, December 22, and good correction was obtained. The plaster was removed, March 12, 1922 and a Thomas caliper brace was applied; this was worn until July 1.
>
> "Nov. 12, 1923, normal use, without pain or limp, had been restored. All movements were normal with the exception of flexion, which was limited at a point slightly beyond a right angle. There was a one-half inch shortening."
>
> (Philip D. Wilson 1924)

restoration" (Wilson and Cochrane 1925). They did note, "However...the great majority of such injuries must perforce be treated by general practitioners...not in the well-equipped hospital [by specialists], but in the physician's office or in the patient's home" (Wilson and Cochrane 1925).

To aid such general practitioners, Wilson and Cochrane (1925) aimed:

> to report as faithfully as possible the practice of a group of surgeons constituting the staff of the Fracture Service of the Massachusetts General Hospital...the later outgrowth of the Fracture Squad...organized by Dr. C. L. Scudder...A wealth of clinical material has been available for free discussions at the weekly staff visits... The staff is composed of six surgeons, two being appointed from each of the two surgical services, and two from the orthopaedic service; from the former, Drs. Arthur W. Allen, Tarr W. Harmer, George A. Leland, Jr., and Henry C. Marble; from the latter, Drs. Zabdiel B. Adams and Philip D. Wilson...
>
> Early in 1922 it was possible for the staff to agree upon and prepare an outline of methods of treatment. Later in the same year a conference of...surgeons...from...the United States and Canada...[met] in Boston for the purpose of discussing standard methods of treatment of fractures...[resulting in a] Syllabus which was finally adopted... The authors have tried to keep in mind the needs of the general practitioner. It is for this reason that we have chiefly stressed non-operative methods of treatment....

They also gave tribute "to Dr. Robert B. Osgood...who has reviewed and criticized the manuscript, given invaluable suggestions for its improvement, and been ready with help at all times when aid was requested," and to whom they owed a "great debt of gratitude" (Wilson and Cochrane 1925).

The same year that Wilson and Cochrane published *Fractures and Dislocations*, Wilson published the paper "Joint Fractures" in the *Boston Medical and Surgical Journal*. In it he discussed the consequences of the difficulties in treating fractures, as they "give rise to long periods of disability...often followed by more or less permanent crippling... Treatment is often unsatisfactory or inadequate"

(Wilson 1925). He presented statistics regarding disability from the state industrial board (he did not name the state), noting that they "are, doubtless, based upon the reports of attending physicians, and there is probably much inaccuracy in the diagnoses" (Wilson 1925). He then discussed fracture types, treatments, and early mobilization. He closed the article by referring to two exceptions to early mobilization—fractures of the carpal scaphoid and of the femoral neck:

> There can be no function in the absence of union...With regard to fracture of the scaphoid, all authorities are in agreement that immobilization is necessary...In respect to the treatment of fractures of the neck of the femur there is no doubt that the Whitman method of reduction, followed by the application of a plaster spica with the hip in the position of wide abduction and internal rotation, marks a great advance...There certainly can no longer be any justification for the old policy of laissez-faire...
> (Wilson 1925)

Wilson (1925) noted that: "It does seem apparent...that such [joint] injuries are responsible for a large amount of disability...that in many cases...is unduly long," but he was "confident that improvement may be brought about by more general recognition of the importance of accurate reconstitution of articular contour and of early mobilization of the injured joint."

Throughout the 1920s, even while working on the Fracture Service, Wilson continued his endeavors in amputations. In 1927, he published the chapter "Amputations" in the multivolume *Nelson Loose-Leaf Living Surgery*. He published three other articles in 1928, the last titled "Major Amputations. Analysis and Study of End Results in Four Hundred and Twenty Cases," which he cowrote with Dr. John Kuhns. In it, they reviewed the outcomes of 420 amputations performed between 1916 and 1926 at MGH. They determined the end results for 253 of the 360 primary amputations (70%) that had been followed up. Data regarding those amputations are presented in **Table 40.5**. The most common reasons for amputation were trauma—almost twice as frequent as any other cause and equal among both upper and lower extremity amputations—and sepsis (most often in the lower extremities). For patients with either of these conditions, the open method of amputation—was safest and allowed a longer stump to be retained. A longer stump, particularly

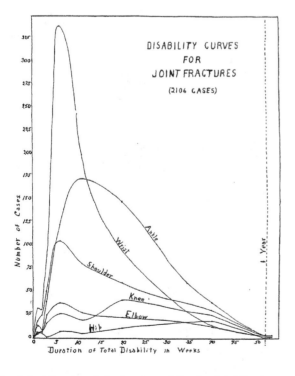

Total disability (weeks) of patients following joint fractures.
P. D. Wilson, "Joint Fractures," *Boston Medical and Surgical Journal* 1925; 193: 339.

Kuhns and Wilson's review of the outcomes of 420 cases of amputations during a ten-year period at MGH. *Archives of Surgery* 1928; 16: 887.

for the lower extremities, was most often associated with better results, though length had little effect on outcomes of upper extremity amputations. Temporary prostheses provided extensive benefit, particularly in patients with amputation at the thigh. Among patients with amputation at the ankle (Syme method), 83% showed satisfactory results.

Results of amputation over time varied among patients with certain disease conditions. In those with thrombo-angiitis and endarteritis, amputations often showed unsatisfactory results because the underlying disease continued to progress. Patients undergoing amputation because of tuberculosis often died within two years because of disease complications. Although a Gritti-Stokes amputation (at the knee) provided the best outcomes related to function in patients with arteriosclerotic gangrene or diabetic gangrene, only a few patients with these conditions survived more than a few years after amputation. Among 30 patients with sarcoma, only 8 (27%) retained good health over years, but even this result seemed to indicate that amputation in this population provides better long-term outcomes than anticipated.

Wilson performed numerous operations to release knee flexion contractures, and in 1929 he published the surgical approach he used in 21 such cases in 15 patients with arthritis at the Robert Breck Brigham Hospital between 1924 and 1927. He described the procedure in detail:

> An incision about five inches long is made over the outer side of the knee…The iliotibial band is sectioned transversely…two inches about the joint…The biceps tendon is split [after retracting the external popliteal nerve] for a distance of two inches, and the two portions divided at different levels and turned back [allowing for a Z-plasty repair]…An incision is made through the capsule…opening into the posterior compartment of the joint. A sharp periosteal dissector is now introduced, and the capsule is stripped upward from the back of the femur…

Table 40.5. Data from 253 Amputations with Evaluated End Results

Procedure	
% of total operations	1%
% of total hospital admissions	0.64%
Reason for amputation	
Trauma	26.9%
Sepsis	10.0%
Thrombo-angiitis/endarteritis	9.5%
Tuberculosis	8.8%
Gangrene (diabetic or arteriosclerotic)	8.5%
Sarcoma	7.1%
Amputation method	
Open flapless	12.4%
Closed	87.6%
In-hospital mortality	13.6%
Postoperative complications	
Operative mortality	11.6%
Wound infection	20.8%
Bronchopneumonia	2.4%
Gangrene (extended)	1.9%
Pulmonary embolism	0.4%
Function	
Use of a prosthesis	
Thigh amputation	65%
Lower leg amputation	85%
Upper extremity amputation	13.3%
Mean time until permanent prosthesis fitted (with temporary prosthesis- without temporary prosthesis)	5.5–13.3 months
Reamputation required	16.4%
First-intention healing	42%

(Adapted from Kuhns and Wilson 1928).

> The outer head of the gastrocnemius is separated, and the subperiosteal dissection carried…three inches above the joint…inward until the midline of the femur is reached. At this point a second incision is made…over the medial aspect of the knee…the capsule at the posterior margin of the joint is incised and the posterior compartment entered. The subperiosteal stripping of the posterior capsule is now

> POSTERIOR CAPSULOPLASTY IN CERTAIN FLEXION
> CONTRACTURES OF THE KNEE*
>
> BY PHILIP D. WILSON, M.D., BOSTON, MASS.
>
> JBJS, 1929, Volume 11, Issue 1

Wilson's article on his results with posterior releases of knee flexion contractures at the RBBH. *Journal of Bone and Joint Surgery* 1929; 11: 40.

repeated from the inner side...until it meets the dissection previously made from the outer side...It is usually impossible even yet to completely extend the knee and it is the tight capsular structures that still remain attached to the femur in the region of the intercondylar notch. These must be completely freed by subperiosteal dissection... (Wilson 1929)

The procedure allowed the knee to "be strengthened by gentle manipulation" (Wilson 1929), and he elaborated the management of the joint after the procedure: "At the end of one week, the plaster casing is removed during the day to permit motion of the knee, but is reapplied at night. Physiotherapy, including baking, massage, and active voluntary exercises, is instituted... At the end of four weeks a knee caliper brace to maintain extension is applied and weight-bearing allowed" (Wilson 1929). He reported full painless extension in all knees with increased range of motion in most; with one death and three cases of transient foot drop, all of which resolved within three months.

In the discussion of the article, Dr. David Silver (1929), who two years earlier had published a paper in which he advocated posterior capsular stripping through a lateral approach and subcutaneously from the medial side, stated: "The free exposure used by Dr. Wilson gives ready access not only to the affected position of the capsule but also to the tendons of the shortened muscles he finds it necessary to lengthen; it further permits ready inspection of the external popliteal nerve... [which] may be advisable in the more severe cases."

That year, Allison left MGH to assume the position of professor of surgery in the Division of Orthopaedic Surgery at the University of Chicago. The hospital leadership, in deciding who would replace Allison as chief of the Orthopaedic Service, "was now faced by the choice between two outstanding men already in the Orthopaedic Department—the brilliant virtuoso Marius Smith-Petersen and the gifted all-rounder Philip Wilson" (H. P. 1969). The trustees ended up appointing Smith-Petersen, who was noted for his original contributions to orthopaedic surgery. Wilson was given the position of orthopaedic surgeon and was appointed co-chief of the Fracture Service (with Dr. Henry Marble). (Drs. Armin Klein and William Rogers became assistant orthopaedic

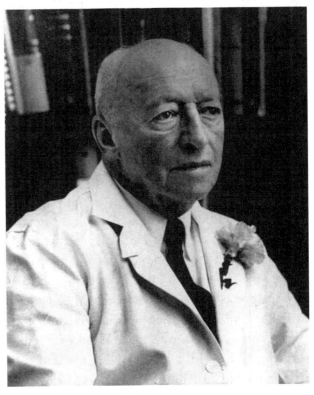

Philip D. Wilson Sr. H.P., "Philip Duncan Wilson, MD 1886–1969," *Journal of Bone and Joint Surgery* 1969; 51: 1445.

surgeons, and Cave became the orthopaedic surgeon to outpatients.)

However, he was extremely disappointed by the trustees' action, i.e., their appointment of Smith-Petersen as chief of orthopaedics. During his 15-year career at MGH, Wilson published ~30 articles—almost half of those for the Report of Progress in Orthopaedic Surgery series in the *Archives of Surgery*. In 1934, Wilson was chosen to be the surgeon-in-chief at the Hospital for the Ruptured and Crippled in New York City. (The hospital had been founded in 1863. Wilson and the hospital's Board of Managers renamed it the Hospital for Special Surgery [HSS] in 1940, and it still operates under that name today). That same year, he was elected the third president of the then still new American Academy of Orthopaedic Surgeons. He was also selected to serve as temporary secretary of the recently organized American Board of Orthopaedic Surgery; he was elected to the board the following year.

In 1938, four years after leaving MGH, Wilson edited a second textbook on fractures, this one titled *Experience in the Management of Fractures and Dislocations*. This huge tome compiled chapters from ~30 contributors. Carter Rowe wrote that Wilson's book was "based on 4,390 fractures treated in the Fracture Clinic while he was on the staff at MGH. It was a remarkable exposition of the treatment of trauma between the years 1923–1930 with follow-up study on patients, one year or more, according to Dr. Codman's recommendations."

Wilson went on to have an illustrious career in his leadership position at HSS, and he became a great statesman for the profession of orthopaedic surgery. In 1954—after 20 years at HSS—he cowrote the book *Human Limbs and Their Substitutes* with Dr. Paul E. Klopsteg. His interest in amputations was evolving even then. Wilson retired as surgeon-in-chief in 1955, and after mandatory retirement at Cornell Medical School, he became emeritus professor of orthopaedic surgery. He died in New York City on May 6, 1969.

EDWIN T. WYMAN JR.

Physician Snapshot

Edwin T. Wyman Jr.
BORN: 1930
DIED: 2005
SIGNIFICANT CONTRIBUTIONS: Restored the MGH Fracture Service and served as its chief for over 20 years

Edwin T. Wyman Jr. was born in 1930, and his father was a physician. Little other information is available about his early years. He graduated from Harvard Medical School in 1955. After two years of training in general surgery at St. Luke's/Roosevelt Hospital in New York City, he entered the three-year Children's Hospital/Massachusetts General Hospital orthopaedic residency program, which he completed in 1960. Thirty years later, Wyman recalled his experience in the Harvard Orthopaedic Program: "At the time of his residency in the late 1950s learning was largely through intimidation. Some teachers used grinding techniques to educate house staff, 'like the way a tin plate assumes the shape of a hubcap when placed in a hubcap press'" (Gross and Tate 1997).

Wyman practiced mainly at MGH, particularly in association with Dr. William R. MacAusland Jr. His primary interest was fractures. Of the five articles Wyman published over his career, three involved the treatment of fractures. His first two

Management of Metastatic Pathological Fractures

WILLIAM R. MACAUSLAND, JR., M.D.,* AND EDWIN T. WYMAN, JR., M.D.

Clinical Orthopaedics and Related Research
Number 73
November–December, 1970

MacAusland and Wyman reported a small series of patients with metastatic disease in whom they argued for patients' comfort by internal stabilization of the fractures.
Clinical Orthopaedics and Related Research 1970; 73: 39.

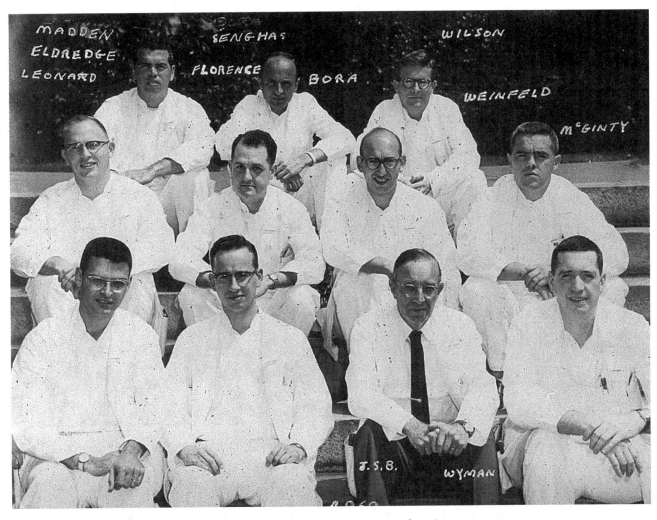

Dr. Barr with MGH residents, 1960. Dr. Wyman is seated in the first row at the far right. MGH HCORP Archives.

articles were published in *Clinical Orthopaedics and Related Research* in 1970. The first was cowritten with Dr. William H. Simon and titled "Femoral Neck Fractures. A Study of the Adequacy of Reduction." Simon and Wyman (1970) noted, "Although most investigators in the past have felt that anteroposterior (AP) and lateral roentgenographic views adequately evaluated the reduction of the femoral neck fracture, it was our feeling that…[these] views gave a false picture of the adequacy of reduction." Over two years (1966–68), they studied 24 patients with cineradiography or fluoroscopy, as well as femurs from cadavers. Using roentgenology they captured scans of the bones in basic AP and lateral views, and with three specific AP views: in maximum internal rotation, in maximum external rotation, and with the hip flexed 60°. "These special [AP] views demonstrated a poor reduction in 8 cases in which [routine] AP and lateral views were interpreted as showing an 'acceptable' reduction…[W]e may be lulled into accepting a reduction as shown in 2 plane roentgenograms which in no way appears acceptable when rotational and flexion views are taken" (Simon and Wyman Jr. 1970).

In the second paper, "Management of Metastatic Pathological Fractures," Wyman and his close associate William MacAusland Jr. reported the outcomes of patients in whom metastatic fractures were not stabilized with internal fixation; e.g., intramedullary rod, plate and screws, or femoral head prothesis; and compared them with outcomes from eight patients in whom a pathological fracture was internally stabilized (see **Case 40.22**). MacAusland and Wyman (1970) concluded: "metastatic fractures…often heal normally…[and that] a major fracture through a metastatic area in bone must not depress the physician into therapeutic nihilism, since this will only increase patient discomfort and loss of function for the remainder of the patient's life…In pathological fractures of the shafts of the femur, tibia and humerus, where rigid internal fixation can be anticipated, a strong plea is made for this vigorous approach in spite of the inevitable prognosis."

After Dr. Henry Mankin arrived at MGH in 1972, Wyman led the charge in "restor[ing] to full and active life" the MGH Fracture Service, "which had all but disappeared over the previous

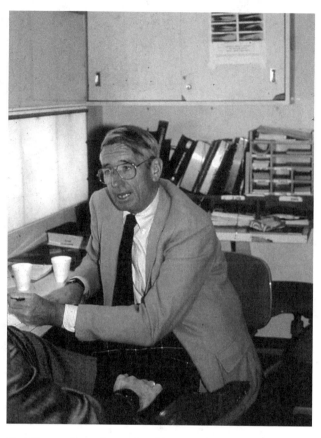

Dr. Wyman discussing patients in a ward work-station.
MGH HCORP Archives.

Case 40.22. Management of Metastatic Pathological Fractures

> "This 67-year-old woman began having pain in the left femur 5 years after the diagnosis of carcinoma of the breast. Roentgenograms at this time revealed a lytic lesion in the left femoral shaft. She was treated with a brace, which gave some relief. Several months later, she slipped while getting out of bed and sustained a fracture through the metastatic area. Five days after the fracture, open reduction and internal fixation with an intramedullary nail was performed. Postoperatively, the patient was given radiotherapy to the involved area. Except for minor incisional pain, this patient was entirely comfortable, requiring no medication after the first postoperative day. She was allowed to walk with crutches on the fifth postoperative day and discharged asymptomatic and weight bearing within two weeks. This patient remained comfortable for the remainder of her life.
>
> "This patient thus achieved the desired goals of early internal fixation of this metastatic fracture: a short stay in the hospital, prompt relief of pain, and early return to fairly normal activity."
>
> (MacAusland and Wyman 1970)

years" (Mankin 1983). Wyman served as chief of that service for 21 years (1973–1994).

Wyman was also interested in teaching orthopaedics, and he had a hand in administering orthopaedic services at MGH, namely in operations improvement. He also became concerned with how physicians and orthopaedic surgeons practice—particularly how they provide high-quality care while lowering costs. In February 1985, a medical malpractice crisis reached a head in Massachusetts: Several hundred physicians in high-liability specialties like orthopaedics refused to care for patients because their malpractice premiums had rapidly risen to include exorbitant fees. Harvard physicians were not involved, however, because they were covered by lower institution-based malpractice insurance. According to Wyman, in 1984 at least 25% of graduating orthopaedic residents in the state stayed in

Massachusetts to practice. Of those graduating in 1985, however, *none* set up practices in the state.

In 1986, Wyman cowrote a paper about medical costs with Dr. Bernard R. Bach Jr., "Financial Charges of Hospitalized Motorcyclists at the Massachusetts General Hospital." They evaluated 47 motorcyclists who had been admitted to MGH during a 1-year period (July 1, 1982–July 1, 1983). Their findings are presented in **Table 40.6**. On the basis of those data, Bach and Wyman emphasized the need for motorcyclists to carry medical insurance as well as disability insurance so they would be covered in the case of an accident or injury.

Table 40.6. Outcomes of 47 Hospitalized Motorcyclists

Mean duration of hospitalization	22 days
Injury	
At least one fracture	85%
Open fracture	55%
Related head, chest, abdominal injury	40%
Hospital charges*	
Mean	$15,114
Total	~$700,000
Charges collected	84%
Insurance	
Yes	55%
No	45%

(Adapted from Bach and Wyman 1986).
*These charges did not include costs for surgeons' fees, rehabilitation, lawsuits, lost wages, and other related costs.

In the mid-1990s, Wyman was focusing his efforts on major medical problems in the Worker's Compensation System, which aimed to both lower costs and retain quality of care. In 1994, he served on the American Academy of Orthopaedic Surgeons Committee on Occupational Health. That year, he and William L. Cats-Baril, PhD, published the results of a national multidisciplinary consensus panel comprising 119 stakeholders from various industry, legal, and health care groups—including insurance companies, physicians and other health care professionals, administrators, attorneys, and unions—that were charged to come to consensus on more than 35 issues facing health care. By use of multiple workshops and Delphi panels, the group advanced mutually beneficial solutions for 14 of those issues. Included among those solutions were:

- Efforts should be made to foster better integration of prevention initiatives on the state government level.
- Employers and employees should be given incentives to work together to develop injury prevention programs.
- State worker's compensation legislation should create incentives for temporary modified work for injured workers.
- Ergonomic principles should be applied in the workplace. (Wyman and Cats-Baril 1994)

Wyman became part of Omni Med, a group of volunteer physicians who work in developing countries that formed in 1998. In 2001, he initiated a program at St. Mary's Hospital in Nairobi, Kenya, as part of a broad range of medical services offered in the sub-Sahara, including Kenya and Uganda. The umbrella program was started in 1998 by Dr. Edward O'Neil Jr. in Auburndale, Massachusetts. Three years later, Wyman retired from practice at MGH in 2004; his career there

Working It Out: Recommendations from a Multidisciplinary National Consensus Panel on Medical Problems in Workers' Compensation

Edwin T. Wyman, MD
William L. Cats-Baril, PhD
JOM • Volume 36, Number 2, February 1994

Wyman and Cats-Baril's report on the results of multiple workshops and Delphi panels concerned with major medical problems in workers' compensation in the United States.
Journal of Occupational Medicine 1994; 36: 144.

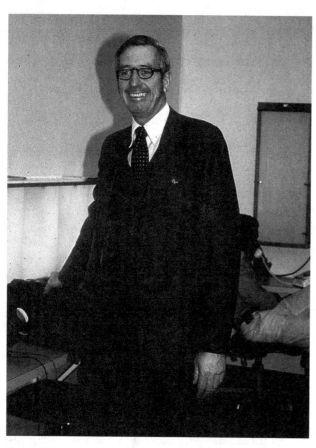

Edwin T. Wyman Jr. MGH HCORP Archives.

had spanned more than 40 years, and at the time he was a visiting orthopaedic surgeon. He also left his duties at Harvard Medical School, where he was an assistant clinical professor of orthopaedic surgery. He died the following year, on July 16, 2005. He lived in Weston and was predeceased by his wife.

CHAPTER 41

Henry J. Mankin
Prolific Researcher and Dedicated Educator

The youngest of three boys, Henry Jay Mankin was born to Hymie and Mary Mankin on October 9, 1928. The family lived in Pittsburgh (Squirrel Hill neighborhood), Pennsylvania, where Hymie Mankin ran the Special Clothing Company. Hymie and Mary were both Jewish, and at the time of Henry's birth they had just immigrated from Lithuania. After graduating from Colfax grade school, Henry attended seventh through twelfth grades at Taylor Allderdice High School; he graduated in 1946. At school, he played the oboe in the orchestra. He worked at numerous jobs throughout his early school years—as a *Pittsburgh Press* daily newspaper and *Pittsburgh Post-Gazette* morning paper delivery boy, an usher at the Nixon Theatre, a soda jerk at the Manor Pharmacy, a mail sorter at the post office during the holiday season, an usher at the Syria Mosque, and a busboy at the Pittsburgh Athletic Club. Henry held a longer job making sandwiches at Polansky's Hebrew National Delicatessen and did odd jobs in his father's Specialty Clothing Company.

Henry lived in his family's home at 6307 Crombie Street, in Squirrel Hill, from the year he was born until 1952, when he was 24 and in his third year of medical school. While growing up, Henry's next-door neighbor and friend was Myron Kopelman—later known as Myron Cope, the famous Pittsburgh sports announcer and commentator and inventor of the famed Terrible Towel. In his memoir, Mankin noted, "Major

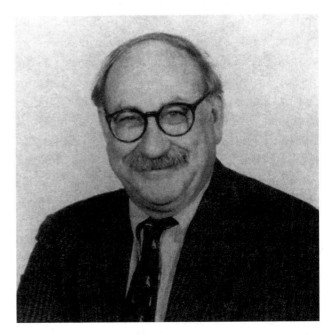

Henry J. Mankin. MGH HCORP Archives.

Physician Snapshot

Henry J. Mankin
BORN: 1928
DIED: 2018
SIGNIFICANT CONTRIBUTIONS: Created an articular cartilage histological-histochemical grading system for osteoarthritis (the Mankin System); overhauled the orthopaedic program at MGH; enthusiastic supporter of the use of allografts in limb-salvage surgery; initiated the annual Boston Pathology Course; supported and facilitated the creation of the MGH Institute of Health Professions

league baseball was one of my favorite activities during the season...We started going to [Pittsburgh Pirates] baseball games before night games were possible...Forbes Field had no lights...it was a great way to spend the day. There is something really exciting about the umpire standing up there and shouting 'play ball!'...It still stirs me" (Mankin and Mankin 2017).

After graduating from high school, Mankin entered the University of Pittsburgh, where he majored in physics and graduated in 1952. That summer he married Carole Pinkney. Even though he received a bachelor of science degree magna cum laude, he was still enrolled in the University of Pittsburgh Medical School and had one more year before graduating with an MD degree at the age of 25. At the university, he was elected into Phi Eta Sigma, a freshman honorary society; Sigma Pi Sigma, an honorary physics society; and Alpha Epsilon Delta, an honorary premedical society. In medical school, he was elected into Alpha Omega Alpha in 1952. As one of the top 5 students in his class of 100, he received the Luba Robin Goldsmith Award at graduation.

Early Career

From 1953 to 1954, Mankin was a rotating intern at the University of Chicago clinics. Two of his fellow interns were Wayne Akeson (who became a leader in orthopaedic research) and Ralph Marcove (who became a bone tumor orthopaedic surgeon). Apparently, he had committed to an internal medicine residency there, but he most enjoyed his final internship rotation in orthopaedics. He worked with Tom Brower (who was later appointed to the orthopaedic faculty at UPMC), Bill Enneking (who became famous for his work as an orthopaedic bone tumor surgeon and was a lifelong friend of Mankin), and Howard Hatcher (who specialized in bone tumors and influenced Mankin's decision to become an orthopaedic surgeon). He became a junior resident in medicine on July 1, 1954.

The first three months of Mankin's medicine residency went well, but, in November 1954, the US Navy sent him a letter. Mankin described it in his memoir:

[The letter stated] Either I accept a position as a Medical Officer in the Navy or I would have to report to Pittsburgh on January 1 to serve as an ordinary seaman. It was the end of the Korean War and I decided to become a Lieutenant Junior Grade in the Navy Medical Corps and see where I would have to go. These were not the happiest days...my assignment... was to the U.S. Naval Ammunition Depot in Hawthorne, Nevada!...At some point during our two years...I decided after my experience in Orthopaedics at the University of Chicago and the amount of orthopaedic care I gave patients in Hawthorne, that I would rather do that then go back into internal medicine. (Mankin and Mankin 2017)

Mankin completed his military service in 1956. In 1957, he asked Hatcher for a position in Hatcher's orthopaedic residency program at the University of Chicago but none was available. He recommended that Mankin contact Dr. Joseph Milgram at the Hospital for Joint Diseases in New York City. Milgram would not have a position open until July, so Mankin spent the next five months there as a resident in pathology with Dr. Henry Jaffe before he started his orthopaedic residency. After Mankin completed his three-year orthopaedic residency at the Hospital for Joint Diseases in 1960, Tom Brower (who had been at the University of Chicago) and Dr. Albert B. Ferguson, chairman of the orthopaedic department at the University of Pittsburgh, offered him a one-year position there as active staff and an instructor of orthopaedic surgery. His annual salary would be $11,000 (a value of almost $97,000 in 2020).

Mankin was busy during his first year of practice and started a research program to investigate articular cartilage structure. In 1962 he received his first grant from the National Institutes of Health (NIH). In that same year, he published his first two basic research publications on growth and repair in immature cartilage of rabbits:

> Tritiated thymidine, when administered intra-articularly, provides a remarkably good tool to study the growth of articular cartilage…thymidine…a precursor of deoxyribonucleic acid…uptake by a cell indicates an imminent division and…serves as a highly specific qualitative index of cellular production… In the immature rabbit, thymidine localization in the cartilaginous epiphysis occurs in two distinct layers, one subjacent to the articular surface and one in relation to the ossific nucleus of the epiphysis…It is suggested that these two layers represent sites of interstitial growth of the cartilaginous epiphysis…to growth of the articular surface and…to growth of the ossific nucleus of the epiphysis. (Mankin 1962a)

In a second publication (part 2), Mankin described his attempts at repairing articular cartilage in rabbits using tritiated thymidine:

> The response of articular cartilage to the types of surgically created wounds in the distal part of the thirty-five femora of immature rabbits. The response of the cartilage was identical in each type of trauma…by marginal necrosis which extended four to six cells from the defect. This disappeared by three weeks…An intense proliferative activity began on the first day and extended eight to twelve cell widths from the necrotic zone. This response…could no longer be observed…by two weeks. There was no evidence in…six weeks…that this proliferation contributed…to wound healing… Articular cartilage…[in response] to trauma… undergoes necrosis and proliferation but lacks the vascular response of inflammation. (Mankin 1962b)

Localization of Tritiated Thymidine in Articular Cartilage of Rabbits
I. GROWTH IN IMMATURE CARTILAGE
BY HENRY J. MANKIN, M.D., PITTSBURGH, PENNSYLVANIA
From the Department of Orthopedic Surgery, University of Pittsburgh, Pittsburgh
THE JOURNAL OF BONE AND JOINT SURGERY
VOL. 44-A, NO. 4, JUNE 1962

Localization of Tritiated Thymidine in Articular Cartilage of Rabbits
II. REPAIR IN IMMATURE CARTILAGE
BY HENRY J. MANKIN, M.D., PITTSBURGH, PENNSYLVANIA
From the Department of Orthopedic Surgery, University of Pittsburgh, Pittsburgh
THE JOURNAL OF BONE AND JOINT SURGERY
VOL. 44-A, NO. 4, JUNE 1962

Mankin's initial publications on growth and repair of articular cartilage. *Journal of Bone and Joint Surgery* 1962; 44: 688.

Mankin was invited to remain at the University of Pittsburgh after his one-year position ended, and Ferguson supported and promoted Mankin during his time there. In 1963, he recommended that Mankin be promoted to associate professor. After six years in Pittsburgh, Mankin had published more than 25 papers. In 1966, he was invited to go back to New York as chief of orthopaedics at the Hospital for Joint Diseases and a professor in and co-chair (with Dr. Robert Siffert) of the Department of Orthopaedics at Mount Sinai Medical School. Ferguson encouraged Mankin to accept the position, which he did.

At the Hospital for Joint Diseases, Mankin continued his basic research on cartilage and expanded his research group to include Louis Lippiello and Antra Zarins. In 1970, he cowrote a paper with Lippiello about their study of the biochemical and metabolic abnormalities in "Articular cartilage of the proximal end of the femur from twenty-four patients with osteoarthritis and twenty 'normal' controls with fractures of the neck of the femur." They found that:

[a] decrease in the intensity of staining with Safranin-O...correlated roughly with the severity of the osteo-arthritic process...[There was] essentially no change in the collagen content in the osteoarthritis-arthritic cartilage...[but there was] a marked increase in the rates of DNA, protein, and polysaccharide synthesis without significant change in the rate of RNA synthesis...[and] an inverse correlation...between the rates of polysaccharide synthesis and the levels of hexosamine. On the basis of these studies, it is postulated that the chondrocyte...in osteo-arthritis-arthritis, seems to revert to a chondroblast and is capable of making new cells and matrix at a much more rapid rate than is normally seen. (Mankin and Lippiello 1970)

The following year he and his colleagues reported part 2 of the 1970 study. Their goal was "to explore the variability of the process further and to define its effect on the biomechanical and metabolic parameters" (Mankin et al. 1971). To this end, they developed a "histologic-histochemical grading system...so that small but representative areas on a single femoral head could be classified according to 'severity'" (Mankin et al. 1971); that is, these grades were considered "an index of severity of the osteo-arthritic process" (Mankin et al. 1971). This grading system is shown in **Table 41.1**.

Using this system, they graded "thirty-two areas of cartilage from nine osteo-arthritic and four 'normal' femoral heads" (Mankin et al. 1971). They used various biomarkers as indicators: "DNA and hexosamine concentrations were determined as indicators of cell density and polysaccharide content...[and] the incorporation rates of ^{3}H-Thymidine and ^{35}SO$_4$ were measured as indicators of synthesis of DNA and polysaccharide" (Mankin et al. 1971). They found that:

osteo-arthritis is a focal disease...[with] considerable variation of the severity...on each...femoral head...There is excellent direct correlation between the severity of the process and the rates of DNA and polysaccharide synthesis... however, the reparative mechanisms seem to "fail" and to decrease with advancing disease... There is a significant inverse correlation with between the severity of the process and the polysaccharide concentration, but...no correlation between the cell density...and the severity of the disease...The cartilage covering osteophytes is less severely involved. (Mankin et al. 1971)

Their histological-histochemical grading system became known as the Mankin System, and investigators used or modified it for years afterward. Despite this wide use, researchers have also questioned the validity of the system, as it was based on an analysis of specimens from patients with advanced osteoarthritis. In 2012, for example, Pauli et al. compared the Mankin System with the Osteoarthritis Cartilage Histopathology

Table 41.1. Histological-Histochemical Grading System for Osteoarthritis in Articular Cartilage

Structure		Cells		Safranin-O staining		Tidemark integrity	
Normal	0	Normal	0	Normal	0	Intact	0
Surface irregularities	1	Diffuse hypercellularity	1	Slight reduction	1	Crossed by blood vessels	1
Pannus and surface irregularities	2	Cloning	2	Moderate reduction	2		
Clefts to transitional zone	3	Hypocellularity	3	Severe reduction	3		
Clefts to radial zone	4			No dye noted	4		
Clefts to calcified zone	5						
Complete disorganization	6						

Adapted from Mankin et al. 1971.

> **Biochemical and Metabolic Abnormalities in Articular Cartilage from Osteo-Arthritic Human Hips*†**
>
> BY HENRY J. MANKIN, M.D.‡, AND LOUIS LIPPIELLO, M.S.‡, NEW YORK, N.Y.
>
> *From the Department of Orthopaedics, Hospital for Joint Diseases—Mount Sinai School of Medicine, New York*
>
> THE JOURNAL OF BONE AND JOINT SURGERY
> VOL. 52-A, NO. 3, APRIL 1970
>
> ---
>
> **Biochemical and Metabolic Abnormalities in Articular Cartilage from Osteo-Arthritic Human Hips**
>
> II. CORRELATION OF MORPHOLOGY WITH BIOCHEMICAL AND METABOLIC DATA*†
>
> BY HENRY J. MANKIN, M.D.‡, HOWARD DORFMAN, M.D.‡, LOUIS LIPPIELLO, M.S.§, AND ANTRA ZARINS, M.S.‡, NEW YORK, N.Y.
>
> *From the Departments of Orthopaedics and Pathology, Hospital for Joint Diseases, Mt. Sinai School of Medicine, New York*
>
> THE JOURNAL OF BONE AND JOINT SURGERY
> VOL. 53-A, NO. 3, APRIL 1971

Mankin and colleagues' articles on articular cartilage biochemical and metabolic abnormalities in human osteo-arthritic hips—in which they reported Mankin's classic grading system commonly used today. *Journal of Bone and Joint Surgery* 1970; 52: 424; *Journal of Bone and Joint Surgery* 1971; 53: 523.

Assessment System (OARSI) using specimens from a large number of adult donors (aged 23–92 years). Both scoring systems were reliable with excellent interobserver agreement (especially Mankin's surface irregularities) and high reproducibility. However, both were also complex and cumbersome to use, and very time consuming when assessing lesion severity. Interobserver disagreements were common for cellularity, Safranin O staining, and tidemark.

As at the University of Pittsburgh School of Medicine, Mankin remained for six years at the Hospital for Joint Diseases and the Mount Sinai Medical School. Mankin highlighted his major accomplishments in New York:

> I devoted myself to improving the quality of care in a number of areas such as hand surgery (by appointing Richard Smith and Bob Leffert), pediatric surgery, (by doing it myself…), and later I added Charlie Weiss and Michael Ehrlich to the teams as well as key players in other disciplines. I really worked hard at residency education, starting my infamous breakfast conferences, grand rounds on Saturdays [same as in Pittsburgh], resident thesis days for their presentations, and anatomy sessions. I really think that the resident education was my best accomplishment…I also did my first allograft… using a distal femur…(Mankin and Mankin 2017)

At the Hospital for Joint Diseases and Mount Sinai Medical School he published another ~30 to 40 articles.

CHIEF OF ORTHOPAEDICS AT MGH

In 1972, Dr. Mankin was recruited to become a professor of orthopaedic surgery at Harvard Medical School and chief of the Orthopaedic Department at Massachusetts General Hospital (MGH). There he succeeded Dr. Melvin Glimcher, who had chaired the department at MGH for six years (1965–1970), and replaced the interim chair, Dr. Thornton Brown. (This was Brown's second stint as interim chair; he had also been in that role briefly after Dr. Joseph Barr retired, before Glimcher was appointed.)

Mankin and his family (his wife, Carole, and their three children) "moved to Brookline…[into] a 100 year old 'mansion'…[with lots] of storage space…[for] vast collections of slides and pathologic material willed to [him] by the esteemed pathologists Crawford Campbell and Henry Jaffe" (Mankin and Mankin 2017). In his memoir, Mankin stated that he "didn't go to Boston alone" professionally, either (Mankin and Mankin 2017): "In March (1972) I drove to Boston…[with] Antra Zarins [and] Lou Lippiello…I [also] took four Jewish boys with me, namely Dick Smith, Bob Leffert, Charlie Weiss and Michael Ehrlich…We all moved in over the next few months, and the hospital gave us office space on the 6th floor of the Gray Building next to the Smith-Petersen Orthopaedic Library…" He went on to describe the roles he and his colleagues took on once in Boston:

> Richard Smith was a hand surgeon and took that service over; Bob Leffert decided to be a shoulder and rehabilitation person and took over the rehab floor of White 9; Charlie Weiss decided that trauma might be good for him [but he left MGH for Miami a short time later]; and Michael became a superb pediatric orthopaedist. I wasn't sure what I should do but it seemed to me that there were no orthopaedic oncologists in Boston, so that's what I became. I also became a bone bank person based on my experience using bone transplants (allografts) and started a very reputable bone bank in cooperation with the Boston Organ Bank Group. With the later help of Bill Tomford and Sam Doppelt [who eventually left MGH, moving to Cambridge City Hospital], we developed the standard at the time and became major contributors to the American Association of Tissue Banks. (Mankin and Mankin 2017)

Upon his arrival at MGH, Mankin enhanced the importance of teaching: "Shortly after I arrived I started the dreaded breakfast conferences with the residents [see chapter 11] and worked very hard to introduce science, pathophysiology and history into their discipline and I think that may have been my most successful educational activity…I brought in some senior people who were very helpful. These included Crawford Campbell, Leroy Lavine and Paul Curtiss" (Mankin and Mankin 2017). Mankin's "attention to academics and more specifically teaching and research" wasn't easily accepted by all of the current staff, some of whom thought it "interfered with their private practice and that bringing four additional full-time physicians really interfered with their lifestyles. I overcame their resistance, but it wasn't always easy and I think there are still some people who really would have been happy if I hadn't joined the staff" (Mankin and Mankin 2017). On the other hand, the staff working in his laboratory "were wonderful. Antra Zarins, Lou Lippiello, and later Ben Treadwell, Carol Trahan, Chris Towle, and all the rest were dedicated and productive" (Mankin and Mankin 2017). "Between 1972 and 1980 we published 78

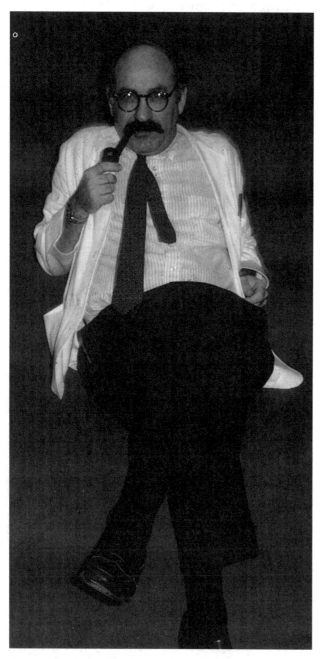

Henry J. Mankin, 1972, shortly after arriving at MGH.
MGH HCORP Archives.

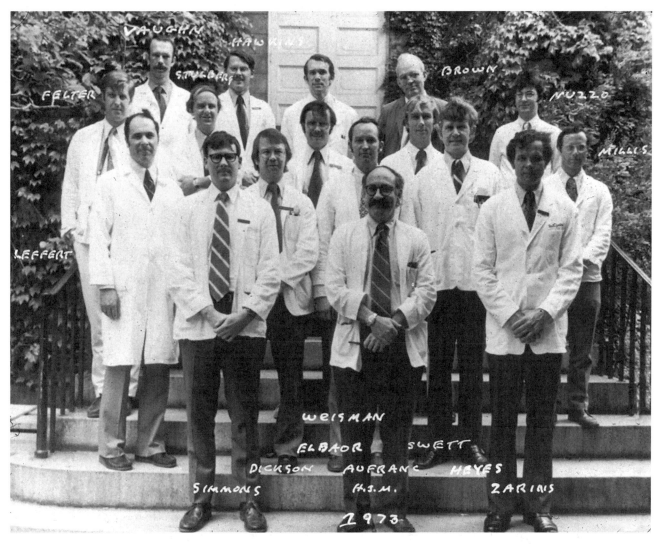

Mankin with MGH residents, 1973. MGH HCORP Archives.

papers…a lot about articular cartilage, cartilage healing and osteoarthritis. We had NIH money for several of these projects" (Mankin and Mankin 2017). He and his team won two awards for their research (see **Box 41.1**).

In his 1996 book about orthopaedics at MGH during the twentieth century, Carter Rowe described Mankin's arrival at MGH as a "dramatic…[and] tremendous transplantation," mainly because he was accompanied by so many others who took on important positions there. At the time, although it had historical significance, orthopaedics was waning at MGH. Mankin refreshed the program and built the service, also improving the renowned Harvard Combined Orthopaedic Residency Program. (See chapter 11 for the history of the HCORP.)

Soon after his arrival, Mankin formalized specialty services in the Department of Orthopaedic Surgery. Each was led by an individual with special interest in a specific field (**Table 41.2**).

Mankin privatized the ward service and reorganized the teaching program (see chapter 11). In 1973, in order to reduce patients' length of stay and open beds for new patients on the Orthopaedic Service at MGH, he formed a liaison with the Massachusetts Rehabilitation Hospital in Boston's West End; founded in 1971. It was renamed in 1983 as the Spaulding Rehabilitation Hospital, a Harvard teaching hospital and a member of

Table 41.2. Specialty Services in the Department of Orthopaedic Surgery at MGH under Mankin

Service	Chief
Hip and Implant	William H. Harris
Hand	Richard J. Smith
Pediatric Orthopaedics	Michael G. Ehrlich
Tumor Service	Henry J. Mankin
Rehabilitation Service (White 9)	Robert Leffert (who succeeded Donald Pierce)
Problem Back Service	Robert Boyd
Sports Medicine	Dinesh Patel, Bertram Zarins, and Carter Rowe
Orthopedic Arthritis Service	William Jones
Fracture Service	Edwin T. Wyman

Adapted from Mankin's writings cited in the 1983 edition of *The Massachusetts General Hospital, 1955–1980*; Castleman, Crockett, and Sutton (eds.)

Partners Healthcare. That same year Mankin asked Dr. Leroy Lavine, the former chief of orthopaedics at SUNY Downstate Medical Center (1964–1981), to lead the orthopaedic rehabilitation service. Lavine remained as the chief of orthopaedic rehabilitation at Spaulding until he retired in 2005, a professor at the Institute of Health Professions at MGH, and a lecturer at Harvard Medical School.

In 1974, Dr. Mankin published in the *Journal of Bone and Joint Surgery* a two-part review titled "Rickets, Osteomalacia, and Renal Osteodystrophy"—a landmark contribution. These articles were written in classic Mankin style and included a detailed explanation of the pathophysiology of these complex metabolic abnormalities:

> Rickets and osteomalacia may result from a wide spectrum of inherited and acquired metabolic abnormalities which produce sufficient decrease in serum calcium, phosphate, or both to impair mineralization of the skeleton and epiphyseal growth. Although these various abnormalities may cause strikingly similar findings in affected patients, the respective disease can usually be separated and identified by careful evaluation of the clinical, roentgenographic, and laboratory data. The prognosis and treatment may vary considerably depending on the cause of the rickets or osteomalacia. Each patient must be carefully studied and treated with the appropriate regimen for his or her particular metabolic abnormality. (Mankin 1972)

While at MGH, Mankin continued to make research contributions in articular cartilage, investigating its healing potential, its protein composition, its water content, and the biochemical and metabolic abnormalities in osteoarthritis. He would study articular cartilage throughout his career and enjoyed continuous funding from the NIH for 40 years.

WIDE-RANGING INTERESTS IN RESEARCH AND EDUCATION

Mankin studied more than articular cartilage. He participated in numerous yearly instructional courses at the Academy (AAOS) meetings, including repeat lectures on cartilage, arthritis, bone disease, and bone tumors. In some papers he described the skeletal abnormalities in patients with, and the pathophysiology and treatment of, Gaucher's disease. In addition to publishing a remarkable number of articles on these and other clinical entities and performing basic research while at MGH, Mankin developed into an orthopaedic oncology surgeon, grew and maintained a very large clinical practice treating musculoskeletal tumors, initiated a successful orthopaedic tumor fellowship program, established (with Dr. Bill Tomford) a bone bank at MGH (see chapter 42), and was an early adopter of flow cytometry to identify bone cancer cells and their response to treatment.

Allografts

Mankin described in his memoir the first allograft he implanted while at the Hospital for Joint Diseases in New York: "[I] did my first allograft… in November of 1971, on a very nice 16-year-old girl from upstate New York, using a distal femur from a 17-year-old girl who had died that morning at Montefiore Hospital (the graft lasted until 1996…25 years!)" (Mankin and Mankin 2017) (see **Case 41.1**). Five years later, Mankin and his colleagues published "Massive Resection and Allograft Transplantation in the treatment of Malignant Bone Tumors." In it they described their first series of "19 allograft transplantations for aggressive or malignant tumors of bone" (Mankin et al. 1976). They were able to follow up on 15 of those 19 patients for approximately two years, and they described their findings:

> An effective allograft replacement for a massive osteoarticular defect has three components: the bones; tendons and ligaments… and articular cartilage…Freezing reduces the immunogenicity of the component portions… For the cartilage, which should remain viable, application of the well-known techniques of glycerinization of the tissue during the freezing process to prevent ice-crystal formation and maintain chondrocyte viability seemed

Mankin and colleagues' classic article on limb salvage using large bone allografts to treat malignant bone tumors.
New England Journal of Medicine 1976; 294: 1247.

Case 41.1. Femoral Allograft Transplantation to Treat Malignant Bone Tumors

"A 16-year-old girl was first seen in September 1971, with a history of pain about the left knee of approximately three months' duration. X-ray examination disclosed a lytic destructive lesion of the distal end of the femur occupying the epiphysis and metaphysis of the bone, with several areas of cortical destruction and evident "breakout" of the lesion associated with a pathologic fracture. A biopsy disclosed an aggressive giant-cell tumor. On November 25 of the same year the left distal femoral segment was harvested from a 17-year-old girl who had died as a result of an automobile accident. Four days later the tumor containing bone and adjacent soft tissues were resected en bloc, and the allograft inserted and held in place with a femoral rod and cerclage wires. The patient's own medial collateral ligament was reattached with a staple, but the donor's posterior capsule and lateral collateral ligament were used since these parts in the patient were resected with the tumor. The patient tolerated the procedure well and was placed in a long leg cast for six weeks and then in a cylinder for the next two months. After discontinuation of immobilization, exercises and non-weight-bearing crutch walking were begun. At nine months, the patient had good healing of the site of anastomosis but had a limited range of motion of the knee, so that an operative procedure was performed. Biopsies of bone and cartilage were obtained at the time of lysis of intra-articular adhesions. The bone showed cortical remodeling and medullary necrosis, and the cartilage appeared viable (it should be noted that this case was performed before the introduction of the use of glycerol to preserve viability of the cartilage). The patient has subsequently retained good stability of the knee joint and has over 90 degrees of flexion and full extension. She has excellent quadriceps power, and walks without support or a limp, x-ray examination shows good bony structure of the distal femur and preservation of the knee-joint space. Her scan remained 'hot' four years after operation."

(Mankin, Fogelson, Zarins, Thrasher, and Jaffer 1976)

reasonable. Experiments in our laboratory… have demonstrated that a 10 percent aqueous solution of glycerol introduced into rabbit articular cartilage before freezing allowed some of the cartilage cells to survive. (Mankin et al. 1976)

In that series, Mankin and his team operated most often on giant-cell tumors. Other tumor types included chondrosarcoma, fibrosarcoma, adamantinoma, metastatic adenocarcinoma, and osteocartilaginous exostosis. Complications varied: three cases of delayed or nonunion; two cases each of hepatitis, infected allograft, transient nerve palsy, error in diagnosis, and ligamentous laxity; and one case of each of cardiac arrest during the procedure, graft fracture, wound hemorrhage, brachial artery laceration, malunion, and shoulder subluxation. Despite the "arduous [and] complex" procedure and the numerous complications they encountered, the group concluded that:

> en bloc resection and massive allograft transplantation appears to have merit, particularly as an experimental approach to the treatment of certain types of lesions for which no other solution is available…[O]f the 15 patients followed for an average of almost two years, none have as yet required amputation, or had local recurrence or metastases and, with the exception of two infected patients, all have retained reasonable function of the extremity…it seems likely that the technique will in the future serve as an important approach to certain neoplastic and possibly even benign disorders of bones and joints. (Mankin et al. 1976)

Chordoma

In his first 20 years at MGH, Mankin and his associates treated 53 patients with a chordoma of the spinal column. Of those, 21 patients with a sacrococcygeal chordoma received primary care at MGH. After biopsy, Mankin and his co-investigators used a posterior approach to resect the lesion. They concluded:

> that sacrococcygeal chordomas are best treated with wide operative resection and, in most cases, with adjuvant radiation…If contamination during the operation is likely (as in patients who have a large tumor or in whom a cephalic sacral resection is planned), preoperative radiation therapy to a maximum dose of fifty gray is recommended. If contamination by tumor occurs during the operation, sixteen gray can be administered after the operation. Good bowel and bladder control were preserved in one-half of our patients in whom the second sacral roots were spared, after resection of roots caudad to that level. (Sampson et al. 1993)

Later, during Dr. Francis Hornicek's tenure as chief of the orthopaedic tumor service, MGH established a chordoma center (2003–2017).

Limb Salvage

Mankin was enthusiastic about limb salvage surgery during his career at MGH. In 1982, he, along with Drs. Thomas Lange and Suzanne Spanier, surveyed 20 members of the Musculoskeletal Tumor Society, inquiring about problems associated with the biopsy procedure in relation to the accuracy of diagnosis and importantly whether the biopsy limited the treatment plan (i.e., a limb salvage procedure). They reported that 64 of the 329 cases (20%) had to be managed with a treatment plan that was less than optimal. Almost 5% of the patients who were candidates for a limb salvage procedure had to undergo amputation instead because the biopsy site had been poorly planned.

Mankin, Lange, and Spanier (1982) made six recommendations for biopsy:

1. Plan the biopsy procedure as carefully as the definitive surgery. It is not a simple procedure.

2. Pay as close attention to asepsis, skin preparation, hemostasis, wound closure… as with any other operation.
3. Place the skin incision in such a manner so as not to compromise a subsequent definitive surgical procedure. (Avoid transverse incisions!)
4. Be certain that an adequate amount of representative tissue is obtained, and that the pathologist prepares the slides in a manner that will allow a definitive diagnosis.
5. If the pathologist cannot make a diagnosis because of unfamiliarity with bone and soft-tissue tumors, urge him or her to seek consultation promptly.
6. If the orthopaedist or the institution is not equipped to perform accurate diagnostic studies or definitive surgery and adjunctive treatment, the patient should be referred to a treating center prior to performance of the biopsy.

In 1994, Mankin and his colleagues reported the long-term results in 227 patients with osteosarcoma of the distal femur that was treated with limb salvage or amputation across 26 institutions. "Eight of the seventy-three patients who had a limb-salvage procedure and nine of the 115 patients who had an above-the-knee amputation had a local recurrence, but…no local recurrence [occurred] in the thirty-nine patients who had a disarticulation of the hip" (Rougraff et al. 1994). They deduced "that, compared with amputation, a limb-salvage procedure for…high-grade osteosarcoma of the distal part of the femur is associated with a higher rate of reoperation but produces a better functional outcome without reducing the chances for long-term survival" (Rougraff et al. 1994). Despite this positive outcome, after a mean follow-up of 11 years they could not "demonstrate…a measurably better quality of life for survivors" (Rougraff et al. 1994).

The MGH Institute of Health Professions

One of Mankin's major accomplishments at MGH was the establishment of the Institute of Health Professions (IHP). Since 1873, the hospital had operated a nursing program. In the early 1970s, a working group proposed a Massachusetts General Hospital University, which would grant graduate degrees in various health professions. As chair of the MGH Committee on Teaching and Education, Mankin was very supportive of this new initiative. According to Dr. Alan Jette, a physical therapist who was among the IHP's first faculty members: "Henry was one of the only physicians at the hospital who was involved early on…Most of the doctors thought the institute could become a distraction, but Henry knew immediately that it could be a great asset to Massachusetts General Hospital as well as be a new kind of health professions school." (quoted in Shaw 2019) Throughout the process, Mankin worked primarily with the hospital's general directors, Dr. Charles Sanders, and later with Dr. J. Robert Buchanan.

In 1977, the Commonwealth of Massachusetts authorized the hospital to grant academic degrees despite objections from other local area universities, and later that year, under Mankin's leadership, the hospital formed the IHP. Mankin was also instrumental in attracting its first students. Jette described him as the IHP's "spirit and energy in those early years," and as "dedicated to the school's mission of developing leaders in the healthcare professions. He frequently gave talks at the hospital, and he held well-attended lectures at Shriners Auditorium to publicize the IHP." (quoted in Shaw 2019) In addition, Mankin served as an early

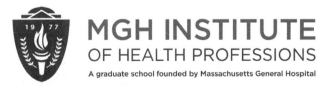

Logo MGH Institute of Health Professions. Courtesy of MGH Institute of Health Professions.

trustee—fulfilling that role for 20 years, and he created the Mary Mankin Prize in remembrance of his mother. Today, the IHP provides education in physical therapy, occupational therapy, physician assistant studies, nursing, communication sciences and disorders, and other health professions. Jette believed, "It's safe to say that without Henry's dedication and commitment, the Institute never would have made it to where it is today…He never wavered in his belief." (quoted in Shaw 2019)

A LEADER IN THE FIELD

Mankin was a prolific researcher. Throughout his career he published more than 670 articles, numerous chapters, and ~7 books. His last book, an autobiography titled *Such a Joy for a Yiddish Boy: A Memoir*, published in 2017—the year before he died.

He was a member or honorary member of 34 organizations, for which he served on many committees. He also held leadership positions in many professional organizations. He served as president of the Orthopaedic Research Society (1969), the American Board of Orthopaedic Surgery (1980), the Academic Orthopaedic Society, the American Orthopaedic Association (1982), and the Musculoskeletal Tumor Society (1983). He was a founding member of the latter organization, which was established in 1974. He was a member of the board of trustees of the Interhospital Organ Bank (1976–1984) and was a trustee of the *Journal of Bone and Joint Surgery* (1985–1987); after a few years, he became chairperson of the *Journal*'s trustees (1988–1990).

Mankin held numerous positions at the NIH, including membership on various study sections and the National Arthritis Advisory Board, and he served as chairperson of the Human Resources and Research Review for the National Institute of Arthritis, Diabetes, Digestive and Kidney Diseases (now defunct; replaced with two institutes: the NIAMS and the NIDDK).

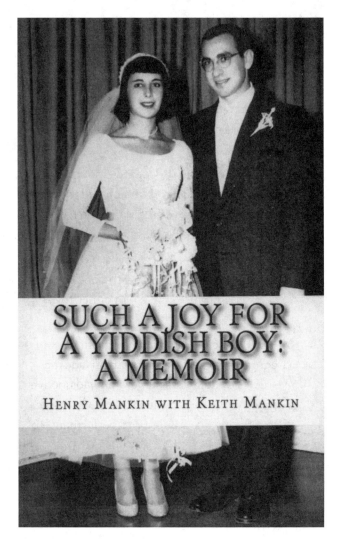

Mankin's autobiography written with his son, Keith.
Courtesy of Keith Mankin.

He served as a member of the Dean's Visiting Committee at the University of Pittsburgh since 1992. In 1992, the University of Pittsburgh School of Medicine endowed a chair in his name: the Henry J. Mankin Orthopaedic Research Professorship. Mankin received more than 45 other honors and awards (**Box 41.1**).

In his retirement years at Massachusetts General Hospital, Dr. Mankin continued to work in his lab office with Carol Trahan digitizing the large pathological collections left to him by Jaffe and Campbell. Mankin noted that during "my last years of clinical practice, I developed a computerized system for recording data for our tumor

Box 41.1. Mankin's Various Honors and Awards

- Philip Hench Distinguished Alumnus Award from the University of Pittsburgh (1974)
- Kappa Delta Award (1975)
- Shand's Award of the American Orthopaedic Association (1977)
- Shand's Award of the Orthopaedic Research Society (ORS) (1987)
- Legacy Laureate Award from the University of Pittsburgh (2001)
- Distinguished Alumnus Award from the University of Pittsburgh (2005)
- Distinguished Investigator Award of the ORS and the Orthopaedic Research and Education Foundation (2010)

Endowed Lectures

- R. I. Harris Lecture, Canadian Orthopaedic Association (1982)
- Bunnell Lecture, American Society for Surgery of the Hand (1984)
- Presidential Guest Speaker, American Academy of Orthopaedic Surgeons (1987)
- Sir John Charnley Lecture British Hip Society; Manchester, England (1995)
- Sir Robert Jones Lecture, Hospital for Joint Diseases (2001)
- Schiff Memorial Lecture, American College of Rheumatology (2001)
- Glen Edwards Day Speaker, University of Calgary (2002)
- The first Greer Lecture, Penn State Medical Center (2004)

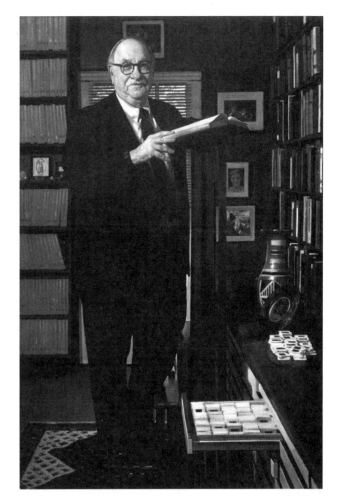

Portrait of Dr. Mankin. Massachusetts General Hospital, Archives and Special Collections.

service that I hope will become a standard in the field, and it now has searchable information for 18,000 patients with bone and soft tissue tumors" (Mankin and Mankin 2017). He was still working at age 90 when he died in his home in Brookline, Massachusetts, on December 22, 2018—"There were still manuscripts in preparation in his home office at the time of his passing" (Gebhardt and Friedlaender 2019). He was predeceased by his wife—Carole Jane (née Pinkey) Mankin—and survived by his three children, Allison (who worked with computers), David (who was a professor of classics at Cornell), and Keith (who was a pediatric orthopaedic surgeon). His colleagues Drs. Mark Gebhardt and Gary Friedlaender (2019) wrote in his obituary, "He will forever be remembered as a dedicated physician…a superb scientist, educator extraordinaire, leader and colorful raconteur…"

CHAPTER 42

MGH
Other Surgeon Scholars (1970–2000)

Dr. Henry Mankin (see chapter 41), chief of orthopaedics at Massachusetts General Hospital (MGH) from 1972 until 1996, transformed the orthopaedic program at MGH. When he first arrived, he brought four orthopaedic surgeons and a few research scientists with him from the Hospital for Joint Diseases. Those surgeons included Drs. Richard J. Smith, Robert D. Leffert, Michael G. Ehrlich, and Charles Weiss. Harvard calls the clinicians who practiced there at the end of the twentieth century "surgeon-scholars." The surgeon scholars covered in this chapter are listed below.

Although I was unable to find any reports of the orthopaedic department at MGH during the 1970s, there are five annual reports from Dr. Mankin on the Orthopaedic Service that he presented to the General Executive Committee (GEC) from 1980 through 1987. In 1980, he wrote, "The Orthopaedic Service at the MGH has a strong commitment to clinical care, education and research in diseases of the musculoskeletal system" (Mankin 1980). The orthopaedic staff consisted of 62 individuals at the time, 11 of whom were not orthopaedic surgeons, i.e., podiatrists and scientists. All had teaching appointments at Harvard Medical School (HMS); four were full professors. Mankin noted that many were distinguished throughout the United States, including current presidents of: the American Academy of Orthopaedic Surgeons (AAOS), the American Board of Orthopaedic Surgery (ABOS), and the Orthopaedic Research Society (ORS); two past presidents and a president-elect of the American Orthopaedic Association (AOA); one past president of the Orthopaedic Research Society (ORS); one president-elect of the American Society for Surgery of the Hand (ASSH); and the editor and

Michael G. Ehrlich	400
Richard H. Gelberman	402
L. Candace Jennings	405
Jesse B. Jupiter	407
Robert D. Leffert	412
David W. Lhowe	416
Frederick L. Mansfield	419
Dinesh G. Patel	421

Francis X. Pedlow Jr.	424
Richard J. Smith	427
Dempsey S. Springfield	431
George H. Theodore	437
William W. Tomford	439
Stephen B. Trippel	444
Bertram Zarins	446

associate editor of the *Journal of Bone and Joint Surgery* (JBJS). The orthopaedic service admitted 3,618 patients to the hospital each year (which was stable for eight years after Mankin's arrival), with an average daily census of 142 patients. Orthopaedic clinic visits averaged 35 patients per day, totaling 20,339 patients annually.

In addition to the specialty services he initiated in 1972 (see chapter 41), Mankin named Dr. Ed Wyman chief of the trauma unit and Drs. Dinesh Patel and Bertram Zarins to the newly formed sports service. A clinical orthopaedic service had recently been started at the Cambridge Hospital with Dr. Roger Emerson in charge. Outreach clinics were opened in Chelsea and Bunker Hill, and a close liaison was established with the Massachusetts Rehabilitation Hospital (later renamed Spaulding Hospital) to manage postoperative patients. There were eight fellows for one to two years: hand (2), hip (2), laboratory (2), tumor (1), and general orthopaedics (1), in addition to the orthopaedic residents (see chapter 11).

Two HMS continuing medical education courses were held yearly: "Hand" and "Hip and Implant" courses. Each were three days in length. Dr. Mankin also organized a two-week course in basic science for orthopaedic surgeons at Salve Regina College in Newport, RI. In 1979, 130 orthopaedists attended the course. The MGH weekly department conferences included hand, trauma, sports, hip and implant, tumor, pathology slide review, morbidity and mortality, as well as a chief's conference. Grand rounds were on Saturday, followed by a basic science conference. The conferences were case oriented with a minimum of didactic presentations. The orthopaedic staff also provided a six-hour weekly course on outpatient orthopaedics for the primary care house officers.

The orthopaedic laboratories (biochemistry and bioengineering) occupied 4,000-square feet on the 10th floor in the Jackson Building. The only growth in the staff of the department by the time of Mankin's next report, in 1981, included two non-orthopaedist positions; total orthopaedic staff was 64. Annual admissions increased slightly to 3,765. Outpatient visits remained unchanged. The orthopaedic clinic was located on the fourth floor of the Ambulatory Care Center (ACC). Mankin reported the following changes: a microvascular team directed by Dr. Jesse Jupiter was included on the hand service; an arthroscopic unit was headed by Dr. Patel; the sports service was headed by Dr. Zarins. A very active podiatry service within the department was led by Dr. Robert J. Scardina; the Massachusetts Rehabilitation Unit was headed by Dr. Samuel Doppelt; a teaching unit for resident rotations under Dr. Ralph Sweetland had been started at Salem Hospital; and orthopaedic outreach clinics were continued in Chelsea and Bunker Hill. A new clinic was opened at Logan Airport. A bone bank for allografts was established by Dr. Mankin and William Tomford with five freezers containing 300 specimens. It was funded by Blue Cross insurance payments. Fellows were increased to 10 with an additional one on the spine service and two on the sports service. The general orthopaedic fellowship was discontinued. A new postgraduate course was initiated—a two-day course called "Orthopaedics for the Nonorthopaedist." Mankin initiated his well-known course in pathology, which was a city-wide program for orthopaedic residents in Boston (Harvard, Tufts, and Boston universities) and others in the region. Six lectures were also given by the staff to the Institute for the Health Professions.

Mankin, in his 1981 report, which he presented to the General Executive Committee on November 12, 1982, noted the following problems facing the orthopaedic service during the next year: 1) The department had several staff members who are approaching or who had passed retirement age. New young staff orthopaedic surgeons were needed in his opinion, including a spine surgeon, a total knee surgeon, and additional surgeons on both the tumor and sports services. At the time, he was negotiating for a combined tumor service with Boston Children's Hospital. 2) The operating time for the department was inadequate. The four designated operating rooms for orthopaedics were very busy, second only to the cardiac service, and the staff often had to delay elective cases until Saturdays. The average orthopaedic daily census was 147 patients; a maximum of 160 beds was designated for orthopaedics. 3) In research, the loss of Dennis Carter, PhD (bioengineering) was significant and, apparently, he was difficult to replace. Mankin commented that HMS and MIT were not interested in giving appropriate joint appointments to researchers working in hospitals.

Dr. Mankin also described the Harvard Combined Orthopaedic Residency Program (HCORP) in great detail, including ongoing changes (see chapter 11). He noted that the residents not only took care of the indigent patients and trauma cases, but were also the major providers of resident education. Partial funding was available for each resident to attend only one course or meeting per year. If they had a paper to present, funding was required from the senior author and would not be covered by the research budget. A stipend of $21,200 ($55,212 in 2014) was provided to the first year orthopaedic residents (PGY 3) and each had three weeks of vacation per year. The average daily bed census for orthopaedics in each hospital in 1981 was: MGH, 145; Children's Hospital, 70; BWH, 90; BIH, 44; Salem, 28; and the West Roxbury VA, 12.

The only growth reported in the department's annual report in 1983 was the addition of nine podiatrists. Annual admissions numbered 3,808, with 135 patients on the Rehabilitation Service. With the managed care movement and, especially the impact of the prospective payment system (PPS) in the 1980s, the orthopaedic service experienced a decrease in patient days by 5% the previous year, by 11% in the past five years. The average length of stay was 10.2 days, reduced from 12.2 days in 1979. The use of allocated beds in 1983 for the orthopaedic service was 76%. Clinic visits increased by 10% to 21,065 for the year, but daily visits remained unchanged at 35. Mankin described the podiatry service as "excellent" with an increase of clinic visits by 32% (total: 5,604) since 1982. One service chief change occurred: Dr. Leroy Levine (former chief of orthopaedics at Downstate) was now in charge of the Orthopaedic Rehabilitation Service at Spaulding Hospital. With the combined efforts of Drs. W. Gerald Austen, Michael Ehrlich, and Donald N. Medearis, and a grant from the Phillips Foundation, a gait laboratory was installed in the basement of Sleeper Hall. It was led by Andrew Hodge and affiliated with Robert Mann at MIT. New research programs included studies on bone growth into implants and studies on chemonucleolysis.

The impact of the PPS was felt in the operating rooms as well. Inpatient operating room cases in Gray decreased from 3,706 in 1982 to 3,456 in 1983. However, there had begun a shift to outpatient surgery, from 1,188 in 1982 to 1,235 in 1983. Fellows increased to 11 with one additional fellow (three in total) added to the laboratory. Dr. Levine taught anatomy to the students in the Institute for the Health Professions. No further changes occurred in the HCORP.

Dr. Mankin continued to express some problems. Even though some staff had been added—Dr. W. Andrew Hodge on hip and implant, Dr. Mark Gebhardt on tumors, and Dr. Frederick Mansfield on spine, introducing chymopapain at both MGH and Cambridge Hospital—there was a deficit approaching in sports medicine with the upcoming planned retirement of Dr. Carter Rowe. Mankin noted a future need to assist Dr. Zarins in providing coverage for both the Patriots and the Bruins. Dr. Crawford Campbell had died, and Mankin wanted to also replace his position on staff. Mankin continued to express a need for additional operating room time, stating that 20% of orthopaedic cases were done on other services' unused time. Younger staff surgeons were apparently also having to operate at the Cambridge, the Deaconess, the Baptist, Sancta Maria, Faulkner, and Boston Children's hospitals.

In his 1984 report to the General Executive Committee, Mankin noted that the staff had increased to 77: 63 orthopaedic surgeons (46 at MGH, Spaulding, and Cambridge Hospitals; 39 geographic full-time), 10 podiatrists, one veterinarian, and two PhDs. There had been no promotions at HMS for several years. Admissions increased by 4% to 4,288 (an increase of 10% since 1979). Patient days decreased 9.5% and the average length of stay was 10 days. The orthopaedic service was the 3rd largest service at MGH (15.3% of patient days). Clinic visits increased 8% (23.6% since 1979). Seventy-five percent of patients at Spaulding came from the MGH. The podiatry service had an increase of 44% in its outpatient department. The department was given an additional operating room one day per week. Primary operating time had increased to 219.5 hours per week. There had been a slight increase in operating room cases (5,051 compared to 4,976 in 1983); 3,298 in Gray and 1,553 in the day care unit. The tumor service saw 350 new patients in 1984. A center to study Gaucher's Disease was established. In the HCORP, a new core curriculum was started on Saturday mornings, each session lasting two hours.

The department's laboratories remained on Jackson 10 during this period. Dr. Samuel Doppelt was studying osteopenia; Drs. William H. Harris and Dennis Burke, the use of centrifugation of cement; and Dr. Murali Jasty was investigating bone upgrowth into metallic implants. Dr. Hodge was studying gait abnormalities in neuromuscular disorders. The following problems were mentioned by Dr. Mankin: a small staff and a low equipment budget in the operating rooms. He identified a need for an additional sports specialist, a replacement for Dr. Thornton Brown (who was planning to retire), and a need for "generalists" to see patients with common problems and "add-ons" in the department's group of specialty practices. Mankin also provided a list of orthopaedic staff at MGH in his 1984 report (see **Box 42.1**)

Mankin's last available annual report was in 1987. The staff consisted of 75 members: 67 orthopaedic surgeons—4 honorary, 3 seniors who

Box 42.1. Orthopaedic Staff at MGH in 1984

Honorary Orthopaedic Surgeons

Drs. Otto Aufranc, Melvin Glimcher, Paul Norton, John Reidy, and Clement Sledge

Senior Orthopaedic Surgeons

Drs. Thornton Brown and Carter Rowe

Visiting Orthopaedic Surgeons

Drs. Joseph Barr Jr., Robert Boyd, Hugh Chandler, Paul Curtiss, Michael Ehrlich, William Harris, William Jones, Leroy Levine, Robert Leffert, William MacAusland, Keith Mankin, Donald Pierce, Richard Smith, Augustus White, and Edwin Wyman

Associate Orthopaedic Surgeons

Drs. William Kermond, Dinesh Patel, William Tomford, and Bertram Zarins

Assistant in Bioengineering

James A. Greer, PhD

Visiting Podiatrist (Orthopaedic Service)

Robert J. Scardina, DPM

Podiatrists (Orthopaedic Service)

Drs. Ioli, Kigner, Soloway, and Yates

Clinical Associates in Podiatry (Orthopaedic Service)

Drs. Donovan, Fritz, and Winer;

Consultants in Podiatry (Orthopaedic Service)

Drs. Bloom and Connolly

Consultant in Engineering Science (Orthopaedic Service)

Robert W. Mann, ScD.

Consultant in Veterinary Medicine (Orthopaedic Service)

William B. Henry Jr.

taught but did not provide patient care—and 55 who cared for patients—32, including 9 fellows and two "chiefs" who were "geographic full-time" (Mankin 1987). Full professors decreased by one, to three, with two promotions to full professor in process. Dr. Richard Smith died a premature death from a brain tumor and was succeeded by Dr. Richard Gelberman. Dr. Rowe retired and was succeeded by Dr. Arthur Boland. Dr. Dempsey Springfield was recruited to the tumor service by Mankin. Regarding clinical care Mankin wrote, "The staff are not great joiners of the various HMOs and for the most part our unit remains unencumbered" (Mankin 1987). Admissions decreased slightly to 3,571 and patient days continued to drop. Cases in the Ambulatory Care Unit (ACU) for outpatients increased, especially in podiatry, which doubled since 1982. On the sports service, Dr. Zarins continued to cover the Patriots and Bruins, and Dr. Boland covered all Harvard teams. The leaders in trauma care included Drs. Edwin Wyman, Jesse Jupiter, John Siliski, and David Lhowe. Jupiter also started a problem foot clinic. Regarding operating-room utilization, Mankin reported that the department continued to "overutilize" facilities, with a modest increase in 1986 in both Gray and same day surgery (SDS) and in operating time, but a decrease in volume of cases (11%) with the loss of Dr. Smith.

The number of fellows increased to 18, including Hand, 3; Hip & Implant, 3; Sports, 3; Tumor, 3; Pediatric Orthopaedics, 1; Microvascular Surgery, 1; Research, 4. Mankin remarked that "none derive their income from general funds" (Mankin 1987). He stated, "The Orthopaedic Service is by standards of other services in the country and abroad, a successful one" (Mankin 1987). However, the following were problems he identified: 1) The lack of volume control, problems in access and competition for scarce resources, associated with fiscal and physical restraints, were having an adverse impact on patient care. Orthopaedics now utilized 23% of the total hours available in the operating room. Average orthopaedic utilization in Gray is 77%; mean overall utilization by other services is 56%. 2) The total malpractice losses of the HCORP "Chiefs" compared to total losses with associated changes in premiums over the previous five years were such that Dr. Mankin "believed we are being inappropriately considered as 'high-risk' by our Insurance Company" (Mankin 1987). 3) Additional space was needed in the clinics, offices and research laboratories. The research budget was very high at $400 per square foot. In the past only, Mankin had grant funding; now other investigators had obtained grants. Approval for an upper extremity service on White 9, approved in 1984, was planned for completion that year. Money had been raised for a Richard J. Smith Learning Center on White 9. 4) Over the past seven years, the Orthopaedic Department had provided an orthopaedic service at Cambridge Hospital, led by Dr. Roger Emerson for the first five years and Dr. David Lhowe the latter two years. Mankin also pointed out that the cost of this service has been carried by the MGH Orthopaedic Department. He alerted the general executive committee that the arrangement might have to be terminated.

Mankin's leadership continued through 1996, when he retired. Afterward, Dr. William Tomford was appointed interim chair from 1996–1998. In 1998, Dr. Harry Rubash was appointed chief of orthopaedics at MGH. The Department of Orthopaedics at MGH continued to have its finger on the pulse of new innovations and advancements as it moved forward into the new millennium. This chapter includes brief biographies of only some of the orthopaedic staff who practiced at MGH from 1970 to 2000. Data on the number and types of publications each surgeon scholar produced are included, however, research for each surgeon was completed over about a 10-year period and such information quickly becomes outdated. These data are representative of the breadth of their work. They may have written many more articles since that time.

MICHAEL G. EHRLICH

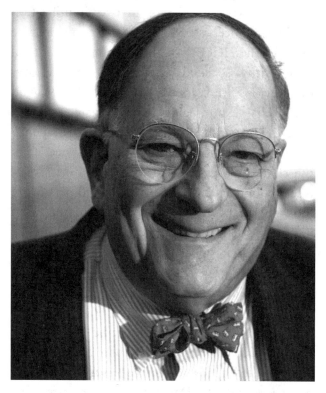

Michael G. Ehrlich. David Del Poio/Brown University. Used with permission.

> **Physician Snapshot**
>
> Michael G. Ehrlich
> BORN: 1939
> DIED: 2018
> SIGNIFICANT CONTRIBUTIONS: Completed basic research in cartilage metabolism and growth plate physiology; permanent member of the NIH Study Section on Orthopaedics and Musculoskeletal Disease; first MGH chief of pediatric orthopaedics; president of the Orthopaedic Research Society; president of the Academic Orthopaedic Society

Michael Gary Ehrlich was born on September 4, 1939, in the Bronx, where he grew up. He graduated summa cum laude from Dartmouth College in 1959 with an AB degree. He received the Thesis Award and was elected into Phi Beta Kappa. In 1963, he received his MD degree from Columbia University College of Physicians and Surgeons and was elected into Alpha Omega Alpha. Following a mixed medical internship at Bellevue Hospital on the First Medical Division/Columbia and a year as assistant medical resident on the same service, he joined the staff at Ohio State Medical School as clinical instructor in preventive medicine for two years. In 1967, he returned to New York as a resident in orthopaedic surgery at Mt. Sinai Hospital. In 1969, he was chief resident in the orthopaedic program. From 1970 to 1972, he was a research/pediatric fellow at the Hospital for Joint Diseases. As a fellow, he held an appointment as a clinical instructor in orthopaedics, was assistant adjunct orthopaedic surgeon at the Hospital for Joint Diseases, and was an assistant attending orthopaedic surgeon at both Mt. Sinai Hospital and City Hospital Center at Elmhurst, New York. Dr. Henry Mankin was Ehrlich's chief during his residency and fellowship years. Ehrlich accompanied Mankin to Massachusetts General Hospital (MGH) in 1972.

Chief of the Pediatric Orthopaedic Service

Mankin named Ehrlich as chief of the pediatric orthopaedic service at MGH; Ehrlich was also appointed instructor of orthopaedics at Harvard Medical School at Mankin's recommendation. In 1975, Ehrlich was promoted to assistant professor and, in 1978, to associate professor and associate orthopaedic surgeon at MGH. He remained at MGH for 18 years. During this period, he served as president of the Orthopaedic Research Society in 1980, received the Elizabeth Winston Lanier Award (Kappa Delta Award) in 1984 for his research, and received the Wood Lovell Award (co-recipient) by the Pediatric Orthopaedic Society in 1989. While at MGH Ehrlich published over 55 articles, one book, about 11 chapters, and one video. **Case 42.1** highlights an example of one of the many cases he reviewed. He received a grant from the Orthopaedic Research and Education Foundation and was co-investigator on several NIH grants on cartilage metabolism.

In 1990 Ehrlich was chosen as professor and chairman of the Orthopaedic Department at

Case 42.1. Idiopathic Subluxation of the Radial Head

> "[The patient] was the product of a 35 week pregnancy and subsequently had retarded psycho-motor development. He was first seen in the Pediatric Clinic of the Massachusetts General Hospital at age 7, where his IQ was measured at 62. He had no specific complaints with respect to his elbows at that time. By age 11, however, he developed pain in his left elbow. There was no history of antecedent trauma or temporary disability. X-rays at that time showed lateral and posterior positioning but not dislocation of the proximal radius compatible with subluxation and mild irregularity of the head on the right. X-rays of the patellae and iliac crests were normal. There was no ligamentous laxity. The nails were normal.
>
> "The discomfort persisted so he was reevaluated in August, 1973. Physical examination then showed a full range of motion of the right elbow except for a 10° fixed flexion contracture. The left elbow had a 30° fixed flexion contracture with further flexion to 135°. Rotation in 90° of flexion showed pronation/supination at 40/25. The radial head was felt to "click" as the elbow moved from flexion to extension. On October 3, 1973, the left radial head was excised through a standard Boyd approach. (The radial head definitely articulated with the capitellum but had an irregular, multi-faceted articular surface covered by smooth glistening articular cartilage.)
>
> "In follow-up at 15 months, he had a 30° flexion contracture and further flexion to 135°. There was no change in pronation and supination, but the pain was gone. He was active in sports and denied symptoms on the right."
>
> (William Southmayd and Michael G. Ehrlich 1976)

Brown University Medical School and surgeon-in-chief of the Department of Orthopaedics at Rhode Island Hospital. (He succeeded me in this role, after I had accepted the position of David Silver Professor and Chairman at the University of Pittsburgh in 1988.) Dr. David Zaleske and Dr. Zeke Zimbler took up the mantle of Ehrlich's work at MGH advancing a curriculum and research program in pediatric orthopaedics. That work was later continued by Dr. Keith Mankin as well.

Partial purification and characterization of a proteoglycan-degrading neutral protease from bovine epiphyseal cartilage.

Authors: Ehrlich MG, Armstrong AL, Mankin HJ

Source: Journal of orthopaedic research : official publication of the Orthopaedic Research Society [J Orthop Res] 1984; Vol. 2 (2), pp. 126-33.

Ehrlich received the 1984 Kappa Delta Award for his research on degradative enzymes in articular cartilage. *Journal of Orthopaedic Research* 1984; 2: 126.

Chairman of the Orthopaedic Department at Brown and Surgeon-in-chief of the Department of Orthopaedics at Rhode Island Hospital

At Brown, Ehrlich continued his basic research in bone and cartilage metabolism and his clinical practice of pediatric orthopaedics, producing over 70 more articles and about 15 book chapters. He was industrious and conscientious, a mentor to many, and had a distinct personality seen in "signature bow ties [and] wry sense of humor" (Naaem 2018). In 1998, he was named the Vincent Zecchino Professor of Orthopaedic Surgery and appointed as surgeon-in-chief in the Department of Orthopaedics at Miriam Hospital. He received additional honors for his research, remained on the orthopaedic study section at NIH for a number of years, and, in 1999, was named president of the Academic Orthopaedic Society.

Dr. Ehrlich died in Providence, RI, on July 21, 2018, at the age of 79. He was predeceased by his wife, Nancy Band Ehrlich. Ehrlich was survived by his sons, Christopher and Timothy Ehrlich. The Michael G. Ehrlich, MD, Fund for Orthopedic Research was formed in his honor.

RICHARD H. GELBERMAN

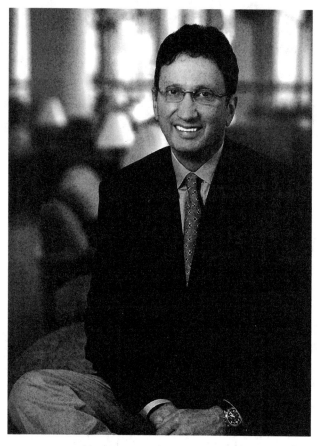

Richard H. Gelberman. Courtesy of the American Orthopaedic Association.

Physician Snapshot

Richard H. Gelberman
BORN: 1943
DIED: —
SIGNIFICANT CONTRIBUTIONS: Established clinical investigator; recipient of the Kappa Delta Award; chief of the MGH orthopaedic hand service 1987–1995; professor and chairman of orthopaedics at Washington University; president of AAOS 2001; president of ASSH 2006; chairman of the *JBJS* board of trustees 2013; member of the National Academy of Medicine 2003

Richard Hugh Gelberman was born in New York City. He graduated from the University of North Carolina, Chapel Hill, in 1965 and the University of Tennessee Medical School in 1969. After an internship at Los Angeles County Hospital, he completed an orthopaedic residency program at the University of Wisconsin Medical Center in 1975. From 1976 to 1977, he was a fellow in Hand and Microvascular Surgery at Duke University Medical Center.

Chief of the Hand and Microvascular Service at the UCSD

In 1977, Dr. Gelberman began his academic career at the University of California in San Diego (UCSD) and at the Veterans Administration Medical Center in La Jolla, California. He was named the chief of the Hand and Microvascular Service and head of the Replantation Surgery Team. In five years, he was promoted from assistant professor of surgery to associate professor. The following year, he was promoted to professor of orthopaedic surgery. In a 10-year period, Gelberman established himself as an expert in hand and microsurgery, asking basic questions about clinical problems and doing the research necessary to answer the questions.

He published about 52 articles and 14 book chapters. Ten articles focused on carpal tunnel syndrome, with important discoveries of the

The vascularity of the lunate bone and Kienböck's disease

Richard H. Gelberman, M.D., Thomas D. Bauman, M.D., Jaysanker Menon, M.D., *and* Wayne H. Akeson, M.D.,
THE JOURNAL OF HAND SURGERY
Vol. 5, No. 3
May 1980

The vascularity of the scaphoid bone

Richard H. Gelberman, M.D., *and* Jaysanker Menon, M.D.
THE JOURNAL OF HAND SURGERY
Vol. 5, No. 5
September 1980

Gelberman's landmark articles on the vascularity of the lunate and carpal scaphoid bones. *Journal of Hand Surgery* 1980; 5: 508.

influence of wrist position on intracarpal pressures as a cause of carpel tunnel syndrome, as well as the value of sensibility testing and treatments of the syndrome. He published landmark papers on the vascularity of the wrist—including the scaphoid and lunate bones—and the vascularity of the talus and the flexor pollicis longus tendon. He published five articles on flexor tendon healing, including three basic research studies in both dogs and pigs. **Case 42.2** also highlights an example of one of the many cases he reviewed. In 1983, he received the Emanuel Kaplan Award for Anatomical Excellence from the American Society for Surgery of the Hand, and in 1985 he received the Elizabeth Winston Lanier/Kappa Delta Award for his research on flexor tendon repair.

Chief of the Hand Service at MGH and Professor of Orthopaedic Surgery at HMS

After 10 years in San Diego, Dr. Gelberman was recruited by Dr. Henry Mankin as the chief of the Hand Service at MGH following the death of Dr. Richard Smith. Gelberman's academic appointment was professor of orthopaedic surgery at Harvard Medical School. He remained at MGH for eight years and was in charge of the hand fellowship program, as he had been at UCSD. He transferred his NIH grant on flexor tendon healing to MGH. His initial grant began in 1977, and it has been renewed throughout his career.

In 1987, he was placed in charge of the Core Educational Curriculum of the Harvard Combined Orthopaedic Residency Program (HCORP)

Case 42.2. Avascular Necrosis of the Lunate in a Patient with Sickle Cell Disease

> "An 18-year-old, right-hand-dominant black man presented in January 1983 with the chief complaint of pain in his right wrist. He described a three-to-four-month period of increasing discomfort and gradual limitation of motion. He had been a patient at the hospital of one of the authors for the previous ten years and had received treatment for a number of sickle cell crises during this period. However, he had received no treatment for skeletal manifestations of sickle cell anemia prior to January 1983 and had no history of trauma to the wrist. Physical examination revealed tenderness dorsally over the radiocarpal articulation. Range of motion of the right wrist was flexion/extension, 10°/40°; radial deviation/ulnar deviation, 10°/10°; and pronation/supination, 75°/80°. Range of motion of the left wrist was flexion/extension, 55°/70°; radial deviation/ulnar deviation, 20°/25°; and pronation/supination, 85°/75°. Grip strength measured 30 lbs on the right and 80 lbs on the left. Review of a skeletal survey performed in October 1979 disclosed decreased bony trabeculae in the distal radius with an apparently normal lunate. Subsequent radiographs of the right wrist obtained in March 1983 demonstrated fragmentation and collapse of the lunate with a widened scapholunate distance and Stage III Kienböck's disease. There appeared to be slight negative ulnar variance although standardized roentgenographic technique for measuring this was not performed. The patient was treated by proximal row carpectomy. The pathologic findings revealed osseous necrosis consistent with advanced Kienböck's disease. In addition, prominent sickling of the red blood cells was seen in the lunate."
>
> (Lanzer, Szabo, and Gelberman 1984)

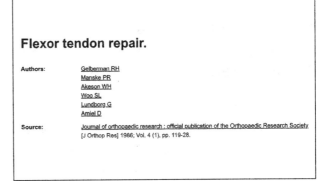

Gelberman received the 1985 Kappa Delta Award for his research on flexor tendon repair. *Journal of Orthopaedic Research* 1986; 4: 119.

> **Kappa Delta Award paper. Tissue fluid pressures: from basic research tools to clinical applications.**
>
> Authors: Hargens AR; Division of Orthopaedics and Rehabilitation, University of California, San Diego.
> Akeson WH
> Mubarak SJ
> Owen CA
> Gershuni DH
> Garfin SR
> Lieber RL
> Danzig LA
> Botte MJ
> Gelberman RH
>
> Source: Journal of orthopaedic research : official publication of the Orthopaedic Research Society
> [J Orthop Res] 1989; Vol. 7 (6), pp. 902-9.

Gelberman received the 1987 Kappa Delta Award for his research on tissue fluid pressures. *Journal of Orthopaedic Research* 1989; 7: 902.

(see chapter 11). In 1990, the residents in the HCORP named him "Teacher of the Year." His commitment to education was unwavering, and in 1994 he was appointed chair of the Council on Education of the American Academy of Orthopaedic Surgeons. He received several national awards for his research in 1989, including the Nicolas Andry Award from the Association of Bone and Joint Surgeons, The Sumner Koch Award from the American Society for Surgery of the Hand, and his second Elizabeth Winston Lanier/Kappa Delta Award for Orthopaedic Research (for his paper "Tissue Fluid Pressures: From Basic Research to Clinical Applications").

Chair of the Department of Orthopaedic Surgery at Washington University School of Medicine

In 1995, Gelberman was recruited to Washington University School of Medicine as the Fred C. Reynolds Professor and chair of the Department of Orthopaedic Surgery and department chair of orthopaedic surgery at Barnes-Jewish and St. Louis Children's Hospital. He was the first chair of the department; previously orthopaedics had been a division in the Department of Surgery. He headed both the orthopaedic residency program and the hand fellowship program.

Dr. Gelberman continued his strong educational and research interests (including asking basic questions about clinical problems) while leading the new department into its new position as one of the country's most excellent academic and training programs. He continued to publish more than 290 articles, four books, and a total of about 32 book chapters. He has received numerous additional awards, including both the Distinguished Clinical Educator Award and the Distinguished Contributions to Orthopaedics Award from the American Orthopaedic Association. In 2003, he was elected to the National Academy of Medicine of the National Academy of Sciences. He served as president of the American Academy of Orthopaedic Surgeons in 2001,

> VOLUME **I**
>
> # OPERATIVE NERVE REPAIR AND RECONSTRUCTION
>
> RICHARD H. GELBERMAN, MD
> Professor of Orthopaedic Surgery
> Harvard Medical School
> Chief of Hand Surgery Service
> Department of Orthopaedic Surgery
> Massachusetts General Hospital
> Boston, Massachusetts
>
> 126 Contributors
> *with illustrations by Elizabeth Roselius*
>
> J. B. LIPPINCOTT COMPANY
> Philadelphia
> New York
> London Hagerstown

Title page of Gelberman's book, *Operative Nerve Repair and Reconstruction*. Philadelphia: J. B. Lippincott, 1991.

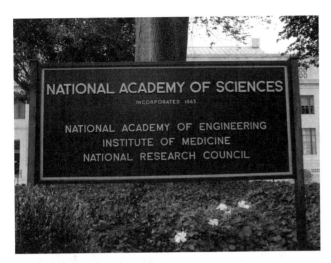

Sign at the entrance to the National Academy of Medicine (renamed from the Institute of Medicine in 2015).
Another Believer/Wikimedia Commons.

president of the American Society for Surgery of the Hand in 2006, and chairman of the trustees of the *Journal of Bone and Joint Surgery* in 2013.

In his 2016 acceptance speech when receiving the American Orthopaedic Association's Distinguished Contributions to Orthopaedics Award, Dr. Gelberman reflected on one of his most prominent achievements: providing the orthopaedic department at Washington University with a unified sense of purpose. During his tenure, the department saw a boost in morale, an overhaul in department funds and finances, and a significant shift in how potential residents viewed an opportunity to work there. The department also obtained important NIH funds and overall established itself as distinguished. In his speech, Dr. Gelberman graciously and humbly took the time to thank his staff for their dedication to accomplishing these changes.

L. CANDACE JENNINGS

Physician Snapshot

L. Candace Jennings
BORN: 1949
DIED: —
SIGNIFICANT CONTRIBUTIONS: Orthopaedic tumor surgeon; specialist in hospice care and palliative medicine

L. Candace Jennings, a distant relative by marriage to Dr. Robert Osgood (see chapter 19), graduated from Tufts University School of Medicine in 1983. After an internship and a year of surgical residency at Beth Israel Deaconess Medical Center, she entered the Harvard Combined Orthopaedic Residency Program (HCORP) in 1985. She completed her orthopaedic residency in 1988 and then a fellowship in orthopaedic oncology with Henry Mankin at MGH.

Orthopaedic Tumor Service at MGH

Dr. Jennings remained on the staff at MGH in a tumor practice with Drs. Mankin, Springfield, and Gebhardt. She published approximately 14 articles. Her first, in 1988, was a report of two cases of compression of the ulnar nerve by a ganglion in canal of Guyon (see **Case 42.3**). Her other papers were coauthored by Dr. Mankin and her colleagues.

Jennings remained in active practice on the tumor service at MGH for about 10 years before becoming ill with cancer herself. She completed chemotherapy and radiation for breast cancer in 1998, but although she attempted to return to practice in 1999, she found it too difficult to overcome the limitations of cancer fatigue. She spent a hiatus volunteering as a part-time high school biology teacher instead. She spoke about her frustrations when she said:

> "Somebody's got to solve cancer fatigue...It really affects your self-esteem," especially if you're used to being productive...

Treatment for the fatigue that can last long after treatment lags far behind...it's a huge, under-recognized problem for many of the 8 million Americans who've had cancer...[in a survey] of 419 patients...fatigue, not pain, was the most common complaint...Even two years after treatment, 76 percent...had debilitating fatigue at least once a week...[Another physician with cancer said] "The adjustment to my energy limitation has been harder than managing many of the other challenges of survivorship." Jennings echoes that. (Foreman 1999)

Despite giving up her practice in 1999, she nevertheless had a significant role in the publication of a paper on chondrosarcoma of bone that same year. She wrote:

The data on 227 patients who had been managed for a chondrosarcoma at one institution were reviewed...Although the data are suggestive...we could not detect a significant difference in the rates of pulmonary metastases and death between the patients who had a grade-3 lesion and those who had a grade-3 lesion that was also dedifferentiated...Overall, patients who had a resection with wide margins...had a longer duration of survival than did those who had a so-called marginal resection. Adjunctive chemotherapy or radiation, or both...did not appear to alter the outcome...It is distressing to note that more recent rates of local recurrence, metastases, and death are no better than those for patients who were operated on twenty years ago. (F.Y. Lee et al. 1999)

Her last known publication with her tumor colleagues was in 2001. She and her colleagues reviewed the case of a patient with multifocal epithelioid hemangioendothelioma. When they followed up with x-rays, the disease appeared to be in remission almost six years after surgical treatment, chemotherapy, and four radiofrequency ablations.

Case 42.3. Ulnar Nerve Compression at the Wrist

"A 46-year-old right hand dominant man was referred for weakness of the left hand of nine months' duration. He complained of difficulty holding dishes and an inability to trim his fingernails while holding a nail clipper in his left hand. Three months before referral the patient complained of pain in the hypothenar region of the left hand, and 2 months later he noted a mass in that region. The past history was remarkable for intermittent mild neck pain and stiffness without radicular symptoms over the past 25 years.

"Physical examination showed a 1 x 1 cm firm mass in the hypothenar region of the left palm. There was atrophy of the hypothenar, first dorsal interosseous, and adductor muscles. There was no atrophy of the extrinsic muscles of the hand. There was a positive Froment's sign. The Allen test showed perfusion of the hand from the ulnar artery in less than 5 seconds. Semmes-Weinstein monofilament testing and two-point discrimination were normal in all digits. Grip strength was 70 pounds on the right and 60 pounds on the left. Nerve conduction studies were consistent with compression of the ulnar nerve in Guyon's canal.

"An exploration of the distal ulnar tunnel was done after the patient was given axillary block anesthetics. The motor branch of the ulnar nerve was followed along its course as it penetrated the interval between the abductor digiti minimi and flexor digiti minimi muscles. At that point the motor branch was noted to be compressed between a fibrous arch at the proximal edge of the hypothenar muscles and a ganglion, which arose from the space between the pisohamate and pisometacarpal ligaments. The sensory branch was spared. The ganglion was traced to its origin at the triquetro-hamate joint and completely excised.

"Histologic examination of the specimen confirmed the diagnosis of ganglion. At follow-up 4 months after surgery the patient noted resolution of symptoms. First dorsal interosseous and adductor muscle strength had returned to normal."

(Kuschner, Gelberman, and Jennings 1988)

Return to Practice

In 2011, Jennings returned to healthcare by completing a one-year fellowship in Hospice and Palliative Medicine at Lehigh Valley Hospital in Allentown, Pennsylvania. The fellowship included several components: 12 months of continuity care with hospice patients, a six-month inpatient experience with one month on the tumor service and one month on long-term care, two months on the inpatient hospice unit and two weeks on pediatrics. She has a Certificate of Added Qualifications (CAQ) from the American Board of Surgery in Hospice and Palliative Medicine and practices in Denver, Colorado.

JESSE B. JUPITER

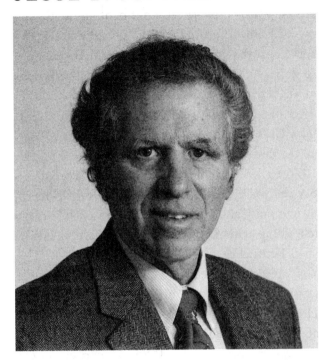

Jessie B. Jupiter. Massachusetts General Hospital.

Physician Snapshot

Jesse B. Jupiter
BORN: 1946
DIED: —

SIGNIFICANT CONTRIBUTIONS: Expert in management of fractures of the upper extremity, prolific speaker and writer, chief of the MGH orthopaedic hand service 1995–2012, coauthor (with Diego L. Fernandez) of *Fractures of the Distal Radius: A Practical Approach to Management*, Hansjörg Wyss/AO Professor at HMS, trustee AO Foundation 1987–1997, president AASH 2012, president ASES 2015

Jesse Barnard Jupiter was born in New York City. He attended Brown University where he played soccer and—several decades later—was elected into Brown University's Athletic Hall of Fame. He graduated from Brown in 1968 with a BA degree and was elected into Phi Beta Kappa. In 1972, he received his MD degree from Yale University School of Medicine. He then completed a surgical internship and one year as an assistant resident in surgery at the Hospital of the University of

Pennsylvania. From 1973 to 1975, he completed his two-year military commitment as a general medical officer in the United States Public Health Service in the Indian Health Branch. In Sacaton, Arizona, he helped develop educational programs in diabetes and arthritis for the Pima Indians. After his discharge, Jupiter entered the Massachusetts General Hospital/Boston Children's Hospital combined orthopaedic residency program from 1976 to 1979. In 1980 and 1981, he completed two fellowships: an AO trauma fellowship in Basel, Switzerland, and a hand and microvascular surgery fellowship with Dr. Harold E. Kleinert in Louisville, Kentucky.

Jupiter returned to Boston in 1981 as an assistant orthopaedic surgeon at Mass. General Hospital and instructor of orthopaedic surgery at Harvard Medical School; he was promoted to assistant professor in 1985. In particular, Dr. Jupiter made major contributions to the management of fractures of the distal radius, especially intra-articular fractures. In 1986, after only five years in practice, he was the lead author on a very frequently quoted paper, "Intra-Articular Fractures of the Distal End of the Radius in Young Adults." This article represents an insight into Dr. Jupiter's contributions.

After observing a clinical, often surgical, problem, and after careful thought, he makes recommendations for new specific approaches to treatment. In this case, it was how to manage an intra-articular fraction of the distal radius. In a retrospective study, 43 patients treated at MGH with intra-articular fractures of the distal radius were followed for an average of seven years. The average age of the patient was 28; yet in 65% of the fractures post-traumatic arthritis resulted. If the radiocarpal joint was incongruent 91% developed arthritis. He concluded:

> As a result of our findings, we now approach the complex fracture in the following manner. An initial attempt at closed reduction...is accomplished...If an anatomical reduction is achieved, external fixation with a frame is applied...if a reduced die-punch fragment is present, additional percutaneous fixation of the fragment with Kirschner wires should be considered...If the surface of the joint remains impacted with an incongruity of more than two millimeters after closed reduction, we now consider open reduction and internal fixation with cancellous bone graft to support the articular surface... This can be further supported with Kirschner wires and external fixation, a cast, or a buttress plate. (Knirk and Jupiter 1986)

Four years later, Jupiter was promoted to associate professor at Harvard Medical School and to associate orthopaedic surgeon at MGH; thereafter, he was promoted at MGH to visiting orthopaedic surgeon in 1994. From 1993 to 1995, he was director of the Orthopaedic Trauma Service and in 1995 became director of the Orthopaedic Hand Service. His scientific publications have been largely in the field of trauma to the upper extremity, especially its treatment. He has published approximately 100 articles involving fractures about the shoulder and elbow (ca. 40), reconstruction of malunion, nonunion or instability/stiffness of the elbow (ca. 60); fractures of the forearm and wrist (ca. 120), with about half on the acute operative treatment of fractures of the distal radius, reconstruction, malunion or instability at the wrist (ca. 20); fractures of the hand (ca. 20); and microsurgery, including free tissue transfer (ca. 10) and replants (ca. 5).

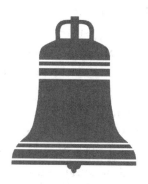

Brown Hall of Fame Logo. Courtesy of Brown University Athletics.

Over about four decades (beginning in 1986), Dr. Jupiter published articles on a variety of treatments for fractures of the distal radius, including casts, Kirschner wires, external fixation, intraoperative distraction, operative treatment with fixation by the pi plate, a dorsal plate, volar plate, percutaneous pinning with limited open fixation, use of structural and nonstructural bone grafts, use of Norian SRS cement, combined dorsal and volar plates, radial column plates, volar fixed angle plate, 2.4-millimeter locking plates, cross-pin fixation with a nonbridging external fixator, volar locking plates, titanium versus stainless steel plates, and the volar rim plate. His extensive experience in treating distal radius fractures resulted in a book, *Fractures of the Distal Radius: A Practical Approach to Management*, coauthored with Dr. Diego L. Fernandez in 1996; a second edition later appeared in 2002. **Case 42.4** highlights an example of one of the many cases he reviewed.

Jupiter was promoted to full professor at HMS in 1998, and, in 2003, he became the first Hansjörg Wyss/AO Foundation Professor of Orthopaedic Surgery. In 2009, 23 years after his seminal publication on distal radius intra-articular fracture with Dr. Knirk, Drs. Brian Haus and Jupiter revisited the earlier work. They wrote that:

> In its day, [it] was arguably one of the most important works on the management of intra-articular fractures of the distal end of the radius...The findings with the greatest impact on treatment algorithms was that accurate articular restoration was the most critical factor in prevention of long-term arthritis in young patients. (Haus and Jupiter 2009)

They went on to point out the flaws in the 1986 article but stated that "an updated critical analysis reveals that its conclusions are still germane in today's treatment of distal radial fracture in young adults" (Haus and Jupiter 2009). However, they called for an updated study:

> that meets rigorous modern criteria [intra-and-inter-observer validation, use of computerized tomography and validated outcome instruments] to answer...questions and to further direct the future management of distal radial fractures. Eventually that study, too, will be transcended by better techniques, newer research, or additional clinical observations—and so the art of medicine, and the progress of science, will go on. (Haus and Jupiter 2009)

In 2013, the Wrist and Radius Injury Surgical Trial (WRIST) was created to answer questions about the treatment of distal radius fractures in response to a systematic review by Margliot et al. 2005 and a Cochrane Report, demonstrating a lack of evidence-based medicine for this condition.

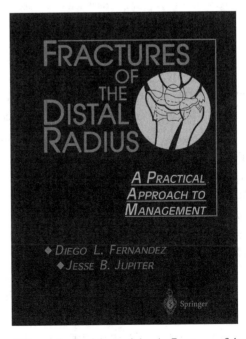

Cover of Fernandez and Jupiter's book, *Fractures of the Distal Radius: A Practical Approach to Management*. New York: Springer Nature, 1996.

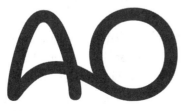

Logo AO Foundation. Courtesy of the AO Foundation.

Case 42.4. Intra-Articular Radial Nerve Entrapment in a Subluxed Elbow

> "A thirty-seven-year-old right-hand-dominant woman presented to our clinic with a four-week history of pain in the left elbow, loss of sensation over the dorsum of the thumb and index finger, and an inability to extend the wrist and fingers.
>
> "Four weeks previously, the patient had fallen onto the outstretched arm while walking outdoors. She felt immediate pain in the left elbow and went to a local emergency room, where she was found to have altered sensation in the radial-nerve distribution in the hand as well as an inability to extend the wrist and fingers. Standard radiographs of the elbow demonstrated posterolateral rotatory elbow subluxation and a manipulative reduction was performed. The limb was placed in an above-the-elbow splint, and the patient was instructed to seek orthopaedic consultation.
>
> "The patient did not seek follow-up evaluation as instructed. Three weeks after the injury, the patient presented to our emergency room because the pain, numbness, and weakness had not resolved. Standard anteroposterior and lateral radiographs of the left elbow revealed an anterior fat-pad sign and widening of the radiocapitellar joint that was suggestive of posterolateral rotatory instability. Closed reduction was not possible. Examination in our clinic one week later revealed swelling of the left elbow, with tenderness over the radial head. The patient had loss of sensation in the distribution of the superficial radial nerve. Assessment of motor function with use of the British Medical Research Council system revealed grade-0 (of 5) strength in the wrist, thumb, and digital extensors. The active and passive ranges of motion of the elbow were from 30° to 95° of flexion. The patient could actively pronate the forearm to 45° but was unable to actively supinate the forearm. The arc of passive forearm supination was 45°. There was no wrist tenderness.
>
> "The patient's medical history included fibromyalgia and discoid lupus. She had a smoking history of fifteen pack-years and used alcohol on a social basis. The patient was scheduled for surgical exploration of the radial nerve and open reduction of the radial head. Preoperative electromyography revealed a complete radial nerve palsy at the level of the elbow.
>
> "With the patient under general anesthesia and with use of a sterile pneumatic tourniquet, the elbow was approached through an extended lateral incision. The radial nerve was identified proximal to the elbow in the interval between the brachialis and the brachioradialis. The nerve was found to be displaced, and it followed a posterolateral, instead of an anterior, course. As the radial nerve was followed distally, it was found to wind posteriorly around

The principle investigator is Kevin C. Chung at the University of Michigan. The study group includes 21 hand centers in the United States, Canada, and Singapore. Members in the HCORP included Jessie B. Jupiter and David Ring, before he moved to Austin, Texas (MGH); Philip Blazer, Brandon Earp, and W. Emerson Floyd (BWH); and Tamara D. Rozental, Paul Appleton, Edward Rodriguez, Lindsay Herder and Katiri Wagner (BIDMC).

As a nationally and internationally well-known hand and upper extremity surgeon, Jupiter has been extraordinarily prolific, having given over 1,500 scientific presentations, served as director or co-director of over 80 postgraduate CME programs, published more than 440 scientific articles and editorials, and authored or coauthored approximately eight books and 115 chapters He has also given more than 45 named lectures. A few of the very prestigious ones include:

- Lee Ramsey Straub Memorial Lecture at the Hospital for Special Surgery
- Harvey Hatcher Lecture at Stanford
- E. Shaw Wilgis Memorial Lecture at Union Memorial Hospital in Baltimore
- Arthur Thibodeau Memorial Lecture at Tufts
- Anthony DePalma Lecture at Jefferson
- Richard J. Smith Lecture at the American Society for Surgery of the Hand
- Richard J. Smith Annual Lecture at MGH
- Alfred Swanson Lecture at the International Federation of Hand Surgery
- Edward E. Nalebuff Lecture at the New England Baptist Hospital

> the lateral musculature and the lateral humeral condyle. It then entered the radiocapitellar joint through the torn posterior and lateral capsule. A few branches of the nerve to the wrist extensors were observed to be avulsed from their muscular innervations. An osteotomy of the lateral epicondyle was performed to facilitate the exposure and to permit easy relocation of the radiocapitellar joint and radial nerve.
>
> "Within the radiocapitellar joint, the radial nerve was found to be encased in granulation tissue. Under a 3.5-power loupe magnification, the nerve was mobilized and was replaced in its anatomic position. The granulation tissue was removed from the radiocapitellar joint, facilitating reduction of the radial head. The osteotomy site was then repaired with use of 24-gauge stainless-steel wire, which was passed through drill-holes in the lateral aspect of the distal part of the humerus and was woven through the origin of the lateral musculature. Anteroposterior and lateral radiographs of the elbow confirmed reduction of the radiocapitellar joint. Full passive elbow flexion and extension and forearm rotation were achieved without subluxation or recurrent dislocation.
>
> "Postoperatively, the limb was immobilized for ten days in a posterior splint with the elbow in 90° of flexion and the forearm in pronation. The wrist was held in 30° of extension, and the metacarpophalangeal joints were supported in 60° of flexion. Active motion of the proximal interphalangeal joints was permitted. No prophylaxis was used to offset heterotopic ossification. Active and active-assisted range of motion of the elbow began at ten days, with the forearm kept in neutral rotation.
>
> "Within two weeks after surgery, the patient began to experience hypersensitivity in the distribution of the superficial radial nerve. By fourteen weeks postoperatively, some return of wrist and digital extensor motor function was observed.
>
> "By eighteen months after surgery, the patient had returned to her job as a filing clerk. Standard radiographs of the elbow demonstrated an anatomically aligned joint. By two years, the patient had regained full strength in the wrist, thumb, and digital extensors. Grip strength was 32 kg, compared with 30 kg for the contralateral hand. The range of motion of the left elbow, including flexion, extension, pronation, and supination, was full and equal to that of the contralateral upper extremity. The elbow was stable to varus and valgus stress in all positions. Sensation to light touch on the dorsum of the first web space was only slightly diminished compared with that in the contralateral hand, but the patient could distinguish between blunt and sharp stimuli."
>
> (Liu and Jupiter 2004)

- Robert E. Carroll Founders Lecture at the American Society for Surgery of the Hand
- Harold E. Kleinert Lecture in Louisville
- Wayne Southwick Lecture at Yale
- Joseph Boyes Lecture at the University of Southern California
- Bernard F. Morrey Oration at the International Shoulder and Elbow Congress

All of his accomplishments were completed while working in a very busy specialty practice and devoting countless hours to teaching orthopaedic residents, fellows, and students.

Dr. Jesse Jupiter belongs to many national and international organizations. In 1988, he was president of the Hand Forum; in 1993, he was chairman of AO/ASIF North America and served as chairman of the International Committee for the American Academy of Orthopaedic Surgeons. From 1989 to 1997, he was a trustee of the AO Foundation and named an honorary trustee in 2009. He was president of the American Association of Hand Surgery in 2012 and president of the American Shoulder and Elbow Surgeons in 2015. He has been given honorary membership in the following organizations: Hellenic Orthopaedic Society, Israel Hand Society, AO Latin America, Brazilian Hand Society, Italian Orthopaedic Society, Cordoba Argentina Academy of Medicine, and the Argentine Shoulder and Elbow Society. He has served as co-editor or editor of many specialty journals. Dr. Jupiter continues to work in his busy practice and lives in Weston, MA, with his wife, Beryl.

ROBERT D. LEFFERT

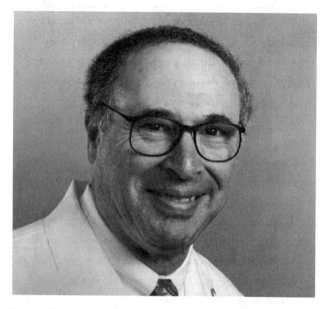

Robert D. Leffert. Courtesy of Lisa Leffert.

Physician Snapshot

Robert D. Leffert
BORN: 1923
DIED: 2008
SIGNIFICANT CONTRIBUTIONS: Specialist in rehabilitation of the upper extremity; shoulder surgeon with expertise in treating brachial plexus injuries and thoracic outlet syndrome; published *Brachial Plexus Injuries*; chief of the MGH Department of Rehabilitation (1972–1989) and of the surgical upper extremity rehabilitation unit (1972–1995); president ASES 1996

Robert David Leffert, the son of a physician, was born in 1923 and grew up in Brooklyn, where he graduated from Erasmus High School. He graduated from Dartmouth College in 1954 with his BS and from Tufts Medical School in 1958 with his MD. He completed "a residency at the Hospital for Joint Diseases in New York City, [and then] served in the United States Navy during the Vietnam War as a Lieutenant Commander in the 3rd Marine Division [from 1964 to 1966]" (Mankin et al. 2009). As a surgeon in Vietnam:

> He said his duty was like "*MASH* [the television show] without the women." "When he was there, he was committed to caring for every patient brought to him to the best of his ability, whether they were American, Vietnamese, or Viet Cong," said [Lee] Schwamm, who is Vice Chairman of the Neurology Department at MGH. "It was a formative experience. It really tested him as an individual and a surgeon, and really helped shape him because they saw hundreds and hundreds of soldiers with debilitating injuries to their arms and legs." (Marguard 2008)

He was decorated for his service.

In 1965, while still serving as a marine, Leffert showed an early interest in the shoulder region and published his second paper, an article on brachial plexus injuries. As a Frauenthal Travel Fellow of the Hospital for Joint Diseases, he collaborated with Sir Herbert Seddon at the Institute of Orthopaedics, University of London. They reviewed 230 cases of closed brachial plexus injuries at the Royal National Orthopaedic Hospital in London and the Nuffield Orthopaedic Centre in Oxford. Between 1940 and 1960, they identified 31 cases of infraclavicular brachial plexus injuries in patients who had sustained a closed injury to the shoulder without a clavicle fracture. In the cases examined, they observed that:

> Except for isolated circumflex nerve injuries the prognosis is generally good whatever part of the plexus is damaged. The treatment is conservative and its two most important features are prevention of stiffness of joints and the control, by regular galvanic stimulation, of denervation

---

INFRACLAVICULAR BRACHIAL PLEXUS INJURIES

R. D. LEFFERT,* NEW YORK, UNITED STATES OF AMERICA, and
SIR HERBERT SEDDON, LONDON, ENGLAND

From the Institute of Orthopaedics, University of London

THE JOURNAL OF BONE AND JOINT SURGERY
VOL. 47 B, NO. 1, FEBRUARY 1965

Title of Leffert and Sir Herbert Sedden's article on infraclavicular brachial plexus injuries. *Journal of Bone and Joint Surgery* [Br] 1965; 47: 9.

atrophy of muscle during the often prolonged period before recovery becomes apparent. (Leffert and Seddon 1965)

After completing his military obligation, Leffert returned to New York City in 1966. He joined the staff at the Hospital for Joint Diseases as an orthopaedic surgeon and had a faculty appointment at the Mt. Sinai Medical School. He remained at the Hospital for Joint Diseases, working with Dr. Richard Smith, for six years. **Case 42.5** highlights an example of one of the many cases he reviewed.

Dr. Leffert was recruited by Dr. Mankin to join him in 1972; along with Drs. Richard Smith, Michael Ehrlich, and Charles Weiss; on the staff of the Massachusetts General Hospital. Leffert was named chief of the Department of Rehabilitation (1972–1989) and chief of the Surgical Upper Extremity Rehabilitation Unit (1972–1995). He also continued to ascend in academic ranks at Harvard Medical School. Joseph Barr Jr. described their role at MGH:

> We worked together on White 9 with amputees, stroke patients, spinal cord injuries and other neuromuscular conditions. Both Physical and Occupational Therapy were under Bob's control. Orthopaedic residents received a good introduction in all these areas. With the advent of Spaulding Rehabilitation Hospital it became evident that a rehabilitation unit was no longer viable at MGH and White 9 was closed. (Barr Jr. 1965)

Leffert had many interests related to the shoulder, and he made major contributions in the diagnosis and treatment of brachial plexus injuries and thoracic outlet syndrome. Dr. Schwamm recalled:

> people came from all over…to be evaluated by him or to be operated upon by him…He was also very much the court of last resort, so people who had had several failed surgeries would come to him for a re-do. (Marquard 2008)

Case 42.5. Diabetes Presenting as a Peripheral Neuropathy

> "[Patient], a sixty-one-year-old right-handed white accountant was seen because of paraesthesias and numbness of the right little finger of one year's duration. These symptoms were inconsistent and often nocturnal. His physician thought they were psychogenic. Past medical history and review of systems revealed essential hypertension, prostatectomy for benign hypertrophy, and some inconsistent burning pain over the anterior aspect of the right thigh of two year's duration that had been diagnosed as meralgia paresthetica. The usual symptoms of diabetes were denied as was the family history of the disease. Alcoholic intake was minimum.
>
> "On physical examination, the head and neck were normal except for Grade II hypertensive retinopathy. The only detectable abnormality in either upper extremity was loss of two-point discrimination in the right little finger. Other positive neurological findings were as follows: The right knee jerk was diminished as compared to the left, and there was diminished position sense in the toes and bilateral loss of deep pain as tested by tendon Achilles compression.
>
> "Roentgenograms of the chest were normal, while those of the cervical spine showed diffuse spondylosis of moderate degree. The roentgenograms of the lumbosacral spine were unremarkable.
>
> "His motor nerve conduction velocity determinations are recorded in Table II. [Ulnar nerve motor nerve conduction velocity: low.]
>
> "The hemogram and urinalysis were within normal limits. The Venereal Disease Research Laboratories test was non-reactive; the blood urea nitrogen was 18 milligrams per 100 milliliters, the one-half-hour value of 187 milligrams per 100 milliliters, the one-hour value of 223 milligrams per 100 milliliters; the two-hour value of 169 milligrams per 100 milliliters, and the three-hour value of 68 milligrams per 100 milliliters.
>
> "In light of the evidence of diffuse peripheral neuropathy and the abnormal glucose tolerance curve, in the absence of other significant causes of neuropathy, the patient was considered to have diabetic peripheral neuropathy."
>
> —Robert D. Leffert "Diabetes Mellitus Initially Presenting as Peripheral Neuropathy in the Upper Limb," *Journal of Bone and Joint Surgery* 1969.

In more than 40 publications, he published eight on issues related to the brachial plexus, including one book, *Brachial Plexus Injuries* (published in 1985), and six articles on the thoracic outlet syndrome. He gave Academy of Orthopaedic Surgeons (AAOS) instructional courses on lesions of the brachial plexus, electrodiagnoses in upper extremity disorders, and frozen shoulder.

Two years after he was appointed chief of the Department of Rehabilitation and chief of the Surgical Upper Extremity Rehabilitation Unit at MGH, Leffert published a paper, in 1974, "Brachial-Plexus Injuries" in the *Medical Progress Series*. He made the following remarks:

> When all diagnostic maneuvers and observations have been performed, assuming that no direct surgical attack on the nerve is indicated, and neurologic recovery has plateaued, the patient may be considered to have entered the chronic phase...For the patient with a frail anesthetic arm there are three possible choices. First...he may retain the extremity if his mode of living and occupation are not unduly prejudiced by being "one-handed." He can then be taught to protect the limb against injury...Second...Hendry in 1949...employed shoulder fusion, posterior bone block at the elbow, and various tenodeses and arthrodeses in the hand...[with] some quite useful results. There has been virtually no enthusiasm for this approach in recent years...Third...dealing with the frail anesthetic limb is by arthrodesis of the shoulder, amputation of the arm above the elbow and fitting with a prosthesis...
>
> For patients with partial functional impairment and adequate emotional stability, a program of staged surgical reconstructive procedures may be the key to rehabilitation...The best results... are in patients with good hands. If the hand is insensitive or will have no prehension, there is little point in attempting to reconstruct the more proximal parts of the limb...Several of the procedures for restoration of elbow flexion have been borrowed from the literature on poliomyelitis...The triceps may in some cases be transferred anteriorly to restore excellent flexion. In our clinic, the transfer of a segment of pectoralis major...on a neurovascular pedicle...has proved most successful and powerful...
>
> As has been implied, shoulder stability is vital for the function of the limb. Stability is most predictably achieved by surgical fusion of the glenohumeral joint...Finally, the problem of intractable pain may be a definite impediment to rehabilitation...Often it is burning and constant...Patients are usually given large doses of narcotic analgesics...often...[without] relief... the occasional patient will become addicted. In some patients, the causalgia is lessened by... stellate-ganglion blocks...Fortunately, in many cases, the pain gradually diminishes spontaneously, often as long as a year or more...surgical therapy has not proved encouraging... Amputation of the arm in a patient with intractable pain is usually not effective in obtaining relief...Unfortunately, for those in whom recurrent ulcerations or infections develop, there may be no alternative to amputation. (Leffert 1974)

In summary, patients with a partial brachial plexus injury may have function improved with surgery; those with intractable pain have not benefitted from surgery; and patients with chronic ulcers and infection may require an amputation as a last resort.

In 1980, Dr. Fred Hochberg (neurologist) and Dr. Leffert began to examine the hands of musicians, especially pianists, who were having difficulty recovering from baffling afflictions of their hands. They consulted on such famous pianists as Gary Graffman and Leon Fleisher. In 1983, Hochberg, Leffert, and coauthors reported on their observations treating 100 musicians with occupational limitations, most of whom were midcareer. The most commonly diagnosed conditions included tenosynovitis, arthritis, or disorders of motor control. The most commonly reported

> ### Hand Difficulties Among Musicians
> Fred H. Hochberg, MD; Robert D. Leffert, MD; Matthew D. Heller, MD; Lisle Merriman
> JAMA, April 8, 1983—Vol 249, No. 14

Hochberg and Leffert's article about hand problems of professional musicians. *Journal of the American Medical Association* 1983; 249: 1869.

symptoms included pain and weakness, and findings upon examination included drooping or inability to elevate the fifth finger.

Leffert's wife, Linda (Garelik) Leffert said his "major interest other than surgery, really, was medical education" (Marguard 2008). Leffert was appointed full professor at HMS in 1991 and, in 1996, was elected president of the American Shoulder and Elbow Surgeons. In 1999, one year before retiring from clinical practice, Leffert and his coauthor, Dr. Gary S. Perlmutter, reviewed 236 patients (282 procedures) treated by transaxillary first rib resection for thoracic outlet syndrome with an average follow-up of 55 months. They reported that:

> of 42 patients who had less than satisfactory results, 41 had persistent postural ptosis of the ipsilateral scapula because of trapezius insufficiency...the percentage of patients who had complications...is high, 45%, [but] the actual incidence of severe or permanent injury to those patients was low. (Leffert and Perlmutter 1999)

Fourteen percent of patients had no relief from the operation and about 70 percent had significant improvement or were completely asymptomatic after surgery. They went on to:

> emphasize that this surgery has no margin of error. The risks are serious and only those surgeons willing to devote considerable time and effort to treatment of these patients and their care should be involved. (Leffert and Perlmutter 1999)

Dr. Leffert was a member of many professional organizations, and he served on the Orthopaedic Study Section of NIH. He retired from clinical practice in July 2000 after he developed a melanoma of his thumb, which required multiple operations and chemotherapy. He nevertheless:

> continued with many activities related to computers and education. He served as Senior Medical Advisor to Partners Telemedicine which provided medical consultation and second opinions for international patients. He was a Founding Member of the Harvard Interfaculty Neuroscience Program...He designed and maintained websites for the MGH Orthopaedics Department and the American Shoulder and Elbow Surgeons. He worked with the Harvard Program for Interdisciplinary Learning on the ICON (Interactive Care-based Online Network). His intellectual curiosity and vigor carried on right to the end of his life. (Barr 2009)

Dr. Leffert died on December 7, 2008, of complications from melanoma. He had lived in Chestnut Hill, and he was survived by his wife Linda and their two children, Adam (who worked in computer software) and Lisa (chief of obstetrical anesthesia at MGH). His family established the Robert Leffert Memorial Fund which supports an annual lecture at MGH in the memory of Dr. Leffert.

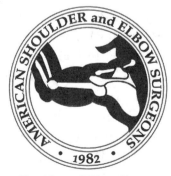

Logo, American Shoulder and Elbow Surgeons. Courtesy of American Shoulder and Elbow Surgeons.

DAVID W. LHOWE

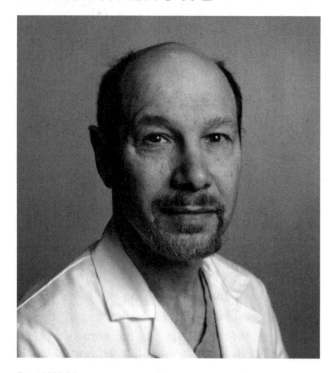

David W. Lhowe. Massachusetts General Hospital.

Physician Snapshot

David W. Lhowe
BORN: 1951
DIED: —

SIGNIFICANT CONTRIBUTIONS: Chief of the MGH orthopaedic trauma service 1995–2001; expert in thigh compartment syndrome; volunteer at AmeriCares, Project HOPE, the International Medical-Surgical Response Team, and Health Volunteer Overseas

---

David W. Lhowe grew up outside New York City. He received his AB degree, magna cum laude, from Harvard College in 1974 and his MD degree from Case Western Reserve University in 1978. He was elected into Alpha Omega Alpha in 1977 and, at graduation, received the Noether Award for Excellence in Therapeutics. Lhowe then returned to Boston where he completed a medical internship followed by a year as a junior resident in surgery at Beth Israel Hospital. From 1981 to 1984, he was an orthopaedic resident in the Harvard Combined Program; followed by six months as an assistant in orthopaedic surgery and chief resident at MGH. In 1985, he was a fellow in orthopaedic trauma at Harborview Medical Center at the University of Washington in Seattle, Washington.

In 1986, Dr. Lhowe returned again to Boston and for about four years was chief of the Department of Orthopedic Surgery at the Cambridge Hospital. He was also a staff physician in the Harvard Community Health Plan, the Massachusetts General Hospital, Brigham and Women's Hospital (1986–1992) and Mt. Auburn Hospital (1986–1998). He focused his practice on trauma. Over the course of his career, he has published 20 articles: 14 on trauma and five on major disasters.

He published his first article on trauma, "Immediate Nailing of Open Fractures of the Femoral Shaft," with Dr. Sigvard T. Hansen in 1988. It was a review of 42 patients treated at Harborview Medical Center between 1980 and 1985. They concluded:

> immediate reamed nailings of open fractures of the femur was not associated with an increased rate of infection…The rates of other complications were low…comparable [to] series of closed fractures…as for all open fractures, prompt debridement, careful handling of the soft tissues, and appropriate antibiotic coverage are essential. (Lhowe and Hansen 1988)

Lhowe later published two articles on retrograde nailing of the femur and one article on management of femoral nonunion.

From 1992 to 1994, Dr. Lhowe was assistant chief of the orthopaedic trauma service at MGH and from 1995 to 2001 was chief of the orthopaedic trauma service. In 2001, he was promoted from instructor to assistant professor of orthopaedic surgery at Harvard Medical School. That same year AmeriCares—an international disaster relief and humanitarian organization—sent a medical team, headed by Dr. Lhowe, to the Department of Orthopaedic Surgery at Pristina Hospital in Kosovo. They provided lectures and performed operative procedures with the goal to advance orthopaedic care in Kosovo. Lhowe was also a member of the International Medical-Surgical Response Team (IMSuRT) that provided orthopaedic emergency care at the World Trade Center, New York City, in 2001. Later, he was also on the staff at Winchester Hospital from 2003 to 2007.

Lhowe's secondary interest in trauma has been management and outcomes of acute compartment syndrome of the thigh (see **Case 42.6**). In 2004, he and his colleagues at MGH described the clinical spectrum of an acute compartment syndrome. They wrote:

> Acute thigh compartment syndrome is characterized by a variable etiology [blunt trauma in motor vehicle accidents or contusion] and presents with features typical for compartment syndrome. Tense swelling, pain with passive stretch, and paresthesias in the distribution of the involved compartment are the most reliable symptoms. Assessment of compartment pressures assumes significant diagnostic relevance in unconscious patients but is of less diagnostic value when assessing alert, cooperative patients. The critical compartment pressure threshold in the thigh has yet to be defined. Fasciotomy provides effective treatment with minimal morbidity. The incidence of short-term complications is related to associated injuries whereas mortality is limited to patients with polytrauma. (Mithoefer et al. 2004)

A compartment syndrome of the thigh had been only occasionally reported and treatment recommendations were variable because only case reports or very small series were found in the literature. The authors studied patients in three level-1 trauma centers and reported 28 patients with a thigh compartment syndrome. They recommended urgent fasciotomy to avoid complications. Overall mortality in these patients was associated with multiple injuries and not the thigh compartment syndrome.

Two articles written by Mithöfer, Lhowe, and colleagues on compartment syndromes of the thigh.
Clinical Orthopaedics and Related Research 2004; 425: 223; *Journal of Bone and Joint Surgery* 2006; 88: 729.

The following year, Llowe was part of Project HOPE of the US Navy, providing medical care for the 2004 tsunami victims in Indonesia. In 2006, two years after publishing a description of the clinical spectrum of an acute compartment syndrome, Lhowe and his colleagues reported on the functional outcomes of 18 patients who survived their injuries after fasciotomies. They wrote:

> Long-term functional deficits were present in eight patients, and only five had full recovery of thigh muscle strength…High injury severity scores, ipsilateral femoral fracture, prolonged intervals to decompression, the presence of myonecrosis at the time of fasciotomy, and an age of more than thirty years were associated with increased long-term functional deficits, persistent thigh-muscle weakness, and worse functional outcome scores. (Mithoefer et al. 2006)

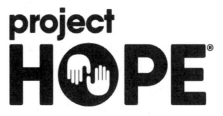

Logo, Project HOPE. Courtesy of Project HOPE.

This was the first long-term detailed outcome study of thigh compartment syndromes.

He was also an active participant in the Orthopaedic Trauma Association Visiting Scholars Program at the US Army Hospital in Landstuhl, Germany in 2008, and, in 2014, with Health Volunteers Overseas, he provided orthopaedic teaching and surgery at the JDW (Jigme Dorji Wangchuk) National Referral Hospital in Thimphu, Bhutan. Dr. Lhowe has maintained a major interest in national and international disasters for over 20 years. He served as the chief orthopaedic officer of the International Medical-Surgical Response Team of the United States for 19 years, until 2018, having held the position since 1999. He continues at MGH as an active member of the orthopaedic trauma service and lives with his wife in Cambridge, Massachusetts.

Case 42.6. Delayed Presentation of Acute Thigh Compartment Syndrome

"A twenty-nine-year-old international-level rugby player received a direct blow to his left anterior thigh by the knee of an opponent during a match. Increasing pain and tightness in his left leg with progressive difficulty with knee flexion and extension prompted presentation to the emergency department two hours after the game. His medical history was negative for bleeding diathesis, and he denied any regular medications. Clinical examination revealed a firm anterolateral swelling of the left thigh without palpable muscle defect. Active range of motion of 30 to 80 degrees with four/five quadriceps strength was maintained. Passive knee flexion produced moderate discomfort. Motor function was normal, and there was no sensory deficit. Distal pulses could be demonstrated by Doppler-ultrasound only. Radiographs demonstrated soft tissue swelling but no fracture. Hematocrit was 34 percent, and creatine-phosphokinase was 876 units per milliliter without evidence of myoglobinuria. His blood pressure was 150/80 millimeters of mercury. Compartment pressures were measured using a Stryker handheld pressure monitoring system (Stryker Surgical, Kalamazoo, MI, U.S.A.) and revealed sixty, thirty-eight, and ten millimeters of mercury in the anterior, medial, and posterior compartments, respectively. The patient was admitted for observation and analgesia. He was discharged two days later after spontaneous return of palpable pulses and marked decrease of thigh swelling and pain with passive motion.

"Eight days later without further trauma, the patient experienced repeated swelling with progressive pain and inability to flex his left knee after ascending stairs. He denied the use of nonsteroidal anti-inflammatory drugs. His examination was remarkable for extreme pain and firm swelling in his left thigh. The patient was unable to actively straight leg raise. Active left knee range of motion was 20 to 80 degrees with significant pain with active and passion motion. Motor strength was normal, distal pulses were palpable, but hypoesthesia was noted in the saphenous nerve distribution. The hematocrit was 23 percent, and creatine-phosphokinase was increased to 560 units per milliliter. Systemic blood pressure was 146/72 millimeters of mercury. Compartment pressures were sixty-four, forty, and fifteen millimeters of mercury for anterior, medial, and posterior compartments, respectively. The patient was taken to the operating room, and a fasciotomy was performed through a lateral thigh incision as described by Tarlow et al. Intraoperatively, a partial defect in the anterior aspect of the vastus medialis was encountered. Active bleeding was present from several perforating vessels, and 750 milliliters of fresh hematoma and old clot was evacuated. The muscle appeared viable with only mild edema. Intraoperative compartment pressure monitoring confirmed adequate surgical decompression. Postoperative neurologic examination showed full recovery of saphenous nerve function. Delayed primary skin closure was successful at second attempt after transient increase of muscular edema ten days after fasciotomy. There were no septic complications. Hematologic evaluation revealed no coagulopathy. The patient recovered full quadriceps and hamstring strength and full active range of motion after three months of intensive physical therapy. Myositis ossificans developed in the vastus medialis with persistent symptoms at three years. After briefly returning to competitive rugby he ended his career after completion of the season."

(Mithoefer, Lhowe, and Altman 2002)

FREDERICK L. MANSFIELD

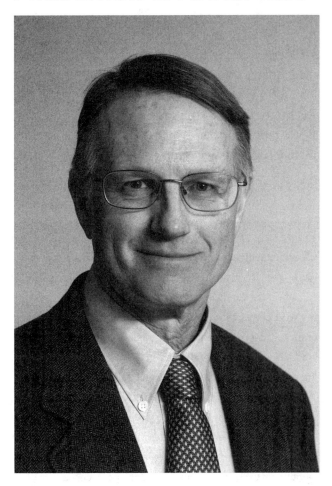

Frederick L. Mansfield. Massachusetts General Hospital.

Physician Snapshot

Frederick L. Mansfield
BORN: 1947
DIED: —

SIGNIFICANT CONTRIBUTIONS: Director of the MGH spine surgery fellowship 1985–1999, chairman of the town of Lincoln Board of Health

Frederick "Fred" L. Mansfield was born in Boston and received his AB degree from Harvard College in 1969. After receiving a Master of Science degree in electrical engineering (MSEE) at Stanford University in 1970, he worked in Silicon Valley as a digital-systems engineer for about two years. He then returned to Boston to attend Harvard Medical School; receiving his MD degree in 1976.

After a surgical internship and an additional year as a junior resident in surgery at the Peter Bent Brigham Hospital, Mansfield entered the Harvard Combined Orthopaedic Residency Program. He finished in 1981 and was chief resident at MGH from January 1, 1982, to June 30, 1982. He then spent six months as a fellow in spine surgery at the Brigham and Women's Hospital followed by six months as a fellow in pediatric orthopaedics at Boston Children's Hospital.

In 1982, Dr. Mansfield was appointed an assistant in orthopaedic surgery at MGH and an instructor in orthopaedic surgery at Harvard Medical School. He has remained at MGH during his entire career as a spine surgeon and has gone on to publish 14 articles about the spine. His first article was a review of the long-term results of the use of chymopapain in a *Clinical Orthopaedics and Related Research* symposium on the use of chymopapain in the treatment of herniated lumbar disks with unrelieved sciatica. He wrote:

> A 10-to-14-year following...of 146 patients treated for sciatica from a herniated nucleus pulposus by chymopapain...injection revealed a durable, satisfactory result in 66%. In the 102 patients rated as excellent or good, 5% required surgical discectomy 50-82 months after injection. One-, two-, and three-level injections were performed [with no] influence [on] the success of the procedure...Robert Boyd and James Huddleston performed 494 chymopapain...injections for disc herniation between 1971 and 1975. (Mansfield et al. 1986)

Eventually, the use of chymopapain was discontinued at the MGH and other institutions as its popularity ceased; its use was discontinued in the United States in 2003.

Two years following his first publication, in 1988, he removed bone from the iliac crest of Kitty Dukakis (the wife of Governor Michael Dukakis) to be used for a two-level anterior cervical spine fusion for degenerative disc disease. Neurospine surgeons Dr. Nicholas T. Zevas (a long-time family friend) and Dr. Larry Borges were the lead surgeons. Later, in the early 1990s, Mansfield was a participant in a prospective study on the safety and efficacy of pedicle screw instrumentation with short-segment fusions in patients with burst fractures of the thoracolumbar spine. He and Drs. W. B. Rogers and D. L. Kramer reported their results in 11 patients with a minimum follow-up of two years. They had a posterior segment fixator (PSF) instrument failure rate of 22% with loss of correction and increased kyphosis; they concluded that a short posterior fusion and instrumentation was inadequate for these anterior column injuries. The following year Dr. Mansfield with Drs. G. R. Rechtine, C. E. Sutterlin, G. W. Wood, and R. J. Boyd reported their experience using the interpedicular segmental fixation (ISF) pedicle screw plate

Case 42.7. Open Anterior Lumbosacral Fracture Dislocation

"A 35-year-old man was bent at the waist when a falling tree struck him across the lumbar region, pinning him in a snow drift. Inclement weather caused delays in rescue and transport, and he was not treated until 28 hours after his injury. There was a jagged, 15-cm laceration through skin, subcutaneous tissue, fascia and paravertebral muscle. The wound was draining cerebrospinal fluid (CSF). Dirt, bark, and clothing fragments were visible among the fracture fragments. The patient also had a closed left ankle fracture (Weber Type B).

"Neurologic examination showed an incomplete cauda equine lesion, with pain impairing precise quantification of muscle function. It appeared that all lower extremity motor groups were working to some degree except the ankle dorsiflexors and evertors on the left. Perianal sensation was present to pin prick testing and rectal tone was good. Radiographs showed a fracture dislocation of the lumbosacral junction, or traumatic spondylolisthesis. Fractures through the posterior arches and pedicles occurred at L3-L5, with spinous process fractures at L1 and L2.

"Initial operative management consisted of thorough debridement of all devitalized tissues, including a large amount of paravertebral muscle. Bilateral laminectomies from L3 to the sacrum permitted inspection of the posterior element fractures and spinal canal contents. The left L5 nerve root was shredded and the left S-1 nerve root severely damaged. Multiple dural lacerations were noted, dorsally and ventrally, and those that were accessible were repaired.

"As the patient was log-rolled to the prone position on the operating table, a marked 'clunk' was felt. Radiographs showed partial reduction of the L5-S1 dislocation. Pedicle screws were used across the fractured pedicles at L3, L4, L5, and S1 with good purchase in the vertebral bodies. Rods were then fixed to the S1 pedicle screws, and threaded reduction clamps were used to realign L5-S1 fully. Because the wound was contaminated and more than 24 hours old, primary closure was not attempted. To avoid persistent CSF leak, and minimize the risk of meningitis, a temporary intraventricular catheter was placed.

"The patient underwent another debridement of the wound and delayed primary closure on the second postoperative day. Fusion was not attempted through the posterior wound for fear of infection. The intraventricular catheter was removed on the seventh postoperative day, and the patient was allowed out of bed. Empirical antibiotic coverage was continued for two weeks.

"Two months later, after uneventful healing of the posterior wound and normalization of the erythrocyte sedimentation rate, the patient underwent anterior interbody fusion from L3 to the sacrum. Multiple fibular autograft struts were used at each intervertebral space. Plain radiographs and lateral flexion – extension views at 2-year and 4-year follow-ups showed maintenance of anterior interbody fusion without loss of alignment.

"At the final follow-up, 4 years after injury, the patient had persistent numbness and foot drop on the left, but normal motor function of the right lower extremity. Bowel and bladder functions were normal. However, the patient continued to experience retrograde ejaculation. He was fully engaged in professional and recreational activities, including golf and hiking."

(Carlson, Heller, Mansfield, and Pedlow 1999)

Long-term Results of Chymopapain Injections

FREDERICK MANSFIELD, M.D., KENNETH POLIVY, M.D., ROBERT BOYD, M.D., AND JAMES HUDDLESTON, M.D.

Clinical Orthopaedics and Related Research Number 206 May, 1986

Mansfield and colleagues' article on long-term outcomes of patients treated with chymopapain. *Clinical Orthopaedics and Related Research* 1986; 206: 67.

system for patients with grade 1 or 2 degenerative spondylolisthesis. All patients were also fused at three or less levels. In 18 patients followed for at least two years, they found a three-fold increase in successful spine fusions in those patients treated with posterior instrumentation (89%) compared to literature controls treated with fusion without instrumentation (average rate: 65%). **Case 42.7** highlights an example of one of the many cases he reviewed during this period as well.

Mansfield was the director of the spine surgery fellowship for 14 years, 1985–1999. He has served on several committees at MGH; for 11 years he was a member of the Utilization Review Committee and its chairman from 1995 to 2000. He was a member of several local professional organizations from 1996 to 2007 and a director of the Massachusetts Orthopaedic Association. He has also been active in his local community, serving since 1996 as chairman of the Town of Lincoln Board of Health. In addition to his busy practice of spine surgery, Mansfield has been active in the teaching program for residents and fellows at MGH and a frequent participant in medical student education (HMS 2 Musculoskeletal Block lecturer, HMS 3 and 4 rotations at MGH, and as an examiner in the HMS 4 OSCE examinations), as well as in the MGH Institute for Health Professions. Dr. Mansfield retired from surgery in 2014 but continues to see patients, conduct independent medical examinations, and teach students and residents.

DINESH G. PATEL

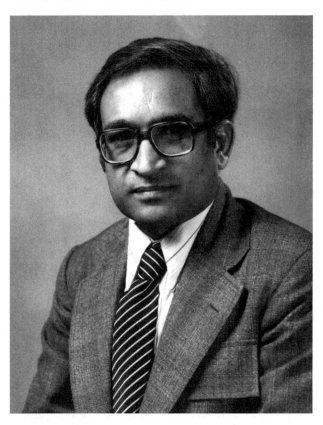

Dinesh G. Patel. Massachusetts General Hospital.

Physician Snapshot

Dinesh G. Patel

Born: 1936

Died: —

Significant contributions: Early advocate for arthroscopic surgery; chief of the MGH arthroscopic surgery unit in 1982; founding member of the Arthroscopy Association of North America and the International Arthroscopic Association; chairman of the Massachusetts Board of Registration in Medicine 1990–1992

Dinesh "Danny" G. Patel was born in Nadiad, India. Also known as Nandgam or "Sakshar Bhumi" (the Land of Educated), Nadiad is a small city in the midwestern area of the state of Gujarat where the summers are very hot, with temperatures averaging 115° F. The city is well-known for the number nine: nine roads in and out of the city, nine step wells around the city, nine lakes in the city, and nine villages or towns located on all nine roads that exit the city. From 1956 to 1962, Patel was a student in the B. J. Medical College of Gujarat University in Ahmadabad, India, just 36 miles north of Nadiad. In 1962, he graduated with a MBBS (Bachelor of Medicine, Bachelor of Surgery) degree. He remained in Ahmadabad as a rotating intern for one year at Gujarat University Affiliated Hospital.

The next year, after completing his internship, Dr. Patel immigrated to the United States. From 1964 to 1965, he was a resident in pathology at the University of Vermont. In 1965, he spent a year as a resident in surgery at Mt. Sinai Hospital in Baltimore, Maryland. He moved again, this time to Boston, where he spent the next four years in the MGH/Boston Children's Hospital combined orthopaedic residency program. He served as chief resident at the MGH from July to December 1971.

Patel's initial appointment at Harvard Medical School was clinical instructor in orthopaedics in 1973, and he joined the staff of the Massachusetts General Hospital in 1974, following a clinical and research fellowship at MGH. He was a founding member of the International Arthroscopic Association that same year. He was an early enthusiast for arthroscopic surgery, and he had begun performing arthroscopic procedures with Dr. Bertram Zarins at the MGH in the mid-1970s. Dr. Robert Jackson described Patel as an early advocate for operative arthroscopy, who quickly began teaching others the procedure as well. Two years later, in 1976, he was appointed codirector of the Sports Medicine Clinic with Zarins. Later, in 1982, Dr. Mankin divided the service into two units: Dr. Patel as chief of the arthroscopic surgery unit and Dr. Zarins as chief of the sports medicine service. In 1981, he was a founding member of the Arthroscopic Association of North America. The following year, at his alma mater, the B. J. Medical College of Gujarat University, he gave his first lecture on arthroscopy, the same year he was the invited speaker on arthroscopic surgery at the meeting of the Indian College of Surgeons in Bombay. Three years later,

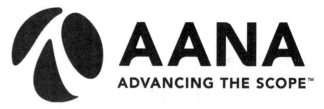

Logo, Arthroscopy Association of North America.
Courtesy of Arthroscopy Association of North America.

he was promoted to associate orthopaedic surgeon at MGH and to assistant clinical professor at HMS in 1985. During this period, he had also been appointed to the staffs of Sancta Maria Hospital (1981–1989) and Somerville Hospital (1988–1999). **Case 42.8** highlights an example of one of the many cases he reviewed.

Case 42.8. Bucket Handle Tear of a Discoid Medial Meniscus

> "A 19-year-old girl presented with right knee pain of 2.5 years duration. Persisting locking and buckling for the last few months had been increasing the patient's discomfort.
>
> "There was no history of trauma. The examination revealed medial joint line tenderness with fullness of the anteromedial portion and there was some patellofemoral subluxation without pain. The McMurray test was positive. The knee was stable in varus valgus and flexion extension position. The clinical impression was torn medial meniscus and mild patellar subluxation, but, an arthroscopy revealed a bucket-handle tear of a large discoid medial meniscus and mild fibrillation of the patella.
>
> "Following the arthroscopy an open partial menisectomy was performed utilizing a medial parapatellar incision. A large portion of the torn meniscus was impinging medially. The anterior horn and the discoid torn portion of the meniscus was removed and a posteromedial and posterior horn rim of the meniscus was left behind.
>
> "The postoperative course was uncomplicated. In two follow up office visits the patient was free of symptoms with full range of motion and good quad strength."
>
> (D. Patel, P. Dimakopoulos, and P. Denoncourt 1986)

Dr. Patel played another major role in healthcare in Massachusetts. He was appointed to the Massachusetts Board of Registration in Medicine in 1987; a position he held for five years, until 1992. He served on and chaired many committees of the board and became its chairman in January 1991. He was appointed by Governor Michael S. Dukakis:

> [It was] at a particularly difficult period. There was a new governor and a new party in power, four new board members [total 5 physicians and 2 public members], and a public angry and upset at what it considered the board's go-soft attitude on physicians. At the same time the state's doctors were upset at what they felt was overly harsh treatment by the board. The atmosphere was so charged, that Secretary of Consumer Affairs…in July 1991 appointed a "Blue Ribbon Task Force" to review policies and operating procedures of the board. "It was an extremely difficult period." Dr. Patel's easy-going personality and consensus-style leadership…helped cool tensions and tone down the rhetoric. "He's a great listener…he likes consensus. It has allowed people on all sides of our issue to trust him. It's quite a balancing act…He was very supportive of the investigation…There was no sense of foot-dragging or whitewashing… He's opened up dialogues with a wide range of groups…He's been a very positive force."
>
> …The task force took six months to complete its investigation and make a number of recommendations…Dr. Patel and current members are in the current process of implementing the recommendations… "It's very confusing to be criticized from opposite poles," noted attorney…and Vice Chairman of the board…"My own view is that when both sides criticize you, it's the strongest indication you can get that you're doing the best job possible." Anything less than perfect harmony can be hard on the ears, but then Dr. Patel has always been a good listener. ("Discord Sometimes Indicates Harmony," n.d.)

Over the course of his career, he would hold workshops and give lectures and courses on operative arthroscopy in countries around the world. At MGH, he started seminars and lab experiences for the HCORP residents, eventually raising funds for a psychomotor skills laboratory in Sleeper Hall, named after Dr. Patel in 2010. In 1996, he not only gave lectures on arthroscopy at Gujarat University, but provided live surgical demonstrations of its use. In 1997, he was appointed visiting orthopaedic surgeon at MGH. That same year (and continuing into 2002), he was the director of an annual arthroscopic surgery course at the meeting of the Indian Orthopaedic Association in Ahmadabad.

In 2001, he established the Center of Healing Arts—Dr. Dinesh G. Patel, Psychomotor Laboratory—the first arthroscopic psychomotor skills lab in Asia—at the Paraplegia Hospital in Ahmadabad, India. He was able to do so after the Endoscopy Division of Smith & Nephew, Inc. donated medical equipment and surgical instruments. The lab's mission was to act as a training facility and fill the gap in arthroscopic psychomotor needs for medical professionals and educators alike, all while simultaneously reducing any need to seek additional training outside of India. Various Indian leaders met for the dedication, including Dr. Patel and Dr. M. M. Prabhakar, who served as director of the Paraplegia Hospital and dean of B. J. Medical College.

From 2002 to 2013, Dr. Patel was a member of the Patient Care Assessment (PCA) Committee of the Quality and Patient Safety Division of the Board of Medicine in Massachusetts. The division provides oversight of quality assurance, risk management, peer review, utilization review and credentialing. During this time, he was also

> Dr. Dinesh Patel, pioneer in arthroscopic surgery joins with Smith & Nephew and leaders from India to create first endoscopic teaching lab in India

2001 Smith and Nephew announcement of the new Arthroscopic Learning Center in India.
Smith and Nephew, 2001.

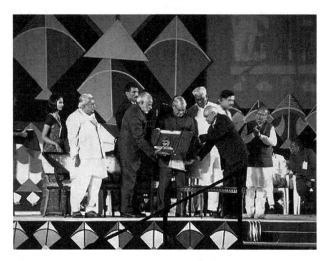

Dr. Patel receiving the 2004 Gujarat Garima Award. Courtesy of Lokvani.

appointed associate clinical professor at HMS in 2005. Throughout his career, he has published about 20 articles and 19 chapters.

For his educational contributions, he has received numerous awards and certificates of appreciation. In India, he has received the silver medal from the Indian Congress of Surgery (1980), a special award from the Indian Arthroscopy Society (1984), a gold medal from the Indian Congress of Surgery (1985), special honors from the V. S. Medical College, Gujarat University (1988), the International Vishwa Gurjari Award from the city of Ahmadabad for public service in education (1988), and, in 2004, he was honored with the Gujarat Garima Award—Outstanding Citizen born in Gujarat for contributions in healthcare.

In October 1996, Governor William Weld's Office of Refugee and Immigration had named Dr. Patel as the Governor's New American Appreciation Award for his contributions to Massachusetts. He also served on the Federation of State Medical Boards (FSMB) for four years and was its director. As a result of his contributions in 2003, Dr. Patel received the John H. Clark Leadership Award from the Federation of State Medical Boards and was recognized by Governor Mitt Romney with a special certificate for his contributions to the regulatory medical board.

FRANCIS X. PEDLOW JR.

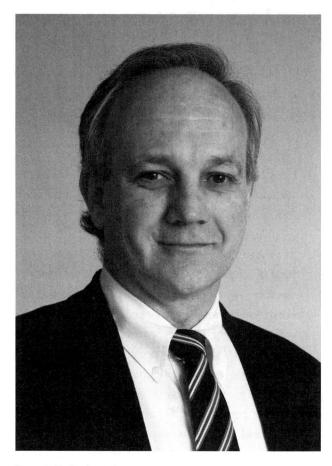

Francis X. Pedlow Jr. Massachusetts General Hospital.

Physician Snapshot

Francis X. Pedlow Jr.
BORN: 1959
DIED: —
SIGNIFICANT CONTRIBUTIONS: Chief of the MGH orthopaedic spine service 1999–2003

Francis "Frank" Xavier Pedlow Jr. was born in Basel, Switzerland. His father, Francis X. Pedlow Sr., was a radiologist from Brooklyn and his mother, Marie T. (Baranello) Pedlow, a nurse was from Queens, New York. They met at Kings County Hospital in Brooklyn while his father was most likely completing a clinical clerkship and still a medical student in Basel, Switzerland, and his mother was a nursing student. They married and then returned together to Basel for his father to complete his medical education. It was during his father's last year in medical school that Frank was born, the first of six children. After graduation, his father completed his training in the United States and was a founding physician for the Putnam Hospital Center in Carmel, New York, in the 1960s. Frank attended the John F. Kennedy High School in Somers, just south of Carmel. In 1981, he received his BS degree in biology from St. Lawrence University and then graduated from New York Medical College in Valhalla, New York, in 1986. He spent the following year as a surgical

Case 42.9. Open Anterior Lumbosacral Fracture Dislocation

"A 15-year-old girl, the unrestrained driver of a motor vehicle, was involved in a collision at high speed. She had back pain and was noted to have a right iliac crest-flank wound. Initial neurologic examination findings indicated decreased rectal tone, decreased sensation on the dorsal and lateral aspects of the right foot, and weak dorsiflexion of both feet, with the right weaker than the left. Plain radiographs showed anterior fracture dislocation with approximately 90% anterolisthesis of L5 on S1. Intravenous methylprednisolone was administered and the patient transferred for further treatment.

"At our institution, again she mentioned back pain, as well as bilateral foot numbness and tingling in the right foot more than in the left. Neurologic examination showed decreased rectal tone and an absent bulbocavernosus reflex. One the right and left lower extremities: the quadriceps, hamstrings, and tibialis anterior exhibited 4/5 strength (based on the Medical Research Council of Great Britain muscle grading scale) with absent extensor hallucis longus function bilaterally and diminished sensation on the dorsal and lateral aspects of both feet. She was taken to the operating room where she underwent irrigation and debridement of the open flank wound and a posterior approach to the spine. The L5 posterior elements were fractured and displaced at the pars interarticularis. The dura was shredded, and CSF flowed freely into the wound. Multiple transected nerve roots were evident. The wound contained necrotic muscle contaminated with dirt and other debris that tracked outward to the flank wound.

"The initial operative session consisted of extensive irrigation and debridement of the wound. All devitalized tissue was removed. A segment of the lumbar fascia was excised and used to fashion a dural graft, which partially stemmed the leaking CSF. Because of the contamination, internal fixation of the fractures was not attempted. Layered primary closure of the operative wound and its communication with the open wound were performed. The flank wound itself was left open.

"After 6 weeks of antibiotic therapy and bed rest, anterior L5-S1 fusion was attempted, with disc excision and a transfixing fibular dowel graft through the L5 body into the sacrum. Bone graft from the hole in the vertebral bodies and from the excess fibula was place around the intervertebral space. A small bowel obstruction developed 6 days after the anterior procedure and a lysis of adhesions was performed. She was fitted with a thoracolumbosacral orthosis with left thigh extension and was allowed out of bed. The thigh extension was removed at 6 weeks, because she was ambulating well without pain.

"She reported increasing back pain 3 months after the anterior fusion. Radiographs showed a fracture of the fibula graft with anterior subluxation of L5. Worsening S1 weakness and paresthesia were noted. She then underwent a posterior fusion from L4 to the sacrum with pedicle screws, intrasacral rods, and iliac crest autograft. Findings in a neurologic examination showed 4/5 muscle strength in the quadriceps, hip flexors, and ankle dorsiflexors bilaterally, 3/5 extensor hallucis longus, 1/5 plantar flexion, a strong anal response, good voluntary rectal tone, and decreased sensation in the L5-S1 distribution.

"She again was immobilized with a thoracolumbosacral orthosis. At last follow-up, 3 years after posterior fusion, her only neurologic deficits included a 4/5 extensor hallucis longus, on both sides and 4/5 peroneal strength on the right. She was walking without leg braces or other aides. Radiographs showed healed posterolateral fusion from L4 to the sacrum."

(Carlson, Heller, Mansfield, and Pedlow 1999)

> **Anterior Spinal Arthrodesis With Structural Cortical Allografts and Instrumentation for Spine Tumor Surgery**
>
> Kai-Uwe Lewandrowski, MD,* Andrew C. Hecht, MD,* Thomas F. DeLaney, MD,†
> Peter A. Chapman,† Francis J. Hornicek, MD, PhD,* and Frank X. Pedlow, MD*
>
> Spine • Volume 29 • Number 10 • 2004

Pedlow and colleagues' article on reconstruction of the spine following anterior resection of spine tumors. *Spine* 2004; 29: 1150.

intern at the Nassau County Medical Center in East Meadow, New York. He demonstrated an early interest in spine surgery, rotating through three hospitals over the next two years: 18 months as a neurosurgery spine fellow at Long Island Jewish Medical Center in New Hyde Park, NY (July 1987–December 1988), and six months in orthopaedics at the Royal National Orthopaedic Hospital in London and the Robert Jones and Agnes Hunt Orthopaedic Hospital in Oswestry, England.

Dr. Pedlow then moved to Boston where he was a resident in general surgery at MGH (1989–1990). In 1990, he began his orthopaedic education in the Edouard Samson Orthopaedic Training Program at the University of Montreal. After two years, he transferred to the Harvard Combined Orthopaedic Residency Program where he graduated in 1994. After his chief residency at MGH, he completed a fellowship in spine surgery at Emory University from 1995 to 1996.

After his spine fellowship, Pedlow returned to MGH as an assistant in orthopaedic surgery and instructor in orthopaedic surgery at Harvard Medical School. He has limited his practice to surgery of the spine with a special interest in primary and metastatic tumors of the spine. From 1999 to 2003, he was the chief of the orthopaedic spine service. As chief, he organized the orthopaedic spine center at MGH—including physiatrists, nurse practitioners, physician assistants, and orthopaedic spine surgeons—to diagnose and manage adults with a variety of spine problems. Since 1999, he had been on the consulting staff in spine surgery at MGH and Spaulding Rehabilitation Hospital; he later joined the attending staffs at Newton-Wellesley Hospital and the New England Baptist Hospital.

Pedlow has published 19 articles and 6 chapters. Of his articles, 17 involved the spine, 9 were on tumors of the spine; 2 on fusion and 1 article on each of the following: cervical spine instrumentation, trauma (see **Case 42.9**), complications of the halo-vest in the elderly, sarcoidosis, epithelioid hemangioma, and lumbar spondylolisthesis. In 2004, he and his colleagues reported on 30 patients with primary bone tumors or metastatic disease to the spine at MGH that were treated by anterior vertebral reconstruction with allograft strut grafts (femur, tibia, or humerus) following anterior resection of the tumor. They reported the technique to be reliable without fracture or collapse. Healing was identical to cortical allografts used in long bone reconstruction with healing at each end of the graft-host junction, but without healing along the shaft of the allograft.

Dr. Pedlow is a member of the America Medical Association, the American Academy of Orthopaedic Surgeons, the Massachusetts Orthopaedic Association, the International College of Surgeons, the North American Spine Society, the American Spinal Injury Association, and the Irish American Orthopaedic Society.

RICHARD J. SMITH

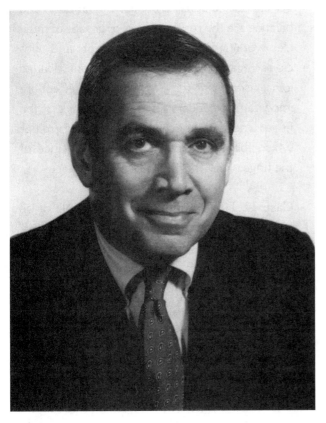

Richard J. Smith. Massachusetts General Hospital, Archives and Special Collections.

Physician Snapshot

Richard J. Smith
BORN: 1930
DIED: 1987
SIGNIFICANT CONTRIBUTIONS: Inspirational teacher; chief of the MGH orthopaedic hand surgery unit; president ASSH 1982

Richard Jay Smith was born to Jacob and Rose Smith in Bronx, New York, in 1930. He had one sibling (Gleniss), with whom he retained a deep friendship. He graduated first from Bronx High School of Science and then from Brown University in 1951. Four years later, he obtained his doctorate in Medicine from New York Medical College in New York City, where he "was elected to Alpha Omega Alpha" (Mankin 1987). He initially completed "a preliminary year of training in general surgery at Bellevue Hospital, [then] he entered the orthopaedic surgical program at the Hospital for Joint Diseases in East Harlem and completed his...program...in 1960" (Mankin 1987). Dr. Henry Mankin recounted Smith's early career progression:

> It was at the Hospital for Joint Diseases that [Smith] became fascinated by the emerging specialty of hand surgery. Richard met and quickly became a disciple of Emmanuel Kaplan, the then reigning authority on anatomy of the hand and one of the early leaders in the evolving new field. The precision, innovation, and technical perfection that were required to solve surgical problems of the hand held tremendous appeal to Richard's sense of order and problem-solving and his innate creativity...Following completion of his residency in 1960 and two years with the Public Health Service in Boston...[he] spent a year of fellowship with Dr. Joseph Boyes in Los Angeles and Mr. Guy Pulvertaft in England. In 1963, he returned to the Hospital for Joint Disease, first to work with Dr. Kaplan, and then in 1968 to succeed him as the Director of Hand Surgery. (Mankin 1987)

During Dr. Smith's nine years on the staff of the Hospital for Joint Diseases, he published about 12 papers on hand surgery; five in the *Bulletin of the Hospital for Joint Diseases*. He wrote about anatomy and clinical topics, including: the radial club hand, boutonniere deformity, camptodactyly, anatomy of a congenitally deformed upper limb, anomalous muscle belly of the flexor digitorum superficialis, as well as surgical treatments such as thumb reconstruction and use of the advancement pedicle flap. During this time, he:

> rapidly became a major force in hand surgery in New York City and...[later] throughout the country and abroad. Those who were fortunate to see his work were impressed by his

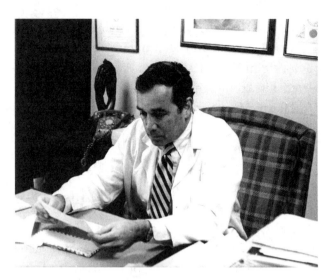

Richard Smith, chief of the Hand and Upper Extremity Service at MGH. Massachusetts General Hospital, Archives and Special Collections.

knowledge and technical skill, and even more so by his extraordinary capacity to impart information. He was an articulate teacher and a spellbinding speaker. His gift of communication extended beyond a clarity of expression; he had the extraordinary and quite unique ability to create an image with words. All who knew him recognized this feature as his most outstanding quality. (Mankin 1987)

By 1972, Smith joined Mankin in his move to the Massachusetts General Hospital in Boston as chief of the Hand Service in the Department of Orthopaedic Surgery. One of his first, often quoted publications after moving to Boston and assuming his new position was his article, "Balance and Kinetics of the Fingers Under Normal and Pathological Conditions." He wrote that:

to understand deformity and abnormality requires an appreciation of normal function in the hand. To study normal function requires an appreciation of anatomy… The anatomical configuration of the muscles, tendons, fascia, and ligaments within the human finger which control its motion, and the relationships of these structures to their function demonstrate that function of any one muscle or tendon to the finger cannot be considered alone, as motion and balance are the result of pairs or groups of muscles working together. The concepts and principles regarding the intercalated bone, loaded joint, viscoelastic force and tenodesis effect are important for understanding the kinetics of the finger and pathomechanics of the deformities which follow disruption of normal balance of the finger. (Smith 1974)

Case 42.10 also highlights an example of one of the early cases he reviewed.

He became very busy in his clinical practice, and in 1980 he was promoted to professor of orthopaedic surgery at HMS. He continued to write about anatomy and clinical topics, several considered classic review articles. During his 15 years on the staff at MGH, he would publish another 50 articles and a book, *Tendon Transfers of the Hand and Forearm* in 1987. He published his personal series of the flexor pollicis longus abductor-plasty for spastic thumb-in-palm deformity, the use of the extensor carpi radialis brevis tendon transfer (adductor-plasty) to improve power pinch and the metacarpal ligament sling tenodesis in patients with an intrinsic paralysis, as well as results and observations on many other conditions of the hand.

Smith was elected president of the American Society for Surgery of the Hand in 1982. His presidential address, "Education of the Surgical

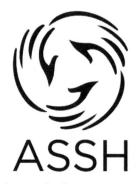

Logo, American Society for Surgery of the Hand.
Courtesy of the American Society for Surgery of the Hand.

Case 42.10. Factitious Lymphedema of the Hand

> "An intelligent thirteen-year-old girl was struck on the dorsum of the right (dominant) hand with a baseball bat while at summer camp. The incident occurred shortly after the birth of her half-brother. The patient had been living with her divorced mother and her stepfather.
>
> "In the days following the injury, the hand became extremely swollen and the patient was seen by local doctors, who recommended that she return home at once. The edema became more severe and extended to the mid-forearm. A biopsy was performed at the dorsum of the hand which was said to reveal fibrosis about the tendons. Swelling persisted intermittently for several months. There was relatively little pain. Six months after its onset, the swelling resolved spontaneously and completely.
>
> "The following summer, approximately one year from the time of the initial injury, edema occurred, with no history of additional trauma. The edema ended abruptly in a circumferential ring of red skin below the elbow. Many medical consultations were sought and the patient was admitted to a minimum of seven hospitals over a period of several months. The diagnoses included juvenile rheumatoid arthritis, synovial cysts, lymphedema praecox, Sécretan's disease, and sympathetic dystrophy. All laboratory tests and roentgenograms were within normal limits. She was forced to stop attending school because of her illness.
>
> "Intermittent edema persisted until two years after the onset of her complaints, at which time a right cervical sympathectomy was performed. The lymphedema cleared completely after surgery. Some months later the right leg became edematous. A right lumbar sympathectomy was performed and again the edema subsided. Within a year lymphedema of the left upper limb developed. A left cervical and then a left lumbar sympathectomy were performed.
>
> "One year later lymphedema again recurred in the right upper limb. The right cervical sympathetic chain was again explored and excised. Shortly thereafter the patient became overtly psychotic and was admitted to a mental hospital after attempting suicide by cutting both wrists. Under psychotherapy she explained that for the preceding years she had applied tourniquets to her limbs in order to cause the edema. There were no further reported incidents of lymphedema following prolonged psychotherapy."
>
> (Richard J. Smith 1975)

Specialist," was no surprise to the members who knew him. He briefly reviewed the history of surgical education, the growth of specialties and subspecialties and the educational efforts of the American Society for Surgery of the Hand. He concluded by noting:

> Perhaps some of our best teachers are our residents and fellows…Surely life would be simpler and easier for many of us if we were to accept our government's advice and spend less time in medical education. But we need only to look around us today and to see how few of us have listened to government officials, state legislators, and television commentators. We know that education of the surgical specialist is our responsibility. It is too important to be left to anyone else. It is as crucial as patient care, for those who we teach today will treat their patients and will be the teachers of other doctors in the decades to come. As educators in the world's most important profession, we have a long and proud heritage. And we do not intend to abandon it. (C. A. Smith 1983)

Smith remained chief of the service until his premature death in 1987, 15 years after his appointment. Dr. Henry Mankin wrote a tribute to Dr. Smith shortly after his passing:

> Perusal of Richard Smith's curriculum vitae discloses that he was not only a "joiner," but also clearly a tireless worker for the organizations within and those allied to his specialty.

PRESIDENTIAL ADDRESS—AMERICAN SOCIETY FOR SURGERY OF THE HAND

Education of the surgical specialist

Richard J. Smith, M.D., *Boston, Mass.*

THE JOURNAL OF HAND SURGERY
Vol. 8, No. 5, Part 1
September 1983

Title of Smith's presidential address, ASSH, 1983.
Journal of Hand Surgery 1983; 8: 509.

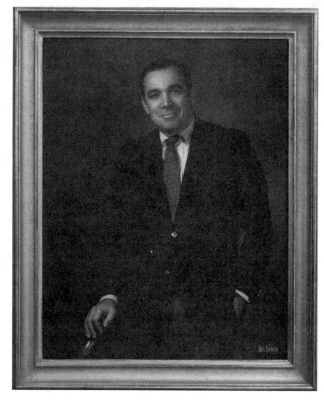

Portrait of Richard J. Smith which hangs in the Richard Smith Library at MGH. Massachusetts General Hospital, Archives and Special Collections.

To mention a few, he was a member of The American Academy of Orthopaedic Surgeons, the American Orthopaedic Association, the American Society for Surgery of the Hand, and the American College of Surgeons; he was awarded honorary membership in the British Society for Surgery of the Hand, Columbian Society for Surgery of the Hand, Peruvian Orthopaedic Association, Western Orthopaedic Association, and Groupe D'Etude de la Main. His list of committee assignments for the various organizations is long and speaks not only to his capability as a statesman and leader, but also to the respect with which he was held ... At the time of his death, he was a member of the Board of Directors of Brown University Medical Association, the Board of Governors of the American College of Surgeons, and the Education Committee of the International Federation of Societies for Surgery of the Hand...

When all the gifts that Richard Smith brought to the world are totaled and weighed, however, the one that will last the longest in the minds of those whom he taught and those whom were fortunate enough to know and work with him were his extraordinary devotion to his family and his warmth and love for his students and friends...He made our world a happier and better place...Richard J. Smith died peacefully at Massachusetts General Hospital on March 30, 1987, at the age of fifty-six. An inoperable glioma of the left temporal lobe had been discovered some thirteen months previously and despite radiation and chemotherapy, he lapsed into a coma in February shortly after returning from the Annual Meeting of the American Academy of Orthopaedic Surgeons.
(Mankin 1987)

Dr. Steven Z. Glickel later wrote of Dr. Smith:

We have some excellent educators in our field...But Dick Smith would have to be at the top of anyone's list. He could communicate to students' level. The word I always come back to is engaging. Of course he was tough at times and demanding. But you know that he was trying to get the best out of you. I just had the feeling that he could be someone I could emulate. (Green 2015)

After his death, the MGH orthopaedic hand service established an annual Richard J. Smith Lecture in his honor. In addition to the guest lecture, faculty, fellows, and residents present papers at a one-day meeting called "Smith Day." To date, these individual lecturers have included:

Thomas J. Fisher
Mark S. Cohen
Joseph Upton III
Graham J.W. King
Douglas Campbell
Amit Gupta
Leonard Gordon
James H. Herndon
A. Lee Osterman
Richard H. Gelberman
Peter C. Amadio
Diego Fernandez
Thomas E. Trumble
Andrew J. Weiland
Neil Jones
Roy Meals
Peter Stern
Barry Simmons
Thomas Bruschart
Terry S. Axelrod

DEMPSEY S. SPRINGFIELD

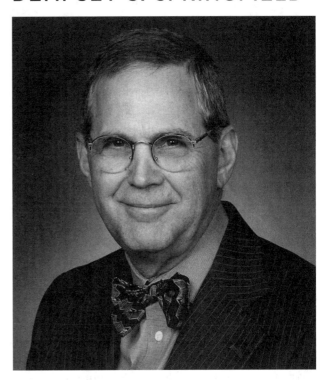

Dempsey S. Springfield. MGH HCORP Archives.

Physician Snapshot

Dempsey S. Springfield
BORN: 1945
DIED: —

SIGNIFICANT CONTRIBUTIONS: Researched improvements in the use of allografts; supported minimum surgical experience in graduate medical education; HCORP Director 2009–2012; president Musculoskeletal Tumor Society 1993 and Association of Bone and Joint Surgeons 1996–1997

Dempsey Stewart Springfield was born and raised in Atlanta, Georgia. He attended Emory University, graduating in 1967 with a bachelor of arts degree. He then attended medical school at the University of Florida, where he received his MD degree in 1971. There he was elected into Alpha Omega Alpha. As an outstanding graduating medical student, he received the W. C. Thomas Award, which is awarded to the student with the best performance during the obstetrics and gynecology clerkship, and the John B. Gorrie Award,

> Instr Course Lect. 1984;33:1-25.
>
> **Principles of tumor management**
>
> D S Springfield, W F Enneking, J R Neff, J T Makley

Springfield et al., AAOS Instructional Course on musculoskeletal tumors. *Instructional Course Lectures* 1984; 33: 1.

given to the student who shows the most potential for becoming an effective physician. Following a surgical internship at the University of Alabama in Birmingham, in 1976 he completed a four-year residency in orthopaedic surgery at the University of Florida Health Shands Hospital in Gainesville, Florida. During his residency, he spent six months of 1974 as a fellow in musculoskeletal pathology.

After completing his residency, Springfield received an American Orthopaedic Association North American Traveling Fellowship. He served a two-year military commitment as a major in the US Army, stationed at Fort Leonard Wood in the Missouri Ozarks. Fort Leonard Wood has historically been a basic training center for noncombat soldiers; combat engineers; military police; and chemical, biological, radiological, and nuclear specialists. At the garrison is the General Leonard Wood Army Community Hospital, a 320-bed hospital that provides a full range of medical services to active-duty and retired military personnel and their families. Tertiary care was available in Springfield, Missouri, and at the University of Missouri in Columbia. In 1977, while Springfield was stationed there in service as an orthopaedic surgeon, the hospital opened a new addition comprising a 180-bed tower (increasing capacity to 500) and a clinic building that effectively doubled the available clinic space.

In 1978, Springfield returned to Gainesville for a one-year musculoskeletal tumor fellowship.

He remained on the staff at Shands Hospital as an assistant professor of orthopaedic surgery; he was awarded an American Cancer Society Junior Faculty Clinical Fellowship that supported him 1978–82, as he began his career. From 1980 to 1987, he served as the chief of orthopaedic oncology at the University of Florida, and from 1981 to 1986 he was the orthopaedic residency program director. In 1983 he was promoted to associate professor of orthopaedic surgery. All told, Springfield remained at the University of Florida for eight years.

While at Shands, Springfield published ~35 papers. As a recognized expert in musculoskeletal tumors, he led an American Academy of Orthopaedics Surgeons instructional course, "Principles of Tumor Management," with Dr. W. F. Enneking and others in 1984.

Move to MGH

In 1987, Dr. Henry Mankin recruited Springfield to Massachusetts General Hospital (MGH) as a visiting orthopaedic surgeon, also appointing him as associate professor at Harvard Medical School. He remained at MGH for nine years. He had a busy practice on the tumor service and published more than 50 papers. Springfield listed his five main research interests in his curriculum vitae: allograft bone transplantation (11 papers), limb-salvage surgery for sarcoma of the extremities (3 papers), effect of preoperative treatment (chemotherapy and irradiation) on sarcomas (6 papers), the relationships between local recurrence and metastases (6 papers), and resident education (2 papers).

Research

One of his first publications while at MGH was titled "Surgical Treatment of Osteosarcoma." In that study: "Fifty-three patients who had a high-grade osteosarcoma had either a limb-salvage resection or an amputation…all received adjuvant therapy…Adriamycin…and whole-limb irradiation…Each patient was followed for at least three years or until death" (Springfield et al. 1988). The authors concluded, "a wide margin is adequate to control a primary osteosarcoma. When a wide surgical margin can be used and a functional limb can be salvaged, an amputation probably is not required" (Springfield et al. 1988).

Case 42.11 provides a report from a 1989 publication about Gaucher's disease cowritten by Springfield, M. Landfried, and Mankin. Two years after that paper, Springfield and Mankin, this time with Mark Gebhardt and Daniel Flugstad, published "The Use of Bone Allografts for Limb Salvage in High-Grade Extremity Osteosarcoma" as part of a symposium in *Clinical Orthopaedics and Related Research*. In that limited review, the authors reported the results of limb-sparing surgery in the treatment of osteosarcoma in 53 patients younger than 30 years of age, with a mean follow-up of just more than 2 years. They found, overall, "the probability of a satisfactory functional result was 73% if local recurrences were excluded. Complications included 16 infections, six fractures, 12 nonunions, and six unstable joints. There were five local recurrences. Eighteen grafts ultimately failed, and...[six] resulted in an above-knee amputation. An additional five received a second graft. The functional 'end results'...were 70% satisfactory" (Gebhardt et al. 1991).

In their discussion, they noted that "the majority...of the osteosarcomas...can be safely resected and that allografts are a reasonable reconstruction option...[but are] not suitable for all patients" (Gebhardt et al. 1991). In fact, they used allografts in only a third of the osteosarcomas they treated, and they applied "rotationplasty for very young patients...and metallic prostheses for elderly patients" (Gebhardt et al. 1991). They believed that "preoperative chemotherapy truly increases the percentage of 'resectable' patients," and, they concluded, "In general, for proximal humerus lesions an allograft-arthrodesis is the preferred method of reconstruction...however about the knee, osteoarticular allografts are preferred" (Gebhardt et al. 1991).

In another *Clinical Orthopaedics and Related Research* symposium dedicated to Marshall R. Urist in 1994; Springfield, John Flynn, and Mankin reported their use of "Osteoarticular Allografts to Treat Distal Femoral Osteonecrosis":

> Since 1980, 21 patients younger than 50 years old...[with] osteonecrosis involving large portions of the distal femur were treated with fresh-frozen osteoarticular surface replacements...15 patients (17 knees)...[were followed] greater than two years...Follow-up time ranged from two to nine years...There were seven excellent results, five good results, one fair result, and four failures...12 (70%) of the 17 knees have been successfully treated. The authors' success rate with frozen allografts is comparable to the results of fresh allograft resurfacings...[and] is more practical, and the allografts are available for use in elective surgery. Failure in this series was principally the result of degeneration of the allografts articular cartilage, or fracture of the allograft.

The musculoskeletal tumor surgeons at MGH reported the long-term (24 years) results of more 870 allografts at the 1995 International Symposium on Bone and Soft Tissue Allografts, which was sponsored by the Musculoskeletal Transplant Foundation in Washington, DC, and was dedicated to the memory of Dr. Mark Coventry. The frozen grafts they had used, from cadavers, had mainly come from the bone bank at MGH, and they were implanted "mostly for the treatment of defects created by the resection of a bone tumor" (Mankin et al. 1996).

> The results show that only stage and type of graft affected outcome predictably. Specifically, grafts for a Stage 2 or Stage 3 tumor had a poorer outcome than those for Stages 0 and 1. The results for allograft arthrodeses were considerably poorer than osteoarticular, intercalary, and allograft plus prosthesis. The

Case 42.11. Gaucher Hemorrhagic Cyst of Bone

"A forty-five-year-old white woman had been diagnosed as having Gaucher Disease when she was thirteen years old, after an aspiration of the bone marrow. The diagnosis was confirmed in 1965, when the patient was twenty-three years old and a splenectomy was done for the treatment of chronic thrombocytopenia. Six months after the splenectomy, the patient began having pain in the left hip. Osteonecrosis and collapse of the left femoral head was identified. The hip was treated non-operatively, and the patient continued to walk without aids.

"In May 1983, the patient sustained a non-traumatic, spontaneous fracture through a previously undetected radiolucent lesion in the distal part of the left femur. The fracture was treated with a cast brace, and it healed in five months. The patient was first seen by one of us (H. J. M.) in August 1983.

"The radiolucent lesion in the distal part of the left femur was initially thought to be a defect in the bone that had been caused by a collection of Gaucher cells. It was also thought that union of the fracture would stimulate healing of the lesion, but it did not.

"The patient continued to walk without aids, but mild pain in the left hip persisted. The right hip also began to be painful, and, in early 1984, radiographs showed osteonecrosis and partial collapse of the femoral head. By May 1987, the radiographic appearance of the lucent lesion in the distal part of the left femur had not changed. However, a large, smooth, non-tender, firm, fixed mass was palpable in the posterior aspect of the distal part of the left thigh. There were no signs of inflammation, and no pulsations or bruit could be detected. Because of the mass, the patient was admitted to the hospital for an incisional biopsy in June 1987.

"On admission to the hospital, the level of serum calcium was 2.42 millimoles per liter, the level of serum phosphorus was 1.03 millimoles per liter, the level of magnesium was 0.80 millimole per liter, the level of creatinine was sixty-two micromoles per liter, the level of alkaline phosphatase was twenty-four units per liter, and the level of 5 nucleotidase was six units per liter. A twenty-four-hour collection of urine contained 7.8 millimoles of creatinine and 3.5 millimoles of calcium, which are normal values. The levels of parathyroid hormone, of 25-hydroxyvitamine D, of 1.25-dihydroxyvitamine D, and of Factor IX were all normal. The prothrombin, partial prothrombin, and bleeding times were normal as well. The platelet count was 110,000.

"Anteroposterior and lateral radiographs of the distal part of the left femur showed an apparently multiloculated radiolucent lesion and expansion of the cortex. The mass extended through the posterior part of the femoral cortex into the thigh. A computerized tomography scan confirmed the posterior extraosseous extension of the mass. The scan also revealed that the lesion was not multiloculated; an irregular inner wall had given that impression.

"The biopsy was done through a lateral femoral approach that included splitting the vastus lateralis muscle. A tourniquet was used. A small opening was made in the thin fibrous wall (which appeared to be periosteum) of the extraosseous mass. A blood-filled cavity was entered, and multiple specimens were taken from the material within and from the lining of the cavity. When the tourniquet was deflated, there was pulsatile bleeding from the cavity; this was controlled by suturing the incision that had been made in the thin, fibrous wall of the cavity. The total loss of blood for the procedure was fifty milliliters.

"Histological examination revealed that the lining of the cavity was composed of reactive bone, organizing blood clot, inflammatory cells, and a few Gaucher cells. There was no evidence of neoplastic tissue. Special stains and culture revealed no organisms.

"The incision for the biopsy healed without difficulty. Nine months postoperatively, the lesion remained unchanged, as seen radiographically. Three months after the biopsy, the patient had a bipolar prosthetic replacement of the right femoral head because of unremitting pain secondary to osteonecrosis, collapse of the femoral head, and degenerative arthritis. At the time of writing, the patient continued to have mild pain in the left hip and used a cane. We were concerned about the defect in the distal part of the left femur, and the patient has remained under observation."

(Springfield, Landfried, and Mankin 1989)

other major factors in results were complications – recurrence, infection, fracture, and nonunion...After the first year of susceptibility to infection (10%) and the third year of increased risk of fracture (19%), the grafts become stable, and approximately 75% are retained by patients and are considered to be successful for >20 years after implantation. Osteoarthritis becomes a problem at approximately 6 years for osteoarticular grafts, and...16% of the patients with distal femoral, proximal tibial, or proximal femoral grafts have required total joint replacements...Reduction or at least control of the immune response will result in a better graft that is less prone to complications and late failure. (Mankin et al. 1996)

In 2000, in an attempt to decrease the rate of infection in allografts, Springfield and his colleagues studied the effects of irradiation (10–30 kGy) on allografts. Between 24 patients with an irradiated graft, who were followed for a mean of five years, and a control group of patients whose grafts were not irradiated, "the outcomes...differed significantly only in the incidence of allograft fracture": in 18% without radiation and in 39% with radiation (Lietman et al. 2000).

In 2002, the tumor group at MGH combined their data on knee fusion with an allograft with data from the Istituto Ortopedico Rizzoli in Bologna, Italy. Among the 92 patients: "Tumor complications were a major problem...Thirty-four percent of the patients died, 47% had metastases develop, and 9% had a local recurrence. Allograft complications included an infection rate of 20%, a fracture rate of 25%, and a nonunion rate of 44%. Repeat surgery was required for more than 50% of the patients" (Donati et al. 2002). In light of these outcomes, when considered against "data for a control series of 880 patients with allografts other than allograft arthrodeses, the complications were greater and the outcome less successful, suggesting that other approaches should be considered" (Donati et al. 2002).

Springfield was recruited to New York City in 1996 as the Robert K. Lippman Professor and chairman of the Leni and Peter W. May Department of Orthopaedics at the Mount Sinai School of Medicine, and as the orthopaedic surgeon-in-chief at the Mount Sinai Hospital. During his nine-year tenure there, he also served as the residency program director of orthopaedic surgery at the Mount Sinai Medical Center.

Thoughts on Graduate Education

Springfield returned to MGH, however, almost a decade later: In 2006, he became a visiting orthopaedic surgeon and in 2008 was named associate director for the Partners Office of Graduate Medical Education. In 2009, he succeeded me as director of the Harvard Combined Orthopaedic Residency Program (HCORP), a position he held for three years.

At a 2005 American Orthopaedic Association Symposium on Critical Issues, Springfield, along with Dr. Michael A. Simon and Dr. Steven P. Nestler (the executive director of the ACGME Orthopaedic Residency Review Committee), discussed the need for a minimal surgical experience for graduating orthopaedic residents. After surveying orthopaedic surgery residents in postgraduate year 4 and residency program directors, and obtaining responses through a survey administered immediately after their presentation at the AOA meeting, Simon, Springfield, and Nestler (2006) determined that: "Given the experience of Residency Review Committees to date, it is appropriate to conclude that quantitative criteria...have been and will become crucial to accreditation decisions...The setting of minimums...make it easier for programs and residents to understand what is expected of them." They qualified this conclusion, however, noting:

neither Residency Review Committees nor certification boards would base their accreditation and certification decisions on quantitative data alone...quantitative evaluation is...required...

> AN AOA CRITICAL ISSUE
>
> SHOULD THERE BE A MINIMAL SURGICAL EXPERIENCE FOR A GRADUATING ORTHOPAEDIC SURGERY RESIDENT?*
>
> BY MICHAEL A. SIMON, MD, DEMPSEY S. SPRINGFIELD, MD, AND STEVEN P. NESTLER, PhD
> THE JOURNAL OF BONE & JOINT SURGERY · JBJS.ORG
> VOLUME 88-A · NUMBER 5 · MAY 2006

Simon, Springfield, and Nestler's article on minimum requirements of surgical cases for orthopaedic residents. *Journal of Bone and Joint Surgery* 2006; 88: 1153.

quantitative minima are now necessary, but still not sufficient, criteria for crucial decisions regarding the competence of surgeons…Documenting residency surgical experience is starting to become a credentialing issue between hospitals and individual surgeons…[and] documentation is likely to have a role in applying for initial hospital privileges…residents…will need to perform certain common orthopaedic surgical procedures to be credentialed… (Simon, Springfield, and Nestler 2006)

They challenged residency review committees to "strengthen orthopaedic education by a variety of changes in the special requirements, especially with more objective and quantitative criteria… With the public drive toward accountability, medicine is moving or being pushed toward more quantitative data to measure quality" (Simon, Springfield, and Nestler 2006). They did, however, caution against relying extensively on surgical volume because although it "seems to be directly related to outcomes in many surgical specialties, surgical volume has not been studied and the resident is almost always supervised" (Simon, Springfield, and Nestler 2006).

Honors and Recognition

While at MGH, Springfield had held two leadership positions in major professional organizations—as president of the Musculoskeletal Tumor Society, in 1993, and as president of the Association of Bone and Joint Surgeons, from 1996–1997. He also received recognition by other universities. He was named the Michael Bonfiglio Professor of Orthopaedic Pathology at the University of Iowa in 1993, and as the Robert H. Pomeroy Musculoskeletal Oncology Visiting Professor at UCLA in 1994. Springfield gave numerous lectures on musculoskeletal tumors between 1996 and 2007 in both the US and abroad—including 11 lectures at the Istituto Ortopedico Rizzoli Bologna, Italy. Springfield stepped down as the HCORP director in 2012 and as associate director of the Partners Office of Graduate Medical Education in 2014. Soon after, he retired and moved to Florida.

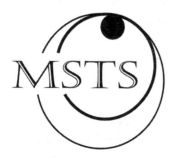

Logo, Musculoskeletal Tumor Society. Courtesy of the Musculoskeletal Tumor Society.

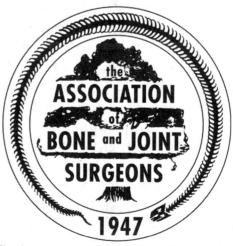

Logo, The Association of Bone and Joint Surgeons. Courtesy of The Association of Bone and Joint Surgeons.

GEORGE H. THEODORE

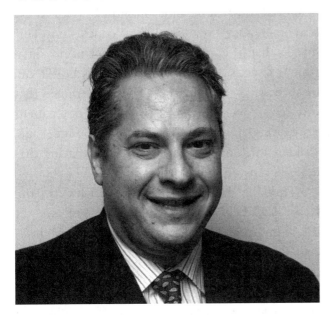

George H. Theodore. Massachusetts General Hospital.

Physician Snapshot

George H. Theodore
BORN: 1965
DIED: —
SIGNIFICANT CONTRIBUTION: Promoted the use and safety of extracorporeal shock wave therapy to treat plantar fasciitis; first chief of the foot and ankle service at MGH

George Harry Theodore, the son of Harry and Marie Theodore, was born and raised in the Jamaica Plain neighborhood of Boston. After graduating from Roxbury Latin High School, he attended Harvard College, and, in 1991, he received an MD degree from Harvard Medical School. He was a surgical intern at MGH in 1991 and completed his orthopaedic training in the Harvard Combined Orthopaedic Residency Program in 1996. From July 1 to December 31, 1996, he was an assistant in orthopaedic surgery (chief resident) at MGH. After a fellowship in foot and ankle surgery at the Brigham and Women's Hospital, he joined the staff at MGH. He is also affiliated with Beth Israel Deaconess Hospital-Milton and Spaulding Rehabilitation Hospital. Theodore is an instructor in orthopaedic surgery at Harvard Medical School.

Research Focusing on Extracorporeal Shock Wave Therapy

Beginning in 2000 and during the subsequent nine years, Theodore published four articles on the use of extracorporeal shockwave therapy (ESWT) to treat plantar fasciitis. In a 2003 letter to the editor of the *Journal of the American Medical Association*, he commented on an article by Buchbinder et al. titled "Ultrasound-Guided Extracorporeal Shock Wave Therapy for Plantar Fasciitis." Buchbinder et al. (2002) had "found no evidence to support a beneficial effect on pain, function and quality of life…12 weeks following treatment" in 79 patients with plantar fasciitis who received ESWT; those patients had been compared with 81 with plantar fasciitis who received a placebo in a double-blind randomized clinical trial. In his letter to the editor, Theodore (2003) wrote, "The results of this study may be a disservice to the future development of ESWT for the treatment of orthopedic conditions." Buchbinder, Forbes, and Ptasznik (2003) responded to Theodore: "We strongly disagree with Dr. Theodore… On the contrary, the negative results of our trial highlight the need to determine the true value of therapeutic interventions by methodically sound randomized clinical trials."

Theodore began using ESWT to treat plantar fasciitis in early 2002. He and his colleagues initially reported its use in 37 patients in the *Orthopaedic Journal* at Harvard Medical School in 2003, then in 150 patients in a multicenter double-blind, placebo-controlled randomized clinical trial in 2004. In that study they reported that, in the study group, ESWT was successful three months (in 56%) and 12 months (in 94%) after treatment. Because a high percentage of cases (53%) in the control group remained symptomatic, they offered treatment at three months; in those patients, success of ESWT was lower (47%) three months after treatment. On the basis of these results, they determined that ESWT was safe in patients with recurring proximal plantar fasciitis.

Theodore et al. Two articles on extracorporeal shock wave therapy for plantar fasciitis. *Foot and Ankle International* 2004; 25: 290; *Journal of Foot and Ankle Surgery* 2009; 48: 148.

They extended their study with results from 225 patients with plantar fasciitis treated with ESWT, which were published in a retrospective review in 2009. Theodore had treated those patients with ESWT between July 2002 and July 2004; the mean follow-up was 30 months (standard deviation, nine months). With these outcomes, they broadened their conclusions, surmising that, if conservative treatment of proximal plantar fasciitis does not achieve results ESWT can be successfully used instead. They determined that various factors reduced the probability of a patient responding positively to ESWT: younger age, walking for long periods each day, or having diabetes or a psychological disorder.

Theodore has published ~12 articles to date. **Case 42.12** highlights an example of one of the many cases he reviewed. He is a team physician for the Boston Red Sox and consultant to the New England Patriots, Boston Bruins, and New England Revolution. He has published several articles on injuries to the foot and ankle and foot/ankle problems in athletes. He continues his work at MGH, with a busy practice in his chosen subspecialty.

Case 42.12. Tenosynovitis of the Flexor Hallucis Longus in a Long-Distance Runner

"A 23-year-old female recreational runner had a 6-month history of left posteromedial ankle pain. She had taken up long-distance running 2 yr. prior, and had no history of prior injuries or medical illnesses. The pain began insidiously after she increased her running schedule from 20 to 30 miles weekly. The pain was initially treated by her family physician with rest (no running), anti-inflammatory medication, and orthotic use. When there was no significant improvement in her symptoms, she received a corticosteroid injection into the affected area. At the time of her referral to the Sports Medicine Clinic, her examination revealed moderate swelling and tenderness over the sheath of the FHL behind the medial malleolus and plantar to the sustenaculum tali. The pain was intensified with active and passive motion of the interphalangeal joint of the great toe. There was no triggering, crepitus, or lateral pain with forced plantarflexion of the foot and ankle. There was no tenderness over the Achilles tendon or pain with resisted inversion of the ankle. Her neurovascular exam was normal, and her plain radiographs were normal. She underwent a course of immobilization (short leg cast) for 3 wk, followed by gentle physical therapy, which included range of motion, ultrasound, and strengthening exercises. Her symptoms recurred as her rehabilitation program progressed. Because of her persistent pain and the absence of a definitive diagnosis, an MRI scan was obtained. It revealed a fluid collection posterior to the medial malleolus in the area of the FHL tendon sheath.

"Operative exploration was elected based on the patient's persistent symptoms, failed response to conservative management, and MRI findings of a well-defined fluid collection. Surgery was performed through a curvilinear posteromedial incision. Exploration of the FHL tendon sheath liberated several cc's of clear fluid and revealed anomalous extension of the muscle belly below the retinaculum with the tenosynovium adherent to the muscle belly. The anomalous muscle belly was excised and the tendon sheath was released. She remained non weight-bearing until her follow-up visit, 1 wk after surgery. The splint was removed, and she began a physical therapy program consisting of progressive weight-bearing and range of motion. Six months after surgery, the patient had returned to her previous running program without ankle discomfort."

(Theodore, Kolletis, and Micheli 1996)

WILLIAM W. TOMFORD

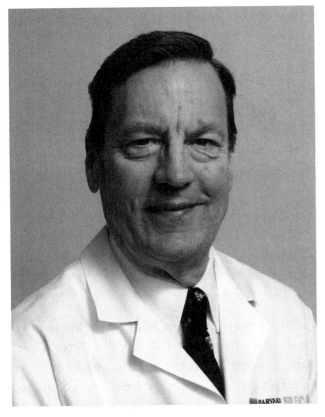

William W. Tomford. Massachusetts General Hospital.

Physician Snapshot

William W. Tomford
BORN: 1945
DIED: —
SIGNIFICANT CONTRIBUTIONS: Studied the use of allografts and articular cartilage preservation; helped pioneer the process of tissue banking in the United States and worldwide; director of the MGH bone bank; president American Association of Tissue Banks; published *Musculoskeletal Tissue Banking*

William Webster Tomford was born and spent his early years in Dallas, Texas, but he was a student at the Choate boarding school in Wallingford, Connecticut, during high school. He entered the University of North Carolina, Chapel Hill, as a Morehead Scholar in 1963, graduating four years later with a bachelor of arts degree. While there, he was a member of Phi Beta Kappa. He went on to medical school at Vanderbilt University in Nashville, Tennessee, graduating with an MD degree in 1971.

While in medical school, he held three clinical and research fellowships. The first, in 1969, was with the United Cerebral Palsy Foundation at the Hospital for Sick Children on Great Ormond Street in London. Then, in 1970, he completed a US Rehabilitation Service Fellowship at Boston Children's Hospital Medical Center. Finally, he was a fellow in surgery at Johns Hopkins University School of Medicine in Baltimore, Maryland, in 1971.

After graduating from medical school, "he started out in General Surgery as an intern and then as a resident at Johns Hopkins from 1971 to 1973" (Mankin 2011). He then entered the MGH/Children's Hospital combined residency program in 1974. In January 1977 he was appointed chief resident and assistant in orthopaedic surgery at MGH; then, "like many of his peers in the Vietnam era, he joined the US Navy and earned the rank of Commander" (Mankin 2011).

Career-long Interest in Tissue Banking and Allografts

After completing his orthopaedic training, Tomford returned to Maryland—this time to Bethesda as an attending physician at the Naval Medical Research Institute. While there, he became engaged with the Naval Tissue Bank, "which started in 1950 under the direction of George Hyatt and subsequently Kenneth Sell, who recruited a number of fellows [including Tomford] to rotate through the system and perform research on graft technology" (Mankin 2011). Tomford eventually created his own tissue bank with Mankin at MGH (1979). His work, and that of Hyatt, Sell, and other fellows, "not only advanced the field in terms of improved success of the implant, but also added greatly to the safety of the host in relation to infections bacterial, and especially viral, transmissions" (Mankin 2011).

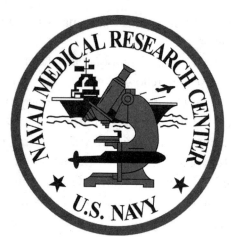

Logo Naval Medical Research Center. Naval Medical Research Center/Flickr.

Box 42.2. Tomford's Appointments at MGH and Harvard

MGH
- 1979   Assistant orthopaedic surgeon
- 1985   Associate orthopaedic surgeon
- 1997   Visiting orthopaedic surgeon

Harvard Medical School
- 1979   Instructor in orthopaedic surgery
- 1982   Assistant professor
- 1989   Associate professor
- 2000   Professor of orthopaedic surgery

Tomford left Bethesda and returned to Boston in 1979; since then, he has served as the director of the MGH Bone Bank, "one of the principal programs in the United States and one of the great contributors to our [MGH's] Orthopaedic Oncology Unit, which has performed a total of over 1,500 allograft transplants—mostly for malignant tumors of bone" (Mankin 2011). Because of the work of Tomford and his staff, MGH has "the lowest complication rate of all the [allograft and tissue-banking] programs, here and abroad" (Mankin 2011)—particularly with regard to virus transmission.

When Tomford returned to MGH he began there as an assistant orthopaedic surgeon. Over the next 20 years he rose through the ranks at MGH and Harvard Medical School (**Box 42.2**). See **Case 42.13** for an example of one of the many cases he reviewed.

Of his more than 65 published articles, approximately 58 discussed: bone banking (5 articles), bone allografts (18), immunogenicity and bone science (19), osteoarticular allografts (3), preservation and use of articular cartilage allografts (7), infection and transmission of disease (5), and soft-tissue allografts (1). He and his colleagues published approximately five articles on infection associated with allografts. In 1981, Tomford, J. E. Ploetz, and Henry Mankin reported on the incidence of infection with use of freeze-dried bone allografts supplied by the US Navy Tissue Bank. Among 303 patients, 21 showed "evidence of infection, of which twelve were considered minor and nine were considered major…In eleven of the twenty-one patients there were positive cultures…[and] in the remaining ten there were not" (Tomford, Ploetz, and Mankin 1981). They concluded "that the allograft was probably not primarily responsible in most of the patients…[and that] the incidence does not appear to be greater than 7 percent and probably is lower" (Tomford, Ploetz, and Mankin 1981).

Two years later, Tomford, along with Dr. Samuel H. Doppelt and Mankin at MGH, and Dr. Gary Friedlaender at Yale, summarized current bone bank procedures including legal issues; donor acquisition and selection; procurement, storage, and retrieval methods; record keeping; and prevention of contamination. With regard to finances, they concluded:

> managing a bone bank can be an extremely expensive endeavor. The Massachusetts General Hospital performed an accounting…of the processing costs from 1979 to 1982…The cost for each procurement was estimated at

more than $2500 per donor…[and] costs for record-keeping supplies…data-processing storage devices…[and] freezers…was estimated at an additional $1200 per donor. Adding administrative and labor costs…[at] an estimated $3000 per donor—the total processing cost came to approximately $6700 per donor…[which] compares favorably with that of a kidney allograft…[at] $8000. Such financial outlay makes the banking of bones very difficult for a small institution, particularly if there is no method for reimbursement. (Tomford et al. 1983)

Case 42.13. Rapid Postoperative Osteolysis in Paget Disease

"A sixty-nine-year-old man was seen because of pain in the right hip that had been increasing for several years and had become intolerable during the previous two to three months. He had extensive Paget disease that involved the pelvis, both femora, and the skull, and he had been treated with injections of Calcimar (calcitonin) for several months before the evaluation. However, about the time that the pain in the hip began to become severe, the patient had stopped taking the Calcimar of his own volition.

"Plain radiographs, made at the initial office visit revealed advanced degenerative osteoarthrosis of the right hip and severe involvement of the right femur with Paget disease. The superolateral portion of the joint space of the hip was markedly narrowed, and there was sclerosis of the femoral head as well as osteophyte formation and cysts within the femoral head and the bone of the acetabulum. A radiolucent horizontal zone of demarcation between the normal and the pagetic bone in the diaphysis of the femur suggested that the Paget disease was in a phase that is usually associated with extensive osteoclastic activity. The course and sclerotic bone trabeculae in the part of the femur proximal to this zone of demarcation were characteristic of osseous repair occurring behind an advancing lytic front in Paget disease. There was also striking intracortical tunneling and thickening of the cortex as well as a varus neck-shaft angle.

"No fractures were visible on the preoperative radiographs. However, at the time of the operation, a pathological fracture of the femoral neck was found. The femoral head was devoid of articular cartilage and had the typical appearance of eburnated bone. When the head was removed and sectioned, a wedge-shaped, soft, yellow area, two centimeters wide, was found under the cortex of the femoral neck. Histological sections revealed hard, thickened bone trabeculae in the center of this area, consistent with Paget disease.

"The operation was uneventful. Postoperatively, the patient had a low-grade fever for three days and then became afebrile. He received narcotic analgesia intramuscularly for two days and thereafter took only acetaminophen orally for relief of pain. He began walking with partial weight-bearing and crutches on the second postoperative day, but he refused to take Calcimar during the postoperative period despite the recommendation of his physician.

"Radiographs made one month after the arthroplasty showed marked rarefaction of the proximal part of the femur compared with the preoperative radiographs. Two months after the operation there was nearly complete resorption of the cortical bone of the femur adjacent to the prosthetic stem, so that only the distal four centimeters of the stem was still surrounded by radiography visible bone.

"During this time, although he continued to walk with partial weight-bearing and the support of crutches, the patient had pain in the right thigh. Physical examination showed no abnormal tenderness or soft-tissue changes around the incision. He was afebrile, and the erythrocyte sedimentation rate and white blood-cell count were normal. About two and one-half months after the operation, the patient agreed to take Calcimar for what was believed to be an increase in the osteolytic activity of the Paget disease following the operation. After he resumed the calcitonin therapy, the pain decreased. Radiographs made eleven months after the arthroplasty showed new bone visible around the prosthetic stem. At this time, the patient followed the advice of the surgeon and began to use a cane when walking outside of the house: he had little or no pain in the thigh."

(Marr, Rosenthal, Cohen, and Tomford 1994)

> **1983 Bone Bank Procedures**
>
> WILLIAM W. TOMFORD, M.D.,* SAMUEL H. DOPPELT, M.D.,**
> HENRY J. MANKIN, M.D.,† AND GARY E. FRIEDLAENDER, M.D.‡
>
> Clinical Orthopaedics and Related Research
> Number 174
> April, 1983

Tomford et al., article on current bone bank procedures.
Clinical Orthopaedics and Related Research 1983; 174: 15.

> **Investigational Approaches to Articular Cartilage Preservation**
>
> WILLIAM W. TOMFORD, M.D.,* AND HENRY J. MANKIN, M.D.**
>
> Clinical Orthopaedics and Related Research
> Number 174
> April, 1983
>
> **Studies on Cryopreservation of Articular Cartilage Chondrocytes***
>
> BY WILLIAM W. TOMFORD, M.D.,† GARY R. FREDERICKS, M.S.,†
> AND HENRY J. MANKIN, M.D.†, BOSTON, MASSACHUSETTS
> *From the Orthopaedic Research Laboratories, Massachusetts General Hospital and Harvard Medical School, Boston*
>
> THE JOURNAL OF BONE AND JOINT SURGERY
> VOL. 66-A, NO. 2, FEBRUARY 1984

Tomford and colleagues' articles on their research to preserve articular cartilage for use in osteoarticular allografts.
Clinical Orthopaedics and Related Research 1983; 174: 22; *Journal of Bone and Joint Surgery* 1984; 66: 253.

Another main interest of Tomford (and of Mankin [chapter 41]) has been the preservation of articular cartilage, especially when using large osteoarticular allografts. They, along with Fredericks, first reported experiments using dimethyl sulfoxide (DMSO) and glycerol in 1981. Three years later, they published "Studies on Cryopreservation of Articular Cartilage Chondrocytes." In that study they "defined limits of concentration of cryopreservatives to which chondrocytes may be exposed and still survive, as well as optimum times and temperatures of exposure for chondrocytes," and they "compared methods of freezing these cells to show that initial slow cooling results in a higher rate of viability than an extremely rapid cooling technique does" (Tomford, Fredericks, and Mankin 1984). They determined "that a cryopreservative is of benefit in preserving viable cells during freezer storage and that chondrocytes, if frozen using dimethyl sulfoxide as a cryopreservative, may survive freezing and synthesize products that will form proteoglycan aggregates in culture" (Tomford, Fredericks, and Mankin 1984).

During the mid- and late-1980s, two large musculoskeletal tissue banks were operating in the US: the US Navy Tissue Bank in Bethesda, and the University of Miami Tissue Bank in Florida. As the popularity of bone allografts increased, orthopaedic surgeons began using banked femoral heads. Tomford and his colleagues at MGH described their experience with banked tissues.

They followed the guidelines of the American Association of Tissue Banks. They stored 76 donated femoral heads during a two-year period (1983–84) and used 58 of them. One implanted femoral head tested positive for *Staphylococcus epidermidis*, which required the patient to be treated with antibiotics; one year after the procedure the patient remained asymptomatic. They recommended shaping and or preparing the femoral head at the time of its use to ensure the specimen does not become contaminated at the time of procurement.

In 1988, Tomford and his colleagues reported their experience with large allografts among 283 patients at MGH: "An infection developed in thirty-three (11.7 per cent)…Gram-positive organisms were the most common cause of infection…[with 36%] being due to staphylococcus epidermidis… The final result in the thirty-three patients who had an infected allograft was poor compared to… [that in] the uninfected patients" (Lord et al. 1988).

He was invited in 1995 to write a current-concepts review to be published in the *Journal of Bone and Joint Surgery*; his review was titled "Transmission of Disease Through Transplantation of Musculoskeletal Allografts." In it, he discussed

Title of Tomford's Current Concepts Review on transmission of diseases via musculoskeletal allografts. *Journal of Bone and Joint Surgery* 1995; 77: 1742.

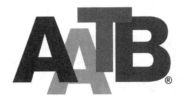

Logo, American Association of Tissue Banks. Courtesy of the American Association of Tissue Banks.

the main concerns related to human immunodeficiency virus and hepatitis A, B, and C; risk of transmission; and methods to reduce transmission (including by properly processing the graft by thoroughly removing blood, bone marrow, and soft tissues; freezing; gamma irradiation; and, for soft-tissue allografts, ethylene oxide and low-dose irradiation). He noted that overall, the risk for transmitting a viral disease "is low, but...not non-existent" (Tomford 1995). In 1993, he published the book *Musculoskeletal Tissue Banking*, in which he reviewed the history of musculoskeletal tissue banking, detailed the procedures used when banking tissues, described procedures for maintaining safety, and enumerated guidelines for surgeons who use allografts.

Not only has he effectively led the MGH Bone Bank, but in 1985–88 and again in 2004–08, Tomford was also a trustee of the New England Organ Bank. He has been the program director there since 1992, and he's chaired the Musculoskeletal Transplant Foundation Board of Directors in New Jersey since 2007. His leadership has extended nationally as well—to the American Association of Tissue Banks, of which he was president for two years (1987–89). "He has also served on many advisory committees for the tissue banks and has consulted for the Food and Drug Administration, the National Institutes of Health and the European Association of Tissue Banks" (Mankin 2011).

He has chaired the MTF Biologics Board of Directors, the world's largest tissue bank, headquartered in Edison, New Jersey. He's also served as chairman of the American Academy of Orthopaedic Surgeons Committee on Biologic Implants. And, as an authority on tissue banking, Tomford has consulted for and helped establish bone banks in various countries including Brazil, China, Israel, Italy, Japan, Korea, Norway, and Spain. "Despite his heavy commitment to many areas in the tissue banking programs...[Tomford has also] been very active in the MGH Orthopaedic Service" (Mankin 2011). He followed Mankin as interim chair of the Department of Orthopaedics at MGH (1996–98). Tomford currently has a clinical practice in adult reconstructive surgery of the hip and knee.

STEPHEN B. TRIPPEL

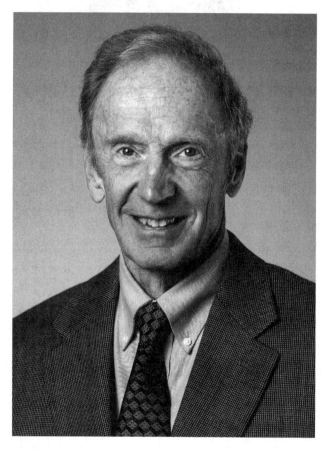

Stephen B. Trippel. Courtesy of Stephen B. Trippel/Indiana University School of Medicine.

Physician Snapshot

Stephen B. Trippel
BORN: 1948
DIED: —
SIGNIFICANT CONTRIBUTION: Researched and published extensively on insulin-like growth factor 1 (IGF-1) and other growth hormones

Stephen B. Trippel was born and raised in Chicago, Illinois. He received a bachelor of arts degree from Swarthmore College in 1970 and an MD degree from Columbia University College of Physicians and Surgeons in 1974. Following a year-long surgical internship and a year as a surgical assistant resident at the Peter Bent Brigham Hospital (1974–76), he spent six months (July through December 1976) in Dr. Henry Mankin's research laboratories at MGH. In January 1977, Trippel entered the three-year Harvard Combined Orthopaedic Residency Program, completing it in 1980. In 1978, well into his residency, he presented the results of his first basic research study, in which he and his colleagues characterized chondrocytes from bovine articular cartilage. They showed "that the chondrocyte population is composed of cells that vary continuously in size and metabolic activity from one unit to another. The largest cells also demonstrated the greatest RNA production while the smallest cells had the least" (Trippel et al. 1980). Trippel went on to serve as chief resident and assistant in orthopaedics at MGH from January 1 to June 30, 1980. He spent the next year as a research fellow in pediatric endocrinology at the University of North Carolina School of Medicine in Chapel Hill.

In 1981, Trippel returned to MGH as assistant in orthopaedics; he also began as an instructor in orthopaedic surgery at Harvard Medical School. He established an active research program on growth factors in growth plate and articular cartilage, focusing specifically on the effects of somatomedin C (insulin-like growth factor 1 [IGF-1]). That same year, he was a North American Traveling Fellow through the American Orthopaedic Association and received his first National Institutes of Health grant to study the role of somatomedin in

Trippel and colleagues research on Somatomedin-C (insulin-like growth-factor 1) in growth plate chondrocytes. *Journal of Bone and Joint Surgery* 1986; 68: 897.

skeletal development and pathology. Throughout his tenure at MGH, he was the principal investigator on numerous National Institutes of Health grants and industry grants to investigate the role of growth factors.

One of these grants funded a study on the regulation of chondrocytes in the growth plate by IGF-1 and basic fibroblast growth factor (bFGF), which Trippel and his colleagues at MGH, in collaboration with investigators from the Karolinska Institutet in Stockholm, Sweden, published in 1993. Regarding the clinical relevance of their findings, they stated: "These results suggest that both IGF-I and bFGF participate in the regulation of skeletal growth and that they differ with regard to…specific cellular functions…IGF-I stimulates both cellular mitotic activity and synthesis of extracellular matrix…consistent with a general anabolic role for IGF-I…IGF-I and bFGF regulate skeletal growth and development" (Trippel et al. 1993).

Trippel was promoted to assistant professor at Harvard in 1989 and to associate professor in 1994. At MGH, he was promoted to associate orthopaedic surgeon in 1996. In 1994, he was chairman of the Gordon Research Conference on Bioengineering and Orthopaedic Sciences. In 2001, after 20 years on the faculty at Harvard Medical School and MGH, Trippel accepted the position of professor and chairman of the Department of Orthopaedic Surgery at the University of Indiana School of Medicine. Many of his grants continued as he moved his work to Indiana. During that transition, his research interests expanded to include gene transfer as treatment of damaged articular cartilage.

To date, Trippel has published more than 70 articles. Approximately 33 of them were published during his two decades at MGH. Of those, ~25 are about IGF-1. Trippel has served on committees for many professional organizations, including as a member of the board of trustees of the Massachusetts chapter of the Arthritis Foundation (1989–99), as chairman of several committees of the Orthopaedic Research Society, as chairman of the research committee of the Academic Orthopaedic Society, and as chairman of the Task Force on Clinical Research of the American Orthopaedic Association. He was president of the Orthopaedic Research Society in 2003 and deputy editor of the *Journal of Orthopaedic Research* from 1993 to 2014. Throughout his career, he also has received several awards, including the Kappa Delta Young Investigator Award in 1989 and the Kappa Delta Ann Dover Vaughn Award (with Dr. L. J. Sandell and others) in 1992.

Logo of the Gordon Research Conference.
The trademarks GRC, GRC (stylized), and GORDON RESEARCH CONFERENCES are trademarks owned by Gordon Research Conferences.

BERTRAM ZARINS

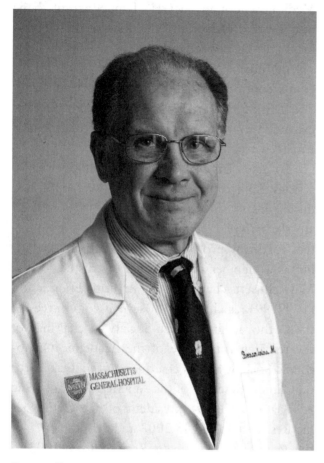

Bertram Zarins. Massachusetts General Hospital.

Physician Snapshot

Bertram Zarins
BORN: 1942
DIED: —

SIGNIFICANT CONTRIBUTIONS: Chief of Sports Medicine at MGH; head physician New England Patriots and Boston Bruins; Augustus Thorndike Jr. Professor; established the Latvian Medical Foundation

Bertram "Bert" Zarins was born in Latvia in 1942. When he was four years old, his family, including his parents and younger brother, escaped the country as the Russian army invaded Latvia for the second time near the end of World War II. They immigrated to New York, where Bert eventually attended Stuyvesant High School. From 1959 to 1963, he attended Lafayette College in Easton, Pennsylvania, graduating with a bachelor of arts degree. After four years at the State University of New York Upstate Medical Center in Syracuse, he received his MD degree cum laude and was elected into Alpha Omega Alpha. In 1967, he interned in surgery at Johns Hopkins Hospital and completed a second year there as an assistant resident in surgery.

Early Training and Career

In 1969, Zarins was accepted into the MGH/Children's Hospital Orthopaedic Residency Program. His residency did not begin until 1970, and during the intervening nine months he worked at the Vail Valley Medical Center in Vail, Colorado—20 years before Dr. Richard Steadman opened the Steadman Clinic there. Zarins recalled that he developed an interest in sports medicine during that time. After completing his orthopaedic residency in 1973 and spending six months as a chief resident/assistant in orthopaedics at MGH, he entered the US Navy, where he served as the chief of orthopaedics at the Navy Regional Medical Center in Guam (Mariana Islands) during the last stages of the Vietnam War. As Saigon fell in April 1975, Zarins was on the USS *Okinawa*, an amphibious assault ship, off the coast of Vietnam during Operation Frequent Wind, the evacuation of Vietnam. He photographed servicemen pushing a helicopter off the deck into the South China Sea to make room on the ship for incoming flights crowded with refugees escaping from Vietnam.

After his discharge from the navy in 1975, Zarins returned to MGH as a clinical fellow in sports, knee, and shoulder surgery. He won a three-month Edwin Cave Traveling Fellowship, during which he visited several medical centers to learn about new concepts in evaluating the knee and using arthroscopes. Dr. Richard O'Connor of Los Angeles had pioneered the arthroscope in North America in the early 1970s; other surgeons—including Dr. Robert W. Jackson in Toronto and Drs. Ward Casscells, Lanny Johnson,

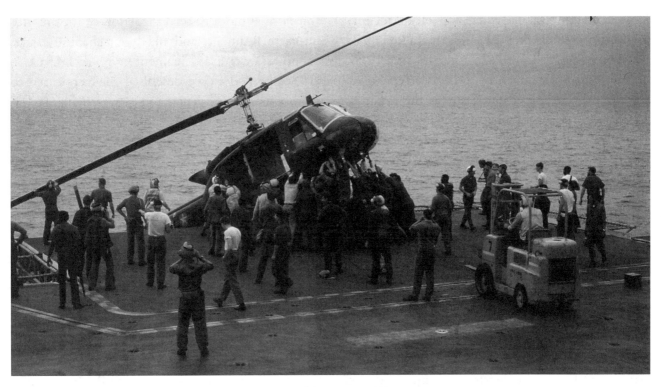
USS *Okinawa* at the fall of Saigon (April 1975) at the end of the Vietnam War. Courtesy of Bertram Zarins.

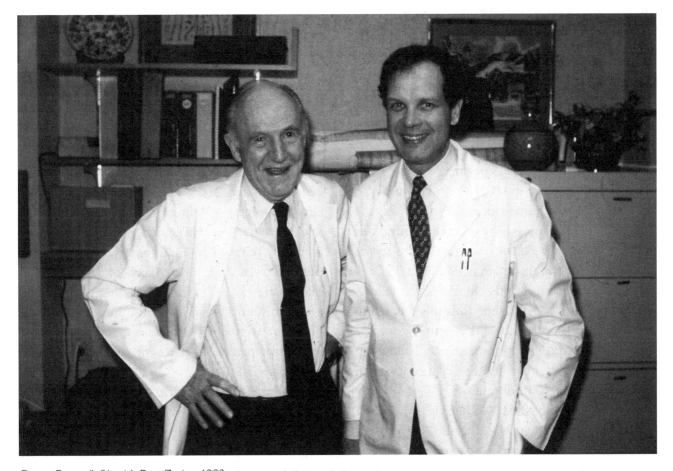
Carter Rowe (left) with Bert Zarins, 1983. Courtesy of Bertram Zarins.

Ken DeHaven, Ralph Lidge, and Jack McGinty in Boston (see chapter 23)—quickly adopted its use. Following his Cave Fellowship, in April 1976, Zarins joined the practice of Dr. Carter Rowe. Cave had been limited physically as the result of a stroke and was no longer practicing with Rowe (see chapter 40); he died in December 1976.

Zarins and Dr. Dinesh Patel started a sports clinic at MGH in 1977. They were codirectors of the clinic until 1982, when Dr. Henry Mankin named Zarins chief of the sports medicine service (a position Zarins held for ~25 years) and Patel chief of the arthroscopic surgery unit. Both began performing arthroscopic surgery in the late 1970s/early 1980s.

Later Orthopaedic Contributions

Zarins specialized in sports medicine, with an emphasis on shoulder and knee injuries. Upon joining Rowe's practice, he began providing orthopaedic care to the Boston Bruins, initially as a consultant. In 1982, Zarins was named head physician for the New England Patriots, and that same year he was promoted to assistant clinical professor of orthopaedic surgery at Harvard Medical School. Two years later, Zarins was head physician for the United States teams at the XIV Winter Olympic Games in Sarajevo. He was promoted to associate orthopaedic surgeon at MGH the following year. By 1986, he was named head physician for the Bruins, after Dr. Early Wilkins retired. During this period, Zarins was named director of the sports medicine fellowship program at MGH in 1979, a position he held until 2004. In 1986, the fellowship merged with Dr. Arthur Boland's fellowship program (see chapter 12) and eventually became the Harvard/MGH Sports Medicine Fellowship Program, accredited by the Accreditation Council for Graduate Medical Education.

Zarins has published ~48 articles, including ~21 on the knee and 12 on the shoulder; co-edited 5 books; and wrote or cowrote ~36 book chapters. His early interest in the knee focused on normal motion, reconstruction of the anterior cruciate ligament, and the biomechanical effects of posterior cruciate ligament injury and repair. In 1986, he and Rowe described their approach to combined intra-articular and extra-articular reconstruction in patients with an anterior cruciate ligament injury:

> The semitendinosus tendon and the iliotibial tract are both routed from opposite directions over the top of the lateral femoral condyle and through the same...drill hole in the proximal... tibia: the [distal] semitendinosus tendon is passed up through the tibia drill-hole [similar to the distally based semitendinous tendon transfer described by Cho], across the knee joint, over the top of the lateral femoral condyle, and deep to the fibular collateral ligament, and the iliotibial tract is passed deep to the fibular collateral ligament, over the top of the lateral femoral condyle [as described by McIntosh], across the knee joint, and down through the drill-hole. Both grafts are...pulled tight...[and] the semitendinosus tendon is sutured to the iliotibial tract laterally and the iliotibial tract is sutured to the semitendinosus tendon medially below the drill hole. (Zarins and Rowe 1986)

They then described the results of the procedure among "106 consecutive patients with chronic instability," the first 100 of whom exhibited the "anterior-drawer sign...[which was] eliminated or reduced to 1+ in eighty knees, and the positive pivot shift was reduced to zero or 1+ in ninety-one knees...[with] significant improvements in strength and normalization of tibial rotation...We were able to achieve functional stability in approximately 90 per cent of knees" (Zarins and Rowe 1986).

His interest in shoulder injuries led to several publications with Rowe, particularly regarding issues related to shoulder instability. **Case 42.14** highlights an example of one of the many cases he reviewed.

Case 42.14. Anterior Interosseous Nerve Palsy after Use of a Sling to Treat an Acromioclavicular Dislocation

"A twenty-eight-year-old professional football quarterback was tackled and was thrown onto the right (dominant) shoulder; this resulted in a Grade-III dislocation of the acromioclavicular joint. The results of a neurological examination were normal. Without anesthesia, a closed reduction was done and a Kenny Howard-type sling was applied and was tightened. Radiographs showed satisfactory reduction of the acromioclavicular joint. The sling was removed after six weeks. Anatomical reduction of the acromioclavicular joint was maintained.

"Several days after the sling was discontinued, the patient noted marked weakness of flexion of the thumb and index finger. He was unsure when the weakness had begun. Examination revealed grade-0 strength of the flexor pollicis longus muscle but an intact flexor pollicis longus tendon, evidenced by passive flexion of the interphalangeal joint of the thumb when the wrist and the first metacarpal were extended. Strength was good (grade 4) for the flexor digitorum profundus muscle to the index finger, trace (grade 1) for the pronator quadratus muscle, fair (grade 3) for the pronator teres muscle, and absent for the flexor carpi radialis muscle. All other muscles of the hand and wrist had normal strength, and there was no weakness proximal to the elbow. There was tenderness at a point two centimeters distal and two centimeters lateral to the medial epicondyle on the volar aspect of the forearm. There was no paresthesia or sensory deficit.

"Within two weeks after the sling was removed, the strength of the flexor pollicis longus muscle improved to poor (grade 2). The strength of pronation improved 30 to 50 per cent, as subjectively determined by the same examiner. The strength of the flexor carpi radialis muscle improved to fair, and the strength of the flexor digitorum profundus muscle to the index finger remained good. The results of electromyographic studies were consistent with a diagnosis of compression syndrome of the anterior interosseous nerve; they revealed a prolonged distal motor latency of 3.6 milliseconds and a conduction velocity of 54.2 meters per second for the median nerve. There was no additional improvement during the next five weeks. Repeat electromyographic studies revealed additional slowing of the conduction of the median nerve, to fifty meters per second, and increased latency of the anterior interosseous nerve, to 4.6 milliseconds. Eighteen weeks after the initial injury, the median nerve, from the mid-part of the arm to the mid-part of the forearm, was explored operatively. The only abnormality that was found was a tight fibrous band that compressed the nerve at the humeral origin of the pronator teres muscle. The band was excised. Intraoperative stimulation of the nerve produced no contraction of the flexor pollicis longus or flexor carpi radialis muscles. All of the other muscles that are innervated by the median nerve contracted on stimulation. Fifteen months after the operation, the patient had recovered full motion and strength of the hand, and he had returned successfully to the starting quarterback position."

(O'Neill, Zarins, Gelberman, Keating, and Louis 1990)

In 1990, he cowrote a publication about the composition of the glenoid labrum:

> Thirty-eight shoulders from cadavers were examined...The labrum appeared to be fibrocartilaginous tissue...a separate anatomical structure...distinguished from the fibrous capsule of the shoulder. Neonatal labra were composed of primitive mesenchymal tissue containing only a few chondrocytes that modulated into fibrocartilage in the first few years of life [not previously appreciated]... [and] contained no elastin, whereas specimens from adults had rare elastin fibers. The labrum was scarcely vascularized throughout its substance...Vascularity decreased with increasing age... (Prodromos et al. 1990)

One of the last articles that Zarins cowrote with Rowe (and Dr. Mark S. McMahon) was about shoulder instability. It was published in a 1993 *Clinical Orthopaedics and Related Research* symposium on instability honoring Dr. A. S. Blundell Bankart. In that article, they described the

Zarins, McMahon, and Rowe's article on management of traumatic anterior instability of the shoulder. *Clinical Orthopaedics and Related Research* 1993; 291: 75.

lesions that commonly arise from anterior glenohumeral joint dislocation:

> Lesions that usually result are avulsion of the anterior capsule and glenoid labrum from the glenoid rim (Bankart lesion), compression fracture of the posterosuperior humeral head (Hill-Sachs lesion), and laxity of the joint capsule. Another common lesion is a lengthwise disruption of the rotator cuff at the interval between the subscapularis and supraspinatus tendons... The aim of the Bankart procedure is to restore stability to the shoulder by repairing the traumatic lesion of the anterior glenoid rim without altering normal anatomy. (Zarins, McMahon, and Rowe 1993)

The authors also reviewed in detail their preferred methods of doing the Bankart procedure and for managing the patient postoperatively.

By 1995, Zarins was promoted to associate clinical professor at HMS, and he joined the courtesy staff at Harvard University Health Services in 1996. That same year, he was appointed head physician for the New England Revolution soccer team. Over the subsequent years he cowrote several articles on the posterior cruciate ligament (PCL), including robotics-assisted research on knees with PCL from cadavers in 2002. That group's results showed that posterior tibial translation and external tibial rotation often occur with PCL deficiency, the latter of which may cause chronic excessive pressure on the patellofemoral joint. Because of this, physicians need to perform an extensive evaluation of knee joint function—including more than just the anterior and posterior drawer tests—to sufficiently identify the consequences of PCL deficiency.

In 2007, through contributions from the family and friends of Dr. Augustus Thorndike, Zarins was named the first Augustus Thorndike Professor of Orthopaedic Surgery. Zarins has also served on many local and national committees (**Box 42.3**). Zarins has continued to practice at MGH throughout his entire career, and he continues to practice and operate there at the time of this publication.

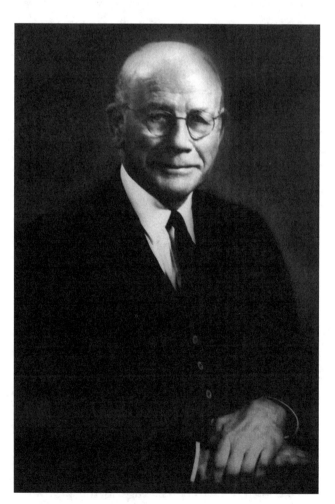

Augustus Thorndike Jr. Courtesy of Joan I. Thorndike.

Box 42.3. Zarins's Various Leadership Roles in Professional Organizations

- President of the North America Trauma Association (1978)
- Sports Medicine Council of the United States Olympic Committee (1981–92)
- President of the Latvian Medical and Dental Association (1990–94)
- Member of the board of directors of the International Arthroscopy Association (1991–94)
- Chairman of the Committee on Sports Medicine of the AAOS (1993–97)
- Massachusetts Governor's Council on Physical Fitness and Sports (2004–8)

Zarins is also unflagging in his devotion to health care in a wider sense. Latvia became an independent country in 1991, and, since then, Zarins has been instrumental in improving health care and education for citizens of his native country. He established the Latvian Medical Foundation to help accomplish these initiatives and to provide traveling fellowships for Latvian physicians. Because of his commitments, Latvia has recognized Zarins with several awards, including the Three Star Medal of Honour, the country's highest civilian honor, which is awarded by the president of Latvia.

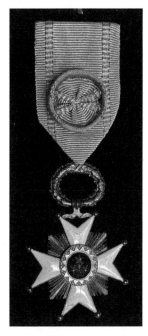

Three Star Medal of Honour, Latvia. Courtesy of Bertram Zarins.

CHAPTER 43

MGH
Modernization and Preparation for the Twenty-First Century

Massachusetts General Hospital (MGH) underwent enormous changes in the middle of the twentieth century, and it had reached a pivotal point in 1946. Although it had a long history in providing outstanding patient care, offering residency training, and shaping the history of orthopaedics, it also experienced severe weaknesses. Dr. Thornton Brown—a graduate of Harvard Medical School (HMS) orthopaedic residency program, lifelong faculty of HMS and MGH, and interim Chief of Orthopaedics—lived through this tumultuous time at MGH into the late 1990s and described it in his own words (see **Box 43.1**). These changes would not have been possible without the leadership of Dr. Joseph S. Barr and the commitment of Dr. Melvin J. Glimcher.

Box 43.1. Dr. Thornton Brown: Dramatic Changes at MGH's Orthopaedic Service

"By 1946 the Orthopedic Service had reached a turning point in its history. Since its beginning in 1900, it had become preeminent in patient care and had established itself as one of the leading orthopedic residency training programs. It was also recognized as an educational center to which postgraduate students and fellows came from many parts of the world. During the 17 years that Marius N. Smith-Petersen had been in charge, there had been outstanding contributions to the advancement of orthopedic surgery.

"Nevertheless, in the mid-forties the Orthopedic Service at MGH had serious weaknesses that endangered its position as a leader in the field. The chief was part-time, and there was no departmental office. In education, the service performed at a rather primitive level; there was little teaching of medical students, while in the realm of resident education the training program took the form of a preceptorship rather than a well-organized educational experience. As for research, there was some clinical investigation by the orthopedic staff, but no basic science investigation of musculoskeletal problems, even though by 1946 this had become an indispensable ingredient of any preeminent academic program...

"Such was the situation when Joseph S. Barr was appointed to succeed Smith-Petersen in December 1946 [chief, 1946–1964] and when he became the John B. and Buckminster Brown Clinical Professor of Orthopedic Surgery at the Harvard Medical School in 1948–a title that in the past had always been held by the Chief of Orthopedic Surgery at Children's Hospital...

"Barr had long been aware of the weaknesses in the orthopedic program at the MGH. In January 1938, he had written Smith–Petersen as follows: 'There is little, or no laboratory work being done. This is an aspect of orthopedic surgery which needs more emphasis, and if our clinic is to maintain its present high position, I feel that it is imperative to establish a program of investigative work and to systematize the teaching of the house officers in the basic fields of anatomy and physiology…I am willing and anxious to curtail my varied duties…in order to devote time to the hospital–laboratory program'.

"Barr had a chance in 1946, but the way was not easy. Barr's professorship was not fully endowed. There were no funds and no space. A clinically oriented residency training program is not likely to produce residents inclined towards a career in research. With no money, there was no chance of attracting a trained investigator from the outside. Thus, the task of converting the Orthopedic Service into a truly academic enterprise that could provide patient care and a stimulating research and educational environment for residents and medical students, consistent with the traditional ideals of the MGH and the HMS, was indeed a formidable one even for someone who could devote full-time to the project. But Barr had no such luxury since, to keep the wolf from his door, he had to maintain a busy private practice on Marlborough Street in association with Frank R. Ober, Brown Professor Emeritus. Despite these many obstacles, during the 17 years before poor health forced him to retire, Barr and his associates managed to lay the foundations for an academic department with space, funds, and personnel…

"In 1951, desperately needed office space was provided by remodeling the north wing of the fifth floor of the White Building adjacent to the orthopedic wards…The Orthopedic Clinic in the basement of the outpatient department had changed little, if any, since the building was constructed in 1905. Its stall-like examining rooms, separated by partial partitions of darkening varnished oak, provided little in the way of privacy and comfort. In 1951, stimulated by a sharp drop in the patient census, the clinic was remodeled to provide more sympathetic surroundings, and scheduling changes were initiated in an effort to reduce patient's waiting time on the long, hard wooden densities in the corridor. In addition, by arrangement with the Boston Police Department, the city was regionalized so that the victims of road accidents in the northern part of the city picked up by the police were brought to the MGH rather than to City Hospital…

"Physical and occupational therapy, located in the basement of the Clinics Building, had been available at the MGH since the turn of the century. Machines for mechano- and electrotherapy imported from Sweden were donated to the hospital, but these activities were terminated for reasons of economy at the outbreak of World War I. Thereafter, physical and occupational therapy apparently came on hard times. In 1929 Smith-Petersen noted that "the outstanding need of the department is the reestablishment of a Physiotherapy Department." However, little was done about the situation until 1940 when Arthur L. Watkins… [neurologist] was appointed chief of the Physical Therapy Department…on the second floor of the Domestic Building. In 1945, physical and occupational therapy were combined under Watkins as the Department of Physical Medicine. With a grant of $1 million from the Baruch Foundation to the MGH and the HMS, a three-year training program in physical medicine and rehabilitation was initiated…

"Gradually the polio patients recovered or were discharged [during the severe epidemic of 1955] to be followed on an ambulatory basis. As a census on White 9 [respiratory center for polio patients] dropped, the

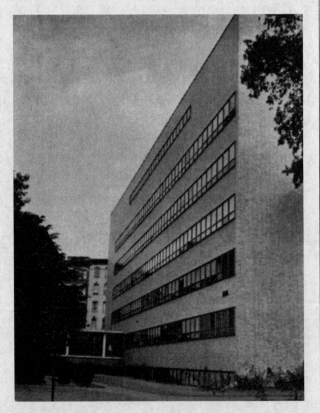

Research Building, 1951. Massachusetts General Hospital, Archives and Special Collections.

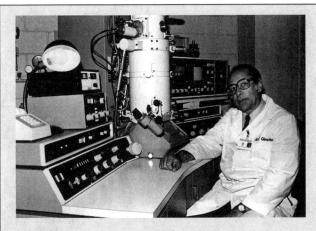

Melvin Glimcher at an electron microscope in his laboratory.
Images of America. Children's Hospital Boston. Charleston, SC: Arcadia Publishing, 2005. Boston Children's Hospital Archives, Boston, Massachusetts.

concept of a multiservice rehabilitation unit again surfaced. [Dr. Thomas] Delorme…with Barr's backing, set about the task of establishing White 9 as the Rehabilitation Unit of the MGH…[with] funding from the Pope Foundation of Chicago…residents now had as one of their rotations time on White 9…[with] other services…As the unit flourished, its 44 beds were filled with a variety of severely disabled patients with spinal cord injuries, persons with neurologic disease such as multiple sclerosis, and amputees. The concept of a special unit to care for them during part of their stay in a General Hospital seem amply justified…

"Residency training had been grossly disrupted during World War II; with the return of peace and a new Chief, the program was reorganized. The orthopedic house staff now consisted of one senior resident (fifth year…) and 5 assistant residents (fourth year…), all coming to the MGH after one year at the Children's Hospital. In addition, there is one third-year surgical resident and one first–year surgical intern who had rotations on the fracture and orthopedic services…Resident seminars were arranged, and orthopedic and fracture rounds were combined…

"By all odds, the most formidable problem that faced Barr when he became chief in 1946 was the need to develop a research program…Because of…[his] interest [spine], he attempted to initiate a multidisciplinary investigation of low back pain and sciatica. With Paul Norton and Thornton Brown…several projects were begun in collaboration with the Department of Structural Engineering at MIT, the American Mutual Liability Insurance Co., and the MGH psychiatric service. However, an ongoing investigation of the low back syndrome failed to materialize because of lack of innovative talent. The problem clearly was to find an orthopedist investigator with the ability and motivation to start a research program of such outstanding promise that it would attract the large-scale financial help needed to build and support the work of orthopedic-research laboratories at the MGH…

"A solution…was in the offing. On the surgical service there was an assistant resident…interested in orthopedic surgery…[with] impressive credentials. He had graduated from Purdue with highest honors in mechanical engineering and physics in 1946 and subsequently from the HMS magna cum laude in 1950. This young man, Melvin J. Glimcher…following completion of his orthopedic residency in July 1956, began postdoctoral studies and a research program at MIT as a fellow of the School for Advanced Studies under tutelage of Francis O. Schmitt, a trustee of the MGH.

"Glimcher's research at MIT concerned the molecular biology of the mineralization of bone and other tissues… The results were exciting, and the concept of a large basic science laboratory staffed mainly by Ph.D.'s trained in the basic biologic and physical sciences evolved. The MGH trustees accepted this concept, and the efforts of all concerned turned to the raising of funds to build an addition to floors 3A and 4 of the White Building to house the laboratories. These funds came from private individuals and foundations, supplemented with matching funds from the federal government…Some of the money was the excess from the funds originally raised by Joel Goldthwait to build Ward I. The money was transferred to the building fund with his blessings; he was 93 years old at the time. In addition, funds were raised to endow a chair of orthopedic surgery at the MGH as well as to support the proposed research…Glimcher and seven full-time Ph.D. investigators were established in the old Allen Street Pathology Building…On September 11, 1960, the new quarters were dedicated. They included the Chemistry Laboratory named after Robert Bagley Osgood, the Histology Laboratory named after Armin Klein, the Physical Chemistry Laboratory honoring Smith–Petersen, and the Biochemistry Laboratory named for Joel Goldthwait.

"From 1960 until his retirement in 1964…[Barr's] tenure as Chief of the Orthopedic Service had seen great and fundamental changes…[During] the Glimcher years (1965–1970)…the Ward Service was reorganized into East and West services, each with its own resident staff. The Fracture Service, which had been administratively separate, was incorporated into Orthopedics. An orthopedic resident was assigned to the Emergency Room full-time. In addition, members of the attending staff were assigned in rotation to supervise the care of patients with musculoskeletal injuries in the Emergency Room whether admitted to the hospital or not…

"[Dr. Glimcher's] conviction [was] that if the East and West services were to provide superior care, closer supervision of the residents by the visiting staff was needed… The rotations of visits on the East and West services were modified so that there was [always] a senior and junior visit…[One] problem in patient care was a shortage of beds and operating time in the Baker Memorial and Phillips House due, in part, to the steadily increasing number of patients with hip disease whom Dr. Aufranc and his associates treated by cup arthroplasty. The patients required four to six weeks of hospitalization after surgery and, since beds and time on the operating schedule were made on a first-come, first-served bases, a large proportion of the beds and operating time was being devoted to them. This difficult situation was finally resolved when Aufranc and his

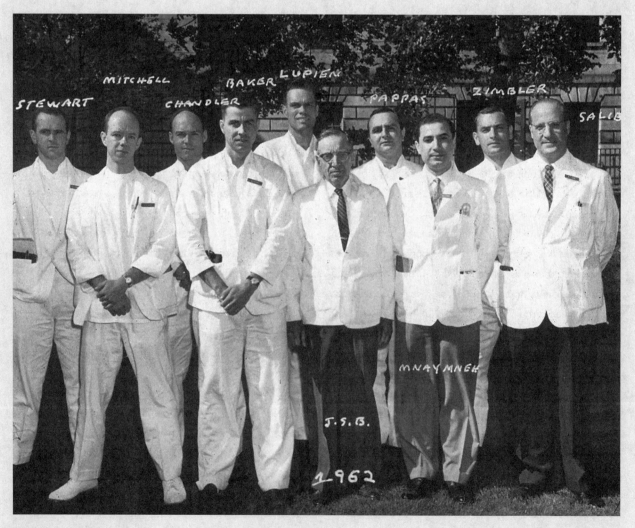

Dr. Barr with MGH residents, 1962. MGH HCORP Archives.

colleagues moved their patients to another hospital [New England Baptist]…in 1969…

"Unlike any of his predecessors, Glimcher involved himself in the activities of the Medical School, especially in connection with the curriculum. In the recently established second-year course in pathophysiology he championed the need for a new section devoted to the hitherto neglected musculoskeletal system, and it was he who organized this 'block'–a multidisciplinary effort in which orthopedics was deeply involved. He persuaded the curriculum committee, on a trial basis, to schedule a portion of the courses on physical diagnosis and introduction to the clinic directly in the Department of Orthopedic Surgery rather than leaving it to General Surgery to apportion the time. He also persuaded the committee to establish a four-week clinical clerkship in orthopedic surgery as a required course.

"To ensure that these clinical courses were first-rate educational experiences, MGH visiting staff men were required to devote more time to medical education. The arrangement after two years resulted in the highest rating from the medical students, a turn of events that capitulated orthopedics from the bottom to the top of the students' rating list…The visiting staff found this additional teaching load a heavy burden…

"Resident education was also extensively remodeled, putting more emphasis on formalized instruction and less on simple experience…gained in a preceptorship. Weekly rounds were changed to two-hour sessions…The traditional format in which problem cases were presented…

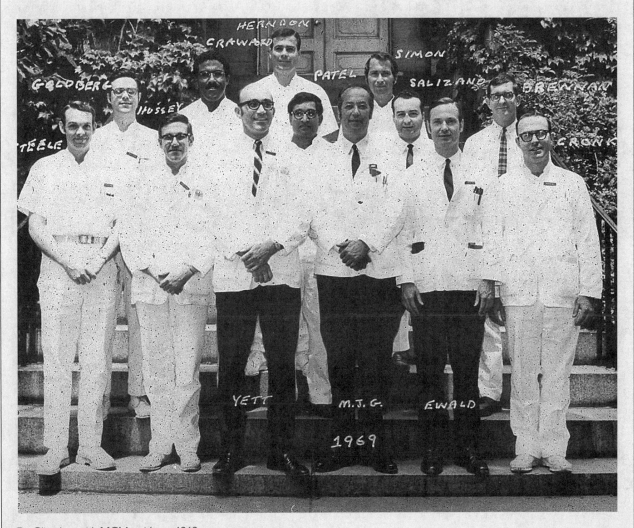

Dr. Glimcher with MGH residents, 1969. MGH HCORP Archives.

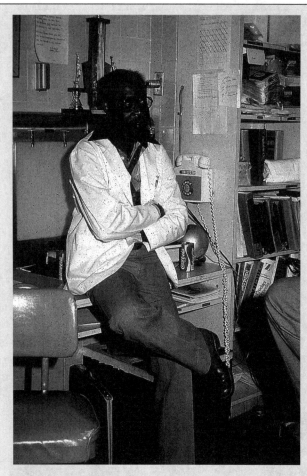

John Burns, supervisor, orthopaedic technicians at MGH. Retired after 48 years (1966–2014). MGH HCORP Archives.

was superseded by a schedule of prearranged topics. A local or invited expert gave a lecture…[and the] residents and visiting staff were urged to prepare in advance for the discussion and presentation of differing views. Problem-solving rounds were held in the wards or the Smith–Petersen Conference Room each week, with the chief and visitors in attendance…Conferences and teaching sessions…[also included] a basic science lecture series, on Wednesday mornings. The faculty for these lectures was drawn from experts in the Boston area. Finally, in an effort to broaden the resident's experience, rotations were arranged at outside hospitals–the Lynn and the Shattuck hospitals locally and Rancho Los Amigos Hospital in Los Angeles.

"The old Children's Hospital–MGH Orthopedic Residency Program had also developed offshoots…Toward the end of Glimcher's tenure, negotiations with the Medical School and the hospitals involved creating the Combined Harvard Orthopedic Residency Program, with orthopedic professors at the MGH, Children's Hospital, and the Peter Bent and Robert Breck Brigham hospitals as well as…the orthopedic services at Beth Israel and the West Roxbury Veterans' Hospital. Glimcher obtained an annual grant from the Camp Corporation for a visiting professor to spend several days each year at the different hospitals in the program, making rounds with the residents and participating in conferences. Finally, the visitor delivered the Samuel Higby Camp lecture on some orthopedic subject…

"After…[Glimcher's] laboratories moved to the new quarters on White 3A and 4 in 1960, research activities expanded like gas in a vacuum. The initial group of seven Ph.D.'s rapidly increased to… as many as eighteen Ph.D.'s and postdoctoral investigators plus three physicians. By 1968 more space was needed, and the orthopedic laboratories were moved to the tenth floor of the recently completed Jackson Tower…Fellows from many countries spent time working in the laboratories. Collaborative efforts with other departments were also undertaken. Glimcher teamed with Stephan Krane of the Arthritis Unit… and with John Burke in General Surgery…

"During Glimcher's five-year tenure at the MGH, approximately 100 papers concerned with basic science were published–a remarkable return of affairs. However, the happy balance of patient care, teaching and research envisaged as the Orthopedic Laboratories were dedicated in 1960 seemed not to be materializing. In one quantum leap the service changed from a purely clinical activity to an academic and scholarly enterprise. In retrospect, it was probably too much to expect such a rapid change to come about without difficulties…In 1970 Glimcher resigned…[to become the] Peabody Professor of Orthopedic Surgery at the Children's Hospital Medical Center."

—B. C. Castleman and D. C. Crockett 1983

ESTABLISHMENT OF ORTHOPAEDIC SUBSPECIALTIES

Following Glimcher's resignation as chairman of the Department of Orthopaedic Surgery at MGH, Dr. Thornton Brown became interim department chair (1970–1972) until Dr. Henry J. Mankin (see chapter 41) arrived as the newly selected department chairman in 1972. In addition to colleagues, he brought with him from New York, Mankin recruited additional orthopaedic surgeons and gave hospital staff privileges to numerous others in private practice during his long tenure. Importantly, he organized the staff into specialties within orthopaedics (see **Box 43.2**).

ORTHOPAEDIC REHABILITATION

When Mankin arrived at MGH, the chief of the orthopaedic rehabilitation unit on White 9 was Dr. Donald Pierce (see chapter 40). Pierce had succeeded Dr. Thomas DeLorme, (see chapter 40) who stepped down in 1955. I was unable to determine if there was another orthopaedic surgeon as chief of the White 9 service between

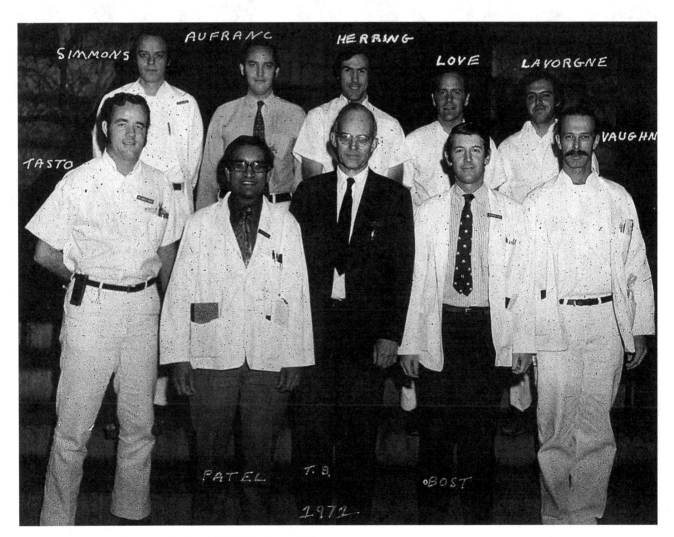

Dr. Thornton Brown (interim chief) with MGH residents, 1972. MGH HCORP Archives.

Box 43.2. Orthopaedic Specialties at MGH

Adult Reconstruction
William H. Harris, Murali Jasty, Dennis W. Burke, Fulton C. Kornack, John M. Siliski, Samuel Doppelt, William Tomford, Philip Salib, and Stephen B. Trippel

Foot and Ankle
George H. Theodore

Hand and Upper Extremity
Richard Smith, Jesse Jupiter, and Sang-Gil P. Lee;

Podiatry
Robert J. Scardina

Shoulder
Robert D. Leffert and Gary S. Perlmutter

Spine
Robert J. Boyd, Joseph S. Barr, Jr., Frederick L Mansfield, Francis X. Pedlow, Stanley Grabias, and Donald Pierce

Sports Medicine
Bertram Zarins, Dinesh Patel, Arthur Boland, and Brian J. Awbrey

Orthopaedic Oncology
Henry Mankin, Mark C. Gebhardt, Dempsey Springfield, and Candice Jennings

Pediatric Orthopaedics
Michael Ehrlich, Keith P. Mankin, and David J. Zaleske

Trauma
David W. Lhowe, Charles Weiss, and Edwin T. Wyman

Research faculty
David E. Krebs, Orhun Moratoglu, Chris McGibbon, Patricia Sullivan, and Lawrence Weissbach

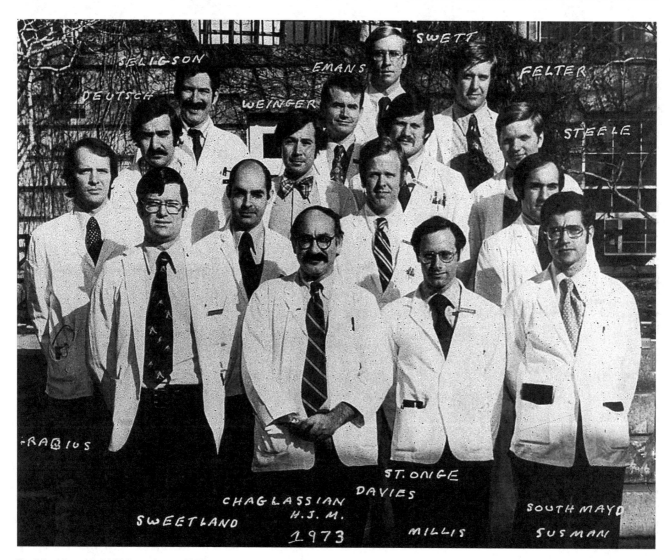

Dr. Mankin with MGH residents, 1973. MGH HCORP Archives.

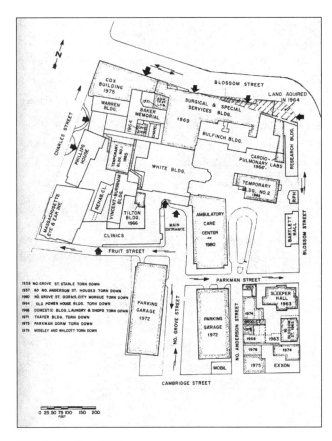

MGH plot plan, 1980.
The Massachusetts General Hospital, 1955–1980 by Benjamin Castleman, David C. Crockett, and S. B. Sutton. Boston: Little, Brown, 1983. Massachusetts General Hospital, Archives and Special Collections.

Dr. DeLorme and Dr. Pierce. Pierce remained chief until Dr. Mankin replaced him with Dr. Robert Leffert in 1972 (see chapter 42). White 9 eventually closed as the orthopaedic rehabilitation unit after Spaulding Rehabilitation Hospital opened in 1971. In 1983, Dr. Mankin recruited Dr. Leroy Levine as Chief of Orthopaedic Rehabilitation at Spaulding.

Transition

In the second decade of Dr. Mankin's tenure as chairman, he added three senior consultant physicians, all of whom were retired chairmen of orthopaedic services:

1. Dr. Paul H. Curtiss Jr., Editor of the *Journal of Bone and Joint Surgery* (1979–1985), former Professor and Chief of the Orthopaedic Division at Ohio State University College of Medicine (1965–1978).
2. Dr. Crawford J. Campbell, former Chief of the Orthopaedic Section at Albany Medical College and an expert in orthopaedic pathology.

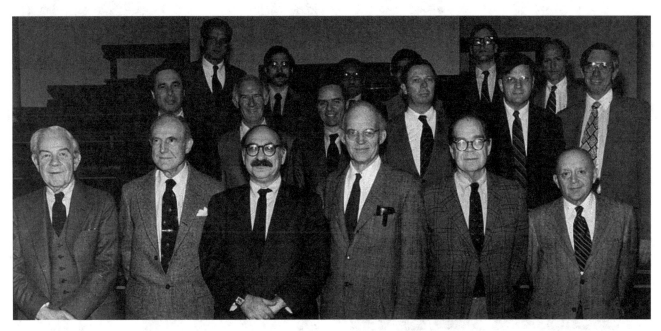

MGH Staff in 1981. Left to right, back row: B. Zarins, S. Doppelt, D. Patel, J. Jupiter, W. Tomford, H. Chandler; second row: R. Leffert, W. Kermond, J. Barr Jr., D. Pierce, M. Ehrlich, E. Wyman; front row: W. Jones, C. Rowe, H. Mankin, T. Brown, P. Curtiss, R. Brendze. MGH HCORP Archives.

3. Dr. Leroy S. Lavine, former Professor and Chief of Orthopaedics at SUNY Downstate Medical Center (1964–1981) who became Professor at the MGH Institute of Health Professions, Lecturer at Harvard Medical School and Chief of Orthopaedic Rehabilitation at Spaulding Hospital (1983–2005).

In 1998, I was recruited as chairman of the Department of Orthopaedics for Partners Healthcare (the parent organization of the MGH and the BWH—later renamed Mass General Brigham [MGB]) and the Partners Professor of Orthopaedic Surgery (later renamed the William H. and Johanna A. Harris Professor) at HMS. I recruited Dr. Harry Rubash (adult reconstruction) to accompany me from the University Pittsburgh to succeed Dr. Mankin as Chief of the Orthopaedic Service at MGH, along with Dr. Jon J. P. Warner (shoulder) and scientists, Dr. Christopher Evans, Dr. Guoan Li and Dr. Arun Shanbhag. Rubash and I recruited the following outstanding orthopaedic surgeons during the transition to the twentieth century: Dr. Francis J. Hornicek (orthopaedic oncology), Dr. Thomas J. Gill (sports medicine), and Dr. Mark Vrahas (trauma); including scientist, Dr. Teresa Morales.

Dr. Rubash, in his first chief's report in 1999, wrote:

> One of our first goals was to reorganize the clinical full-time staff into a more centralized practice model. The current practice sites include the fourth floor of the Professional Office Building (POB), offices of the fifth floor of the Ambulatory Care Center (ACC) and the White/Gray 6 area. At each of the sites, a task-oriented staff model has been instituted… [which] includes…

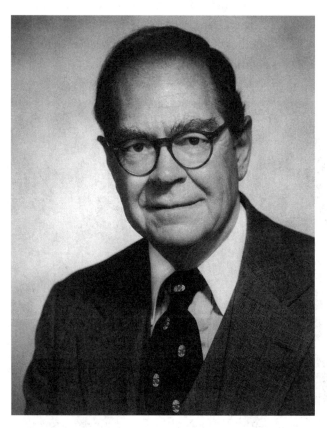

Paul H. Curtiss Jr. "Paul H. Curtiss, Jr., MD 1920–2007," *Journal of Bone and Joint Surgery* 2008; 90: 459.

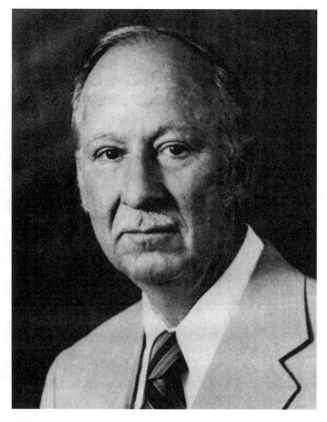

Crawford J. Campbell. H.J.M. and J.C., "Crawford Jennings Campbell, M.D. 1914–1983," *Journal of Bone and Joint Surgery* 1983; 65: 1209.

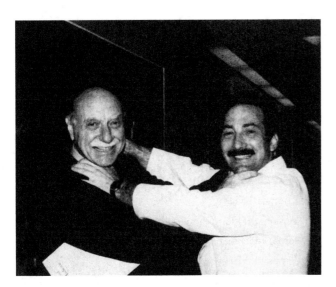

Leroy S. Lavine (left). MGH HCORP Archives.

academic support, surgical and test scheduling, patient reception, and a new phone operating system... In addition...we will develop a new Orthopaedic Billing Office... of the MGH Physicians Organization (MGPO)... [in which] the MGH surgeons will have control over the revenue cycle. (Rubash 1999)

Office relocations occurred, and new faculty continued to be recruited. Orthopaedic research laboratories were also reorganized, including the: Orthopedic Biomechanics Laboratory (later named the Harris Orthopaedic and Biomaterials laboratory), the Biomaterials and Innovative Technologies Laboratory, the Biomotion Laboratory, the Joint Kinematics Laboratory (originally located at BIDMC), the Knee Biomechanics and Biomaterials Laboratory and the Orthopaedic Biology and Oncology Laboratories.

In 2000, Dr. Rubash reported that he had hired David Gaynor as the new department administrative director and Tom Amuralt as the director of the new Orthopaedic Billing Office. He said, "Last year I reported that the clinical volume at the MGH had plateaued. After a series of strategic moves and additional staff recruitment...our clinical activities have grown" (Rubash 2000). Several new faculty members were added, including: Dr. James Heckman (Editor of JBJS) on the foot/ankle service, Dr. James Sarni (physiatrist) on the spine service, and Dr. David Ring on the hand/upper extremity service. A generous gift from Fred E. and Joan Brengle provided funding for the Frederick and Joan Brengle Learning Center, which incorporated the Smith Conference Room and Library, the Smith-Petersen Library, and the Rowe Conference Room into one area on White 5, which was dedicated to use by the residents. In 2008, when I retired as the HCORP Director, the residents created a yearly award—the James H. Herndon Resident Teaching and Mentoring Award. It is awarded yearly to the graduating resident, selected by her/his peers, who has given the most back to other residents as a teacher, mentor and advocate (see **Box 43.3**).

Box 43.3. Recipients of the James H. Herndon Resident Teaching and Mentoring Award

Mark D. Price	2008
Michael J. Weaver	2009
Arnold B. Alqueza	2010
John J. Kadzielski	2011
Matthew Salzler	2012
Natalie E.J. Casemyr	2013
Xavier C. Simcock	2014
Jacob W. Brubacher	2015
Lauren Ehrlichman	2016
Forrest Schwartz	2017
Erik T. Newman	2018
Hai V. Le	2019
Abhiram R. Bhashyam	2020

The Department of Orthopaedic Surgery continued to expand its clinical and research programs as it transitioned into the early twenty-first century (see **Box 43.4**), and it is well-prepared for the challenges of today.

Box 43.4. MGH Clinical and Research Programs

Professorships

John Ball and Buckminster Brown Professor:
- Joseph S. Barr (1947–1964)

Edith M. Ashley Professor:
- Melvin J Glimcher (1966–1970)
- Henry J. Mankin (1972–2002)
- Harry Rubash (2002–2018)

William H. and Johanna A. Harris Professor:
- James H. Herndon (1998—)

Alan Gerry Clinical Professor of Orthopaedic Surgery:
- William H. Harris (1997—)

Hansjorg Wyss/AO Foundation Professor:
- Jesse B. Jupiter (2003—)

Augustus Thorndike Professor:
- Bertram Zarins (2007—)

Research Laboratory Centers

Orthopaedic Biomechanics and Biomaterials Laboratory
- Director: William H. Harris

Biomaterials Research Laboratory
- Director: Arun Shanbhag

Knee Biomechanics and Biomaterials Laboratory
- Directors: William H. Harris; Harry E. Rubash

Joint Kinematics Laboratory
- Director: Guoan Li

Orthopaedic Biologic and Oncology Laboratories
- Director: Henry J. Mankin

Sarcoma Molecular Biology Laboratory
- Director: Francis Hornicek

Orthopaedic Biochemistry and Osteoarthritis Therapy Laboratory
- Director: Teresa Morales

Biomotion Laboratory
- Director: David Krebs

Clinical faculty (at the turn of the Century):
- Harry E. Rubash (Chair)
- Brian J. Awbrey
- Joseph S. Barr Jr.
- Arthur Boland
- Dennis W. Burke
- Mark C. Gebhardt
- Thomas J. Gill
- William H. Harris
- James Heckman
- James H. Herndon
- Francis J. Hornicek
- Murali J. Jasty
- Fulton C. Kornack
- Jesse B. Jupiter
- Sang-Gil P. Lee
- Robert D. Leffert
- David W. Lhowe
- Henry J. Mankin
- Keith P. Mankin
- Frederick L. Mansfield
- Dinesh Patel
- Francis X. Pedlow
- Gary S. Perlmutter
- Donald S. Pierce
- James Sarni
- Robert J. Scardina
- John M. Siliski
- George H. Theodore
- William Tomford
- Stephen B. Trippel
- Mark Vrahas
- John J. P. Warner
- Edwin T. Wyman
- David J. Zaleske
- Bertram Zarins

Index

Illustrations are indicated by page numbers in *italics*. Page numbers followed by t and b indicate tables and boxes.

Page numbers are formatted as: Volume: page

A

AAOS. *See* American Academy of Orthopaedic Surgeons (AAOS)
AAOS Council on Education, 4: 173
AAOS Diversity Committee, 1: 239
AAST. *See* American Association for the Surgery of Trauma (AAST)
Abbott, Edward Gilbert, 1: 59; 2: 87–88
Abbott, Josephine Dormitzer, 2: 97
Abbott, LeRoy C., 1: 189, 197; 2: 77, 110, 160, 183; 3: 180, 229; 4: 473
Abbott Frame, 4: 232, *232*
"Abscesses of Hip Disease, The" (Lovett and Goldthwait), 2: *52*
abdominal surgery, 1: 81; 3: 18, 108
Abe, Isso, 2: 279
Abraham, John, 4: 190b
absorbable animal membrane research, 3: 166, *166*, 167, *171*
Academy of Medicine, 4: 324
Accreditation Council for Graduate Medical Education (ACGME), 1: 200, 213, 217, 237–239
acetabular dysplasia, 2: 389, *389*, 390
"Acetone" (Sever), 2: 84
ACGME. *See* Accreditation Council for Graduate Medical Education (ACGME)
Achilles tendon
    club foot and, 2: 25, 29, 145
    gastrocnemius paralysis and, 2: 150
    injury in, 3: 272
    sliding procedure and, 2: *198*
    subcutaneous release of, 2: 29, 36
    tenotomy, 1: 100–101, 106; 2: 25
achillobursitis, 2: 89
Ackerman, Gary, 1: 217b
acromioclavicular joint dislocation, 1: 268, 277
acromioplasty, 3: 191, 239
ACS Committee on Fractures, 3: 64; 4: 324
activating transcription factor-2 (ATF-2), 2: 330
acute ligament injuries, 1: 277
acute thigh compartment syndrome, 3: 417, *417*, 418
Adams, Frances Kidder, 3: 228
Adams, Helen Foster, 3: 228, 236
Adams, Herbert D., 3: 275
Adams, John, 1: 8–10, 14, 18
Adams, John D.
    back pain treatment, 4: 358
    Boston Dispensary and, 4: 358–359
    education and training, 4: 357–358
    HMS appointment, 4: 360
    Massachusetts Regional Fracture Committee, 3: 64
    Mt. Sinai Hospital and, 4: 204
    New England Medical Center and, 4: 360
    occupational therapy and, 4: 358–359
    patellar turndown procedure, 4: 373–374
    private medical practice, 4: 358
    professional memberships, 4: 360
    publications and research, 4: 359, *359*
    scaphoid fracture treatment, 4: 359–360
    Tufts Medical School appointment, 4: 360
Adams, John Quincy, 1: 10
Adams, M., 3: 133
Adams, Nancy, 3: 236
Adams, Samuel, 3: 236
Adams, Samuel (1722–1803), 1: 13, 15–17
Adams, Zabdiel B. (1875–1940), 3: *228*
    AOA Commission on Congenital Dislocation of the Hip and, 3: 232, *232*, 233–234
    Base Hospital No. 6 and, 4: 433–434
    Boston Children's Hospital and, 2: 247; 3: 228
    Boston City Hospital and, 4: 305b
    CDH treatment, 3: 233–235
    death of, 3: 236
    early life, 3: 228
    education and training, 3: 228
    fracture management and, 3: 61
    HMS appointment, 3: 232
    Lakeville State Sanatorium and, 3: 235
    marriage and family, 3: 228, 236
    Medical Reserve Corps and, 3: 232
    memberships and, 3: 235–236
    as MGH house officer, 1: 189
    as MGH orthopaedic surgeon, 3: 228, 235, 266, 268
    military surgeon training and, 2: 42
    New England Deaconess Hospital and, 4: 225

publications and research,
3: 228–232
scoliosis treatment and, 2: 84,
86; 3: 229–232
World War I and, 3: 232; 4: 412
Adams, Zabdiel B. (father), 3: 228
Adam's machine, 2: 86
Affiliated Hospitals Center, Inc.,
4: 42, 113–114, 118, 120, 127,
132
Agel, Julie, 1: 287
Agency for Healthcare Research and
Quality, 2: 371
Aitken, Alexander P. (1904–1993),
4: *350*
BCH Bone and Joint Service,
4: 353, 356, 380*b*
Boston City Hospital and, 4: 350
Boston University Medical School
appointment, 4: 350
Chelsea Memorial Hospital and,
4: 350
classification of epiphyseal fractures, 4: 355–356
death of, 4: 356
education and training, 4: 350
epiphyseal injury treatment,
4: 350–352, 355–356
fracture of the proximal tibial epiphyseal cartilage case,
4: 355
fracture research and, 4: 354
hospital appointments, 4: 356
legacy of, 4: 356
Liberty Mutual Insurance Rehabilitation Clinic and, 4: 352–353, 356
Massachusetts Regional Fracture
Committee, 3: 64
Monson State Hospital and,
4: 350
private medical practice, 4: 356
professional memberships,
4: 352, 356
publications and research,
4: 350–355
rehabilitation of injured workers
and, 4: 350, 352–354
ruptured intervertebral disc treatment, 4: 350, 352–353
Tufts Medical School appointment, 4: 353
workers' compensation issues,
4: 353–354
Aitken, H. F., 1: *89*
Akbarnia, Behrooz, 2: 359, 361
Akeson, Wayne, 3: 382
Akins, Carlton M., 1: 217*b*
Alais, J., 1: *34*

Alan Gerry Clinical Professor of
Orthopaedic Surgery, 3: 224, 464*b*
Albee, F. H., 3: 157; 4: 406
Albert, E., 3: 95
Albert, Todd J., 4: 266*b*
Albert Einstein College of Medicine,
2: 408
Alden, Eliza, 2: 231
Alden, Louise, 2: 241
Alder Hey Hospital (Liverpool),
4: 401
Aldrich, Marion, 3: 164
Allen, Arthur W., 3: 60*b*, 315;
4: 208
Allen, John Michael, 2: 438
Allen, L., 3: 133
Allen Street House (MGH),
3: 17–18
Allgemeines Krankenhaus, 1: 81
Allgöwer, Martin, 2: 406
Allied Relief Fund, 4: 363
Allison, Addie Shultz, 3: 163
Allison, James, 3: 163
Allison, Marion Aldrich, 3: 164
Allison, Nathaniel (1876–1932),
3: *163, 174*; 4: *417*
absorbable animal membrane
research, 3: 166, *166*, 167, *171*
adult orthopaedics and, 2: 157
AEF splint board, 4: 416–417
American Ambulance Hospital
and, 2: 119
animal research and, 3: 165–167,
170, *171*
AOA Committee on war preparation, 2: 124
AOA preparedness committee,
4: 394
as AOA president, 3: 172
army manual of splints and appliances, 2: 126
arthroplasty research,
3: 165–166
as BCH house officer, 3: 163
on bone atrophy, 3: 170
Chicago University orthopaedics
department, 3: 175
death of, 3: 176
Department for Military Orthopedics and, 4: 405–406
Diagnosis in Joint Disease,
3: 175, 289, *290*
early life, 3: 163
education and training, 3: 163
*Fundamentals of Orthopaedic Surgery in General Medicine and
Surgery*, 2: 135–136
on hip dislocations, 3: 164, 175
HMS appointment, 3: 173

knee derangement treatment,
3: 165
legacy of, 3: 176–177
on Legg-Calvé-Perthes disease,
3: 165–166
low-back pain research, 3: 175
marriage and, 3: 164
memberships and, 3: 176, 176*b*
MGH Fracture Clinic and,
3: 60*b*, 314, 371
MGH house officers and, 1: 189
as MGH orthopaedics chief,
1: 152; 2: 133–134; 3: 11*b*,
173–174, 227
military orthopaedics and, 2: 128
New England Peabody Home for
Crippled Children and, 2: 270;
3: 174
orthopaedic research and,
3: 164–167, 170, 174–175
on orthopaedics education,
2: 134; 3: 170–173
private medical practice, 2: 146
"Progress in Orthopaedic Surgery" series, 2: 297
publications and research,
4: 102, 225–226, 372
on sacroiliac joint fusion, 3: 185
on splints for Army, 3: 167–168,
168, 169, 169*b*
synovial fluid research, 3: 174,
174, 175
Walter Reed General Hospital
and, 4: 452
Washington University orthopaedic department and, 3: 163–165, 170; 4: 419
World War I and, 3: 157,
166–169; 4: 417
Allison, Nathaniel (grandfather),
3: 163
allografts
bone banks for, 3: 386, 396,
433, 440–441
distal femoral osteonecrosis and,
3: 433
femoral heads and, 3: 442
infection and freeze-dried,
3: 440
irradiation and, 3: 435
knee fusion with, 3: 435
long-term study of, 3: 433, 435
malignant bone tumors and,
3: 389
osteoarticular, 3: 442
osteosarcomas and, 3: 433
transmission of disease through,
3: 442–443, *443*
Alman, B. A., 2: 212
Alqueza, Arnold, 4: 190*b*

Index

Alqueza, Arnold B., 3: 463*b*
Altman, Greg, 4: 285–286
Altschule, Mark D., 1: 171, 239
AMA Committee on the Medical Aspects of Sports, 1: 274, 280
AMA Council on Medical Education and Hospitals, 1: 146, 196–197, 199, 211
Amadio, Peter C., 3: 431
Ambulatory Care Center (ACC) (MGH), 3: 396
Ambulatory Care Unit (ACU) (MGH), 3: 399
American Academy for Cerebral Palsy, 2: 176, 196–198
American Academy of Arts and Sciences, 1: 29, 61
American Academy of Orthopaedic Surgeons (AAOS), 1: xxv, 213; 2: 176, 201–203; 3: 90; 4: 337
American Ambulance Field Service, 2: 118
American Ambulance Hospital (Neuilly, France), 2: *119*; 4: *386*
    Harvard Unit and, 2: 118–120; 3: 166, 180, *180*; 4: 386, *387*, 389*b*, 391
    Osgood and, 2: 117–120; 4: 386, 391–393
    Smith-Petersen and, 3: 180
American Appreciation, An (Wilson), 3: 369
American Association for Labor Legislation, 4: 325–326
American Association for the Surgery of Trauma (AAST), 3: 65, 315, *315*; 4: *319*, 349
American Association of Medical Colleges (AAMC), 1: 168–169
American Association of Tissue Banks, 3: 386, 442–443, *443*
American Board of Orthopaedic Surgery (ABOS), 1: xxv, 197–200, 211, 213, 215–216, 231; 2: 317; 4: 173, 377–379
American British Canadian (ABC) Traveling Fellow, 3: 218
American College of Rheumatology, 4: 57–58
American College of Sports Medicine, 2: *387*
American College of Surgeons (ACS), 2: 158; 3: 112, *112*, 113*b*, 131, 310, 367; 4: 102, 324, 354
American College of Surgeons Board of Regents, 3: 62–63
American Expeditionary Forces (AEF)
    base hospitals for BEF, 4: 420, 426

    Division of Orthopedic Surgery, 4: 410*b*, 417, 439, 453–454
    Goldthwait and, 4: 416
    Johns Hopkins Hospital Unit and, 2: 221
    medical care in, 4: 417
    orthopaedic treatment and, 4: 409, 410*b*
    Osgood and, 2: 124, 126, 128; 4: 417, 421*b*
    physician deaths in, 4: 425
    Shortell and, 4: 338
    splint board and, 4: 416
    standardization of splints and dressings for, 2: 124; 3: 168
    Wilson and, 3: 370
American Field Service Ambulance, 4: 386, *386*, 387, *387*, 388
American Hospital Association, 1: 211
American Jewish Committee, 4: 203
American Journal of Orthopedic Surgery, 4: 226
American Medical Association (AMA), 1: xxv, 69, 189–191, 211, 213; 2: 42, 124; 3: 35, 131
American Mutual Liability Insurance Company, 3: 314, 316
American Orthopaedic Association (AOA), 4: 463
    Barr and, 1: 158
    Bradford and, 2: 24–26, 34, 43
    Buckminster Brown and, 1: 111
    Committee of Undergraduate Training, 2: 183
    founding of, 1: 114; 2: 48, *48*, 49
    graduate education study committee, 1: 196–197
    investigation of fusion on tubercular spines, 3: 157–158
    Lovett and, 2: 51
    military surgeon training and, 2: 65
    orthopaedic surgery terminology, 1: xxiv, xxv
    orthopaedics residencies survey, 2: 160–161
    Osgood and, 1: xxii; 2: 137
    Phelps and, 1: 193
    preparedness committee, 4: 394
    scoliosis treatment committee, 2: 87–88
    World War I and, 2: 64, 124
American Orthopaedic Foot and Ankle Society (AOFAS), 2: 316
American Orthopaedic Foot Society (AOFS), 2: 316–317; 3: 295, 298

American Orthopaedic Society of Sports Medicine (AOSSM), 1: 286, 289; 2: 163, 375; 3: 360
"American Orthopedic Surgery" (Bick), 1: 114
American Pediatric Society, 2: 15
American Public Health Association, 4: 439
American Radium Society, 1: 275–276
American Rheumatism Association, 2: 137; 4: 41*b*, 57–58, 63, 169
American Shoulder and Elbow Surgeons (ASES), 2: 380; 3: 415, *415*
American Society for Surgery of the Hand (ASSH), 2: 251; 3: 316, 428, *428*, 429, *430*; 4: 168, 186
American Society for Testing and Materials (ATSM), 3: 210
American Society of Hand Therapists, 4: 168
American Surgical Association, 1: 87; 2: 43; 3: 58
American Surgical Materials Association, 3: 210
American Whigs, 1: 11
AmeriCares, 3: 416
Ames Test, 4: 171
Ammer, Christine, 2: 277
amputations
    blood perfusion in, 3: 287
    economic importance and, 4: 419
    ether and, 1: 61
    fractures and, 1: 50, 54
    geriatric patients and, 3: 330
    Gritti-Stokes, 3: 374
    guillotine, 4: *469*
    John Collins Warren and, 1: 52–53, 61
    kineplastic forearm, 4: 360
    kit for, 1: *60*
    length and, 3: 374
    malpractice suits and, 1: 50
    military wounds and, 1: 23; 4: 418–419
    mortality rates, 1: 65, 74, 84
    osteosarcoma and, 3: 391
    research in, 3: 373, *373*
    results of, 3: 374*t*
    sepsis and, 3: 373
    shoulder, 1: 23
    skin traction and, 4: *419*
    suction socket prosthesis and, 1: 273
    temporary prostheses and, 3: 374
    transmetatarsal, 4: 276
    trauma and, 3: 373
    tuberculosis and, 3: 374

without anesthesia, 1: 10, 36, 65
wounded soldiers and,
4: 446–447
Amputees and Their Prostheses (Pierce and Mital), 3: 320
AMTI, 3.224
Amuralt, Tom, 3: 463
Anatomical and Surgical Treatment of Hernia (Cooper), 1: 36
Anatomy Act, 1: 52
Anatomy of the Breast (Cooper), 1: 36
Anatomy of the Thymus Gland (Cooper), 1: 36
Anderson, Gunnar B. J., 4: 266*b*
Anderson, Margaret, 2: 170, 191–194, 264, 304, 350
Anderson, Megan E., 4: 287
Andrews, H. V., 3: 133
Andry, Nicolas, 1: xxi, xxii, xxiii, xxiv; 3: 90; 4: 233
anesthesia
　acetonuria associated with death after, 3: 305
　bubble bottle method, 4: 323
　charting in, 3: 95, 96
　chloroform as, 1: 62–63, 82
　Cotton-Boothby apparatus, 4: 320, 323
　ether as, 1: 55–58, 60–62, 63, 64–65, 82
　hypnosis and, 1: 56, 65
　nitrous oxide as, 1: 56–59, 63
　orthopaedic surgery and, 2: 15
　surgery before, 1: 6, 10, 23, 36, 74
　use at Boston Orthopedic Institution, 1: 107, 118
　use at Massachusetts General Hospital (MGH), 1: 57–62, 118
anesthesiology, 1: 61
ankle valgus, 2: 212
ankles
　arthrodesis and, 3: 330
　astragalectomy and, 2: 93–94
　athletes and, 3: 348
　central-graft operation, 3: 368
　fractures, 4: 313–315, 315, 316
　gait analysis and, 2: 406–407
　instability and Pott's fracture, 4: 317, 318
　lubrication and, 3: 324
　sports injuries and, 1: 281
　stabilization of, 2: 148
　tendon transfers and, 2: 148
　tuberculosis and, 1: 73
　weakness and, 2: 150
ankylosis, 4: 64
Anna Jacques Hospital, 2: 269, 272

Annual Bibliography of Orthopaedic Surgery, 3: 261
anterior cruciate ligament (ACL)
　direct repair of, 2: 91
　growth plate disturbances, 2: 379
　intra-articular healing of, 2: 439
　intra-/extra-articular reconstruction, 3: 448
　outpatient arthroscopic reconstructions, 4: 255
　reconstruction of, 2: 91, 378–379, 386
　skeletally immature patients and, 2: 378–379
　Tegner Activity Scale and, 2: 380
　young athletes and, 2: 385, 385, 386
Anthology Club, 1: 29
antisepsis
　acceptance in the U.S., 1: 118
　carbolic acid treatment, 1: 82–83
　Coll Warren promotion of, 1: 85
　discovery of, 1: 55
　Lister and, 1: 55, 81, 84; 3: 45
　orthopaedic surgery and, 2: 15
　prevention of infection and, 1: 84–85
　surgeon resistance to, 1: 85
　trench warfare and, 4: 385
Antiseptic surgery (Cheyne), 1: 83
AO Foundation, 3: 409, 409
AOA. *See* American Orthopaedic Association (AOA)
apothecary, 1: 184
Appleton, Paul, 3: 410; 4: 288
Arbuckle, Robert H., 4: 163, 193
Archibald, Edward W., 3: 26, 50
Archives of Surgery (Jackson), 3: 35
Arlington Mills, 2: 267
Armed Forces Institute of Pathology, 4: 126
arms
　Bankart procedure and, 3: 359–360
　Boston Arm, 2: 326
　carpal tunnel syndrome, 2: 375
　compartment syndrome, 2: 249–250
　cubitus varus deformity, 2: 229
　dead arm syndrome, 3: 359–360
　distal humerus prosthesis, 2: 250
　kineplastic forearm amputation, 4: 360
　Krukenberg procedure, 2: 425
　tendon transfers and, 3: 428
　Volkmann ischemic contracture, 2: 200–201, 249–250
　x-ray of fetal, 3: 97, 97
Armstrong, Stewart, 4: 41*b*

Arnold, Benedict, 1: 19, 33
Arnold, Horace D., 1: 250; 3: 122
arthritis. *See also* osteoarthritis; rheumatoid arthritis
　allied health professionals and, 4: 28
　experimental septic, 2: 79
　femoroacetabular impingement, 3: 189
　forms of chronic, 4: 55
　Green and, 2: 171
　growth disturbances in children, 4: 56
　hand and, 4: 96
　hip fusion for, 3: 156*b*
　hips and, 2: 380
　juvenile idiopathic, 2: 171, 350
　Lovett Fund and, 2: 82
　MGH and, 2: 82
　nylon arthroplasty and, 4: 65–66, 66*b*, 69
　orthopaedic treatment for, 2: 171; 4: 32–33
　pauciarticular, 2: 171, 350
　pediatric, 2: 349–350
　prevention and, 4: 60–61
　psoriatic, 4: 99
　rheumatoid, 2: 82, 171, 350; 3: 239
　roentgenotherapy for, 4: 64, 64
　sacroiliac joint fusion for, 3: 184–185
　synovectomy in chronic, 4: 102, 371–372
　treatment of, 4: 32–33, 43, 54–55
　Vitallium mold arthroplasty and, 3: 239
Arthritis, Medicine and the Spiritual Law (Swaim), 4: 58, 58
Arthritis and Rheumatism Foundation, 4: 39
Arthritis Foundation, 3: 279
arthrodesis procedures
　ankles and, 3: 330
　central-graft operation, 3: 368, 368
　joints and, 3: 165
　MCP joint, 4: 97
　Morris on, 2: 282
　rheumatoid arthritis and, 4: 166
　rheumatoid arthritis of the hand research, 4: 167
　sacroiliac joint and, 3: 183–185
　wrists and, 3: 191, 239; 4: 166–167
arthrogram, 3: 99
arthrogryposis multiplex congenita, 2: 274–275, 287

Index

arthroplasty. *See also* mold arthroplasty
  absorbable animal membrane research, 3: 165–167
  advances in, 4: 43
  of the elbow, 3: 64, 341; 4: 63
  hip and, 3: 181, 242, 242*t*, *242*, 243
  implant, 4: 99–100
  of the knee, 4: 64, 70*b*–71*b*, 93–94, 103, 179*t*
  metacarpophalangeal, 4: 97
  nylon, 4: 64, 65, 66, 66*b*, 93
  release of contractures, 4: 166
  silicone flexible implants, 4: 166, *167*, *168*
  total knee, 4: 129–130, 131*t*
  using interpositional tissues, 4: 64
  volar plate, 2: 248
  wrist and, 3: 191
Arthroscopic Surgery Update (McGinty), 2: 279
arthroscopy
  cameras and, 2: 279
  knee injuries and, 1: 279; 4: 129
  knee simulator, 4: 173
  McGinty and Matza's procedure, 2: 279, 280*b*, 281
  operative, 3: 422–423
  orthopaedics education and, 1: 220, 230
Arthroscopy Association of North America, 2: 281; 3: 422, *422*
arthrotomy, 3: 165, 165*b*, 166, 351
Arthur H. Huene Award, 2: 403
Arthur T. Legg Memorial Room, 2: *106*, 107
articular cartilage
  allografts and, 3: 389–390
  chondrocytes and, 3: 444
  compression forces and, 3: 326
  cup arthroplasty of the hip and, 3: 244
  degradative enzymes in, 3: *401*
  dimethyl sulfoxide (DMSO) and glycerol, 3: 442
  gene transfer treatment, 3: 445
  histologic-histochemical grading system for, 3: 384, 385*t*, *385*
  lubrication and, 3: 326–327
  osteoarthritis and, 3: 387–388
  preservation of, 3: 442, *442*
  repair using tritiated thymidine, 3: 383
  sling procedure and, 3: 296
Aseptic Treatment of Wounds, The (Walter), 4: 106, *106*, 107*b*
Ashworth, Michael A., 4: 22
assistive technology, 2: 408

Association of American Medical Colleges (AAMC), 1: 211; 2: 158
Association of Bone and Joint Surgeons, 3: 436, *436*
Association of Franklin Medal Scholars, 1: 31
Association of Residency Coordinators in Orthopaedic Surgery, 1: 238
astragalectomy (Whitman's operation), 2: 92–94
Asylum for the Insane, The, 1: 294
athletic injuries. *See* sports medicine
Athletic Injuries. Prevention, Diagnosis and Treatment (Thorndike), 1: 265, 266
athletic training. *See also* sports medicine
  dieticians and, 1: 258
  football team and, 1: 248, 250–253, 255–256, 258
  over-training and, 1: 251, 265
  scientific study of, 1: 250–251, 265–266
athletics. *See* Harvard athletics
Atsatt, Rodney F., 1: 193; 2: 140
ATSM Committee F-4 on Medical and Surgical Materials and Devices, 3: 210
Attucks, Crispus, 1: 14
Au, Katherine, 2: 425
Aufranc, Otto E. (1909–1990), 3: *236*, *245*, *273*, *300*
  AAOS and, 2: 215
  accomplishments of, 3: 241–242
  Boston Children's Hospital and, 3: 237
  Boston City Hospital internship, 3: 237
  Bronze Star and, 3: 240, 240*b*, *240*
  Chandler and, 3: 277
  Children's Hospital/MGH combined program and, 3: 237
  Constructive Surgery of the Hip, 3: 244, *246*
  on Coonse, 4: 372–373
  death of, 3: 247
  early life, 3: 236–237
  education and training, 3: 237
  Fracture Clinic and, 3: 60*b*, 241–242, 245
  "Fracture of the Month" column, 3: 243, *243*
  hip nailing and, 3: 237
  hip surgery and, 3: 238–243; 4: 187
  HMS appointment, 3: 241–242
  as honorary orthopaedic surgeon, 3: 398*b*

  honors and awards, 3: 245*b*
  Knight's Cross, Royal Norwegian Order of St. Olav, 3: *245*
  kyphosis treatment, 3: 239–240
  legacy of, 3: 247
  MGH Staff Associates and, 3: 241
  as MGH surgeon, 1: 203–204; 2: 325; 3: 74, 192, 217, 238–239, 241, 246
  mold arthroplasty and, 3: 192, 218, 238–239, 241–243, 243*b*, 244, 292*b*, 456*b*
  New England Baptist Hospital and, 3: 246–247
  Newton-Wellesley Hospital, 3: 240
  patient care and, 3: 244
  PBBH and, 4: 373
  private medical practice, 3: 238–240; 4: 158
  publications and research, 1: 286; 3: 191–192, 218, 239–244, 246, 302; 4: 161, 373
  rheumatoid arthritis research, 2: 137; 3: 239
  6th General Hospital and, 4: *476*, 482, 483*b*
  Smith-Petersen and, 3: 237–240
  Tufts appointment, 3: 247
  World War II service, 3: 239–241
Aufranc, Randolph Arnold, 3: 247
Aufranc, St. George Tucker, 3: 247; 4: 163, 193
Augustus Thorndike Professor of Orthopaedic Surgery, 3: 450, 464*b*
Augustus White III Symposium, 4: 265, 266*b*
Austen, Frank F., 4: 42, 114, 119, 128, 132
Austen, R. Frank, 4: 68–69
Austen, W. Gerald, 3: 256, 287, 397
Austin Moore prosthesis, 3: 213, 241, 354*b*
Australian Civil Constitution Corps (CCC), 4: 489
Australian Orthopaedic Association, 3: 360
Avallone, Nicholas, 4: 190*b*
Avicenna Hospital, 2: 421
Awbrey, Brian J., 3: 460*b*, 464*b*
Axelrod, Terry S., 3: 431
Aycock, W. Lloyd, 2: 82
Ayres, Douglas K., 4: 287

469

B

Babcock, Warren L., 4: 429, 433, 437
Bach, Bernard R., Jr., 1: 284, 288–289; 3: 379
back disabilities. *See also* sciatica
   industrial accidents and, 2: 92; 4: 358
   laminectomy and, 3: 204, 206–208
   low-back pain, 2: 371–372, 396; 3: 175, 204–206, 250*b*–252*b*
   lumbago and, 3: 203
   lumbar spinal stenosis, 2: 373–374
   MRI and, 3: 255
   Norton-Brown spinal brace and, 3: 318, *318tg*, 319
   Ober Test and, 2: 151–152
   psychiatric investigation and, 3: 258
   ruptured intervertebral disc, 3: 204, *204*, 205–207, *207*, 208; 4: 352–353
   sacroiliac joint and, 3: 184
   Sever on, 2: 92
   spine fusion and, 3: 207–208
   treatment of, 3: 203
Back Problems Guideline Panel, 2: 371
"Back Strains and Sciatica" (Ober), 2: 151–152
Bader Functional Room, 2: *106*
Bae, Donald S., 2: *417*, 418–419, *419t, 419*; 4: 190*b*
Baer, William S., 2: 126; 3: 158, 166–167; 4: 416
Baetzer, Fred H., 3: 87
Bailey, Fred Warren, 2: 78
Bailey, George G., Jr. (unk.–1998)
   Boston City Hospital and, 4: 360
   death of, 4: 360
   education and training, 4: 360
   kineplastic forearm amputation case, 4: 360
   Mt. Auburn Hospital and, 4: 360
   professional memberships, 4: 360
   publications and research, 4: 360
Baker, Charles, 2: 39
Baker, Frances Prescott, 3: 308
Balach, Franklin, 4: 41*b*
Balch, Emily, 3: 142
Balch, Franklin G., Jr., 4: 193
Balkan Frame, 3: 317, 357*b*
Ball, Anna, 1: 95
Ballentine, H. Thomas, 3: 314
Bancroft, Frederic, 3: 316
Bankart, A. S. Blundell, 3: 449

Bankart procedure, 3: 351–354, 357–358, 358*t, 359*, 360, 450
Banks, Henry H. (1921–), 1: *202*, 205, 207; 4: 72, *342*
   AAOS and, 2: 314
   Aufranc and, 3: 247
   on BCH residencies, 4: 377
   BIH Board of Consultants, 4: 262–263
   Boston Children's Hospital and, 1: 204–206; 2: 233, 301; 4: 72
   Boston City Hospital and, 4: 297
   on Carl Walter, 4: 108
   cerebral palsy research and treatment, 2: 196–200; 4: 74, 76–77
   education and training, 4: 72
   flexor carpi ulnaris transfer procedure, 2: 188
   on Green, 2: 168, 204–205
   Grice and, 1: 206
   hip fracture research, 4: 74–78
   Little Orthopaedic Club and, 4: 74
   on Mark Rogers, 4: 229–230
   metastatic malignant melanoma fracture case, 4: 77–78
   MGH and, 1: 203–204
   on Ober, 2: 149
   Orthopaedic Surgery at Tufts University, 4: 77
   on osteochondritis dissecans, 2: 195
   PBBH and, 1: 204–205; 4: 19–20, 22, 72, 73*b*–74*b*, 128
   as PBBH chief of orthopaedics, 4: 22, 43, 76, 116*b*, 196*b*
   on PBBH research program, 4: 75*b*
   professional memberships, 4: 76–77
   publications and research, 4: 72, 75–77
   on Quigley, 1: 276–277, 282
   RBBH and, 4: 36, 40
   residency training under Green, 1: 202–203
   as Tufts University chair of orthopaedics, 4: 22, 76–77, 116
   US Army Medical Corps and, 4: 72
   on Zimbler, 4: 250
Bar Harbor Medical and Surgical Hospital, 2: 312
Barber, D. B., 2: 172
Barlow, Joel, 1: 292–293
Barnes Hospital, 3: 165; 4: 125
Barr, Dorrice Nash, 3: 247

Barr, Joseph S. (1901–1964), 1: *205*; 2: 249, 278, 286, 290, 320; 3: 142, 201, 213
   as AAOS president, 3: 210
   appointments and positions, 3: 202*b*
   on audio-visual aids in teaching, 1: 161
   back pain and sciatica research, 3: 203–208
   Brigham and Women's Hospital and, 4: 195*b*
   as chair of AOA research committee, 3: 209, *209*
   as clinical professor, 1: 158
   Committee of Undergraduate Training, 2: 183
   death of, 3: 214
   development of research at MGH, 1: 180
   early life, 3: 201
   education and training, 3: 201
   Ferguson and, 2: 188
   Glimcher and, 2: 321–322
   on herniated disc and sciatica, 3: 184
   HMS appointment, 2: 223; 3: 202; 4: 61
   John Ball and Buckminster Brown Professorship, 3: 202, 453*b*, 464*b*; 4: 195*b*
   Joint Committee for the Study of Surgical Materials and, 3: 210
   leadership of, 3: 453, 453*b*–456*b*
   legacy of, 3: 212–214
   Marlborough Medical Associates and, 2: 146, 269, 299
   marriage and family, 3: 214
   memberships and, 3: 212–213
   as MGH orthopaedics chief, 3: 11*b*, 202, 227, 241, 277
   MGH residents and, 3: *212*, 217, 238, 254, 278, 285, 323, 377, 456; 4: *161*, 245
   MGH Staff Associates and, 3: 241
   as MGH surgeon, 3: 187, 201
   New England Peabody Home for Crippled Children and, 3: 209
   New England Society of Bone and Joint Surgery, 4: 347
   orthopaedic research and, 3: 210–212
   on orthopaedics curriculum, 1: 207
   PBBH 50th anniversary, 4: 21
   polio research, 3: 209, 331–333
   private medical practice, 3: 454*b*
   as professor of orthopaedic surgery, 1: 158, 179–180

Index

publications and research, 2: 152, 250; 3: 202–211, 302, 331
rehabilitation planning and, 1: 272
resident training by, 1: 199, 203, 206–207
retirement of, 2: 325
ruptured intervertebral disc research, 3: 204; 4: 352
scoliosis treatment, 2: 396; 3: 208–209
on shoulder arthrodesis, 2: 154
slipped capital femoral epiphysis research, 4: 237
on the surgical experiment, 3: 210
US Navy and, 3: 201
Barr, Joseph S., Jr. (1934–), 3: *247*, *461*
   ankle arthrodesis case, 3: 330
   Boston Interhospital Augmentation Study (BIAS) and, 3: 248–249
   Boston Prosthetics Course and, 1: 217
   Children's Hospital/MGH combined program and, 3: 248
   early life, 3: 247
   education and training, 3: 248
   Faulkner Hospital and, 3: 248
   Glimcher and, 3: 248
   Halo Vest, 3: 321
   HMS appointment, 3: 248
   on Leffert, 3: 413
   on low-back pain, 3: 250*b*–252*b*
   as MGH clinical faculty, 3: 464*b*
   as MGH surgeon, 3: 214, 248, 398*b*
   professional memberships and, 3: 249
   publications and research, 3: 249
   sailing and, 3: 249, 252
   Schmidt and, 3: 248
   spine treatment and, 3: 460*b*
   US Naval Medical Corps and, 3: 248
Barr, Mary, 3: 214
Barrell, Joseph, 3: 9
Barrett, Ian, 2: 400
Barron, M. E., 4: 199
Bartlett, John, 1: 41; 3: 3, 5
Bartlett, Josiah, 1: 293
Bartlett, Marshall K., 3: 241; 4: 475, 482*b*
Bartlett, Ralph W., 2: 34
Barton, Lyman G., Jr., 2: 119; 4: 389*b*
Baruch, Bernard M., 1: 272
Baruch Committee, 1: 272–273

base hospitals. *See also* military reconstruction hospitals; US Army Base Hospitals
   AEF and, 4: 417, 419–420
   amputations and, 4: 418
   Boston-derived, 4: 420*t*
   Camp Devens, 4: 452
   Camp Taylor, 4: 452
   field splinting and, 4: 408
   Harvard Units and, 4: 419–420, 437–438
   injuries and mortality rates in, 4: 424
   organization of American, 4: 419–420
   orthopaedics surgery and, 4: 406, 412, 417–419, 440, 443, 445, 451–453
   training in, 4: 420–421
   US and British medical staff in, 4: 422
   wounded soldiers and, 4: 385, 414, 416–417
basic fibroblast growth factor (bFGF), 3: 445
Bateman, James E., 2: 317; 3: 295
Bates, Frank D. (1925–2011)
   Boston Children's Hospital and, 2: 301
   Brigham and Women's Hospital and, 4: 193
   Korean War and, 2: 218
   PBBH and, 4: 20, 22, 116, 128
   Winchester Hospital and, 3: 299
Battle of Bunker Hill, 1: *17*, 18, *18*, 19, 22
Battle of Lexington and Concord, 1: 17–18, 22
"Battle of the Delta, The," 1: 245–247
Baue, Arthur, 1: 90
Bauer, Thomas, 4: 174
Bauer, Walter, 2: 82, 171; 3: 335
Bayne-Jones, Stanhope, 4: 405*b*
Beach, Henry H. A., 2: 24; 3: 40
Bean, Harold C., 2: 230
Bearse, Carl, 4: 208
Beattie, George, 2: 300
Beauchamp, Richard, 2: 351, *351*
Bedford Veterans Administration Hospital, 3: 314
Beecher, Henry K., 1: 171, 239; 3: 96
Begg, Alexander S., 1: 88
Bell, Anna Elizabeth Bowman, 2: 219
Bell, Emily J. Buck, 2: 220
Bell, Enoch, 2: 219
Bell, J. L., 1: 24
Bell, John, 1: 37

Bell, John F. (1909–1989)
   Boston Children's Hospital and, 2: 299
   club foot treatment, 2: 208
   Crippled Children's Clinic and, 2: 221
   Crotched Mountain Foundation, 2: 221
   death of, 2: 221
   disabled children and, 2: 221
   education and training, 2: 219, 220*b*
   Journal of Bone and Joint Surgery editor, 2: 221
   marriage and family, 2: 220
   Ober and, 2: 220
   Palmer Memorial Hospital and, 2: 219–220
   PBBH and, 2: 220
   pediatric orthopaedics and, 2: 221
   publications of, 2: 208, 220–221
   University of Vermont and, 2: 220–221
   Vermont Department of Health and, 2: 221
Bell, Joseph, 1: 84
Bell, Sir Charles, 1: 37, 73, 76
Bellare, Anuj, 4: 194
Bellevue Medical College, 2: 63
Bemis, George, 1: 307, 317
Bender, Anita, 4: 81
Bender, Ralph H. (1930–1999), 4: *80*
   on back pain, 4: 80
   Beth Israel Hospital and, 4: 247
   death of, 4: 81
   education and training, 4: 80
   hospital appointments, 4: 80
   marriage and family, 4: 81
   private medical practice, 4: 80
   professional memberships, 4: 81
   RBBH and, 4: 41*b*, 68, 80, 102
   US Air Force and, 4: 80
Benet, George, 4: 389*b*
Bennet, Eban E., 2: 72, 74–75
Bennett, G. A., 3: 335
Bennett, George E., 2: 77–78, 119; 4: 473
Benz, Edward, 2: 331
Berenberg, William, 2: 196, 213, 354, 406, 408
Bergenfeldt, E., 4: 356
Berlin, David D.
   Beth Israel Hospital and, 4: 361
   Boston City Hospital and, 4: 361
   education and training, 4: 361
   publications and research, 4: 361
   scaphoid fracture treatment, 4: 361

Tufts Medical School appointment, 4: 361
Bernard, Claude, 1: 82; 3: 142
Bernard, Francis, 1: 8, 13
Bernese periacetabular osteotomy, 2: 391–392
Bernhardt, Mark, 4: 263
Bernstein, Fredrika Ehrenfried, 4: 220
Bernstein, Irving, 4: 220
Bernstein, J., 1: 168
Berry, George P., 1: 180; 2: 183, 324; 3: 202, 334; 4: 113, 303
Bertody, Charles, 1: 60
Berven, Sigurd, 3: *278*
Beth Israel Deaconess Medical Center (BIDMC)
    Augustus White III Symposium, 4: 265, 266*b*
    Bierbaum and, 1: 233–234
    CareGroup and, 4: 281
    Carl J. Shapiro Department of Orthopaedics, 4: 288
    East Campus, 4: *213*, *287*
    Emergency Department, 4: 286
    financial difficulties, 4: 283–284
    formation of, 4: 214, 223, 270, 281, 283
    HCORP and, 4: 284, 288
    as HMS teaching hospital, 4: 214
    Kocher and, 2: 377
    orthopaedics department, 1: 171; 4: 284–288
    orthopaedics department chiefs, 4: 289*b*
    orthopaedics residencies, 1: 223–224, 234, 236, 242; 4: 285–288
    West Campus, 4: *213*, *280*
Beth Israel Hospital Association, 4: 204–205
Beth Israel Hospital (BIH)
    affiliation with Harvard Medical School, 4: 213–214, 251
    affiliation with Tufts Medical School, 4: 213–214, 214*b*, 228
    Brookline Avenue location, 4: 211, *211*, 228
    continuing medical education and, 4: 208
    establishment of new location, 4: 210, 210*b*, 211
    facilities for, 4: 207–208, 210
    financial difficulties, 4: 210–211, 281
    founding of, 4: 199
    growth of, 4: 209–210
    HCORP and, 1: 218; 4: 247–248
    HMS courses at, 1: 158
    house officers at, 4: 209*b*
    immigrant care in, 4: 283
    infectious disease fellowship, 1: 91
    internships at, 1: 196
    Jewish patients at, 4: 199, 205–206, 223
    Jewish physician training at, 1: 158; 4: 199, 283
    leadership of, 4: 206–211
    medical education and, 4: 213
    merger with New England Deaconess Hospital, 4: 214, 223, 270, 281, 283
    Mueller Professorship, 4: 263
    non-discrimination and, 4: 199
    opening of, 4: 205, 223
    operating room at, 4: *212*, *228*
    Orthopaedic Biomechanics Laboratory, 4: 262
    orthopaedic division chiefs, 4: 223, 289*b*
    orthopaedic residencies at, 4: 247–248, 251
    orthopaedics department at, 4: 213, 247, 262–263
    orthopaedics department chiefs, 4: 289*b*
    orthopaedics surgery at, 2: 377; 3: 325; 4: 208, 208*b*
    sports medicine and, 4: 255
    surgeon-in-chiefs at, 4: 283, 283*t*
    surgical departments at, 4: 208
    Townsend Street location, 4: 205, *205*, *206*, *207*
Beth Israel Medical Center (NY), 2: 408; 4: 206
Bettman, Henry Wald, 3: 86
Bhashyam, Abhiram R., 3: 463*b*
Bianco, Anthony, Jr., 2: 304
Bick, Edgar M., 1: 101, 114; 4: 88
Bicknell, Macalister, 3: 192
BIDMC. *See* Beth Israel Deaconess Medical Center (BIDMC)
Bierbaum, Benjamin
    as BIDMC chief of orthopaedics, 1: 233–234, 236; 4: 284–286, 289*b*
    Boston Children's Hospital and, 2: 286, 438
    Brigham and Women's Hospital and, 4: 193
    Crippled Children's Clinic and, 2: 314
    hip surgery and, 4: 284
    HMS appointment, 4: 284–285
    New England Baptist Hospital and, 1: 233; 4: 284
    PBBH and, 4: 22, 116, 128, 163
    Tufts Medical School appointment, 4: 284
Biesiadecki, Alfred, 1: 82
Bigelow, Henry Jacob (1818–1890), 1: *137*; 3: *23*, *30*, *32*, *46*
    as accomplished surgeon, 3: 39–41
    bladder stones treatment, 3: 41–42
    cellular pathology and, 3: 34
    Charitable Surgical Institution, 3: 30
    Chickahominy fever and, 3: 44
    Civil War medicine and, 3: 43–44
    code of conduct, 3: 47*b*, 48
    controversy over, 3: 44–45
    disbelief in antisepsis, 3: 45
    discounting of Warren, 3: 32–34, 36
    "Discourse on Self-Limited Diseases, A," 3: 12–13
    drawings of femur malunions, 3: *42*
    early life, 3: 23
    education and training, 3: 23–25
    ether and anesthetics, 3: 27–29, 31–34
    European medical studies, 3: 25
    excision of the elbow, 3: 34
    femoral neck fractures, 3: 38–39, *39*
    hip dislocations and, 3: 34–36, 38
    hip joint excision, 3: 34
    as HMS professor of surgery, 1: 137; 3: 34, 42–43, *43*, 44
    home in Newton, 3: *48*
    house on Tuckernuck Island, 3: *49*
    on the importance of flexion, 3: 38
    injury and death of, 3: 49–50
    "Insensibility During Surgical Operations Produced by Inhalation," 3: 27, *27*
    legacy of, 3: 45–48
    Manual of Orthopedic Surgery, 3: 25–26, *26*
    marriage and family, 3: 30, 34
    Mechanism of Dislocation and Fracture of the Hip, 3: 35, *35*, 38
    memberships and, 3: 48
    as MGH surgeon, 1: 84; 3: 15, 25–27, 30–31, *31*
    as MGH surgeon emeritus, 3: 45–46
    New England Peabody Home for Crippled Children and, 2: 230

Index

nitrous oxide and, 1: 56
orthopaedic contributions, 3: 34–36, 37*b*, 38–39
orthopaedics curriculum and, 1: 140
posthumous commemorations of, 3: 50, 50*b*, 51, 51*b*
reform of HMS and, 1: 139; 3: 44–45
resistance to antisepsis techniques, 1: 85
as senior surgeon at MGH, 1: 86; 2: 20
on spinal disease, 2: 57
support for House of the Good Samaritan, 1: 124
surgical illustrations and, 3: 25
surgical instruments and, 3: 40–41
Tremont Street Medical School and, 3: 26, 42
ununited fractures research, 3: 34–35
on use of ether, 1: 57, 59, 61–62
Bigelow, Jacob, 1: 60, 296, 299–300, 302; 3: 12, 23, 42
Bigelow, Mary Scollay, 3: 23
Bigelow, Sturgis, 1: *61*
Bigelow, Susan Sturgis, 3: 30, 34
Bigelow, W. S. (William Sturgis), 3: 23, 34, 40–41, 47*b*, 48, 50
Bigelow Building (MGH), 3: 15–17
Bigelow Medal, 3: *49*, 50
Bigelow's septum, 3: 39
Bigos, Stanley, 2: 371
BIH/Camp International Visiting Lecture, 4: 263
Billroth, Theodor, 1: 81–82
Binney, Horace, 3: 237; 4: 420
Biochemistry and Physiology of Bone (Bourne), 3: 337
bioethics, 4: 324
Biography of Otto E. Aufranc, A, 3: *246*
Biomaterials and Innovative Technologies Laboratory, 3: 463, 464*b*
biomechanics
    backpack loads and, 2: 408
    bone structure property relations, 2: 410
    collagen in the intervertebral discs and, 2: 328
    CT arthrography and, 2: 410
    early study of, 1: xxii
    Harrington rods and, 2: 325
    hips and, 2: 407
    laboratory for, 3: 220
    orthopaedics education and, 1: 220, 230, 241
    osteoarthritis and, 3: 322, 326–328, 383–384
    posterior cruciate ligament injury and, 3: 448
    subchondral bone with impact loading, 3: 326–327
"Biomechanics of Baseball Pitching" (Pappas), 2: *288*
Biomotion Laboratory, 3: 463, 464*b*
biopsy, 3: 390–391
Bird, Larry, 2: 369
birth abnormalities, 2: 275, 334, *334*
birth fractures, 2: 172. *See also* congenital pseudarthrosis of the tibia
birth palsies research, 2: 415, 417, *417*, 418–420
Black, Eric, 4: 190*b*
Blackman, Kenneth D., 1: 178
bladder stones, 3: 41–42
Blake, John Bapst, 4: 291
Blake, Joseph A., 2: 118; 4: 416
Bland, Edward, 4: 482*b*
Bland, Edward F., 3: 241; 4: 22
Blazar, Philip, 3: 410; 4: 194
Blazina, M. E., 1: 279
blood poisoning, 2: 299
blood transfusions, 1: 23; 3: 313
Bloodgood, Joseph C., 3: 137
bloodletting, 1: 9, 23, 74
Bloomberg, Maxwell H., 4: 208*b*
Blount, Walter, 2: 176, 335
Blumer, George, 2: 158
Boachie-Adjei, Oheneba, 4: 266*b*
Bock, Arlie V., 1: 265; 2: 253
Bock, Bernard, 1: 217*b*
body mechanics, 3: 81, 91; 4: 82–83, 233, 236
Body Mechanics in Health and Disease (Goldthwait et al.), 3: 91; 4: 53, 62
Body Snatchers, 1: *32*
Bohlman, Henry H., 4: 266*b*
Böhm, Max, 3: 67, 71, 265–266
Boland, Arthur L. (1935–), 1: *283*, 285
    awards and honors, 1: 288–289
    Brigham and Women's Hospital and, 1: 284; 4: 163, 193
    Children's Hospital/MGH combined program and, 1: 283
    on concussions, 1: 286–287
    education and training, 1: 283–284
    Harvard University Health Service and, 1: 284
    as head surgeon for Harvard athletics, 1: 284–288; 3: 399
    as HMS clinical instructor, 1: 166, 284
    knee injuries and, 1: 287
    as MGH clinical faculty, 3: 464*b*
    as MGH surgeon, 3: 399
    PBBH and, 4: 116, 128, 163
    publications of, 1: 286, 288
    sports medicine and, 1: 284–289; 2: 384; 3: 448, 460*b*
    women basketball players and, 1: 285–286
Boland, Jane Macknight, 1: 289
Bonar, Lawrence C., 2: 324
bone and joint disorders
    arthrodesis and, 3: 165
    atypical multiple case tuberculosis, 2: 257
    bone atrophy and, 3: 170
    chondrosarcoma, 3: 406
    conditions of interest in, 3: 82*b*
    fusion and, 3: 368
    Legg and, 2: 110
    lubrication and, 3: 324–327
    mobilization of, 4: 27*b*
    PBBH annual report, 4: 13, 13*t*, 16
    sacroiliac joint treatment, 3: 183–184
    schools for disabled children, 2: 37
    subchondral bone research, 3: 326–327, *327*
    total disability following fractures, 3: *373*
    tubercular cows and, 2: 16
    tuberculosis in pediatric patients, 2: 308–309
    tuberculosis of the hip, 3: 148
    tuberculosis treatment, 2: 11, 25; 3: 166, 289
    use of x-rays, 3: 101–103
bone banks, 3: 386, 388, 396, 433
bone cement, 4: 129, 133, 171
bone grafts
    arthrodesis procedures, 3: 368
    Boston approach and, 2: 392
    chemotherapy and, 2: 423
    chronic nonunions of the humerus and, 2: *96*
    early study of, 1: xxiii
    flexion injuries and, 3: 348
    Grice procedure and, 2: 209–210
    injured soldiers and, 3: 336, *337*
    kyphosis and, 2: 343
    modified Colonna reconstructive method, 3: 194
    non-union fractures and, 2: 238; 3: 59
    posterior spinal fusion and, 2: 341
    radioactive calcium tracers in, 2: 237, 240
    spinal fusion and, 3: 208, 425

tibial pseudarthrosis in neurofibromatosis case, 2: 175–176
   total hip replacement and, 3: 279
bone granuloma, 2: 171
bone growth
   activating transcription factor-2 (ATF-2) and, 2: 330
   Digby's method for measuring, 2: 170, 170*t*
   distal femur and proximal tibia, 2: 191–192, *192*, 193
   effects of irradiation on epiphyseal growth, 3: 331
   epiphyseal arrest and, 2: 192, 192*t*, 193
   Green and, 2: 170, 191–194
   Green-Andersen growth charts, 2: 193, *193*, 194
   Moseley's growth charts, 2: 194
   orthoroentgenograms and, 2: 192–193
   Paley multiplier method, 2: 194
   research in, 2: 191–194
   skeletal age in predictions, 2: 192
bone irradiation, 2: 237
Bone Sarcoma Registry of the American College of Surgeons, 4: 102
bone sarcomas, 3: 136–137, 137*t*, 138–140, 140*b*, 141–142
bones and teeth
   apatite crystals and, 2: 321
   collagen in, 2: 327–328
   electron microscopes and, 2: 323, *324*
   Haversian systems in, 2: 241
   hydroxylysine and, 2: 327–328
   mineralized crystals, 2: 325–326
   research in, 2: 322–324
   research in lesions, 2: 236
Bonfiglio, Michael, 3: 303
Boothby, Walter M., 4: 216, 323, 389*b*, 422*b*
Boott, Francis, 1: 59
Borden Research Award, 2: 319
Borges, Larry, 3: 420
Boron Neutron Capture Synovectomy, 4: 136
Bosch, Joanne P., 4: 183
Bost, Frederick C., 2: 274; 4: 60
Boston, Mass.
   annual Christmas tree from Halifax, 3: 135, *135*
   cholera epidemic, 1: 295; 4: 293
   colonial economy in, 1: 10
   Committee of Correspondence in, 1: 16
   Fort Warren, 1: 20
   Halifax Harbor explosion aid, 3: 134–135
   infectious disease in, 1: 7–9; 2: 4
   inoculation hospitals, 1: 8–9
   Irish Catholics in, 4: 200
   Irish immigration to, 4: 293
   Jewish immigration to, 4: 199–200, 220
   Jewish physicians in, 4: 199–200
   Jewish Quarter, 4: 200, *200*
   malnutrition in, 2: 4
   maps, 1: *7*, *114*, *296*
   military reconstruction hospital and, 4: 444
   need for hospital in, 1: 41; 3: 3; 4: 293–294, 294*b*
   orthopaedics institutions in, 1: 189–190
   Stamp Act protests in, 1: 11–13
   tea party protest and, 1: 15–16
   Townshend Act protests, 1: 13–14
   Warren family and, 1: 4*b*
Boston Almshouse, 1: 29; 3: 3
   HMS clinical teaching at, 1: 28, 40; 3: 4–5
   house pupils at, 1: 80
   inadequacy of, 1: 41; 3: 3–4
   John Ball Brown and, 1: 96
   medical care at, 2: 20; 3: 3–4
Boston Arm, 2: 326, *326*; 3: 287
Boston Association of Cardiac Clinics, 1: 129
Boston Ballet, 2: 384, *384*
Boston brace, 2: 339–340, *340*, 358–359, *359–360*, *361*, 423, *424*
Boston Brace Instructional Courses, 2: 358
Boston Bruins, 3: 348, 356–357, 357*b*, 397, 399, 448; 4: 342
Boston Children's Hospital (BCH), 1: *194*; 2: 177, 437, 438
   Act of Incorporation, 2: 7, *7*
   astragalectomy at, 2: 93–94
   bedside teaching at, 2: *435*
   Berlin polio epidemic team, 2: 260, 264
   Boston brace and, 2: 339–340, 423
   Boston Concept and, 2: 392
   cerebral palsy cases, 2: 171–172
   Cerebral Palsy Clinic, 2: 402, 406, 409
   charitable surgical appliances, 2: *14*
   children with poliomyelitis and, 1: 191; 2: 163
   children's convalescence and, 2: 9
   clinical service rotations, 1: 198
   clinical surgery curricula at, 1: 141, 143, 147, 151, 155–157, 162
   cows and, 2: *429*
   decline in skeletal tuberculosis admissions, 2: 16, 16*t*
   Department of Medicine, 2: 427
   Department of Orthopaedic Surgery, 1: 171–172, 189–190; 2: 10–13, 15–16, 40, *98*, *133*, *156*, *177*, *200*, *222*, *252*, *255*, *283*, *293*, 354–355, 427, 434, 438–439, 439*b*; 3: 67
   Department of Surgery, 2: 427
   endowed professorships, 2: 438, 439*b*
   founding of, 1: 123; 2: 3–9
   Growth Study (Green and Anderson), 2: 193
   HCORP and, 1: 213, 215
   hip disease and, 2: 52
   House of the Good Samaritan merger, 1: 130; 2: 433
   house officers at, 1: 184, 189
   house officer's certificate, 2: *41*
   impact of World War II on, 4: 468
   Infantile Paralysis Clinic, 2: 79
   innovation and change at, 2: 427–428, 430–434, 436–439
   internships at, 1: 196
   Massachusetts Infantile Paralysis Clinics, 2: 188–189
   military surgeon training at, 1: 151, 191; 4: 396
   Myelodysplasia Clinic, 2: 359, 402
   named funds, 2: 436, 439*b*
   nursing program at, 2: 13–14
   objections to, 2: 8–9
   organizational models, 2: 436–437
   orthopaedic admissions at, 2: 15*t*, 40, 40*t*
   orthopaedic chairpersons, 2: 15*b*
   orthopaedic surgeries, 2: 9–12, 12*t*, 13, *13*, 14–15, 39–40, 337–338, 338*t*
   orthopaedics residencies, 1: 186–187, 199, 202–207, 211, 217–218, 224–225; 2: *413*
   outpatient services at, 1: 190; 2: 11–12
   patient registry, 2: *10*
   PBBH and, 4: 10, 14
   pediatrics at, 2: 3
   polio clinics at, 2: 78–79, 188
   private/public system in, 2: 313, 337, 339
   psoas abscesses and, 2: 54
   radiology at, 2: 16, *16*, 17, 17*t*, *431*
   Report of the Medical Staff, 2: 9

Index

resident salaries, 1: 206, *206*
scoliosis clinic at, 2: 35–36, 84–86
Sever-L'Episcopo procedure, 2: 417
Spanish American War patients, 4: *311*
specialization in, 2: 11
Spinal Surgery Service, 2: 359
spinal tuberculosis and, 2: 11, 308–309
sports medicine and, 2: 287, 384
Statement by Four Physicians, 2: 6–7
surgeon-scholars at, 2: 217, 357
surgical procedures for scoliosis, 2: *369*
surgical training at, 1: 188–189
teaching clinics at, 1: 194; 2: *62*
teaching fellows, 1: 192–193
tuberculosis patients, 2: 275
20th century overview of, 2: 427–428, 430–434, 436–439
use of radiographs, 2: 54
Boston Children's Hospital (BCH). Facilities
  appliance shop at, 2: 22, *22*, *431*
  Bader building, 2: 432, *432–433*
  Bader Solarium, 2: *432*
  Boy's Ward, 2: *14*
  expansion of, 2: 9–11, 13, *433*, 434*t*
  Fegan building, 2: *433*
  Functional Therapy Room, 2: *432*
  gait laboratory, 2: 107, 406
  Girl's Surgical Ward, 2: *15*
  gymnasium, 2: *433*
  Hunnewell Building entrance, 2: *429*
  on Huntington Ave., 2: 11, *11*, 12, *12*, 427–428, *428*
  Ida C. Smith ward, 2: *431*
  Infant's Hospital, 2: *431*
  lack of elevators in, 2: 430, *430*
  on Longwood Avenue, 2: 64, 428, 430–431
  Medical Center and Prouty Garden, 2: *436*
  orthopaedic research laboratory, 2: 234
  Pavilion Wards, 2: *435*
  research laboratories, 2: 234–236, 285, 434, 438–439
  standard ward in, 2: *144*, *429*
  Ward I, 2: *434*
  at Washington and Rutland Streets, 2: *11*
  in the winter, 2: *430*

Boston Children's Hospital/Massachusetts General residency program, 1: 210; 2: 144
Boston City Base Hospital No. 7 (France), 4: 301–302
Boston City Hospital (BCH), 4: *306*, *379*
  affiliation with Boston University Medical School, 4: 296–297, 303, 380
  affiliation with Harvard Medical School, 4: 296, 298, 302–303, 379–380
  affiliation with Tufts Medical School, 4: 228, 296–297, 303
  Base Hospital No. 7 and, 1: 256; 4: 301–302, 420*t*, 438–439
  Bone and Joint Service, 4: 306–307, 328, 333–334, 357, 377, 377*t*, 380*b*
  Bradford and, 2: 21; 4: 298, 303, 307
  Burrell and, 4: 298–299, *299*, 300–301, 307
  Centre building, 4: *295*
  clinical courses for Harvard students at, 4: 380*t*–381*t*
  compound fracture therapy at, 4: *335*, 337
  construction of, 4: 295
  end of Harvard Medical School relationship, 4: 380
  ether tray at, 4: *298*
  examining room, 4: *300*
  fracture treatment and, 4: 362
  Harvard Fifth Surgical Service at, 4: 275, 277, 297, 302–303, 305–306
  Harvard Medical Unit at, 4: 296–297, 303
  house officers at, 4: 305, 305*b*
  intern and residency training programs, 4: 303–306
  internships at, 1: 189, 196
  Joseph H. Shortell Fracture Unit, 4: *342*, 342, 357
  medical school affiliations, 4: 370–371
  merger with Boston University Medical Center Hospital, 4: 297
  Nichols and, 1: 174, 252; 4: 301–302
  opening of, 4: 295–296
  operating room at, 4: *298*, *301*
  orthopaedic residencies at, 1: 186, 199; 3: 237; 4: 377–380
  orthopaedic surgery at, 4: 307

  Outpatient Department, 4: *300*, 357
  Pavilion I, 4: *295*
  physical therapy room, 4: *308*
  planning for, 4: 293–295
  plot plan for, 4: *293*, *307*
  Relief Station, 4: *305*
  specialty services at, 4: 306–307
  staffing of, 4: 296
  surgeon-scholars at, 1: 174; 4: 333, 357
  Surgical Outpatient Department Building, 4: *295*
  surgical services at, 4: 297–303, 307, 370–371
  Surgical Ward, 4: *295*
  teaching clinics at, 1: 141, 143
  Thorndike Building, 4: *296*
  Thorndike Memorial Laboratory, 4: 297
  treatment of children in, 2: 4
  Tufts University Medical Service and, 4: 297
  undergraduate surgical education, 4: 303
  Ward O, 4: *296*
  wards in, 4: *301*
  West Roxbury Department, 4: 447–448
  women in orthopaedics at, 1: 200
Boston City Hospital Relief Station, 2: 269
Boston Concept, 2: 391, *391*, 392
Boston Dispensary, 1: 40, 96; 2: 20, 306; 3: 3; 4: 48, 311, *311*, 358
Boston Dynamics, 4: 173
Boston Hospital for Women, 4: 42–43, 69, 113–114, 119
Boston Infant's Hospital, 2: 242
Boston Interhospital Augmentation Study (BIAS), 3: 248–249
Boston Lying-in-Hospital, 1: 123; 4: 113–114
Boston Massacre, 1: 14–16
Boston Medical and Surgical Journal, 4: 293, 294*b*
Boston Medical Association, 1: 25, 38; 3: 25
Boston Medical Center (BMC), 4: 89, 297
Boston Medical Library, 1: 39, 59; 2: 271
Boston Medical Society, 4: 200, 202
Boston Organ Bank Group, 3: 386
Boston Orthopaedic Group, 4: 251, 285–286, 288
"Boston Orthopaedic Institution, The" (Cohen), 1: 114

Boston Orthopedic Club, 2: 171, 230, 294, 329; 3: 289; 4: 66
Boston Orthopedic Institution
    attraction of patients from the U.S. and abroad, 1: 99
    Buckminster Brown and, 1: 107, 118, 120–122
    closing of, 1: 121–122; 3: 30
    founding of, 1: xxiv, 99
    John Ball Brown and, 1: 99–100, 107, 113–114, 118–122
    long term treatment in, 2: 25
    origins and growth of, 1: 114–118
    scholarship on, 1: 114
    treatment advances in, 1: 118–120
    use of ether, 1: 107, 118
Boston Orthopedique Infirmary, 1: 99–100, 113. *See also* Boston Orthopedic Institution
Boston Pathology Course, 1: 216, 218
Boston Prosthetics Course, 1: 220
Boston Red Sox, 1: 258; 2: 288; 3: 348; 4: 345
Boston Rugby Football Club, 2: 383, *383*, 400
Boston School of Occupational Therapy, 4: 30, 32
Boston School of Physical Education, 3: 84
Boston School of Physical Therapy, 4: 30, 32
Boston Shriner's Hospital, 1: 123
Boston Society for Medical Improvement, 1: 61; 3: 44, 48, 150
Boston Surgical Society, 2: 69; 3: 50, 65
Boston University School of Medicine, 1: 239; 2: 273–274; 4: 67–68, 296
Boston Veterans Administration Hospital, 1: 71, 90; 3: 298
Bottomly, John T., 3: 116
Bouillaud, J. B., 4: 93
Bourne, Geoffrey, 3: 337
Bouvé, Marjorie, 4: 444
Bouvier, Sauveur-Henri Victor, 1: 106
Bowditch, Charles Pickering, 1: 82; 3: 142
Bowditch, Henry I., 1: 53, 73, 82, *82*; 2: 306; 3: 9, 97–98; 4: 3
Bowditch, Henry P., 2: 48; 3: 94
Bowditch, Katherine Putman, 3: 142
Bowditch, Nathaniel, 3: 15, 142, 146
Bowen, Abel, 1: *29*
Bowker, John H., 3: 299

Boyd, A. D., Jr., 4: 136
Boyd, Robert J. (1930–), 3: *254, 256*
    Barr and, 3: 255
    Children's Hospital/MGH combined program and, 3: 253
    education and training, 3: 253
    hip surgery and, 3: 253
    HMS appointment, 3: 254
    Lemuel Shattuck Hospital and, 3: 253
    Lynn General Hospital and, 3: 253
    MGH Staff Associates and, 3: 256
    as MGH surgeon, 3: 253, 256, 398*b*
    private medical practice, 3: 256
    Problem Back Clinic at MGH and, 3: 254
    problem back service and, 3: 388*t*
    publications and research, 3: 253–255, *255*
    Scarlet Key Society and, 3: 253
    Sledge and, 4: 127
    spine and trauma work, 3: 254–255, 420, 460*b*
    Trauma Management, 3: 62, 253
Boyes, Joseph, 3: 427
Boylston, Thomas, 3: 5
Boylston Medical School, 1: 138
Boylston Medical Society, 3: 25–26, 48
Bozic, Kevin J., 1: 225; 4: 266*b*
brachial plexus injuries, 2: 90–91, 96; 3: 412–414
Brachial Plexus Injuries (Leffert), 3: 414
brachioradialis transfer, 2: 153–154, *154*
Brackett, Elliott G. (1860–1942), 3: *147, 157*; 4: *394*
    Advisory Orthopedic Board and, 3: 157
    AOA meeting and, 2: 137
    Beth Israel Hospital and, 4: 208*b*
    Boston Children's Hospital and, 2: 13, 34, 40, 247, 264; 3: 147–148, 153
    Boston City Hospital and, 4: 305*b*, 308*b*, 406
    Bradford and, 3: 147, 150–151
    on Buckminster Brown, 3: 150
    chronic hip disease and, 3: 147, 151
    Clinical Congress of Surgeons in North America and, 3: 116

Department for Military Orthopedics and, 4: 405–406
    early life, 3: 147
    education and training, 3: 147
    on functional inactivity, 2: 110
    on fusion in tubercular spines, 3: 148–149, 157–158, 158*b*
    on gunshot injuries, 3: 156, 156*b*
    HMS appointment, 3: 154
    HMS Orthopaedic surgery and, 1: 171
    hot pack treatment and, 2: 264
    House of the Good Samaritan and, 2: 114; 3: 148
    interest in the hip, 3: 148
    Journal of Bone and Joint Surgery editor, 3: 157–159, 160*b*, 161, 344
    legacy of, 3: 161–162
    marriage and, 3: 154
    memberships and, 3: 161
    as MGH orthopaedics chief, 2: 129–130; 3: 11*b*, 155, 227
    as MGH surgeon, 2: 99; 3: 153
    military surgeon training and, 2: 42; 4: 393, 395–396
    pathological findings in tubercular spine specimens, 3: 154–155
    Pott's Disease treatment, 3: 148–150
    private medical practice, 3: 154
    publications and research, 2: 56, 61; 3: 148, 151, 153–155
    RBBH and, 4: 406
    rehabilitation of soldiers and, 4: 396, 439, 444
    on sacroiliac joint fusion, 3: 185
    schools for disabled children, 2: 36; 3: 151, 161
    scoliosis treatment and, 2: 35, 56; 3: 151–152
    Section of Orthopaedic Surgery and, 4: 412
    treatment by Bradford, 3: 147
    US Army Medical Corps and, 4: 405
    use of orthopaedics apparatus, 3: 150–151
    Volunteer Aid Association and, 3: 152–153
    World War I and, 3: 156–157; 4: 404–405, 411
Brackett, Katherine F. Pedrick, 3: 154
Bradford, Charles F., 2: 19
Bradford, Charles Henry (1904–2000)
    Battle of Corregidor, 4: 363–364

Index

BCH Bone and Joint Service, 4: 367
Boston City Hospital and, 4: 362
Boston University Medical School appointment, 4: 366
Britten hip fusion technique and, 4: 363
civil defense and, 4: 364–366
Combat Over Corregidor, 4: *364*
Cotting School and, 4: 367
death of, 4: 368
education and training, 4: 361–362
Faulkner Hospital and, 4: 362
fracture treatment and, 4: 362
hospital appointments, 4: 364
legacy of, 4: 366–368
marriage and family, 4: 361
Massachusetts Medical Society lecture, 4: 365, 366b, 367, 367b
Mt. Auburn Hospital and, 4: 362
poetry writing and, 4: 364
professional memberships, 4: 368
publications and research, 4: 352, 363, 365, *365*, 368
tibial spine fracture case, 4: 365
Tufts Medical School appointment, 4: 366
US Army Medical Corps and, 4: 363–364
World War II medical volunteers and, 4: 362–363
Bradford, Charles Hickling, 2: 42–43
Bradford, Edith Fiske, 2: 42; 4: 361
Bradford, Edward H. (1848–1926), 2: *19*, *39*, *44*
AOA address, 2: 24–26
as AOA president, 2: 43
as BCH surgeon-in-chief, 2: 39–40, *41*
Boston Children's Hospital and, 2: 10–11, 13, 15–16, 21, 29, 39–40
Boston City Hospital and, 4: 298, 303, 307
Boston City Hospital appointments, 2: 21, 24
Bradford Frame and, 2: 27, *27*, 30–31, *31*, 32
Buckminster Brown and, 2: 20; 3: 150
on Burrell, 4: 298–299
CDH treatment, 2: 32–33, *33*, 34
club foot apparatus, 2: 22–23, *23*
club foot treatment, 2: 22–24, 28, *28*, 29
curative workshops and, 4: 403
as dean of HMS, 1: 172–174; 2: 15, 41–42; 4: 324
death of, 2: 43–44
early life, 2: 19
education and training, 2: 19–20
European medical studies, 1: 186; 2: 20
first craniotomy performed, 2: 24–25
FitzSimmons and, 2: 255
general surgery and, 2: 24
hip disease treatment, 2: 21–22, 32
HMS appointment, 2: 21, 40–41, 428; 4: 213
House of the Good Samaritan and, 1: 128–130; 2: 21
influences on, 2: 20, 22
knee flexion contracture appliance, 2: *20*, *21*
knee valgus deformity, 2: *21*
legacy of, 2: 42–44
loss of eyesight, 2: 43
Lovett and, 2: 49
marriage and family, 2: 42
on medical education, 4: 299–301
memberships and, 2: 43
method of reducing the gibbus, 3: *149*
as MGH surgeon, 3: 266
nose and throat clinic creation, 2: 40–41
orthopaedic brace shop, 2: 22, *22*
as orthopaedic chair, 2: 15b
Orthopaedic Journal Club, 3: 369
orthopaedic surgery advances, 2: 27, 36, 39–40
Orthopedic Surgery, 4: 318
osteotomies and, 2: 29, 34
poliomyelitis treatment, 2: 264
on Pott's Disease, 3: 148
on preventative measures, 2: 36
private medical practice and, 1: 176
as professor of orthopaedic surgery, 1: 69, 111, 141, 143, 171
"Progress in Orthopaedic Surgery" series, 2: 43, 297
schools for disabled children, 2: 36–39, 67, 97, 308; 3: 151
scientific study and, 1: 256
scoliosis treatment, 2: 35, *35*, *36*, 58
Sever and, 2: 92
Soutter and, 2: 292, 297
as surgical house officer at MGH, 2: 20
teaching hospitals and, 1: 174, 187–188
Treatise on Orthopaedic Surgery, A, 1: 108, 143; 2: 29–30, 43, 50, *50*, 51
treatment of Brackett, 3: 147
tuberculosis treatment, 2: 32
Bradford, Edward H., Jr., 2: 42
Bradford, Edward, Jr., 4: 361
Bradford, Eliza Edes Hickling, 2: 19
Bradford, Elizabeth, 2: 42; 4: 361, 368
Bradford, Gamaliel, 1: 96
Bradford, Mary Lythgoe, 4: 361
Bradford, Robert Fiske, 2: 42
Bradford, William, 2: 19
Bradford Frame, 2: 27, *27*, 30–31, *31*, 32
Bradlee, Helen C., 3: 18
Bradlee, J. Putnam, 3: 18
Bradley, Alfred E., 4: 416
Bradley, John, 3: 289
Braintree HealthSouth Hospital, 4: 194
Brase, D. W., 4: 167
Braswell, Margaret, 2: 349
Braunwald, Eugene, 4: 119
Brazelton, T. Berry, 2: 385
Breed's Hill (Bunker Hill), 1: 18, *18*
Breene, R. G., 4: 93
Bremer, John L., 4: *6*
Brendze, R., 3: *461*
Brengle, Fred E., 3: 463
Brengle, Joan, 3: 463
Brewster, Albert H. (1892–1988), 2: *222*
AAOS and, 4: 337
Boston Children's Hospital and, 2: 222–223, 231, 252, 274; 4: 60, 338
countersinking the talus, 2: 228, 283
Crippled Children's Clinic and, 2: 230, 287
death of, 2: 231
donations to Boston Medical Library, 2: 271
education and training, 2: 221
foot deformity treatment, 2: 228–229
grand rounds and, 2: 230
HMS appointment, 2: 222–223; 4: 60
Marlborough Medical Associates and, 2: 269, 299
marriage and family, 2: 231
New England Peabody Home for Crippled Children and, 2: 230–231
Osgood tribute, 2: 136

PBBH and, 2: 222; 4: 16–18, 20, 110
private medical practice, 2: 146, 230, *230*
professional memberships and, 2: 230
publications of, 2: 79, 223, 225, 227–229; 4: 240
scoliosis treatment, 2: 223–228
on supracondylar fractures of the humerus, 2: 229
turnbuckle jacket and, 2: 223–224, *224*, 225, 227
World War I service and, 2: 221–222
Brewster, Albert H., Jr., 2: 231
Brewster, Elsie Estelle Carter, 2: 231
Brewster, Nancy, 2: 231
Brezinski, Mark, 4: 194
Brick, Gregory W., 4: 193, 195*b*
Brickley-Parsons, D., 2: 328
Bridges, Miss, 3: 133
Brigham, Elizabeth Fay, 4: vii, 1*b*, 23*b*, 24, 39*b*
Brigham, John Bent, 4: 1*b*
Brigham, Peter Bent, 4: 1, 1*b*, 2, 2*b*, 4–5, 22
Brigham, Robert Breck, 4: vii, 22, 23*b*, 24, 39*b*
Brigham, Uriah, 4: 1*b*
Brigham and Women's Hospital (BWH), 4: vii, *120*, *122*, *192*, *196*
　acute rehabilitation service, 4: 191
　Administrative Building, 4: *191*
　Ambulatory building, 4: *193*
　Ambulatory Care Center, 4: *193*, 194
　Bornstein Family Amphitheater, 4: *191*
　capitellocondylar total elbow replacements, 4: 146–147
　Carl J. and Ruth Shapiro Cardiovascular Center, 4: *195*
　carpal tunnel syndrome study, 2: 375
　Cartilage Repair Center, 4: 195*b*
　Center for Molecular Orthopaedics, 4: 194, 195*b*
　clinical and research faculty, 4: 195*b*
　Faulkner Hospital, 4: 194, *194*
　Foot and Ankle Center, 4: 194
　formation of, 4: 43, 113–114, 119–120, 127
　fundraising for, 4: 118
　HCORP and, 1: 213, 215
　Mary Horrigan Conner's Center for Women's Health, 4: *194*
　modernization of, 4: 191–196
　Musculoskeletal (MSK) Research Center, 4: 195*b*
　naming of, 4: 119, 123
　new facility construction, 4: 118–119, 122, 132
　opening of, 4: 121, *123*
　Orthopaedic and Arthritis Center, 4: 121, 123, 195*b*
　orthopaedic biomechanics laboratory, 4: 137–138
　orthopaedic chairmen at, 4: 196*b*
　orthopaedic grand rounds in, 4: 191
　orthopaedic research laboratory and, 4: 194
　orthopaedic surgery department, 1: 171; 4: 43, 113–115, 121
　orthopaedics fellowships, 1: 241
　orthopaedics residencies, 1: 217–218, 223–224, 241–242
　professional staff committee, 4: 132
　professorships at, 4: 195*b*
　RBBH as specialty arthritis hospital in, 4: 122–123
　research at, 4: 121
　Skeletal Biology Laboratory, 4: 195*b*
　staffing of, 4: 193–196
　surgeon-scholars at, 4: 143, 163, 193–194, 195*b*
　surgical caseloads at, 4: 194–195
　Tissue Engineering Laboratory, 4: 195*b*
　Total Joint Replacement Registry, 4: 141, *172*, 173
　transition period at, 4: 113–118, 132
　work with prosthetic devices at, 4: 122
Brigham and Women's Physician Organization (BWPO), 4: 192
Brigham and Women's/Mass General Health Care Center (Foxboro), 4: 194
Brigham Anesthesia Associates, 4: 22
Brigham Family, 4: 1*b*
Brigham Orthopaedic Foundation (BOF), 4: 123, 172, 191–192
Brigham Orthopedic Associates (BOA), 4: 123, 172, 191–192
British 31st General Hospital, 4: 485
British Base Hospital No. 12 (Rouen, France), 3: 166
British Expeditionary Forces (BEF)
　American Medical Corps and, 4: 420
　American medical volunteers and, 4: 405*b*, 425
　Base Hospital No. 5 and, 4: 420
　Harvard Unit and, 1: 256; 4: 10, 391, 438
　physician deaths in, 4: 425
　use of AEF base hospitals, 4: 420
British hospitals
　American surgeon-volunteers in, 4: 409
　documentation and, 4: 407
　general scheme of, 4: *414*
　increase in military, 4: 454
　orthopaedic surgery and, 4: 409
　registrars in, 4: 12
　World War I and, 4: 407, 409, 454
British Orthopaedic Association, 1: xxiv; 2: 137; 3: 345, 360; 4: 363, *404*
British Red Cross, 4: 399, 401
British Royal Army Medical Corps, 4: 393
British Society for Surgery of the Hand, 4: 95
Broderick, Thomas F., 3: 209, 332–333
Brodhurst, Bernard Edward, 1: 83, 106
Brodie, Sir Benjamin Collins, 1: 106
bronchitis, 2: 4
Bronfin, Isidore D., 4: 206, 209
Brooks, Barney, 3: 165–167, 170, *171*; 4: 178
Brooks, Charles, 1: 239
Brostrom, Frank, 2: 78, 110
Browder, N. C., 1: 259
Brower, Thomas D., 1: 162; 3: 382
Brown, Anna Ball, 1: 95
Brown, Arnold Welles, 1: 98
Brown, Buckminster (1819–1891), 1: *105*
　advancement of Harvard Medical School and, 1: 111
　advocacy for disabled children, 1: 107, 109, 126
　Boston Dispensary and, 2: 306
　Boston Orthopedic Institution and, 1: 107, 118, 120–122
　congenital hip dislocation treatment, 1: 108
　death of, 1: 111
　Edward H. Bradford and, 2: 20, 22
　European medical studies, 1: 105–106, 186
　forward-thinking treatment of, 1: 107–108
　House of the Good Samaritan and, 1: 107, 121–122, 125–128; 2: 49
　long-term treatment and, 2: 25
　marriage and, 1: 107

Index

orthopaedic specialization of, 1: 99, 107–108
orthopaedic treatment advances, 1: 118; 2: 26–27, 32
Pott's Disease and, 1: 97, 105, 109
publications of, 1: 110*b*, 120, *120*, 121
scoliosis brace and, 1: 109
Brown, Charles H., Jr., 4: 193, 195*b*
Brown, Douglas, 2: 163
Brown, Francis Henry
Boston Children's Hospital and, 2: 5, *5*, 6, 9–10, 21
on hospital construction, 2: 5
orthopaedics expertise, 2: 9
Brown, George, 1: 98
Brown, Jabez, 1: 95
Brown, John Ball (1784–1862), 1: *95*, 102
apparatus used for knee contracture, 1: *98*
Boston dispensary and, 1: 293
Boston Orthopedic Institution and, 1: 99–100, 107, 113–122; 3: 30
club foot treatment, 2: 36
correction of spine deformities, 1: 97–98, 100
death of, 1: 103, 122
early telemedicine by, 1: 100
education and training, 1: 95–96
establishment of orthopaedics as specialty, 1: 95–96, 98–99, 119
founding of Boston Orthopedic Institution, 1: xxiv
George Parkman and, 1: 296
legacy of, 1: 102–103
marriage and family, 1: 96–98
opening of orthopaedic specialty hospital, 1: 99
orthopaedic surgery and, 1: 99–102, 113; 2: 25–26
publications of, 1: 102*b*, 120, *120*, 121
Remarks on the Operation for the Cure of Club Feet with Cases, 1: 100
Report of Cases in the Orthopedic Infirmary of the City of Boston, 1: *120*
surgical appointments, 1: 96–97
Brown, John Warren, 1: 97
Brown, Larry, 4: 364
Brown, Lloyd T. (1880–1961), 4: *81*
on body mechanics and rheumatoid disease, 4: 82–83
Boston Children's Hospital and, 4: 82

Boston City Hospital and, 4: 406
Burrage Hospital and, 4: 226
Children's Island Sanitorium and, 4: 87
chronic disease treatment and, 4: 52
club foot treatment, 4: 84
congenital club foot and, 4: 81–82, *83*, 87
death of, 4: 39, 87*b*
education and training, 4: 81–82
HMS appointment, 2: 223; 4: 60, 86
hospital appointments, 4: 83
marriage and family, 4: 83, 87
medical officer teaching, 4: 84
MGH and, 4: 82, 84, 86
military surgeon training and, 2: 42
orthopaedics surgery and, 2: 66; 3: 268
Orthopedics and Body Mechanics Committee, 4: 235
posture research and, 4: 84, *84*, 85–86, 233
private medical practice, 4: 82
professional memberships, 4: 87, 87*b*
publications and research, 2: 297; 3: 91; 4: 82–84, 87
RBBH and, 3: 257; 4: vii, 25, 31–34, 36, 45, 79, 86–87, 93, 111, 406
RBBH Emergency Campaign speech, 4: 32, 32*b*
rehabilitation of soldiers and, 4: 444
retirement and, 4: 36
Brown, Marian Epes Wigglesworth, 4: 83
Brown, Percy E., 2: 16, 54; 3: 99
Brown, Rebecca Warren, 1: 96, 98
Brown, Sarah Alvord Newcomb, 1: 107
Brown, Sarah Tyler Meigs, 3: 257, 263
Brown, T., 3: 209, 214
Brown, Thornton (1913–2000), 1: *203*; 3: *257*, 263, 461
as AOA president, 3: 262, *262*, 263
back pain research and, 3: 257–258, *258*, 259–260
on Boston and orthopaedics, 1: 93; 2: 324
on changes at MGH Orthopaedic Service, 3: 453*b*–458*b*
Children's Hospital/MGH combined program and, 3: 257
death of, 3: 263

early life, 3: 257
education and training, 3: 257
Journal of Bone and Joint Surgery editor, 3: 260–262, 346
marriage and family, 3: 257
Massachusetts General Hospital, 1955–1980, The, 3: 299
as MGH orthopaedics chief, 3: 11*b*, 202, 227, *259*, 459
MGH residents and, 3: *259*, *260*, *459*
as MGH surgeon, 3: 257, 398*b*
Milton Hospital and, 3: 257
on Mt. Sinai Hospital, 4: 201–202
Norton-Brown spinal brace, 3: 317–319
"Orthopaedics at Harvard," 1: 195; 2: 271
private medical practice, 1: 203
publications and research, 3: 257–260, 317, 455*b*
RBBH and, 4: 37, 40
World War II service, 3: 257
Brown University Medical School, 3: 400–401
Browne, Hablot Knight, 1: *21*
Browne & Nichols School, 2: 83, 97
Brubacher, Jacob W., 3: 463*b*
Brugler, Guy, 2: 214
Brunschwig, Hieronymus, 4: 469
Bruschart, Thomas, 3: 431
Bryant, Henry, 3: 30
Bryant, Thomas, 1: 83
Buchanan, J. Robert, 3: 391
Buchbinder, Rachelle, 3: 437
Buchman, Frank N. D., 4: 57
Buchmanism, 4: 57
Bucholz, Carl Hermann (1874–unk.), 3: *264*
back pain research and, 3: 203
education and training, 3: 264
on exercise treatment of paralysis, 3: 265
HMS appointment, 3: 265
legacy of, 3: 269
as MGH surgeon, 3: 268
publications and research, 2: 136, 297
Therapeutic Exercise and Massage, 3: *269*
World War I and, 3: 268
Zander's medico-mechanical department and, 3: 71, 264–266, 266t, 267, 268*b*
Buck, Emily Jane, 2: 220
Buck's traction, 1: 80
Budd, J. W., 4: 102
Bulfinch, Charles, 1: 28, 41; 3: 10–11

Bulfinch Building (MGH), 1: *41*; 3: *9*, *13*, 15, *16*, 22, *60*, 70*b*
Bull, Charles, 3: 77
Bullard, S. E., 2: 244
Bunker Hill Monument Committee, 1: 68
Bunnin, Beverly D., 4: 101
Burgess, Earnest M., 3: 248
Burke, Dennis W., 3: 398, 460*b*, 464*b*
Burke, John, 3: 62, 253, 458*b*
burn care, 3: 336
Burne, F., 2: 98
Burnett, Joseph H. (1892–1963)
    BCH Bone and Joint Service, 4: 307, 328, 369, 371
    Boston City Hospital and, 4: 347, 368, 370–371
    Boston University Medical School appointment, 4: 368
    carpal scaphoid fracture case, 4: 368
    death of, 4: 371
    education and training, 4: 368
    football injury research, 4: 370, *370*
    HMS appointment, 4: 368
    marriage and, 4: 371
    professional memberships, 4: 371
    publications and research, 4: 368–370, *370*
    scaphoid fracture research, 4: 360, 368–369
    sports medicine and, 4: 368–370
Burnett, Margaret Rogers, 4: 371
Burns, Frances, 2: 260, 264
Burns, John, 3: *458*
Burns, Mary, 2: 214
Burrage Hospital, 4: 226, *227*
Burrell, Herbert L., 4: 298–299, *299*, 300–301, 307
Burrell-Cotton operation, 4: 329
Burwell, C. Sidney, 1: 131, 158, 179, 272; 4: 362
Burwell, Sterling, 4: 472
Buschenfeldt, Karl W., 3: 317
Butler, Allan M., 3: 301
Butler, Fergus A., 4: 53
BWH. *See* Brigham and Women's Hospital (BWH)
Bygrave, Elizabeth Clark, 2: 92, 97
Byrne, John, 2: 250
Byrne, John J., 4: 303

C

Cabot, Arthur Tracy, 2: 11; 3: 53–54, 56
Cabot, Richard C., 2: 320
Cabot, Samuel, 3: 25, *31*

Cadet Nursing Corps, 4: 467
calcaneal apophysitis (Sever's Disease)
    case study of, 2: 89
    characteristics of, 2: 89
    heel pain in children, 2: 89
    Sever's study of, 2: 88–90, 100
    x-ray appearance of, 2: *88*
calcaneovalgus deformity, 2: 92
calcar femorale, 3: 39, *39*
Calderwood, Carmelita, 3: 303
Calderwood's Orthopedic Nursing (Larson and Gould), 3: 303
Caldwell, Guy A., 1: 162; 2: 183
Calhoun, John C., 1: 307
Calvé, Jacques, 2: 103–104
Cambridge Hospital, 1: 220; 3: 396–397, 399
Camp, Walter, 1: 248, *248*
Camp Blanding Station Hospital, 4: 475
Camp Devens (Mass.), 4: 426, 437, 452
Camp Kilmer (N.J.), 4: 475
Camp Taylor (Kentucky), 4: 452
Camp Wikoff (Montauk Point, LI), 4: 310–311
Campbell, Crawford J., 1: 216; 3: 385–386, 392, 461, *462*
Campbell, Douglas, 3: 431
Campbell, W., 2: 91
Campbell, Willis, 2: 105, 294
Campbell Clinic, 4: 356
Canadian Board of Certification for Prosthetics and Orthotics, 2: 347
Canadian Orthopaedic Association, 2: 137, 183
Canadian Orthopaedic Research Society, 3: 262
Cannon, Bradford, 3: 336
Cannon, Walter B., 4: *6*, 299, 420
Cannon, Walter W., 3: 97
capitellocondylar total elbow prosthesis, 4: 145, *145*, 146–147
carbolic acid treatment, 1: 82–83, *84*
CareGroup, 1: 233; 4: 281, 284
Carlos Otis Stratton Mountain Clinic, 3: 311
Carnett, John B., 4: 235–236
Carney Hospital, 3: *78*
    adult orthopaedic clinic at, 2: 101; 3: 78
    Goldthwait and, 3: 78, 80; 4: 45
    internships at, 1: 186, 189
    Lovett and, 2: 49
    MacAusland and, 3: 308; 4: 45
    orthopaedics residencies, 4: 378
    Painter and, 4: 44–45, 224
    posture clinic at, 4: 86
    Rogers (Mark) and, 4: 224
    Sullivan and, 4: 343

    testing of foot strength apparatus, 2: 102
    treatment of adults and children in, 2: 4
    Tufts clinical instruction at, 4: 45
Carothers, Charles O., 4: 356
carpal bones, 3: 101–102
carpal tunnel syndrome
    computer use and, 4: 186
    familial bilateral, 3: 321
    genetics in, 4: 186
    research in, 2: 375; 3: 402
    self-assessment of, 4: 184–185
    wrist position and, 3: 403
Carpenter, G. K., 2: 438
Carr, Charles F., 3: 363–364
Carrie M. Hall Nurses Residence, 4: 20
Carroll, Norris, 2: 305
Carroll, Robert, 2: 251
Carter, Dennis, 3: 397
cartilage transplantation, 2: 294
Case Western Reserve University School of Medicine, 3: 337
Casemyr, Natalie E.J., 3: 463*b*
Casino Boulogne-sur-Mer, 4: 426, *427*, *428*
Caspari, Richard B., 2: 279
Casscells, Ward, 3: 446
Cassella, Mickey, 2: 178–180, 182
Castle, A. C., 1: 314–317
Castleman, Benjamin, 2: 320; 3: 205, 259
Catastrophe, The, 1: 78
Catharina Ormandy Professorship, 2: 438, 439*b*
Cats-Baril, William L., 3: 379, *379*
Cattell, Richard B., 4: 275–276
Cave, Edwin F. (1896–1976), 1: *270*; 3: *270*, *271*, *273*; 4: *491*
    on Achilles tendon injury, 3: 272
    AOA presidential address and, 3: 274, *274*
    Bankart procedure and, 3: 351, *351*
    on Barr's orthopaedic research, 3: 211
    Children's Hospital/MGH combined program and, 3: 270
    death of, 3: 276, 448
    early life, 3: 270
    education and training, 3: 270
    endowed lectures and, 3: 275
    femoral neck fracture treatment, 3: 185–186, *186*
    5th General Hospital and, 4: 484
    as Fracture Clinic chief, 3: 60*b*, 241, 272

Index

Fractures and Other Injuries, 3: 273, *273*; 4: 356
hip nailing and, 3: 237
HMS appointment, 2: 223; 3: 272; 4: 60–61
Joint Committee for the Study of Surgical Materials and, 3: 210
knee arthrotomy research, 3: 351
marriage and family, 3: 271, 276
on measuring and recording joint function, 3: 270
as MGH surgeon, 3: 187, 192, 270–271
New England Peabody Home for Crippled Children and, 2: 270
105th General Hospital and, 4: 489
orthopaedics education and, 3: 272–274
private medical practice, 3: 271–272
professional honors, 3: 275*b*, 276
publications and research, 2: 297; 3: 270, 272, 366
Scudder Oration on Trauma, 3: 63
Smith-Petersen and, 3: 270
34th Infantry Division and, 4: 484
torn ligaments in the knee research, 3: 272
on trauma, 3: 275–276
Trauma Management, 3: 62, 253, 273
on Van Gorder, 3: 368
World War II service, 1: 270; 3: 271; 4: 17
Cave, Joan Tozzer Lincoln, 3: 276
Cave, Louise Fessenden, 3: 271, 276
cavus feet, 2: 228–229
CDH. *See* congenital dislocated hips (CDH)
celastic body jackets, 2: 178
Center for Human Simulation, 4: 173
Center of Healing Arts, 3: 423
Central States Orthopedic Club, 4: 393
cerebral palsy
  Banks and, 2: 196–200
  Boston Children's Hospital and, 2: 171–172
  children and, 2: 171–172, 196–198, 300–301
  experimental approaches to, 3: 164
  foot surgery in, 2: 229
  Green and, 2: 171–172, 196–200
  Grice procedure and, 2: 212
  hamstring lengthening and, 2: 172
  Lovett and, 2: 51
  research in, 2: 196, 401
  sensory deficits in children's hands, 2: 300–301, *301*
  spinal deformities in, 2: 370
  surgery for, 2: 197–198
  treatment of, 2: 172, 196–200, 300–301
  triple arthrodesis (Hoke type) and, 2: 172
Cerebral Palsy and Spasticity Center (Children's Hospital), 2: 406
Cerebral Palsy Clinic (Children's Hospital), 2: 402, 406, 409
cerebrospinal meningitis, 2: 4
"Certain Aspects of Infantile Paralysis" (Lovett and Martin), 2: *70*
Cervical Spine Research Society, 3: *249*, 321; 4: 265, 269
Chandler, Betsy McCombs, 3: 280
Chandler, Fremont A., 2: 176, 183
Chandler, Hugh P. (1931–2014), 3: *277–278*, 280, *461*
  Aufranc Fellowship and, 3: 277
  Bone Stock Deficiency in Total Hip Replacement, 3: 278–279
  Children's Hospital/MGH combined program and, 3: 277
  death of, 3: 280
  direct lateral approach to the hip and, 3: 277–278, *278*
  early life, 3: 277
  education and training, 3: 277
  marriage and family, 3: 280
  as MGH surgeon, 3: 244, 277, 398*b*
  pelvic osteolysis with acetabular replacement case, 3: 279
  publications and research, 3: 278
  recognition of, 3: 279–280
  sailing and, 3: 280
Channing, Walter, 1: 296, 299, 302
Chanoff, David, 4: 265
Chapin, Mrs. Henry B., 1: 129
Chaplan, Ronald N., 4: 163, 193
Chapman, Earle, 3: 241
Chapman, Mabel C., 3: 304
Charcot, Jean-Martin, 3: 142
Charitable Surgical Institution, 3: 30
Charleston Naval Hospital, 3: 191; 4: 246
Charnley, John, 2: 239
Charnley, Sir John, 3: 218–220
Chase, Henry, 3: 101
Cheal, Edward, 4: 263
Cheever, Charles A., 1: 96
Cheever, David W., 4: *297*
  on Bigelow, 3: 39, 44
  Boston City Hospital and, 4: 298, 303–304
  as Boston City Hospital surgeon-in-chief, 4: 298, 306–307
  British Expeditionary Forces and, 4: 9–10
  on Goldthwait, 3: 79
  HMS appointment, 3: 94; 4: 298, 307
  PBBH and, 4: 5, 10–11, 17
Chelsea Memorial Hospital, 2: 102; 3: 314
Chelsea Naval Hospital, 4: 47–48, 97
chemotherapy, 2: 422–423
Chen, Chien-Min, 3: 368
Chernack, Robert, 4: 194, 195*b*
Cheselden, William, 1: 6, 36
Chessler, Robert, 1: xxii
Chest Wall and Spinal Deformity Study Group, 2: 361–362
Cheyne, W. Watson, 1: *83*
Chicago Polyclinic, 2: 50
Chicago Shriner's Hospital, 2: 355
Chicago University, 3: 175
Chickahominy fever, 3: 44
Child, C. Gardner, 4: 303
children
  bone granuloma and, 2: 171
  cerebral palsy and, 2: 171–172, 196–198, 300–301
  club foot and, 1: xxii, 118–119; 2: 12*t*, 15*t*, 22–23, 145
  development of hospitals for, 2: 3–4
  early treatment of, 1: xxii
  growth disturbances with chronic arthritis, 4: 56
  heel pain in, 2: 89
  hip disease and, 2: 52
  juvenile idiopathic arthritis and, 2: 164, 171, 350
  kyphosis and, 2: 343–345
  mortality, 2: 4–5, 15
  muscle atrophy in, 2: 110
  national health initiatives, 4: 235–236
  orthopaedic rehabilitation and, 1: 107, 121
  osteochondritis dissecans in, 2: 194–195
  osteomyelitis in, 2: 169
  physical therapy and, 2: 61, 107
  poliomyelitis and, 1: 191; 2: 61, 189–191, 210, 213
  posture and, 4: 233–234, *234*, 235, *236*
  rheumatic heart disease and, 1: 130

schools for disabled, 2: 36–39, 97
spinal deformities and, 1: xxi, xxii, 97–98, 123
spinal tuberculosis and, 1: 108
Sprengel deformity, 2: 195, *196*
state clinics for crippled, 2: 107, 221
trauma and, 2: 359, 365, 368, 378, 385
use of ether, 1: 63
children, disabled. *See* disabled children
Children's Convalescent Home, 2: 84
Children's Hospital (Boston, Mass.), 2: 4–16. *See also* Boston Children's Hospital (BCH)
Children's Hospital Medical Center, 4: 113–114. *See also* Boston Children's Hospital (BCH)
Children's Hospital of Philadelphia (CHOP), 2: 3–5, 424
Children's Infirmary, 2: 3
Children's Island Sanitorium, 4: 87
Children's Medical Center (Wellesley), 2: 314
Children's Memorial Hospital (Chicago), 2: 302
Children's Sports Injury Prevention Fund, 2: 439*b*
Children's Sunlight Hospital (Scituate), 3: 307
Childress, Harold M., 4: 335
Chiodo, Christopher, 4: 190*b*, 194
Chipman, W. W., 3: 113*b*
chloroform, 1: 62–63, 82; 3: 15, 31
Choate, Rufus, 1: 307
Choate Hospital, 2: 256
cholera epidemic, 1: 295; 4: 293
chondrocytes, 3: 327, 442, 444–445, 449
chondrodysplasia, 4: 218–220
chondrosarcoma, 2: 237; 3: 390, 406
Christian, Henry A., 1: 173–174, 176; 4: 4, 6, 9, 16, 79, 104
Christophe, Kenneth, 4: 40, 89
chronic diseases
  anatomy and, 3: 91
  body mechanics and, 3: 81, 91
  bone and joint disorders, 1: 153; 3: 85, 90
  faulty body mechanics and, 3: 91
  Goldthwait and, 4: 39*b*, 52
  orthopaedic surgeons and, 4: 46, 53
  posture and, 4: 52, 86
  prevention of, 3: 90

RBBH and, 4: 25*b*, 27, 30, 30*b*, 32*b*, 33, 36, 39*b*, 45, 86
rheumatoid arthritis and, 4: 36
travel abroad and, 1: 72
chronic regional pain syndrome (CRPS), 2: 68
Chronicle of Boston Jewry, A (Ehrenfried), 4: 220
Chuinard, Eldon G., 1: 162
Chung, Kevin C., 3: 410
Church, Benjamin, 1: 15–16
Churchill, Edward D., 1: 198–199; 2: 322; 3: 1; 4: 302, 470–471, *472*
Churchill, Edward H., 2: 79
Churchill, Winston, 4: 479
chymopapain, 3: 254–255, 397, 419, *421*
Civale, Jean, 3: 41
Clark, Charles, 4: 174
Clark, Dean A., 4: 158
Clark, H. G., 3: *31*
Clark, John G., 3: 113*b*, 122, 355
Clarke, Joseph Taylor, 4: 448
Clay, Lucius D., 2: 260, 264
Clayton, Mack, 4: 243
cleidocranial dysostosis, 2: 254
Cleveland, Grover, 2: 72
Cleveland, Mather, 3: 196
Clifford, John H., 1: 307
Clifton Springs Sanatorium, 3: 88; 4: 52–53
Cline, Henry, 1: 33–34, 37
Clinical Biomechanics of the Spine (White and Panjabi), 4: 262
Clinical Congress of Surgeons in North America, 3: 116, 123
Clinical Orthopaedic Examination (McRae), 1: 167
Cloos, David W., 4: 163, 193
clover leaf rod, 3: 272
club foot
  apparatus for, 1: 98, 100, 106; 2: 23, 24; 4: 83
  Bradford and, 2: 22–24, 28–29
  correction of, 1: 98, 100, *100*, *101*, 106; 2: 36
  correction of bilateral, 2: *29*
  Denis Browne splint, 2: 208
  early diagnosis and treatment for, 1: 100; 2: 28–29
  medial deltoid ligament release, 2: 145
  nonoperative treatment of, 2: 28; 4: 216
  Ober and, 2: 145
  osteotomies and, 2: 29
  pathological findings and, 3: 54
  plantar fasciotomy and, 2: 24

Stromeyer's subcutaneous tenotomy for, 1: 118, *118*
tarsectomy and, 2: 23
tenotomy and, 1: 106, 118; 2: 25–26
Cobb, John, 2: 225–226
Cochran, Robert C., 4: 438–439
Cochrane, William A., 3: 244, 302, 371, *371*, 372
Codman, Amory, 2: 182
Codman, Catherine, 1: 50, *129*, 130
Codman, Elizabeth Hand, 3: 93
Codman, Ernest A. (1869–1940), 3: *93*, *103*, *105*, *115*, *143*
  abdominal surgery and, 3: 108
  as anatomy assistant at HMS, 2: 114
  anesthesia and, 3: 95, *95*, 96
  bone sarcomas and, 3: 136–140, 140*b*, 141–142, 145; 4: 102
  on brachial plexus injury, 2: 96
  Camp Taylor base hospital and, 4: 452
  cartoon of Back Bay public, 3: 121, *121*, 122, *122*
  clinical congress meeting, 3: 116
  Committee on Standardization of Hospitals and, 3: 112, 113*b*, 115–116, 123–124
  death of, 2: 116; 3: 145–146
  dedication of headstone, 3: *145*, 146
  on diagnosis with x-rays, 3: 99
  duodenal ulcer and, 3: 108
  early life, 3: 93
  education and training, 3: 93–95
  End-Result Idea, 1: 194; 2: 135; 3: 110–111, *111*, 112, 114, 116, *116*, 118–119, 119*b*, 120, 122–126, *126*, 127*b*, 128–131, 136; 4: 12, 141
  fluoroscope and, 2: 307
  forward-thinking of, 3: 135–136
  Fracture Course and, 3: 62
  fracture treatment and, 3: 101–102
  Halifax Harbor explosion and, 3: 132–135
  Harvard Medical Association letter, 3: 119*b*
  HMS appointment, 3: 96, 99
  Hospital Efficiency meeting, 3: 120–122
  interest in hunting and fishing, 3: 94, 143–145
  interest in sprains, 3: 100–102
  interest in subacromial bursitis, 3: 104–105, 107–109

Index

interest in subdeltoid bursa, 3: 95, 98, 103–104, *104*, 105, 108
legacy of, 3: 145–146
life history chart, 3: *106*
marriage and, 3: 142–143
memberships and, 3: 65
MGH internship and, 3: 95–96
as MGH surgeon, 1: 190, 194; 3: 99, 112, 118, 142, 266
on monetary value of surgeon services, 3: 129–130
operating in the Bigelow Amphitheatre, 3: *107*
personal case documentation, 3: 126, 128–130
Philadelphia Medical Society address, 3: 117*b*–118*b*
private hospital ideals, 3: 114*b*, 115
private hospital of, 3: 112, 114, 116, 118, 135
private practice and, 3: 136
publication of x-rays, 3: 97, *97*, 98, *99*
publications and research, 3: 99–104, *104*, 108–112, 115–116, 125, 136, 139–142
resolution honoring, 3: 144*b*, 146
on safety of x-rays, 3: 99–100
Shoulder, 2: 239; 3: 105, 115, 122, 140*b*
shoulder and, 3: 103–105, 107–110, 354
as skiagrapher at BCH, 2: 16, 114; 3: 96–99, 142
Study in Hospital Efficiency, 3: 125, *125*, 127*b*, 128–131
surgical scissor design, 3: *138*
Treatment of Fractures, 3: 56
World War I and, 3: 132, 135
Codman, John, 3: 94, 108, 142
Codman, Katherine Bowditch, 3: 142–143, 144*b*, 145
Codman, William Combs, 3: 93
Codman Center for Clinical Effectiveness in Surgery, 3: 146
Codman Hospital, 3: 112, 114, 116, 118, *126*, 135
Codman's Paradox, 3: 105
Cohen, Jonathan, 1: 114
Cohen, Jonathan (1915–2003), 2: *179*
as assistant pathologist, 2: 234
on Barr, 3: 206–207
bone irradiation research, 2: 237, *237*
bone lesions and tumor research, 2: 236
book reviews by, 2: 239, 240*b*
Boston Children's Hospital and, 2: 233–236, 301; 4: 126, 245
Boston Orthopedic Institution and, 1: 121
death of, 2: 241
education and training, 2: 231
Farber and, 2: 235–236
Fourth Portable Surgical Hospital (4PSH) and, 2: 232–233
Fourth Portable Surgical Hospital's Service in the War against Japan, 2: 232–233
Green and, 2: 234–235
HMS appointment, 2: 233
Jewish Hospital (St. Louis) and, 2: 231
Journal of Bone and Joint Surgery editor, 2: 238–240; 3: 346
marriage and family, 2: 241
metal implants and, 2: 237–238
MGH and, 2: 233
mobile army surgical hospitals (MASHs) and, 2: 231
105th General Hospital and, 4: 489
orthopaedic research laboratory and, 2: 234
orthopaedic surgery and, 2: 235
professional memberships, 2: 240–241
publications and research, 2: 233–234, 236, 239, *239*; 3: *216*; 4: 102
publications of, 2: 236*b*
World War II service, 2: 231–233
Cohen, Louise Alden, 2: 241
Cohen, Mark S., 3: 431
Cohnheim, Julius, 1: 82
Coleman, Sherman, 2: 302
college athletes. *See also* Harvard athletics
Arthur L. Boland and, 1: 286
Augustus Thorndike and, 1: 274
Bill of Rights for, 1: 274, 280, 280*b*
Coller, Fred A., 2: 119; 4: 389*b*
Colles fracture, 2: 47; 3: 99
Collins, Abigail, 1: 24
Collins, John, 1: 24, 31
Collis P. Huntington Memorial Hospital for Cancer Research, 1: 87
Colonna, Paul C., 2: 183; 3: 208
Colton, Gardner Quincy, 1: 56
Colton, Theodore, 3: 253
Combat Over Corregidor (Bradford), 4: *364*
Combined Jewish Philanthropies (CJP), 4: 168
Committee F-4 on Surgical Implants, 3: 210
Committee for International Activities (POS), 2: 425
Committee of Correspondence, 1: 16
Committee of the Colonization of Society, 1: 239
Committee of Undergraduate Training (AOA), 2: 183
Committee on Education of the American Medical Association, 2: 41
Committee on Industrial Injuries, 3: 63
Committee on Recording Lateral Curvature, 2: 247
Committee on Staff Reorganization and Office Building (King Committee). *See* King Report (MGH)
Committee on Standardization of Hospitals, 3: 112, 113*b*, 115–116, 123–125, 131
Committee on Surgical Implants, 2: 238
Committee on Trauma, 2: 131; 3: 63
compartment syndrome, 2: 249–250; 3: 417–418
Compere, Edward, 2: 300
compound fractures
amputation and, 1: 54, 68
Boston City Hospital outcomes, 4: 335, 337
Committee on Fractures and, 3: 64
fracture boxes and, 1: 80
immobilization methods, 4: 399
Lister's antisepsis dressings and, 1: 84–85; 3: 59
military orthopaedics and, 2: 120; 3: 64; 4: 391, 399, 409, 423*b*, 434
orthopaedic treatment for, 4: 464
surgery and, 4: 320, 321*b*–322*b*
computed tomography (CT), 2: 365, 389, 410–411; 3: 254
Conant, William M. (1856–1937), 1: 248
Concord, Mass., 1: 17–18
concussions
athletes and, 2: 385
football and, 1: 247, 254, 274–275
signs and symptoms of, 1: 287*t*
three knockout rule, 1: 275
treatment of, 1: 286–287
congenital dislocated hips (CDH)
Allison and, 3: 164, 175
AOA Commission on, 3: 234

Bradford and, 2: 32–34
Buckminster Brown and, 1: 108
closed manipulation, 2: 33–34
Guérin's method for, 1: 106–107
open reductions, 2: 33; 3: 233–234
reduction procedures, 3: 234–235
reductions reviewed by the AOA Commission, 3: 232–233, 233*t*
treatment of, 2: 32–33
use of shelf procedure, 2: 151
congenital pseudarthrosis of the tibia, 2: 172–176
congenital torticollis, 2: 256, 258
Conn, A., 2: 334–335
Conn, Harold R., 4: 473
Conquest of Cancer by Radium and Other Methods, The (Quigley), 1: 275
Conservational Hip Outcomes Research (ANCHOR) Group, 2: 392, *393*
Constable, John D., 3: 321
Constructive Surgery of the Hip (Aufranc), 3: 244, *246*
Continental Hospital (Boston), 1: 24
Converse, Elizabeth, 3: 339
Converse, Frederick S., 3: 339
Conway, James, 2: 305
Conwell, H. Earle, 3: 191
Cook, Robert J., 2: 438
Cooke, John, 3: 193*b*, 238
Cooksey, Eunice, 2: 247
Coonse, G. Kenneth (1897–1951)
 Aufranc and, 4: 372–373
 BCH Bone and Joint Service, 4: 373
 death of, 4: 375
 education and training, 4: 371
 HMS appointment, 3: 237; 4: 371, 373
 hospital appointments, 4: 371
 humerus fracture treatment, 4: 372
 legacy of, 4: 375–376
 marriage and family, 4: 375
 Massachusetts Regional Fracture Committee, 3: 64
 MGH and, 4: 371–372
 Newton-Wellesley Hospital and, 4: 371, 373, 375
 patellar turndown procedure, 4: 373–374
 PBBH and, 4: 373
 professional memberships, 4: 371, 375, 375*b*
 publications and research, 4: 371–374
 synovectomy in chronic arthritis research, 4: 102, 371–372
 treatment of shock, 4: 373, *373*
 University of Missouri appointment, 4: 372–373
 World War I service, 4: 371, 373
Coonse, Hilda Gant, 4: 375
Cooper, Maurice, 4: 373
Cooper, Reginald, 1: 234; 3: 303
Cooper, Sir Astley, 1: *34*
 anatomy lectures, 1: 34–35, 37
 Bigelow on, 3: 36
 dislocations and, 1: 44–45
 as Guy's Hospital surgeon, 1: 35–36
 influence on John Collins Warren, 1: 36–37
 publications of, 1: 35–36
 surgical advances by, 1: 35
 Treatise on Dislocations and Fractures of Joints, 1: *35*, 42, *43*
Cooper, William, 1: 33–34
Coordinating Council on Medical Education (CCME), 1: 211
Cope, Oliver, 3: 336
Cope, Stuart, 4: 116, 128, 163, 193
Copel, Joseph W. (1917–1985), 4: *88*
 Beth Israel Hospital and, 4: 89, 247, 262
 Boston University appointment, 4: 89
 Brigham and Women's Hospital, 4: 163
 death of, 4: 89
 education and training, 4: 88
 HMS appointment, 4: 89
 marriage and family, 4: 88–89
 private medical practice, 4: 89
 publications and research, 4: 88–89
 RBBH and, 4: 35, 38, 68, 89, 93
 US Army and, 4: 88
Copel, Marcia Kagno, 4: 89
Copley, John Singleton, 1: *3*, *11*
Corey Hill Hospital, 3: *88*, 89; 4: 224
Corkery, Paul J., 4: 295
Corliss, Julie, 4: 183
Cornell Medical School, 4: 109
Cornwall, Andrew P., 3: 268
Cotrel, Yves, 2: 342
Cotting, Benjamin E., 2: 10
Cotting, Frances J., 2: 38
Cotting, W. F., 4: 338
Cotting, W. P., 2: 438
Cotting School, 2: 38, 308, *312*; 3: 151; 4: 367
Cotton, Frederic J. (1869–1938), 1: 202; 4: *309*, *323*, *331*
 ACS founder, 4: 324
 ankle fractures and, 4: 313–315
 bacteriology research, 4: 310
 BCH Bone and Joint Service, 4: 307, 328, 333, 380*b*
 BCH residencies and, 4: 377
 Beth Israel Hospital and, 4: 207, 220
 board certification efforts, 4: 324
 bone and joint treatment, 4: 313, 323, 328
 book of x-ray photographs and, 3: 57
 Boston Children's Hospital and, 4: 311
 Boston Children's Hospital skiagrapher, 3: 56
 Boston City Hospital and, 4: 217, 242, 307, 312–313, 328
 Boston Dispensary and, 4: 311
 bubble bottle anesthesia method, 4: 323
 calcaneus fracture treatment, 4: 313, *313*, 314*b*
 clinical congress meeting, 3: 116
 as consulting surgeon, 4: 323–324
 Cotton's fracture and, 4: 313–315, *315*, 316
 death of, 4: 330
 Dislocations and Joint Fractures, 3: 371; 4: 307, 314, 316–317, *317*, 318
 education and training, 4: 309
 on fracture management, 4: 320, *320*, 321*b*–322*b*, 339*b*–340*b*
 George W. Gay Lecture, 4: 324
 hip fracture treatment, 4: 318–320
 HMS appointments, 4: 323, 323*b*, 329
 honors and awards, 4: 312, 324, 329
 on industrial accidents, 4: 325–327, 338
 lectures of, 4: 329
 legacy of, 4: 329–331
 marriage and family, 4: 330
 Massachusetts Regional Fracture Committee, 3: 64
 medical illustration, 3: 56, *58*
 as mentor, 3: 237
 MGH and, 4: 310
 military reconstruction hospitals and, 4: 444–445, 449–451
 Mt. Sinai Hospital and, 4: 204, 220, 312
 named procedures, 4: 329

Index

New England Regional Committee on Fractures, 4: 341
orthopaedics education and, 4: 323
Orthopedic Surgery, 4: 318
os calcis fracture research, 4: 313
PBBH teaching and, 4: 10
Physicians' Art Society and, 4: 329–330
professional memberships, 4: 324, 329–330
publications and research, 4: 310–313, 316–320, 323, 325–326, 329
Reverdin method and, 4: 216
roentgenology and, 2: 56
sling device to reduce kyphosis, 4: *317*
Spanish American War service, 4: 310–311
test to determine ankle instability, 4: *317*, 318
Treatment of Fractures, 4: 312
trigger knee research, 4: 311–312
Tufts Medical School appointment, 4: 329
US General Hospital No. 10 and, 4: 452
worker health care advocacy, 4: 325–327
workers' compensation advocacy, 4: 325, 444
World War I service, 4: 327
Cotton, Isabella Cole, 4: 309
Cotton, Jane Baldwin, 4: 330
Cotton, Jean, 4: 330
Cotton, Joseph Potter, 4: 309, 316
Cotton advancement operation, 4: 329
Cotton osteotomy, 4: 329
Cotton-Boothby anesthesia apparatus, 4: *320*, 323
Cotton's Fracture, 4: 313–315, *315*, 316
Cotton's Hammer, 4: *319*, 320
Council of Medical Specialty Societies, 1: 211
Council of Musculoskeletal Specialty Societies (AAOS), 4: 186
Councilman, William T., 2: 32; 4: 4, 6
Coventry, Mark, 3: 261–262, 433
Cowell, Henry, 2: 239
Cox, Edith I., 4: 389*b*
coxa plana, 2: 102–106. *See also* Legg-Calvé-Perthes disease
Cozen, Lewis N., 3: 70*b*, 74, 187; 4: 383, 471
Cracchiolo, Andrea, 2: 317

Craig, John, 2: 234
Crandon, LeRoi G., 4: 207, 216, *217*
Crane, Carl C., 3: 266
craniotomy, 2: 24–25
Crawford, Alvin, 4: 246, 266*b*
Crawford, Dorothy, 2: 313
Crenshaw, Andrew H., Jr., 4: 168, 356
crew, 1: 250–251, 258
Crile, George, 3: 104
Crippled Children's Clinics (Massachusetts Dept. of Health), 2: 221, 230, 287, 299, 314; 4: 376
Crippled Children's Service (Vermont Dept. of Health), 2: 208, 220–221; 3: 209
Crockett, David C., 2: 322; 3: 259
Cronkhite, Leonard, 2: 285
Crosby, L. M., 3: 133
Crotched Mountain Foundation, 2: 221
Crothers, Bronson, 2: 171–172
Crowninshield, Annie, 1: 76
cubitus varus deformity, 2: 229
Cudworth, Alden L., 2: 326
Cullis Consumptive Home, 4: 275
curative workshops
    King Manuel II and, 4: 400–403
    rehabilitation of soldiers and, 4: 401–403, *403*, 404, 442, 448, *448*, 449
    Shepherd's Bush Military Hospital and, 4: 399, 401
    trades practiced in, 4: 402*b*
    US Army and, 4: 403–404
Curley, James M., 3: 120
Curran, J. A., 1: 185
Curtis, Burr, 2: 351
Curtiss, Paul H., Jr., 2: 238; 3: 398*b*, 461, *461–462*
Cushing, Ernest W., 4: 23
Cushing, Harvey W., 3: *180*
    American Ambulance Hospital and, 4: 9–10, *388*, 389*b*, *390*
    anesthesia charting and, 3: 96
    Base Hospital No. 5 and, 4: 420, 420*t*, 422*b*, *422*
    Boston Children's Hospital and, 2: 12
    Codman and, 3: 94–95
    on Dane's foot plate, 2: 245
    development of orthopaedics department, 1: 177
    Harvard Unit and, 2: 119, 125; 3: 369, *370*; 4: 419
    honors and awards, 3: 94
    as MGH surgeon, 3: 95
    on organization of surgery, 4: 13–14

PBBH and, 1: 174, 204; 2: 168, 269; 4: 4–6, *6*, 8–9, 12–13, 16, 79
Quigley and, 1: 276
Sever and, 2: 92
Surgeon's Journal, 3: 369
Thorndike and, 1: 263
Cutler, Elliott C., 4: *106*, *472*
    American Ambulance Hospital and, 4: 389*b*, 390–391
    Base Hospital No. 5 and, 4: 420, 422*b*
    Carl Walter and, 4: 104–105
    death of, 4: 18
    Harvard Unit and, 2: 119; 4: 17
    HMS appointment, 1: 179
    on medical education, 4: 16
    Moseley Professor of Surgery, 1: 268
    as PBBH chief of surgery, 1: 269–270; 4: 8, 10, 15–16, 18, 79, 110
    publications and research, 1: 153–154
    specialty clinics and, 4: 15–16
    support for orthopaedic surgery specialization, 4: 16–17
    Surgical Research Laboratory, 3: 237
    on wounded soldier care, 4: 389–390
    as WWII surgery specialist, 4: 471
Cutler, Robert, 4: 20
Cutler Army Hospital (Fort Devens), 2: 358

D

Dabuzhaky, Leonard, 4: 279
Daland, Florence, 3: 159, 347
Dalton, John Call, Jr., 1: 60
Dana Farber Cancer Institute, 1: 91; 2: 331
Dandy, Walter, 3: 204
Dane, Eunice Cooksey, 2: 247
Dane, John H. (1865–1939), 2: *241*
    Boston Children's Hospital and, 2: 242, 307
    Boston Dispensary and, 2: 247
    Boston Infant's Hospital and, 2: 242
    clinical congress meeting, 3: 118
    death of, 2: 247
    education and training, 2: 241–242
    flat feet research and treatment, 2: 242, *242*, 243, *243*, 244–246
    foot plate, 2: 244–246

485

HMS appointment, 2: 242, 247
House of the Good Samaritan
 and, 2: 242
Lovett and, 2: 242, 246–247
Marcella Street Home and,
 2: 242, 247
marriage and family, 2: 247
professional memberships, 2: 246
publications of, 2: 246–247
Thomas splint modification,
 2: 247, *247*
US General Hospital No. 2 and,
 4: 452
World War I service, 2: 247
Dane, John H., Jr., 2: 247
Danforth, Murray S.
 on importance of examination
  and diagnosis, 3: 185
 Journal of Bone and Joint Surgery
  editor, 3: 161, 344; 4: 50
 MGH and, 3: 268
 military orthopaedics and,
  4: 406, 444
 publications and research,
  2: 136, 297
 rehabilitation of soldiers and,
  4: 444
 Walter Reed General Hospital
  and, 4: 452
Danforth, Samuel, 1: 15, 25, 40
D'Angio, G. J., 2: 237
Darling, Eugene A. (1868–1934),
 1: 250–251
Darrach, William, 4: 473
Darrach procedure, 3: 191
Darrow, Clarence, 1: 276
*Dartmouth Atlas of Health Care in
 Virginia, The* (Wennberg et al.),
 2: 374, *374*, 375
Dartmouth Medical School, 2: 371;
 3: 363
Dartmouth-Hitchcock Medical Center, 2: 371
David S. Grice Annual Lecture,
 2: 215–216, 216t
Davies, John A. K., 4: 194, 195b,
 263
Davies, Robert, 4: 262
Davis, Arthur G., 3: 344
Davis, G. Gwilym, 3: 157; 4: 406
Davis, Henry G., 2: 22–23, 26
Davis, Joseph, 2: 219
Davis, Robert, 4: 286
Davy, Sir Humphrey, 1: 56
Dawbarn, Robert H. M., 3: 105
Dawes, William, 1: 17
Dawson, Clyde W., 3: 74
Dawson, David M., 4: 168
Day, Charles, 1: 169; 4: 287
Day, George, 4: 307

Day Nursery (Holyoke), 2: 256
De Forest, R., 3: 210
De Machinamentis of Oribasius,
 3: *149*
De Ville, Kenneth Allen, 1: 47
Deaconess Home and Training
 School, 4: 273
Deaconess term, 4: 274b
dead arm syndrome, 3: 359–360
*Death of General Warren at the Battle
 of Bunker's Hill, The* (Trumbull),
 1: *19*
Deaver, George, 4: 76
DeBakey, Michael, 4: 469
debarkation hospitals, 4: 451–452
deep vein thrombosis (DVT),
 3: 218; 4: 251–252
DeHaven, Ken, 3: 448
Deland, F. Stanton, Jr., 4: 114, 120
Deland, Jonathan, 1: 217b
Delano, Frederick, 2: 72
DeLorme, Eleanor Person, 3: 281,
 287
DeLorme, Thomas I., Jr. (1917–
 2003), 3: *281*, 285
 awards and, 3: 281–282
 blood perfusion research, 3: 287
 Children's Hospital/MGH combined program and, 3: 285
 death of, 3: 287
 early life, 3: 281
 education and training, 3: 281
 Elgin table and, 3: *287*
 expansion of MGH orthopaedics
  and, 3: 286
 Fracture course and, 3: 273
 Gardiner Hospital and, 3: 282,
  284
 heavy-/progressive resistance
  exercises and, 3: 282, *282*,
  283–286
 HMS appointment, 3: 287
 legacy of, 3: 287
 Legon of Merit medal, 3: 284,
  284
 as Liberty Mutual Insurance
  Company medical director,
  3: 286–287
 Marlborough Medical Associates
  and, 2: 146, 269, 299
 marriage and family, 3: 281
 as MGH surgeon, 3: 285
 Milton Hospital and, 3: 287
 physical therapy and, 3: 284
 PRE (Progressive Resistance Exercise), 3: *286*
 publications and research,
  3: 282–283, 285–286; 4: 91
 rehabilitation and, 3: 459, 461

resistance training in recovery,
  3: 282
 spinal surgeries and, 3: 287
 US Army Medical Corps and,
  3: 282
 weightlifting and, 3: 281
 West Roxbury Veterans Hospital
  and, 3: 285
DeLorme table, 3: 284
Delpech, Jacques-Mathieu, 1: xxiii,
 106
Delta Upsilon fraternity, 4: 258, *258*
Denis Browne splint, 2: 208
dentistry, 1: 56–57
Denucé, Maurice, 3: 233–235
Derby, George, 4: 307
Description of a Skeleton of the Mastodon Giganteus of North America
 (J. C. Warren), 1: *52*
Deshmukh, R. V., 4: 178
Detmold, William Ludwig, 1: 100–
 101; 2: 25–26
DeWolfe, C. W., 3: 133
Dexter, Aaron, 1: 25, 95–96
Deyo, Richard, 2: 371
diabetes, 3: 408, 413, 438
Diagnosis in Joint Disease (Allison
 and Ghormley), 3: 175, 289, *290*
Diao, Edward, 1: 217b
diarrheal disease, 2: 4
diastematomyelia, 2: 236, 399–400
Dickinson, Robert L., 3: 120, 123
Dickson, Frank D., 2: 78
Dickson, Fred, 2: 77
Dieffenbach, Johann Friedrich, 1: 76
Digby, Kenelm H., 2: 170
Diggs, Lucy, 4: 492
Dignan, Beth A., 2: 277
Dillon Field House, 1: 274, *284*,
 285
Dines, Robert, 4: 247
Dingle, J., 4: 127
diphtheria, 2: 4
disabled adults
 back problems and, 3: 207
 hip disease and, 2: 294; 3: 155
 MGH rehabilitation clinic and,
  1: 273; 3: 455
 orthopaedic care for, 2: 132
 polio and, 3: 286
 soldiers and veterans, 1: 271–
  273; 2: 65, 67; 3: 44
disabled children. *See also* cerebral
 palsy; club foot
 advocacy for, 1: 107
 Crippled Children's Clinic and,
  2: 221
 House of the Good Samaritan
  and, 1: 123
 industrial training and, 2: 97

orthopaedic care for, 2: 132
  polio and, 2: 191
  schools for, 2: 36–41, 67–68, 97, 308, 310–311, *312*
"Discourse on Self-Limited Diseases, A" (Bigelow), 3: 12–13
Diseases of the Bones and Joints (Osgood, Goldthwait and Painter), 2: 117; 3: 81–82; 4: 45
dislocations. *See also* congenital dislocated hips (CDH); hip dislocations
  chronic posterior elbow, 3: 366
  patella and, 2: 294–296; 3: 79, *79b*, *80*, *81*
  shoulders and, 3: 352, *352*, 353, 355–356, *356*
  Treatise on Dislocations and Fractures of Joints, 1: 35, *42*, *43*
  use of ether, 1: 62
  voluntary, 3: 355–356, *356*
Dislocations and Joint Fractures (Cotton), 3: 371; 4: 307, 314, 316–317, *317*, 318
distal humerus, 2: 250
Division of Orthopaedic Surgery in the A.E.F., The (Goldthwait), 4: 473
Dixon, Frank D., 3: 173
Dixon, Robert B., 4: 23
Doctor's Hospital, 1: 276
Dodd, Walter J., 2: 114, 116; 3: 20, *20*, 21, 96, 99, 192, 266; 4: *389b*
Dodson, Tom, 3: 1
Donaghy, R. M., 3: 205
Doppelt, Samuel, 1: 167; 3: 386, 396, 398, 440, *460b*, *461*
Dowling, John Joseph, 4: *420t*, 438
Down syndrome, 2: 368, 370
Dr. John Ball Brown (Harding), 1: *95*
Dr. Robert K. Rosenthal Cerebral Palsy Fund in Orthopaedics, 2: *439b*
Draper, George, 2: 72, 75–76, 78
Drew, Michael A., 4: 163, 193, 279
Drinker, C. K., 2: 81
Drinker, Philip, 2: 78, *78*, 191
Dubousset, Jean, 2: 342
Dudley, H. Robert, 4: 102
Duggal, Navan, 4: 288
Duhamel, Henri-Louis, 1: xxi
Dukakis, Kitty, 3: 419
Dukakis, Michael, 3: 419, 423
Dunlop, George, 4: 279
Dunn, Beryl, 2: 180–181
Dunn, Naughton, 2: 92–94, 150, 181
Dunphy, J. Englebert, 2: 220; 4: 303
Dunster House (Harvard University), 2: *388*
Duocondylar prostheses, 4: 178

duodenal ulcer, 3: 108
duopatellar prosthesis, 4: 130
Dupuytren, Guillaume, 1: 73–75
Duthie, J. J. R., 4: 33
Dwight, Edwin, 4: *302*
Dwight, Thomas, 1: 87–88, 127; 2: *97*, 247, 296; 3: 33, 94, 231; 4: 82, 310
Dwyer, Allen, 2: 336
Dwyer instrumentation, 2: 336, *336*, 342
Dwyer procedure, 2: 328
Dyer, George, 4: *190b*

E

Eames, Charles, 4: *470*
Eames, Ray, 4: *470*
Eames molded plywood leg splint, 4: *470*
early onset scoliosis (EOS), 2: 360–361
Early Orthopaedic Surgeons of America, The (Shands), 1: 114
Earp, Brandon, 3: 410; 4: *190b*
Easley, Walter, 3: 282
East Boston Relief Station, 2: 254
Eastern States Orthopaedic Club, 4: 87
Eaton, Richard G. (1929–), 2: *200*, 249
  animal model of compartment syndrome, 2: 248
  Boston Children's Hospital and, 2: 248, 250
  Children's Hospital/MGH combined program and, 2: 248
  education and training, 2: 248
  hand surgery education, 2: 248, 250–251
  HMS appointment, 2: 248
  on ischemia-edema cycle, 2: 200–201, *201*
  Joint Injuries of the Hand, 2: 250, *250*
  Peter Bent Brigham Hospital and, 4: 22
  professional memberships, 2: 251
  publications and research, 2: 248–250; 3: 309
  Roosevelt Hospital and, 2: 248, 250–251
  US Army active duty, 2: 248
Ebert, Robert H., 1: 210–211; 2: 203; 4: 113, 119, 123
École de Médicine (University of Paris), 1: 73
Eddy, Chauncey, 1: 103
Edison, Thomas, 3: 96

Edith M. Ashley Professorship, 3: 202, *464b*
Edsall, David L., 4: *6*
  Allison and, 1: 152
  Beth Israel Hospital and, 4: 213
  clinical research at MGH and, 3: 211
  as dean of HMS, 1: 174–177; 2: 81–82; 4: 213, 275, 297, 302
  on departmental organization, 1: 176–178
  on faculty governance, 1: 175–178
  on faculty rank, 1: 178
  HMS reforms and, 1: 147
  on MGH and HMS relations, 1: 174
  postgraduate education and, 2: 160
Edwards, Thomas, 4: 262–263
Effects of Chloroform and of Strong Chloric Ether as Narcotic Agents (J. C. Warren), 1: 62
Ehrenfried, Albert (1880–1951), 4: *215*
  attempts at resignation from Beth Israel, 4: 209, *209b*, 210
  Beth Israel Hospital and, 4: 205–210, 220
  Boston Children's Hospital and, 4: 215
  Boston City Hospital and, 4: 217–218
  Chronicle of Boston Jewry, 4: 220
  civic and professional engagements, 4: *221b*
  clinical congress meeting, 3: 116
  club foot research and, 4: 216
  death of, 4: 221
  education and training, 4: 215
  hereditary deforming chondrodysplasia research, 4: 218–219, *219*, 220
  HMS appointment, 4: 218
  insufflation anesthesia apparatus, 4: 215–216
  Jewish Memorial Hospital and, 4: 215
  on military service, 4: 220–221
  military surgeon training and, 4: 218
  Mt. Sinai Hospital and, 4: 202–205, 215
  on need for total Jewish hospital, 4: 205
  publications and research, 4: 216–219, *219*, 220–221
  pulmonary tuberculosis treatment, 4: 215

Reverdin method and,
4: 216–217
Surgical After-Treatment,
4: 217, *217*
vascular anastomosis and, 4: 216
Ehrenfried, George, 4: 215, 220
Ehrenfried, Rachel Blauspan, 4: 215
Ehrenfried's disease (hereditary deforming chondrodysplasia), 4: 218–220
Ehrlich, Christopher, 3: 401
Ehrlich, Michael G. (1939–2018), 3: *400*, *461*
   Brown University Medical School appointment, 3: 400–401
   death of, 3: 401
   early life, 3: 400
   education and training, 3: 400
   gait laboratory and, 3: 397
   honors and awards, 3: 400
   idiopathic subluxation of the radial head case, 3: 401
   marriage and family, 3: 401
   as MGH surgeon, 3: 385–386, 395, 398*b*, 413
   Miriam Hospital and, 3: 401
   pediatric orthopaedics and, 3: 388*t*, 400–401, 460*b*
   publications and research, 3: 400–401
   Rhode Island Hospital and, 3: 401
Ehrlich, Nancy Band, 3: 401
Ehrlich, Timothy, 3: 401
Ehrlichman, Lauren, 3: 463*b*
Eiselsberg, Anton, 1: 264
elbow
   arthroplasty of, 3: 64, 341; 4: 63
   basket plaster treatment, 2: 122
   brachioradialis transfer and, 2: 153
   capitellocondylar total prosthesis, 4: 145, *145*, 146–147
   chronic posterior dislocations, 3: 366
   early arthrogram of, 3: *99*
   excision of, 3: 34, 309, 368
   external epicondyle fracture of, 2: 46
   flexion contracture of, 2: 418
   fusion and, 3: 368
   hinged prostheses, 4: 147
   idiopathic subluxation of the radial head, 3: 401
   intra-articular radial nerve entrapment, 3: 410–411
   nonconstrained total prosthesis, 4: 145

   non-hinged metal–polyethylene prosthesis, 4: 145–146
   total replacement of, 4: 129
electromyogram, 3: 320
electron microscopes, 2: 323, *324*, *325*
Elgin table, 3: *287*
Eliot, Charles W., 1: *139*
   educational reforms and, 1: 139, 140*b*, 146–147; 2: 19, 41; 3: 44–45, 94
   medical education and, 1: 141; 4: 2
   on medical faculty organization, 1: 173
   on medical leadership, 4: 4
   on medical student caliber, 1: 131, 140
   opposition to football, 1: 253
Elks' Reconstruction Hospital, 4: 447–448
Ellen and Melvin Gordon Professor of Medical Education, 4: 264
Elliott, J. W., 2: 306
Elliott G. Brackett Fund, 3: 161
Ellis, Daniel S., 3: 241
Elliston, Harriet Hammond, 4: 90, 92
Elliston, William A. (1904–1984), 4: 41*b*, *90*
   Boston Children's Hospital and, 2: 313
   Brigham and Women's Hospital and, 4: 193
   death of, 4: 92
   education and training, 4: 90
   hip arthroplasty follow-up, 4: 40
   HMS appointment, 4: 90
   life and community service in Weston, 4: 91–92
   marriage and family, 4: 90, 92
   on nylon arthroplasty of the knee, 4: 91
   PBBH and, 4: 18, 20
   publications and research, 4: 90–91
   RBBH and, 4: 32, 35, 38, 41, 68, 89–90, 93, 132
   US Army Medical Corps and, 4: 90
   Veterans Administration Hospital and, 4: 90–91
Elliston, William Rowley, 4: 90
Emans, John (1944–), 2: *357*
   Boston brace and, 2: 358–359, *359*
   Boston Children's Hospital and, 2: 338, 354, 358–359
   Brigham and Women's Hospital and, 4: 163, 193

   Chest Wall and Spinal Deformity Study Group, 2: 361–362
   Core Curriculum Committee and, 1: 216
   Cutler Army Hospital and, 2: 358
   education and training, 2: 358, 388
   Hall and, 2: 347, 358
   HMS appointment, 2: 358
   honors and awards, 2: 363
   Myelodysplasia Program, 2: 359
   nutritional status research, 2: 361–362
   Parker Hill Hospital and, 2: 358
   professional memberships, 2: 363, 363*b*
   publications and research, 2: *358*, 359–363
   scoliosis treatment, 2: 339, 344
   Spinal Surgery Service, 2: 359
embarkation hospitals, 4: 451–452
Emergency Care and Transportation of the Sick and Injured (MacAusland), 3: 310, *311*
Emerson, Ralph Waldo, 1: 57
Emerson, Roger, 3: 396, 399
Emerson Hospital, 3: 317, 319
Emmons, Nathaniel H., 2: 6
Emory University Hospital, 4: 158
Enders, John, 2: 189
End-Result Idea (Codman)
   accountability and, 3: 119*b*
   bone sarcomas and, 3: 136–138
   Boston Children's Hospital and, 1: 194
   cards recording outcomes, 3: *111*, 113*b*
   Codman Hospital and, 3: 112, 114, *126*
   Codman's personal cases, 3: 126, 128–129
   Codman's promotion of, 3: 126
   as experiment, 3: 119–120
   filing system for, 3: *116*
   Halifax YMCA Emergency Hospital and, 3: 134
   hospital efficiency and, 3: 127*b*
   opposition to, 3: 118–120, 122–123
   PBBH and, 4: 12
   performance-based promotions and, 3: 123–124
   promotion of, 3: 116, 118, 123
   Robert Osgood and, 2: 135
   spread of, 3: 125
   treatment outcomes reporting, 3: 110–111
   young surgeons and, 3: 130–131

Enneking, William, 1: 218–220; 3: 382
Entrapment Neuropathies (Dawson, et al.), 4: 168
Epidemic Aid Team, 2: 260
epiphyseal arrest, 2: 170–171, 192, 192*t*, *192*, 193
epiphyseal injuries, 2: 321; 4: 350–351, *351*, 352, 355
Erickson, A. Ingrid, 1: 217*b*
Ernest A. Codman Award, 3: 146
Ernst, Harold C., 1: 171; 4: *6*
Erving, W. G., 4: 394
Esposito, Phil, 3: 357, 357*b*
Essentials of Body Mechanics (Goldthwait et al.), 3: *90*, 91
Estok, Dan M., II, 4: 193, 195*b*
ether
  asthma and, 1: 56
  commemoration of first use, 1: *61*, *64*, 65; 3: 32
  composition of, 1: 61
  deaths and, 3: 31
  discovery rights of, 1: 60
  ethical use of, 1: 58
  Morton's inhaler, 1: *58*
  use as anesthesia, 1: 55–62, *63*, 64–65, 82
  use at MGH, 1: 57–63, 85; 3: 15, 22, 27–28, 28*b*, 29, 29*b*, 30–34
  use at social events, 1: 56
  use on children, 1: 63
  use outside the U.S., 1: 59
Ether Day 1846 (Prosperi and Prosperi), 1: *59*
Ether Dome (MGH), 1: *59*, *63*, 84; 3: *14*, 16
Ether Monument, 1: *64*, 65; 3: 32, 32*b*
Etherization (J. C. Warren), 1: 62, *62*; 3: 33
Evans, Christopher, 2: 82, 166; 3: 462; 4: 194, 195*b*
Evans, D. K., 2: 211
Evans, Frances, 4: 41*b*
Evarts, C. M. "Mac," 1: 234
Ewald, Frederick C. (1933–), 4: *144*
  Brigham and Women's Hospital, 4: 163
  Brigham Orthopedic Associates (BOA) and, 4: 123
  capitellocondylar total elbow prosthesis, 4: 145, *145*, 146, *146*, 147
  Children's Hospital/MGH combined program and, 4: 144
  education and training, 4: 144
  giant cell synovitis case, 4: 148
  Helen Fay Hunter orthopaedic research fellowship, 4: 144
  HMS appointment, 4: 144
  Knee Society president, 4: 150
  legacy of, 4: 150
  PBBH and, 4: 116, 129, 144–145, 161
  professional memberships, 4: 150
  publications and research, 4: 130, *130*, 134, 144–146, *146*, 147, *147*, 148–149, *149*, 150, 189
  RBBH and, 4: 129, 132, 144–145, 150
  roentgenographic total knee arthroplasty-scoring system, 4: 150
  total knee arthroplasty and, 4: 130–131, 131*t*, 145
  total knee prosthesis research, 4: 147–148, *148*, 149–150
  West Roxbury Veterans Administration Hospital and, 4: 144
Ewing, James, 3: 137
Experience in the Management of Fractures and Dislocations (Wilson), 3: 376
"Extra-Articular Arthrodesis of the Subastragalar Joint" (Grice), 2: *208*, 209
extracorporeal shockwave therapy (ESWT), 3: 437–438

F

Fahey, Robert, 4: 341
Fallon, Anne, 2: 260, *260*
Falmouth Hospital, 4: 89
Faraday, Michael, 1: 56
Farber, Sidney, 2: 171, 215, 234–236; 4: 72
Farnsworth, Dana, 1: 277, 284
fasciotomies, 1: 35; 2: 201, 250; 3: 417–418. *See also* Ober-Yount fasciotomy
fat embolism syndrome, 2: 397, *397*, 398
Faulkner Hospital, 3: 248, 314, 331; 4: 194, *194*
Faxon, Henry H., 4: 482
Faxon, John, 1: 42, 44
Faxon, Nathaniel W., 3: 70*b*; 4: 475, 482
Fearing, Albert, 2: 5
Federated Jewish Charities, 4: 205
Federation of Jewish Charities, 4: 200
Federation of Spine Associations, 4: 265
Federation of State Medical Boards (FSMB), 3: 424
Felch, L. P., 3: 269
Feldon, Paul, 4: 98
Fell, Honor B., 4: 126
femoral heads
  acetabular dysplasia case, 2: 390
  acetabular replacement and, 3: 279
  avascular necrosis of, 4: 154–156, 238
  blood supply to, 1: 36; 2: 392
  bone allografts and, 3: 442
  excision of, 3: 155
  flattening of, 2: *103*
  fractures of, 1: 49; 3: 38–39
  hip dislocations and, 2: 352–353, 401, 418
  hip joint excision and, 3: 34
  histologic-histochemical grading system for, 3: 384
  Legg-Calvé-Perthes disease, 2: 105, 351
  osteoarthritis and, 3: 221
  osteonecrosis of, 2: 328–329, 394; 3: 434; 4: 156–157
  palpating, 1: 48
  replacement of, 3: 213
  sclerosis of, 3: 441
  slipped capital femoral epiphysis (SCFE) and, 2: 176
  tuberculosis and, 2: 108
  wear on, 3: 224
femoral neck fractures. *See also* hip fractures
  AAOS study of, 3: 191
  Bigelow and, 3: 38–39
  calcar femorale and, 3: 39, *39*
  experience among AAOS members, 3: 190*t*
  fracture research and, 3: 377
  osteoarthritis and, 3: 383–384
  roentgenology and, 3: 377
  Smith-Petersen and, 3: 62, 181, 185–186, *186*, 189, 189*b*, 190
  tissue response at, 4: 76
  treatment of, 3: 367
  triflanged nail for, 3: 62, 185–186, *186*, 189, 189*b*, 190
femoral spurs, 3: 39
femoroacetabular impingement, 3: 188–189
femur fractures
  Buck's traction and, 1: 80
  Gaucher's disease, 3: 434
  growth disturbances in, 2: 400
  immediate reamed nailings of, 3: 416
  malunions, 3: *42*

sepsis after intramedullary fixation, 2: 248; 3: 309–310
triflanged nail for, 3: 62, 185, *186*, 189, 189*b*
wartime treatment of, 4: 408
Ferguson, Albert B., Jr. (1919–2014), 4: *109*
death of, 4: 111
education and training, 4: 110
HMS appointment, 4: 111
muscle dynamics research, 4: 111
Orthopaedic Surgery in Infancy and Childhood, 2: 188, 239, 303
PBBH and, 1: 204; 2: 188; 4: 19, 21, 36, 79, 110–111
professional memberships, 4: 111
publications and research, 4: 102
RBBH and, 4: 93, 111
spiral femur fracture case, 4: 110
University of Pittsburgh appointment, 2: 188; 3: 382–383; 4: 73*b*, 111
US Marine Corps and, 4: 110
Ferguson, Albert B., Sr., 4: 109–110
Ferguson, Jeremiah, 4: 109
Fernandez, Diego L., 3: 409, 431
Fessenden, Louise, 3: 271
Fifth Portable Surgical Hospital, 4: 489
Fine, Jacob, 4: 283*t*
Fink, Edward, 4: 279–280
Fink, Mitchell P., 4: 283*t*
Finkelstein, Clara, 2: 319
Finney, John M. T., 4: 324
Finton, Frederick P., 1: *80*
First Operation Under Ether (Hinckley), 1: *55*, 59
Fischer, Josef E., 4: 287, 289*b*
Fisher, Bob, 1: 255
Fisher, Josef E., 1: 234; 2: 397
Fisher, Roland F., 3: 167
Fisher, Thomas J., 3: 431
Fiske, Eben W., 4: 389*b*, 394
Fiske, Edith, 2: 42
Fiske Prize, 2: 52
Fitchet, Seth M. (1887–1939), 2: *252*
Boston Children's Hospital and, 2: 222, 252, 274; 4: 338
cleidocranial dysostosis, 2: 254
death of, 2: 254
education and training, 2: 251
Harvard Department of Hygiene and, 2: 253
HMS appointment, 2: 252
MGH and, 2: 252
military service, 2: 251
Morris and, 2: 282
private medical practice, 2: 252

public health and, 2: 253
publications and research, 1: 263; 2: 253–254
ruptures of the serratus anterior, 2: 253
Stillman Infirmary and, 2: 253
Fitton-Jackson, Sylvia, 4: 126
Fitz, Reginald Heber, 1: 179; 3: 94
Fitz, Wolfgang, 4: 194
FitzSimmons, Elizabeth Grace Rogers, 2: 258
FitzSimmons, Henry J. (1880–1935), 1: *187*; 2: *254, 255, 258*
on atypical multiple bone tuberculosis, 2: 257
Boston Children's Hospital and, 1: 187; 2: 252, 254–256, 258, 274, 282; 4: 338
Boston University and, 2: 258
Camp Devens base hospital and, 4: 452
congenital torticollis research, 2: 256, 258
death of, 2: 258
East Boston Relief Station and, 2: 254
education and training, 2: 254
European medical studies, 2: 255
HMS appointment, 2: 223, 256, 258; 4: 59–60
marriage and family, 2: 258
military surgeon training and, 2: 42
Ober on, 2: 256, 258
orthopaedics internship under Bradford, 2: 255
orthopaedics internship under Lovett, 2: 144
Osgood on, 2: 258–259
professional memberships, 2: 258, 258*b*
publications and research, 2: 256, 258
ton Children's Hospital and, 1: 188
World War I service, 2: 258
5005th USAF Hospital (Elmendorf), 3: 215
Flagg, Elisha, 3: 67
Flatt, Adrian, 4: 97
Fleisher, Leon, 3: 414
Flexner, Abraham, 1: 146–147; 3: 165
Flexner Report, 1: 146–147
flexor carpi ulnaris transfer procedure, 2: 172, 188, 198–199, *199*, 200
Fliedner, Theodor, 4: 274*b*
Flier, Jeffrey, 1: 242
Floating Hospital for Children, 2: 306, 370

flow cytometry, 3: 388
Floyd, W. Emerson, 3: 410
Floyd, W., III, 2: 417
Flugstad, Daniel, 3: 433
fluoroscope, 2: 307; 3: 96–97
Flynn, John, 3: 433
Foley, T. M., 4: 451
Folkman, Judah, 4: 182
Foot and Ankle, The (Trott and Bateman), 2: 317
foot problems. *See also* club foot
ankle valgus, 2: 212
arches and, 2: 317
arthritis and, 4: 61
astragalectomy (Whitman's operation), 2: 92–93
athletes and, 3: 348
Batchelor technique, 2: 212
Brewster and, 2: 228–229
calcaneovalgus deformity, 2: 92–93
cavus feet, 2: 229
cerebral palsy treatment, 2: 229
congenital flatfoot, 4: 63
correction of fixed deformities, 4: 62, 62*t*, 63
countersinking the talus, 2: 228–229, 283
Dane and, 2: 242–246
design of shoes for, 2: 54–56
evaluation through glass, 2: 54–55, *55*
extra-articular arthrodesis of the subtalar joint, 2: 210–211, *211*, 212
flat feet, 2: 54–56, 101–102, 107–108, 242–243, *243*, 244–246
gait analysis and, 2: 407
Green-Grice procedure, 2: 212
heel cord contractures, 2: 265
hindfoot pain, 4: 188
Hoke's stabilization requirements, 2: 282–283
John Brown's device for, 1: 106
Lambrinudi stabilization, 2: 229
Morton's neuroma, 2: 287
nurses and, 2: 54–56
Osgood on, 2: 123–124
paralytic flat foot deformities, 2: 210–212
planovalgus deformity, 4: 188
poliomyelitis and, 2: 210
radiography and, 2: 56
rheumatoid arthritis and, 4: 188
shoe fit and design, 2: 293, 317, 407
skeletal anatomy and, 2: 247
sling procedure and, 3: 294, *294*, 295, 296*b*–297*b*

Index

stabilization of, 2: 282–284
treatment of, 2: 54–56, 107–108
triple arthrodesis, 2: 172, 228–229
valgus deformity treatment, 2: 197, 209–212
weakness/paralysis in, 2: 150–151
wire drop foot splints, 2: *123*
football
acromioclavicular joint dislocation in, 1: 268, 277
athletic training and, 1: 248, 250–253, 255–256, 258
Bloody Monday game, 1: 245
Boston Game, 1: 247
collegiate reform and, 1: 253–254
concussions in, 1: 247, 254, 274–275
establishment of rules in, 1: 247–248
Hampden Park, Springfield, 1: *249*
Harvard game, 1906, 1: *257*
Harvard Rose Bowl game, 1920, 1: *259*
injuries in, 1: 247–248, 252–255, 255t, 256, 258–262, 288
preventative strappings, 1: *269*
protective padding and helmets in, 1: 255, *267*
ruptures of the serratus anterior, 2: 253
secondary school injuries in, 4: 370, *370*
sports medicine and, 1: 248, 250, 254–256
team photo, 1890, 1: *249*
Forbes, A. Mackenzie, 2: 87–88; 3: 231; 4: 233, 394
Forbes, Andrew, 3: 437
Forbes, Elliot, 2: 277
Fort Bragg (Fayetteville, N.C.), 4: 484
Fort Leonard Wood (Missouri), 3: 432
Fort Oglethorpe (Georgia), 4: 338
Fort Ord US Army Hospital, 4: 259
Fort Riley (Kansas), 4: 452–453
Fort Totten (Queens, NY), 4: *422*
Fort Warren (Mass.), 1: 20
Foster, Charles C., 1: 109, 111
Foster, Charles H. W., 3: 123
Foster, Helen, 3: 228
Foultz, W. S., 2: 237
Fourth Portable Surgical Hospital (4PSH), 2: 232–233; 4: 489
Fourth Portable Surgical Hospital's Service in the War against Japan, The (Cohen), 2: 232–233

fracture boxes, 1: 80–81
Fracture Clinic (MGH), 2: 130; 3: 60, 60b, 61–62, 241–242, 245, 273, *273*, 313–315, 371, 373, 378, 456b
Fracture Committee of the American College of Surgeons, 2: 131; 3: 61
fractures. *See also* compound fractures; femoral neck fractures; femur fractures; hip fractures
amputations and, 1: 50, 54
ankle, 4: 313–315, *315*, 316
Austin Moore prosthesis, 3: 213
bandaging care and, 1: 76
basket plasters for, 2: *122*
bilateral comminuted patellar, 3: 56b
birth, 1: 264
calcaneus treatment by impaction, 4: 313, 314b
cervical spine, 3: 340–341
clinics for, 2: 130–131
conference on treatment for, 2: 131
Cotton's, 4: 313–315, *315*, 316
displaced supracondylar humerus, 2: 379
distal femoral physeal, 2: 400
distal radius treatment, 3: 408–409
elderly patients and, 3: 353, 354, 354b; 4: 341
fender, 4: 242
Gartland type 3 supracondylar humeral, 2: 368
general and orthopaedic surgeon collaboration on, 4: 463–465
hip nailing and, 3: 237
hips and, 3: 213; 4: 74–75, 159b–160b, 318–320, 341
of the humerus, 3: 323–324; 4: 372
impaction treatment for, 4: 319–320
increase in, 1: 63
intercondylar T humeral, 2: 397, *397*
intra-articular, 3: 408
lateral tibial plateau, 4: *312*
leg length and, 2: 350
long-bone, 3: 60–61
malpractice suits and, 1: 50–51; 3: 63
managing pediatric, 2: 379
metastatic breast disease and, 2: 411
metastatic pathological, 3: 376, 377–378
olecranon, 3: 309

open anterior lumbosacral dislocation, 3: 420
open treatment of, 3: 55–56, 58–62, 64
open-bone, 4: *400*
orthopaedic treatment of, 4: 463
os calcis, 4: 313, 314b, 335–336
outcomes of, 1: 50; 3: 339
plaster casts for, 2: *122*
portable traction device, 2: 297
Pott's, 4: *317*, 318
proximal humerus, 2: 96, *122*
pseudofracture of tibia, 3: 341, *342*
of the radial head, 2: 396–397; 3: 322–323
risk prediction research, 2: 411, *411*
scaphoid, 3: 101–102; 4: 359–361
scientific study of, 1: 264
shoulders, 3: 339
supracondylar humerus, 2: 229, 345, 379
Swiss method of treating, 2: 406
table for, 2: *121*
tibial spine, 4: 365
tibial tuberosity, 2: 91
total disability following joint, 3: *373*
traction treatment for, 2: 23
treatment for compound, 4: 335, 337, *392*
treatment of, 1: 80–81; 3: 35, 60, 101; 4: 339b–340b, 362
triflanged nail for, 3: 62, 185–186, *186*, 189, 189b
ununited, 3: 34–35
vanadium steel plates and, 4: 340, *342*
wire arm splint for, 2: *122*
Fractures (Wilson), 3: 315
Fractures and Dislocations (Stimson), 1: 147
Fractures and Dislocations (Wilson and Cochrane), 3: 371, *371*
Fractures and Other Injuries (Cave), 3: 273, *273*; 4: 356
Fractures of the Distal Radius (Fernandez and Jupiter), 3: 409, *409*
Francis A. Countway Library of Medicine, 1: 59, 66; 2: 271; 4: 20
Frank R. Ober Research Fund, 2: 165
Franklin, Benjamin, 1: 12, 14
Fraser, Somers, 4: 438–439
Frazier, Charles H., 4: 299
Frederick and Joan Brengle Learning Center, 3: 463

Frederick W. and Jane M. Ilfeld Professorship, 2: 438, 439*b*
Fredericks, G. R., 3: 442
Free Hospital for Women, 4: 113–114
Freedman, K. B., 1: 168
Frei, Emil, III, 2: 422
Freiberg, Albert H., 2: 77–78, 87; 3: 157, 229; 4: 406, 451
Freiberg, Joseph A., 1: 193; 2: 79; 4: 59
Friedenberg, Z., 2: 214
Friedlaender, Gary, 3: 393, 440; 4: 266*b*
Friedman, Richard, 1: 217*b*
Frost, Eben H., 1: 60
Frost, Gilbert, 3: 97
frozen shoulder, 1: 277–278
Frymoyer, J. W., 3: 205
Fuldner, Russell, 3: 74
Fundamentals of Orthopaedic Surgery in General Medicine and Surgery (Osgood and Allison), 2: 135–136
Funsten, Robert, 3: 303
Furbush, C. L., 4: 439, 440*b*

G

Gage, M., 3: 210
Gage, Thomas, 1: 16
gait
    backpack loads and, 2: 408
    cerebral palsy and, 2: 406–407
    clinical analysis and, 2: 408
    hip abductor weakness and, 2: 33
    impact of shoes on, 2: 293, 407
    low back disorders and, 2: 408
    nonmechanical treatment of, 2: 244
    nonoperative treatment of, 2: 271
    Ober-Yount fasciotomy and, 2: 153
    physical therapy and, 2: 107
    shelf procedure and, 2: 151
    stroke and, 2: 408
    total knee replacement and, 2: 408
    Trendelenburg, 2: 33, 108, 151
    use of cameras to analyze, 2: 406
gait laboratory, 2: 107, 406, 424; 3: 397
Galante, Jorge, 3: 220, 222
Galeazzi method, 2: 227
Gall, Edward, 3: 331
Gallie, William E., 1: 197; 2: 160; 4: 443
Galloway, Herbert P. H., 3: 233; 4: 411, 426, 454, 464
Gambrill, Howard, Jr., 4: 40
Gandhi, Mohandas Karamchand, 4: 262
Ganz, Reinhold, 2: 390–392
Garbino, Peter, 2: 438
Gardiner Hospital, 3: 282, 284
Gardner, George E., 2: 215
Garg, Sumeet, 2: 378
Garland, Joseph E., 3: 12
Garrey, W. E., 1: 267
Gartland, John, 3: 308–309
Gates, Frank D. (1925–2011), 2: *218*
    Boston Children's Hospital and, 2: 218
    death of, 2: 218–219
    education and training, 2: 218
    HMS appointment, 2: 218
Gates, Frederick T., 1: 146
Gatton Agricultural College, 4: 489, *489*
Gaucher's disease, 3: 433–434
Gauvain, Sir Henry, 4: 363, 367
Gay, George H., 1: 308; 3: *31*
Gay, George W., 4: 324
Gay, Martin, 1: 306
Gay, Warren F., 3: 68, 266
Gaynor, David, 3: 463
Gebhardt, Mark C.
    as Beth Israel chief of orthopaedics, 4: 289*b*
    as BIDMC chief of orthopaedics, 4: 287
    Boston Children's Hospital and, 2: 439*b*
    Boston Pathology Course and, 1: 216
    Frederick W. and Jane M. Ilfeld Professorship, 2: 439*b*
    HCORP and, 1: 218, 224–225, 227
    on Mankin, 3: 393
    as MGH clinical faculty, 3: 464*b*
    orthopaedic chair at BIDMC, 1: 234, 242
    orthopaedic oncology and, 3: 460*b*
    publications and research, 3: 433
    tumor treatment and, 3: 397
Geiger, Ronald, 2: 277, 290
Gelberman, Richard H. (1943–), 3: *402*
    avascular necrosis of the lunate case, 3: 403
    Core Curriculum Committee and, 1: 216
    education and training, 3: 402
    flexor tendon research, 3: 403, *403*
    hand and microvascular service, 3: 402–403
    HCORP and, 3: 403–404
    HMS appointment, 3: 403
    honors and awards, 3: 403–405
    as MGH chief of Hand Service, 3: 403
    as MGH surgeon, 3: 399
    Operative Nerve Repair and Reconstruction, 3: 404
    publications and research, 3: 402, *402*, 403–404
    Smith Day lectures, 3: 431
    tissue fluid pressures research, 3: 404, *404*
    University of California in San Diego and, 3: 402
    Washington University School of Medicine and, 3: 404–405
gene therapy, 2: 82
General Leonard Wood Army Community Hospital, 3: 432
General Leonard Wood Gold Medal, 4: 337
genu valgum, 1: *117*
genu varum, 1: *117*
George III, King, 1: 11
George W. Gay Lecture, 4: 324
George Washington University, 2: 351
Georgia Warm Springs Foundation, 2: 77–78, 107, 264, *264*, 270
Gerald, Park, 2: 234
Gerbino, Peter, 2: 439*b*
Gerhart, Tobin, 1: 217*b*; 4: 251, 262–263, 286, 288
German Orthopaedic Association, 2: 43
Ghivizzani, Steve, 4: 194
Ghogawala, Zoher, 4: 272*b*
Ghormley, Jean McDougall, 3: 288, 290
Ghormley, Ralph K. (1893–1959), 3: *288*
    death of, 3: 290
    Diagnosis in Joint Disease, 3: 175, 289, *290*
    early life, 3: 288
    education and training, 3: 288
    HMS appointment, 3: 288; 4: 59
    on joint disease, 3: 288–289, *289*
    as joint tuberculosis expert, 3: 289
    leadership of, 3: 289–290
    marriage and family, 3: 288
    Mayo Clinic and, 3: 289
    memberships and, 3: 290, 290*b*
    as MGH surgeon, 3: 288
    military orthopaedics and, 4: 453

Index

New England Peabody Home for Cripped Children and, 2: 270; 3: 288
private medical practice, 2: 146; 3: 288
publications and research, 3: 288–289
triple arthrodesis and, 2: 150
tuberculosis research and, 3: 288–289
US Army Medical Corps and, 3: 288
Giannestras, Nicholas, 2: 317; 3: *293*
Gibney, Virgil P., 2: 27, 43, 48, 52; 4: 463
Gilbreth, Frank B., 3: 120
Gill, A. Bruce, 2: 78, 183
Gill, Madeline K., 4: 59
Gill, Thomas J., 1: 167; 3: 462, 464*b*
Gilles, Hamish G., 4: 163, 193
Giza, Eric, 1: 217*b*
glanders, 2: 46
Glaser, Robert J., 4: 113
Glazer, Paul, 4: 286
Gleich operation, 4: 313
glenohumeral deformity, 2: 418–419, 419*t*
Glick, Hyman, 4: 251, 262–263, 286, 288
Glickel, Steven Z., 3: 430
Glimcher, Aaron, 2: 319
Glimcher, Clara Finkelstein, 2: 319
Glimcher, Laurie, 2: 330–331
Glimcher, Melvin J. (1925–2014), 1: *208, 210,* 285; 2: *319, 320, 330*; 3: 455
  activating transcription factor-2 (ATF-2) and, 2: 330
  BIH Board of Consultants, 4: 262–263
  bone research, 2: 321–330
  Boston Arm development, 2: 326
  Boston Children's Hospital and, 1: 180; 2: 320, 327, 329; 4: 127
  Brigham and Women's Hospital and, 4: 163, 193
  Children's Hospital/MGH combined program and, 2: 320
  as Children's orthopaedic surgeon-in-chief, 2: 15*b*, 286, 326–327, 337, 406, 422, 434
  death of, 2: 331
  on DeLorme's blood perfusion research, 3: 287
  as Edith M. Ashley Professor, 3: 464*b*

education and training, 2: 319–321
electron microscopes and, 2: 323, *324,* 325
epiphyseal injuries after frostbite case, 2: 321–323
gait laboratory, 2: 406
Hall and, 2: 336
as Harriet M. Peabody Professor, 2: 327, 337, 439*b*
HCORP and, 4: 247
HMS appointment, 2: 321, 327
as honorary orthopaedic surgeon, 3: 398*b*
honors and awards, 2: 319, 324–325, 327–331
leadership of, 3: 453, 455*b*–457*b*
legacy of, 2: 330–331; 3: 458*b*
marriage and family, 2: 331
MGH Orthopaedic Research Laboratories and, 2: 321–324
as MGH orthopaedics chief, 1: 210; 2: 325; 3: 11*b,* 202, 228, 245, 385, 458*b,* 459; 4: 126
MGH residents and, 2: *327*; 3: *457*
orthopaedic research and, 3: 211
orthopaedics curriculum and, 1: 164; 3: 457*b*
osteonecrosis of the femoral head research, 2: 328, *328,* 329; 4: 156
PBBH and, 4: 163
professional memberships, 2: 329, 331
publications and research, 2: 321, *321,* 322, 324–330
research laboratories, 2: 434, 439; 3: 455*b,* 458*b*
Glowacki, Julie, 4: 194, 195*b*
gluteus maximus
  modification of use of sacrospinalis, 2: 146–147
  Ober operation and, 2: 148, 153
  paralysis of, 2: 146–147
  posterior approach to the hips, 2: 353
Goddu, Louis A. O., 3: 268; 4: 204
Godfrey, Ambrose, 1: 56
Godfrey, Arthur, 3: 198–199
Goethals, Thomas R., 4: 474, 482*b*
Goetjes, D. H., 2: 91
Goff, C. F., 4: 313
Gokaslan, Ziya L., 4: 272*b*
Goldberg, Michael, 2: 368
Goldring, Steve, 4: 280
Goldstone, Melissa, 3: 328
Goldthwait, Ellen W. R., 4: 27
Goldthwait, Francis Saltonstall, 3: 89

Goldthwait, Jessie Sophia Rand, 3: 79, 89
Goldthwait, Joel C., 4: 37–38
Goldthwait, Joel E. (1866–1961), 3: *77, 89, 91*; 4: *24,* 398
  adult orthopaedics and, 2: 101; 3: 78–79
  AOA preparedness committee, 4: 394
  back pain research and, 3: 203–204
  Beth Israel Hospital and, 4: 247
  Body Mechanics in Health and Disease, 3: 91
  Boston Children's Hospital and, 1: 187; 2: 13, 40, 247; 3: 78
  Boston City Hospital and, 1: 187; 4: 305*b*
  Boston School of Physical Education and, 3: 84
  Brigham Hospital and, 3: 81, 84, 91–92
  Carney Hospital and, 3: 78, 80; 4: 45, 86
  chronic disease treatment and, 4: 52
  clinical congress meeting, 3: 118
  Corey Hill Hospital and, 3: 89; 4: 224
  curative workshops and, 4: 402–403
  death of, 3: 92; 4: 38
  Diseases of the Bones and Joints, 2: 117; 3: 81–82
  dislocation of the patella case, 3: 79, 79*b,* 80, *81*
  Division of Orthopedic Surgery in the A.E.F., 4: 473
  early life, 3: 77
  education and training, 3: 77–78
  Essentials of Body Mechanics, 3: *90,* 91
  etiology of orthopaedic impairments and diseases, 3: 81–82
  on faulty body mechanics, 3: 91
  founding of AAOS, 3: 90
  on hip disease, 2: 52, *52*
  HMS appointment, 3: 80, 84
  Hospital Efficiency meeting, 3: 120
  House of the Good Samaritan and, 2: 114; 3: 78
  on importance of posture, 3: 81, 83, 87–89; 4: 53, 62, 82, 233
  interest in visceroptosis, 3: 83–84, 84*b,* 86–88
  iron bars, 3: 89, *89, 149*
  legacy of, 3: 91–92
  Marcella Street Home and, 2: 247

marriage and family, 3: 79, 89
on medical research, 3: 2
memberships and, 3: 92
MGH biochemistry laboratory, 2: 322; 3: 455*b*–456*b*
as MGH orthopaedics chief, 3: 11*b*, 67–68, 80–81, 227
military orthopaedics and, 2: 127–128; 3: 156; 4: 406, 443
military reconstruction hospitals and, 4: 440, 444–445
military surgeon training and, 2: 65
New England Deaconess Hospital and, 3: 78; 4: 274
orthopaedic surgery, 2: 116
patellar tendon transfer, 2: 294
on patient evaluation, 3: 90
on polio, 2: 77
private medical practice, 4: 62
publications and research, 3: 78–84, 90, *90*, 91
RBBH and, 3: 81, 84, 91–92; 4: 23–25, 25*b*, 26–28, 31, 36–38, 39*b*, 79, 93, 111
rehabilitation of soldiers and, 4: 396, 402, 411
resolution in honor of, 4: 38, 39*b*
Robert Jones Lecture, 3: 90
Shattuck Lecture, 3: 84–85, *85*, 86
surgical records from, 2: 115*b*
US Army Distinguished Service Medal, 3: 83, *83*
US Medical Reserve Corps, 3: 89
on variations in human anatomy, 3: 85–86, 86*t*
World War I and, 2: 124–125; 4: 402–403
World War I volunteer orthopaedic surgeons and, 4: 398–399, *399*, 404, 406–407, 411
Goldthwait, Mary Lydia Pitman, 3: 77
Goldthwait, Thomas, 3: 77
Goldthwait, William Johnson, 3: 77
Goldthwait Research Fund, 4: 27–28
Goldthwait Reservation, 3: 92, *92*
Good Samaritan Hospital, 1: 107. *See also* House of the Good Samaritan
Goodnow, Elisha, 4: 293
Goodridge, Frederick J., 3: 266
Goodsir, John, 1: xxii
Gordon, Leonard, 3: 431
Gordon Hall, 1: *86*

Gordon Research Conference on Bioengineering and Orthopaedic Sciences, 3: 445, *445*
Gorforth, Helen R., 3: 365
Gorgas, William C., 4: 411, 429, 447
Gould, Augustus Addison, 1: 60
Gould, Marjorie, 3: 303
Gould, Nathaniel D., 1: 309; 3: *293*
Grabias, Stanley L., 1: 217*b*; 3: 460*b*
Graffman, Gary, 3: 414
Graham, Henry, 2: 168
Grand Palais (Paris), 4: 401
Grandlay, J., 3: 210
Great Britain, 1: 11–16; 4: 393, 399, 432, 476. *See also* British Expeditionary Forces (BEF); British hospitals
Great Ormond Street Hospital, 2: 5
Greater Boston Bikur Cholim Hospital, 4: 212
Greater Hartford Tuberculosis Respiratory Disease Association, 2: 267
Green, Daniel, 4: 239
Green, David, 4: 98
Green, Elizabeth, 2: 168
Green, Gladys Griffith, 2: 168
Green, Janet, 2: 168
Green, Jean, 2: 167
Green, Neil, 2: 351, *351*
Green, Robert M., 1: 89
Green, Samuel A., 3: 46
Green, William T. (1901–1986), 1: *200*, *204*, *207*; 2: 167, *169*, *177*, *179*, *180*, *204*
as AAOS president, 2: 201–202, *202*, 203
on arthritis, 2: 171
birth palsies research, 2: 415, 417
on bone granuloma, 2: 171
on bone growth and leg length discrepancy, 2: 170, 191–193
Boston Children's Hospital and, 1: 158, 179–180; 2: 168–169, 176–178, 191, 274, 301; 3: 277, 293; 4: 72
CDH treatment, 3: 235
cerebral palsy treatment, 2: 171–172, 196–200, 229
Children's Hospital/MGH combined program and, 4: 68, 158
on clinical staff, 1: 201
Cohen and, 2: 234–235
on congenital pseudarthrosis of the tibia, 2: 172–176
contributions to pediatric orthopaedics, 2: 168

Crippled Children's Clinic and, 2: 287
death of, 2: 205
early life, 2: 167
education and training, 2: 167–168
Epidemic Aid Team, 2: 260
as first Harriet M. Peabody Professor, 2: 183, 203, 439*b*
flexor carpi ulnaris transfer procedure, 2: 172, 188, 198–200
grand rounds and, 2: 178–181, *181*, 182, 230, 271
on Grice, 2: 215
Growth Study, 2: 193, *193*, 194, 304, 432
hamstring contractures and, 2: 198
Harriet M. Peabody Professor of Orthopaedic Surgery, 3: 202
Harvard Infantile Paralysis Clinic and, 2: 176, 188
HCORP and, 1: 200–210
HMS appointment, 2: 168, 176, 183, 223, 270; 4: 61
honorary degrees, 2: 203
Infantile Paralysis Clinic and, 2: 79
on Kuhns, 4: 66
legacy of, 2: 203–205
marriage and family, 2: 168
McGinty and, 2: 279
meticulousness and, 2: 178–179, 182–183
on muscle grades, 2: 180
Ober and, 2: 163, 168
as orthopaedic chair, 2: 15*b*
orthopaedic research laboratory and, 2: 234
on orthopaedics curriculum, 1: 159, 162–164, 200–201; 2: 202
orthopaedics education and, 2: 183–186, 188, 203, 205
orthopaedics leadership, 2: 176–178, 191, 197
on osteochondritis dissecans, 2: 194–195
on osteomyelitis, 2: 169–170
PBBH and, 4: 16, 18–22, 73*b*, 79, 108, 110
as PBBH chief of orthopaedic surgery, 4: 196*b*
Pediatric Orthopaedic Society and, 2: 351
polio research and, 2: 189–190; 3: 332
polio treatment, 2: 188–191
private medical practice and, 1: 179; 2: 313

Index

professional memberships, 2: 204
as professor of orthopaedic surgery, 1: 158, 176, 198; 2: 176
publications and research, 2: 169, 188, 194–200, 229, 249, 264, 350
RBBH and, 4: 40, 68
rehabilitation planning and, 1: 272
on residency program, 1: 208
resident training by, 1: 199, 202–203, *203*, 204–206
on slipped capital femoral epiphysis (SCFE), 2: 176
on Sprengel deformity, 2: 195
surgery techniques, 2: 177
Tachdjian and, 2: 301–304
tibial osteoperiosteal graft method, 2: *228*
Trott and, 2: 317–318
Unit for Epidemic Aid in Infantile Paralysis (NFP), 2: 188–189
on Volkmann ischemic contracture, 2: 200–201, *201*
Green, William T., Jr., 2: 168, 182, 204–205
Green Dragon Tavern, 1: *11*, 12, *12*, 17, 24
Green-Andersen growth charts, 2: 193, *193*, 194, 304
Greenberg, B. E., 4: 199
Green-Grice procedure, 2: 212
Greenough, Francis, 2: 9
Greenough, Robert B., 2: 119, 157–158; 3: 118; 4: 389*b*
Greer, James A., 3: 398*b*
Gregory, Ernest, 4: 226
Grenfell, Sir William, 3: 91
Grenfell Mission, 2: 111
Grice, David S. (1914–1960), 2: *207*
  AAOS and, 2: 215
  Banks and, 1: 202, 205
  Boston Children's Hospital and, 2: 208, 299
  club foot treatment, 2: 208
  education and training, 2: 207–208
  extra-articular arthrodesis of the subtalar joint, 2: *208*, 209–212
  HMS appointment, 2: 208, 210, 213
  legacy of, 2: 214–216
  marriage and family, 2: 214
  Massachusetts Infantile Paralysis Clinic and, 2: 208, 212, 314
  memorial funds for, 2: 215
  orthopaedics education and, 2: 213–214
  orthopaedics leadership, 2: 191
  paralytic flat foot operative technique, 2: 210–212
  PBBH and, 2: 208; 4: 18–19, 110
  poliomyelitis treatment, 2: 208, 212–213, 213*b*, 315
  private medical practice and, 2: 313
  professional memberships, 2: 215
  publications of, 2: 189, 208, 220
  residency training by, 2: 213–214
  Simmons College and, 2: 213
  University of Pennsylvania and, 2: 213–214
  University of Vermont and, 2: 208
  valgus deformity treatment, 2: 198, 209–210
Grice, Elizabeth Fry, 2: 207
Grice, John, 2: 207
Grice, Mary Burns, 2: 214
Griffin, Bertha Mae Dail, 2: 349
Griffin, Jesse Christopher, 2: 349
Griffin, Margaret Braswell, 2: 349
Griffin, Paul P. (1927–2018), 2: *349*, *350*, 356
  arthritis treatment, 2: 350
  BIH Board of Consultants, 4: 262
  Boston Children's Hospital and, 2: 301, 338, 349, 351, 354–355, 434
  Chicago Shriner's Hospital and, 2: 355
  Crippled Children's Clinic and, 2: 314
  death of, 2: 356
  education and training, 2: 349
  George Washington University and, 2: 351
  HMS appointment, 2: 349–351, 354
  Laboratory for Skeletal Disorders and Rehabilitation and, 2: 413
  as orthopaedic chair, 2: 15*b*, 286
  orthopaedics appointments, 2: 351
  PBBH and, 4: 20, 22
  Pediatric Orthopaedic International Seminars program, 2: 304
  Pediatric Orthopaedic Society and, 2: 351
  pediatric orthopaedics, 2: 354–355
  private medical practice and, 2: 313
  publications and research, 2: 349–351, *351*, 354
  traumatic hip dislocation case, 2: 352–353
Griffith, Gladys, 2: 168
Griffiths, Maurice, 4: 92
Grillo, Hermes C., 1: 184
Gritti-Stokes amputation, 3: 374
Gross, Richard, 2: 354–355, 438
Gross, Robert E., 2: 215
Gross, Samuel D., 1: 79
Gross, Samuel W., 3: 142
Groves, Ernest W. Hey, 2: 91; 3: 209
Gucker, Harriet, 2: 266
Gucker, Thomas III (1915–1986), 2: *259*, *260*
  Berlin polio epidemic and, 2: 260, 264
  Boston Children's Hospital and, 2: 260, 264
  contributions to orthopaedic rehabilitation, 2: 266
  death of, 2: 266
  education and training, 2: 259–260
  Georgia Warm Springs Foundation and, 2: 264
  marriage and family, 2: 266
  on patient reaction to polio, 2: 261*b*–263*b*
  poliomyelitis and, 2: 259, 264, 266
  professional memberships, 2: 264–265
  publications and research, 2: 264–266
  on pulmonary function, 2: 265–266
  tendon transfers and, 2: 265
  University of Pennsylvania and, 2: 265
  University of Southern California and, 2: 266
Guérin, Jules, 1: 54, 98, 106; 3: 26
gunshot injuries, 2: 66, 119, 161, 233; 3: 43, 156, 156*b*; 4: 437, 441
Gupta, Amit, 3: 431
Guthrie, Douglas, 1: 183
Guy's and Old St. Thomas hospitals, 1: *34*
Guy's Hospital (London), 1: 6, 33–35, 37, 83

H

Haggert, G. Edmund, 2: 165; 4: 344–345, 378
Hale, Worth, 1: 176–177
Hale Hospital, 3: 331

Halifax Harbor explosion, 3: 132, *132*, 133–135
Halifax YMCA Emergency Hospital, 3: *133*, 134
Hall, Caroline Doane, 2: 267
Hall, Col. John, 3: 282, 284
Hall, Emmett Matthew, 2: 333
Hall, Francis C., 3: 338
Hall, Francis N. Walsh, 2: 333, 337, 348
Hall, H. J., 2: 55
Hall, Isabelle Mary Parker, 2: 333
Hall, John E. (1925–2018), 2: *333*, 346
   as BCH Orthopaedic chair, 2: 15*b*, 338–339, 384, 434, 436
   BIH Board of Consultants, 4: 262
   Boston Children's Hospital and, 2: 61, 279, 337–339, 399, 439*b*
   Brigham and Women's Hospital and, 2: 337; 4: 163, 193
   Cerebral Palsy Clinic and, 2: 402
   as clinical chief, 2: 286, 422
   death of, 2: 348
   Dwyer instrumentation and, 2: 342
   education and training, 2: 333
   Harrington Lecture, 2: 344, *344*
   Hospital for Sick Children and, 2: 334–336
   kyphosis and, 2: 343–345
   marriage and family, 2: 333, 337
   as mentor, 2: 345–347
   military service, 2: 333
   New England Baptist Hospital and, 2: 338
   orthopaedics leadership, 2: 347
   orthopaedics residents and, 2: *413*
   PBBH and, 4: 163
   pediatric orthopaedics, 2: 345, *345*
   private medical practice, 2: 338
   professional memberships, 2: 347
   Prosthetic Research and Development Unit, 2: 335
   publications and research, 2: *336*, 340–344, *344*, 345, 385, 391–392
   Relton-Hall frame, 2: 334–335, *335*
   Royal National Orthopaedic Hospital and, 2: 333–334
   scoliosis treatment, 2: 328, 334–336, 339–340, *340*, 341–345; 4: 127
   Seal of Chevalier du Tastevin, 2: 348
   spinal surgery at BCH and, 2: 337–338
   sports medicine and, 2: 287
   Tachdjian and, 2: 304
   Toronto General Hospital and, 2: 334
Hall, Leland, 3: 364
Hall, Llewellyn (ca.1899–1969), 2: 267, *267*
Hall, Marshall, 1: xxii
Hallett, Mark, 4: 168
hallux valgus deformities, 4: 40, 94
Halo Vest, The (Pierce and Barr), 3: 321
halo-vest apparatus, 4: 153
Halsted, William, 1: 185–186; 4: 105
Hamann, Carl A., 3: 104
Hamilton, Alice, 3: 142
Hamilton, F. A., 4: 204
Hamilton, Frank H., 1: 50–51
Hamilton, Steward, 4: 482*b*
Hamilton Air Force Base, 3: 337
Hammersmith Hospital, 4: *398*, 401
Hammond, Franklin, 4: 90
Hammond, George, 3: 275
Hammond, Harriet, 4: 90
Hampden Park (Springfield, Mass.), 1: *249*
hamstring contractures, 2: 197–198, *198*
Hancock, John, 1: 17–18
Hand, The (Marble), 3: 316
Hand Division of the Pan American Medical Association, 2: 251
Hand Forum, 3: 411
Handbook of Anatomy Adapted for Dissecting and Clinical References from Original Dissections by John Warren (Green), 1: 89
Handbook of Anatomy (Aitken), 1: 89
hands. *See also* wrists
   arthritis and, 4: 96
   boutonniere deformities, 4: 98
   epiphyseal injuries after frostbite, 2: 321–323
   extensor tendon ruptures, 4: 97
   factitious lymphedema of, 3: 429
   focal scleroderma of, 4: 183
   IP joint hyperextension, 4: 97
   neuromas in, 2: 248
   opera-glass deformity, 4: 99
   osteochondritis in a finger, 3: 363
   pianists and, 3: 414
   proximal interphalangeal joint and, 2: 251
   reconstructive surgery of, 4: 98–99
   rheumatoid arthritis and, 4: 96–98, *98*
   sarcoidosis, 4: 98
   soft tissues and, 4: 98
   swan neck deformity, 4: 98
   systemic lupus erythematosus (SLE), 4: 98
   systemic sclerosis, 4: 98
   tendon transfers and, 3: 428
   treatment of, 2: 248
   volar plate arthroplasty and, 2: 248
Hands (Simmons), 4: 183
Hand-Schüller-Christian disease, 2: 171
Hanelin, Joseph, 3: 294; 4: 91, 237–238
Hanley, Daniel F., 2: 372
Hanley, Edward, 3: 249
Hannah, John, 3: 357
Hansen, Robert L., 3: 258, 317
Hansen, Sigvard T., 3: 416
Hansjörg Wyss/AO Foundation Professor of Orthopaedic Surgery, 3: 409, 464*b*
Harborview Medical Center, 3: 416
Harding, Chester, 1: 95
Harmer, Torr W., 1: 264; 3: 60; 4: 208
Harold and Anna Snider Ullian Orthopaedic Fund, 2: 439*b*
Harrast, J. J., 4: 173
Harriet M. Peabody Professor of Orthopaedic Surgery (HMS), 2: 183, 203, 327, 337, 438, 439*b*; 3: 202
Harrington, F. B., 2: 245; 3: 96, 110–111
Harrington, Paul, 2: 316, 335
Harrington, T. F., 1: 23
Harrington rods, 2: 316, *317*, 325, 335, 340
Harris, C. K., 2: 285
Harris, Mathew, 2: 439
Harris, Mitchel, 4: 194
Harris, Robert, 1: 204
Harris, W. Robert, 4: 351, 355–356
Harris, William H. (1927–), 3: 215, *217*
   adult reconstruction and, 3: 460*b*
   AMTI and, 3:224
   as Alan Gerry Clinical Professor of Orthopaedic Surgery, 3: 464*b*
   awards and, 3: 224, 224*b*
   biomechanics laboratory director, 3: 464*b*

Index

biomechanics research and, 3: 220
bone-ingrowth type prostheses, 3: 222–223
Children's Hospital/MGH combined program and, 3: 215
early life, 3: 215
education and training, 3: 215
fellowships and, 3: 216, 218
Harris Hip Score and, 3: 219, *219*
on Haversian systems in bone, 2: 241; 3: *216*
hip research and surgery, 3: 217–225, 244, 388*t*
HMS appointment, 3: 216–217, 219–220, 224
innovation and, 3: 216–217, 224
knee arthroplasty and, 4: 129
Knee Biomechanics and Biomaterials Laboratory, 3: 464*b*
legacy of, 3: 224–225
memberships and, 3: 224–225
as MGH clinical faculty, 3: 464*b*
as MGH surgeon, 3: 216, 219–220, 398*b*; 4: 126
MIT appointment, 3: 219–220
mold arthroplasty and, 3: 218–219
on osteolysis after hip replacement, 3: 220, *220*, 221
publications and research, 3: 215–216, 218–220, 243, 398; 4: 135, *135*
on Smith-Petersen, 3: 216–217
Vanishing Bone, 3: 225, *225*
Harris Hip Score, 3: 219, *219*
Harris Orthopaedic Biomechanics and Biomaterials Laboratory, 3: 220, 463
Harris S. Yett Prize in Orthopedic Surgery, 4: 251
Harris-Galante Prosthesis (HGP), 3: 222
Hartwell, Harry F., 3: 68
Harvard Athletic Association, 1: 253, 258–259, 263
Harvard Athletic Committee, 1: 250; 4: 85
Harvard athletics
athlete heart size, 1: 262, 267, 288
Athlete's Bill of Rights and, 1: 279, 280*b*, 281
basketball and, 1: 285–286
crew team, 1: 250–251, 258
dieticians and, 1: 258
fatigue and, 1: 264–265
football development, 1: 245, 247–248
football injuries and, 1: 247–248, 252–262
football team, 1: *249*, 251, *257*
ice hockey, 1: 275, 286
injury prevention and, 1: 279, 285–286
knee joint injuries in, 1: 267–268, 268*t*
musculoskeletal injuries, 1: 288
physical therapy and, 1: 258
protective padding and helmets in, 1: 255, *267*, 275
sports medicine and, 1: 245–269, 274–282, 284–286; 2: 287; 3: 399
Varsity Club logo, 1: *274*
women athletes, 1: 285–286
Harvard Cancer Commission, 1: 256
Harvard Club, 1: 181, *181*
Harvard College. *See also* Harvard University
anatomical society at, 1: 21, 133
faculty in 1806, 1: 40
football at, 1: 245
medical examination of freshmen, 4: *84*
normal and abnormal posture in freshmen, 4: *84*
Spunkers and, 1: 21, 32, 133
vote to send Harvard Medical School surgeons to WWI service, 4: 386
Harvard Combined Orthopaedic Residency Program (HCORP)
accreditation of, 1: 232–233, 239–241
ACGME Orthopaedic RRC Committee review of, 1: 217–220
Beth Israel Deaconess Medical Center and, 4: 284, 288
Boston Pathology Course, 1: 216, 218
Boston Prosthetics Course, 1: 220
case sessions in, 1: 229*t*
clinical curriculum, 1: 223–225
combined grand rounds, 1: 232
conference schedule for, 1: 221*t*
core curriculum and, 1: 215–217, 227–232, 241–242
development of, 1: 192–200
directors of, 1: 243*b*
distribution of residents and staff, 1: 227*t*
diversity in, 1: 239
early surgical training, 1: 183–186
educational resources for, 1: 217
evolution of, 1: 183
funding for, 1: 206
Green and, 1: 200–210
growth of, 1: *240*
Herndon and restructuring, 1: 222–243
independent review of, 1: 234–237
leadership of, 1: 181, 210–211
Mankin and, 1: 211–220, 239; 3: 387, 397
orthopaedic research in, 1: 218
Pappas and, 1: 208–209
program length and size, 1: 214–215, 218–220, 222–223, 239
program review, 1: 238, 242–243
reorganization of, 1: 211–216
resident evaluations and, 1: 237–238
resident salaries, 1: 206
rotation schedule, 1: 225–226, 226*t*, 227, 227*t*
specialty blocks in, 1: 228, 229*t*
weekly program director's conference, 1: 230*b*
women in, 1: 239; 3: 208
Harvard Community Health Physicians at Beth Israel Hospital, 4: 263
Harvard Community Health Plan, 1: 225
Harvard Corporation, 1: 25, 27, 40, 133, 178; 3: 4
Harvard Department of Hygiene, 2: 253
Harvard Fifth Surgical Service, 4: 275, 277, 279, 297, 302–303, 305–306
Harvard Fourth Medical Service, 4: 296
Harvard Hall, 1: 25, 134, *135*
Harvard Health Services, 3: 310
Harvard Infantile Paralysis Clinic, 2: 79, 107, 109, 176, 191, 432
Harvard Infantile Paralysis Commission, 2: 68, 70, 72, 99, 189
Harvard Medical Alumni Association, 1: 264; 2: 306
Harvard Medical Association, 3: 116, 119*b*
Harvard Medical Faculty Physicians (HMFP), 4: 214
Harvard Medical Meetings, 1: 174
Harvard Medical School (HMS), 1: *135*, 298. *See also* Holden Chapel; orthopaedics curriculum
admission requirements, 1: 138, 141
admission tickets to lectures, 1: *27*, *300*
Almshouse and, 3: 4

attendance certificates, 1: *28*
Beth Israel Hospital and, 4: 213–214
Bigelow and, 1: 137; 3: 34, 42–44
Boylston Medical Society, 3: 25–26
Brigham Orthopaedic Foundation staff and, 4: 192
budget and, 1: 158, 174
calendar reform, 1: 140
Cheever Professor of Surgery, 4: 303
classes and faculty, 1834, 1: *297*
clinical courses at BCH, 4: 380*t*–381*t*
Coll Warren and, 1: 85
construction in 1904, 1: *86*
continuing medical education and, 3: 396
curricular reform, 1: 140
deans of, 1: 68–69
departmental organization, 1: 172–175
diversity in, 1: 239
educational reforms and, 1: 139, 140*b*, 141, 146–147; 2: 41; 3: 44–45, 94
Ellen and Melvin Gordon Professor of Medical Education, 4: 264, 266
Epidemic Aid Team, 2: 260
faculty at, 1: 40, 176
faculty salaries, 1: 178–179
financial structure reform, 1: 140
floor plan, 1: *304*
founding of, 1: 6, 25–29, 133–134
George W. Gay Lecture, 4: 324
human dissections and, 1: 26, 38
Jack Warren and, 1: 21, 25–29, 40
John Ball and Buckminster Brown chair, 2: 63–64
John Collins Warren and, 1: 38–40, 66, 68–69; 3: 30
John Homans Professor of Surgery, 4: 298
Laboratory for Skeletal Disorders and Rehabilitation, 2: 413
Laboratory of Surgical Pathology and, 2: 90
locations of, 1: 134*t*, *135*, 141
military hospitals and, 1: 270
military orthopaedic surgery course, 4: 455–462
military surgeon training at, 2: 42, 65–66
minority admissions to, 1: 138*b*

move from Cambridge to Boston, 1: 40–41; 2: 3
musculoskeletal medicine in, 1: 169
nose and throat clinic, 2: 40–41
orthopaedic clinic, 1: 173–174
orthopaedic curriculum, 1: 133–170
orthopaedic research and, 1: 193
orthopaedics as specialty course, 1: 141–143
PBBH and, 4: 1–4, 12, *12*, 13–14
postgraduate education and, 2: 157
preclinical and clinical departments, 1: 182*b*
qualifications for professors, 1: 26
radiology at, 2: 16
School for Health Officers, 2: 42, 65–66
Sears Surgical Laboratory, 4: 303
student evaluation of curricula, 1: 157–158, 167
surgery curriculum, 1: 140–141
surgical illustrations and, 3: 25
Surgical Research Laboratory, 4: 105, *106*, 107–108
teaching departments, 1: 157
Warren family and, 1: 71
women students and, 1: 138, 138*b*, 239; 3: 44
World War I volunteer orthopaedic surgeons, 2: 117–119, 124–127, 145; 3: *180*
World War II surgeons, 2: 232
Harvard Medical School (HMS). Department of Orthopaedic Surgery. *See also* Harvard Combined Orthopaedic Residency Program (HCORP)
advisory councils, 1: 182
as branch of Division of Surgery, 1: 171
chairperson of, 1: 180–182
curricular reform and, 1: 177
evolution of, 1: 171–182
faculty governance and, 1: 175–178
faculty rank and, 1: 178
faculty salaries, 1: 178–180
Harriet M. Peabody Professor of Orthopaedic Surgery, 2: 183, 203, 327, 337
John Ball and Buckminster Brown Chair of Orthopaedic Surgery, 1: 111, 177; 2: 63–64

John E. Hall Professorship in Orthopaedic Surgery, 2: 347
Lovett as chief of, 2: 64
organization of, 1: 171–182, 182*b*
teaching hospitals and, 1: 172–176, 180–181
Harvard Orthopaedic Journal, 1: 231–232
Harvard Orthopaedic Residency Program, 1: 167
Harvard Second Medical Service, 4: 296
Harvard Unit (1st), 3: 180, *180*
Harvard Unit (5th General Hospital), 1: 270, 277; 3: 271; 4: 17, *17*, 484–485
Harvard Unit (105th General Hospital), 1: 270–271; 2: 231–232; 3: 271, 351; 4: 488–489
Harvard Unit (American Ambulance Hospital), 2: 119–121, 123–124; 3: *180*, 369, *370*; 4: 388, *388*, 389*b*, *390*, 391, 393. *See also* American Ambulance Hospital (Neuilly, France)
Harvard Unit (Base Hospital No. 5), 1: 270; 2: 125, 145; 4: 405, 419–421, 421*b*, *421*, 422–424, *428*
Harvard Unit (Walter Reed General Hospital), 4: 488
Harvard University. *See also* Harvard athletics; Harvard College
Dunster House, 2: *388*
establishment of medical school, 1: 6, 25–29, 133–134
Kirkland House, 2: 358, *358*
posture research and, 4: 84, *84*, 85–86, 234, *234*
public service ideal and, 2: 64
World War I and, 2: 64
Harvard University Health Services, 1: 274, 277, 284; 3: 450
Harvard Vanguard Medical Associates, 4: 194, 195*b*, 288
Harvard Varsity Club, 1: 272, 282, 289
Harvard/MGH Sports Medicine Fellowship Program, 3: 448
Hasty Pudding Club, 1: 32
Hatcher, Howard, 3: 382
Hatt, R. Nelson, 3: 368; 4: 378
Hauck, Charles, 4: 41*b*
Haus, Brian, 3: 409
Haverhill Clinic, 2: 107
Haversian system, 1: xxii
Hawkes, Micajah, 1: 42, 44, 49
Hayes, Helen, 2: 315
Hayes, Mabel, 4: 97

Hayes, Wilson C. (Toby), 4: 262–264, 271, 284–285
Hayward, George, 1: 54, 60, *60*, 61–62, 65, 137, 296, 302; 3: 12, 27, 34, 112
HCORP. *See* Harvard Combined Orthopaedic Residency Program (HCORP)
Head, William, 4: 116, 129, 161–162, 193
head surgery, 3: 18
Health, William, 1: 18
health care
    disparities for minorities, 4: 264–265
    humanitarianism and, 2: 413, 421
    injured workers and, 4: 327
    issues in, 2: 375
    managed care movement, 3: 397
    medical costs, 3: 379, 379*t*
    physician profiling and, 2: 373–374
    policy and, 2: 371
    polio courses for, 2: 189
    prospective payment system (PPS), 3: 397
    resource utilization, 2: 372
Health Security Act, 2: 374–375
Heard, J. Theodore, 4: 23
Heary, Robert F., 4: 272*b*
heavy-resistance exercise, 3: 282, *282*, 283–285
Hebraic debility, 4: 203
Heckman, James, 1: 233; 2: 240; 3: 463, 464*b*; 4: 173–174
Hedequest, Daniel, 2: 344
Hektoen, Ludvig, 2: 78
Helems, Don, 4: 129
Helen Hallett Thompson Fund, 2: 107
Helmers, Sandra, 2: 342
Henderson, M. S., 3: 166; 4: 394
Hendren, Hardy, 2: 182, 399
Henry, William B., Jr., 3: 398*b*
Henry Ford Hospital, 2: 167–168; 3: 328
Henry J. Bigelow Medal, 2: 69; 3: 135
Henry J. Bigelow Operating Theater, 1: 84
Henry J. Mankin Orthopaedic Research Professorship, 3: 392
Hensinger, Robert, 2: 302
heparin, 3: 362
Hérard, Françoise, 3: 48
Herder, Lindsay, 3: 410
Hermann, Otto J. (1884–1973), 4: *334*
    AAOS and, 4: 337

BCH Bone and Joint Service, 4: 307, 328, 333–334, 337, 380*b*
BCH compound fracture therapy research, 4: *335*, 337
BCH residencies and, 4: 377–378
Boston City Hospital and, 3: 237; 4: 242, 333–334
Boston University Medical School appointment, 4: 335
Cotton and, 4: 334
death of, 4: 337
education and training, 4: 333
HMS appointment, 4: 334–335
honors and awards, 4: 337
lectures and presentations, 4: 334–335, 337
Massachusetts Regional Fracture Committee, 3: 64
New England Regional Committee on Fractures, 4: 341
os calcis fractures research, 4: 335–336
professional memberships, 4: 334
publications and research, 4: *335*, 335, 337
Scudder Oration on Trauma, 3: 63
Tufts Medical School appointment, 4: 335
Herndon, Charles, 2: 195
Herndon, James H., 1: *222*
    Brigham and Women's Hospital and, 4: 195*b*
    congenital kyphosis case, 2: 399
    dedication of Codman's headstone, 3: *145*
    fat embolism syndrome research, 2: 397
    on Frank R. Ober, 2: 149
    on Glimcher, 2: 325
    on Hall, 2: 347
    Harvard Orthopaedic Journal, 1: 232
    leadership of, 1: 236
    as MGH clinical faculty, 3: 464*b*
    military service, 2: 399
    Pittsburgh Orthopaedic Journal, 1: 232
    as residency program director, 1: 222
    restructuring of HCORP, 1: 222–243
    on Riseborough, 2: 398–399
    Scoliosis and Other Deformities of the Axial Skeleton, 2: 398, *398*
    Smith Day lectures, 3: 431
    on Watts, 2: 421–422
    William H. and Johanna A. Harris Professor, 3: 464*b*

    on William T. Green, 2: 169, 178–179
Herndon, William, 2: 359
Herodicus Society, 2: *387*
Herring, Tony, 2: 346, 438
Hersey, Ezekiel, 1: 25, 133
Heuter, Carl, 3: 181
Hey, William, 1: xxii
Heymann, Emil, 4: 215
Heywood, Charles Frederick, 1: 60
Hibbs, Russell A., 3: 155, 203; 4: 343, 394
Hibbs spinal fusion procedure, 2: 164; 3: 155; 4: 343
Hickling, Harriet Fredrica, 1: 299
Hildreth, Dr., 1: 97
Hilibrand, Alan S., 4: 266*b*
Hill, Walter, 4: 401
Hillman, J. William, 1: 162
Hinckley, Robert C., 1: *55*, 59; 3: *30*
hip abduction splint, 1: *127*
hip dislocations. *See also* congenital dislocated hips (CDH)
    bilateral, 1: 126–127; 3: 235
    diagnosis of, 1: 46
    Henry J. Bigelow and, 3: 34–36
    hip joint excision, 3: 34
    J. Mason Warren and, 1: 75
    John Collins Warren and, 1: 42, 44–46, *46*, 47–50, 68; 3: 13, 13*b*, 36
    Lorenz technique and, 3: 164
    relaxing the Y-ligament, 3: 35–36, 38
    traction treatment for, 1: 108, *108*; 2: 32
    traumatic hip dislocation case, 2: 352–353
    treatment of, 1: 68, 74–75
hip disorders. *See also* total hip replacement
    abduction contracture, 2: 153, *153*
    acetabular dysplasia, 2: 389, *389*, 390
    anterior supra-articular subperiosteal approach to, 3: 181, 182*b*
    antisepsis technique, 2: 52
    bacterial infections and, 2: 108
    bilateral bony ankylosis, 3: *196*
    biomechanics research, 2: 407
    Bradford and, 2: 21–22, 32
    congenital hip dysplasia, 2: 302
    direct anterior approach to, 3: 181
    direct lateral approach and, 3: 277–278
    displacement of proximal femoral epiphysis, 3: 372

Down syndrome and, 2: 368
fascia lata arthroplasty and, 3: 181
femoroacetabular impingement, 3: 188–189
flexion/adduction contractures, 2: 293–294
hip abductor paralysis treatment, 2: 149–150
hip fusion for severe disabling arthritis, 3: 156b
importance of anticoagulation in, 3: 218
lateral approach, 3: 219
Legg-Calvé-Perthes disease, 2: 351
Lovett and, 2: 32, 53
Lovett and Shaffer's paper on, 2: 49, 49, 52
metastatic malignant melanoma fracture case, 4: 77–78
Millis and, 2: 392
mold arthroplasty and, 3: 196, 218–219, 241, 244
nailing fractured, 3: 237
Ober-Yount fasciotomy, 2: 172
osteoarthritis and, 2: 389; 3: 155, 222
poliomyelitis contracture treatment, 2: 294, 295b
posterior approach to, 2: 146
prophylactic antibiotics in surgery, 3: 253
prostheses and, 2: 407
radiography in, 2: 54
septic arthritis of, 2: 380
slipped capital femoral epiphysis (SCFE), 2: 176
splints for, 2: 247
subtrochanteric osteotomy, 2: 293–294
traction treatment for, 2: 21–22, 53, 54; 3: 148
transient synovitis of, 2: 380
Trendelenburg gait and, 2: 33
Trumble technique for fusion of, 3: 367
tuberculosis and, 2: 21–22, 52–53, 54; 3: 148
vastus slide and, 3: 278
hip fractures. *See also* femoral neck fractures
antibiotic use, 3: 253, 255
anticoagulation in, 3: 218
Austin Moore prosthesis for, 3: 213
Banks and, 4: 74–75
Britten hip fusion technique, 4: 363
elderly patients and, 4: 341

hospitalization for, 2: 372
MGH approach to, 4: 159b–160b
mold arthroplasty and, 3: 218
pathophysiology and treatment of, 4: 43
reduction and impaction of, 4: 318–320, 322b
Hip Society, 2: 407; 3: 224; 4: 141
Hippocratic Oath, 2: 1
Hirohashi, Kenji, 4: 145
Hirsch, Carl, 4: 259–260
History of the Massachusetts General Hospital (Bowditch), 3: 15
History of the Orthopedic Department at Children's Hospital (Lovett), 2: 247
HMS. *See* Harvard Medical School (HMS)
Ho, Sandy, 2: 405
Hochberg, Fred, 3: 414
Hodge, Andrew, 3: 397–398
Hodgen, John T., 1: 188
Hodges, Richard M., 3: 44, 51
Hodgkins, Lyman, 2: 244
Hodgson, Arthur R., 2: 336, 398
Hoffa, Albert, 2: 33
Hogan, Daniel E., 4: 263
Hoke, Michael, 2: 77–78, 282–283
Holden Chapel, 1: 135
anatomy lectures in, 1: 26, 29, 38
floor plan, 1: 26
human dissections and, 1: 26, 38
medical instruction in, 1: 134
Holland, Daniel, 3: 241
Holmes, Donald, 4: 117
Holmes, George, 3: 192
Holmes, Oliver Wendell, 1: 291
as anatomy professor at HMS, 1: 66; 4: 298
on anesthesia, 1: 56, 61
on Bigelow, 3: 13, 27, 38, 51
Boston Dispensary and, 2: 306
European medical studies, 1: 73
on George Hayward, 1: 302
on George Parkman, 1: 291, 294, 296
on hip dislocation case, 1: 46
on invention of stethoscope, 1: 74
on J. Mason Warren, 1: 77
on John Warren, 1: 27, 69; 3: 33–34
on medical studies, 1: 138
as MGH consulting surgeon, 3: 14
as MGH surgeon emeritus, 3: 46
on need for clinics, 3: 3

reform of HMS and, 1: 139–140; 3: 45
Tremont Street Medical School, 3: 42
trial of John Webster and, 1: 308–309
Holmes, Timothy, 1: 81, 83
Holyoke, Augustus, 1: 95
Holyoke, Edward A., 1: 21
Homans, John, 2: 10, 306; 3: 38, 94, 118, 145; 4: 5, 9
Hooton, Elizabeth, 1: 9
Hoover, Herbert, 4: 235
Hôpital de Bicêtre, 1: 73
Hôpital de la Charité, 1: 37, 73–74
Hôpital de la Pitié, 1: 73–74
Hôpital de la Salpêtrière, 1: 73
Hôpital des Enfants Malades, 1: 73, 106
Hôpital Saint-Louis, 1: 73, 82
Hormell, Robert S. (1917–2006), 4: 92
Boston Children's Hospital and, 4: 93
chronic arthritis research, 4: 92–93
on congenital scoliosis, 4: 65, 93
death of, 4: 94
education and training, 4: 92
HMS appointment, 4: 93
knee arthroplasty and, 4: 93–94
PBBH and, 4: 35
publications and research, 4: 92–94
RBBH and, 4: 38, 41b, 68, 89, 93–94
study of hallux valgus, 4: 40, 94
Horn, Carl E., 2: 271
Hornicek, Francis J., 3: 390, 462, 464b
Hosea, Timothy, 4: 262
Hospital for Joint Diseases, 3: 382–383, 385, 389, 413, 427
Hospital for Sick Children (Toronto), 2: 334–336
Hospital for Special Surgery, 1: 89; 2: 27; 3: 376; 4: 130, 134
Hospital for the Ruptured and Crippled, 2: 27, 43, 52, 225–226; 3: 376
Hospital of the University of Pennsylvania, 4: 465
hospitals. *See also* base hospitals; military reconstruction hospitals
Boston development of, 3: 3–7, 9–12
consolidation of, 4: 20
debarkation, 4: 451–452
embarkation, 4: 451–452
end results concept, 1: 112

Index

exclusion of poor women from, 1: 123
F.H. Brown on construction of, 2: 5
government and, 2: 138*b*–139*b*
internships in, 1: 186
military field, 1: 272; 2: 118; 4: *414*, 468
military hospitals in Australia, 4: 488–489
mobile army surgical hospitals (MASHs), 2: 231–232; 4: 468–469, *470*
orthopaedics services in, 4: 451
portable surgical, 4: 468–469, 489
prejudice against Jewish physicians in, 1: 158
reserve units for army service, 4: 429
standardization of, 3: 112, 113*b*, 115–116, 123–125, 131
unpopularity of, 1: 41
Hôtel-Dieu, 1: 37, 73–74, 82
Hough, Garry de N., Jr., 2: 230
House of Providence, 2: 256
House of the Good Samaritan, 1: *128*; 2: *4*
Anne Smith Robbins and, 1: 123–125; 2: 114
attraction of patients from the U.S. and abroad, 1: 125
BCH merger, 1: 130; 2: 433
Bradford and, 2: 21, 25, 28–29
Buckminster Brown and, 1: 107, 121–122, 125–128; 2: 28
Children's Ward, 1: *123*
closure of orthopaedic wards, 1: 129–130
disabled children and, 2: 306
founding of, 1: 123–124
hip disease treatment at, 1: 128–129
Lovett and, 2: 49
orthopaedic wards in, 1: 123, 125–126, 129; 2: 20
orthopaedics residencies, 1: 186
Osgood and, 2: 114
poor women and, 1: 123–124
rheumatic heart disease treatment at, 1: 130
surgical records from, 2: 114, 115*b*
training of orthopaedic surgeons, 1: 127, 129
treatment of adults and children in, 2: 4
house pupils (pups), 1: 80, 184, *185*; 2: 20; 3: 4, 16
Howard, Herbert B., 3: 120

Howard University, 1: 239
Howorth procedure, 4: 243
Hresko, M. Timothy (1954–), 2: *364*
Boston Children's Hospital and, 2: 364, 366–368, 439*b*
education and training, 2: 364
HMS appointment, 2: 364
latent psoas abscess case, 2: 365
Medical Student Undergraduate Education Committee, 1: 166
orthopaedics appointments, 2: 364
orthopaedics curriculum, 1: 167
pediatric orthopaedics, 2: 365
publications and research, 2: 366, *366*, 367, *367*, 368
scoliosis and spinal deformity research, 2: 364–367
on trauma in children, 2: 365, 368
University of Massachusetts and, 2: 364
Hse, John, 2: 266
Hsu, Hu-Ping, 4: 194
Hubbard, Leroy W., 2: 77–78
Huddleston, James, 3: 254, 256
Huffaker, Stephen, 4: 190*b*
Hugenberger, Arthur, 2: 268
Hugenberger, Elizabeth, 2: 268
Hugenberger, Franklin, 2: 268
Hugenberger, Gordon, 2: 272
Hugenberger, Helen, 2: 268
Hugenberger, Herman, 2: 268
Hugenberger, Janet McMullin, 2: 272
Hugenberger, Joan, 2: 269, 271–272
Hugenberger, Paul W. (1903–1996), 2: *268*, *271*
Boston Children's Hospital and, 2: 233, 269–272, 301
Boston City Hospital and, 2: 269
donations to Boston Medical Library, 2: 271
education and training, 2: 268
famous patients of, 2: 271–272
Georgia Warm Springs Foundation and, 2: 270
grand rounds and, 2: 271
HMS appointment, 2: 269–270
Marlborough Medical Associates and, 2: 146, 269, 299
marriage and family, 2: 272
MGH and, 2: 268
New England Peabody Home for Crippled Children and, 2: 269–270
Ober and, 2: 269, 271
orthopaedics appointments, 2: 270

orthopaedics internships, 2: 269
PBBH and, 2: 269; 4: 16, 18–20, 22, 110, 116, 128
private medical practice, 2: 269
professional memberships, 2: 270, 272
publications and research, 2: 268–269, 271
Salem Hospital and, 2: 270–272
Hugenberger Orthopaedic Library, 2: 272
Huggins Hospital (Wolfeboro, NH), 2: 218
Hughes, Mable, 3: 362
human anatomy
anatomical atlas and, 1: 89
Astley Cooper and, 1: 34
Harvard courses in, 1: 6, 25, 133–134, 136–138, 140–141
HMS courses in, 1: *229*, 230
legalization of human dissection, 1: 52
military surgeon training and, 2: 66
orthopaedic chronic disease and, 3: 85
skeleton, 1: *136*
variations in, 3: 85–86, 86*t*
human dissections
grave robbing and, 1: 32, 34
legalization of, 1: 52
in medical education, 1: 26–27, 34, 38, 40, 51–52
in military hospitals, 1: 24
Human Limbs and Their Substitutes (Wilson and Klopsteg), 3: 376
humeral fractures
displaced supracondylar, 2: 379
Gartland type 3 supracondylar, 2: 368
intercondylar T fractures, 2: 397, *397*
nonunion of the humerus, 2: 96, *96*, 250
pins used in, 2: 379
proximal, 2: 96, *122*
resorption of the humerus, 2: 97, *97*
supracondylar, 2: 229, 345, 379
Hunter, John, 1: xxi, 33, 36–37
Hunter, William, 1: 6, *133*
Hussey, Phyllis Ann, 4: 153
Hussey, Robert W. (1936–1992), 4: *151*
Brigham and Women's Hospital, 4: 163
Children's Hospital/MGH combined program and, 4: 151
death of, 4: 153
education and training, 4: 151

HMS appointment, 4: 152
marriage and family, 4: 153
Medical College of Virginia
  appointment, 4: 153
PBBH and, 4: 116, 128–129,
  151, 163
publications and research, 4: 151,
  152–153
Rancho Los Amigos fellowship,
  4: 129, 151
spinal cord injury research and
  treatment, 4: 151, *151*,
  152–153
US Navy and, 4: 151
VA Medical Center (Richmond,
  VA), 4: 153
West Roxbury Veterans Administration Hospital and, 4: 129,
  152
Hutchinson, Thomas, 1: 16
Hyatt, George, 3: 439
hydroxylysine, 2: 327–328
Hylamer metal-backed polyethylene acetabular components, 4: 172
Hynes, John, 4: 303
hypnosis, 1: 56

I

ice hockey, 1: 275, 286
Ida C. Smith ward (BCH), 2: 431
Ilfeld, Fred, 3: 317
iliofemoral ligament, 3: 35–36, 38
iliotibial band
  ACL reconstruction and, 2: 378–379, *386*; 3: 448
  contractures and, 3: 209
  hip abductor paralysis treatment,
    2: 149–150
  knee flexion contracture and,
    3: 374
  modification of sacrospinalis and,
    2: 147
  Ober Operation and, 2: 153
  tendon transplantations and,
    2: 109
  tightness in, 2: 151–152
IMSuRT. *See* International Medical-Surgical Response Team (IMSuRT)
inclinometers, 2: 366, *367*
industrial accidents
  back disabilities and, 2: 92;
    4: 358
  BCH Relief Station and, 4: 305,
    305
  carpal tunnel syndrome and,
    4: 184–186
  Cotton and, 4: 323, 325, 327
  defects in patient care, 4: 325,
    352–354

fracture care and, 4: 338,
  339*b*–340*b*
insurance and, 2: 92; 4: 325,
  339*b*, 341
intervertebral disc surgery in,
  3: 316
kineplastic forearm amputation
  case, 4: 360
Maria Hospital (Stockholm) and,
  1: 263
os calcis fractures and, 4: 325
ruptured intervertebral discs and,
  4: 352
Sever and, 2: 92
workers' compensation issues,
  4: 184–186, 253, 325,
  352–353
Industrial School for Crippled and
  Deformed Children (Boston),
  2: 36–37, *37*, 38, 97, 308; 3: 151,
  161
Industrial School for Crippled Children (Boston), 2: 38, *38*
infantile paralysis (poliomyelitis). *See*
  poliomyelitis
infections
  allografts and, 3: 435, 440, 442
  amputations and, 1: 23, 74, 84
  antisepsis dressings and,
    1: 84–85
  carbolic acid treatment,
    1: 82–83, *83*, *84*
  hand-washing policy and, 1: 193
  infantile paralysis (poliomyelitis)
    and, 2: 261
  mortality due to, 1: 74, 81, 84
  postoperative, 3: 253
  resection and, 1: 81
  Revolutionary War deaths and,
    1: 22
  tubercular cows and, 2: 16
  use of ultraviolet light for,
    4: 164, 164*t*
infectious diseases, 1: 7–9; 2: 4–5,
  15
influenza, 1: 4, 7; 3: 135
Ingalls, William, 1: 32; 2: 5, 9, 11
Ingersoll, Robert, 4: 376
Ingraham, Frank, 2: 215
Insal, John, 4: 130
insane, 3: 3–4, 6
"Insensibility During Surgical Operations Produced by Inhalation"
  (Bigelow), 3: 27, *27*
Inside Brigham and Women's Hospital, 4: *123*
Institute for Children with Thalidomide Induced Limb Deformation,
  2: 413
Institute Pasteur, 1: 91

institutional racism, 3: 15–16
Instituto Buon Pastore, 4: *480*, 481
insufflation anesthesia apparatus,
  4: 215–216
"Interior of a Hospital Tent, The"
  (Sargent), 4: *424*
International Arthroscopic Association, 3: 422
International Association of Industrial Accident Boards and Commission, 2: 92
International Federation of Societies
  for Surgery of the Hand, 2: 251
International Hip Society, 3: 224
*International Journal of Orthopaedic
  Surgery*, 2: 80
International Knee Documentation
  Committee (IKDC), 1: 287;
  2: 381
International Medical-Surgical
  Response Team (IMSuRT),
  3: 417–418
International Pediatric Orthopedic
  Think Tank (IPOTT), 2: 304, *304*
International Society of Orthopaedic Surgery and Traumatology
  (SICOT), 2: 80–81, *81*, 137
interpedicular segmental fixation (ISF) pedicle screw plate,
  3: 420–421
Interurban Orthopaedic Club,
  2: 230
Ioli, James, 4: 193, 195*b*
Iowa Hip Score, 3: 219
Ireland, Robert, 1: 317
iron lung, 2: 79
  Berlin polio epidemic and,
    2: 260, 264
  Boston polio epidemic and,
    2: 314
  Drinker and, 2: 78, *78*
  infantile paralysis (poliomyelitis)
    and, 2: 261*b*–262*b*, 266
  invention of, 2: 191
  Massachusetts Infantile Paralysis
    Clinic and, 2: 212
  poliomyelitis and, 2: 78, *190*
ischemia-edema cycle, 2: 200–201,
  201
ISOLA implants, 2: *370*, 371
Isola Study Group, 2: 371
Istituto Ortopedico Rizzoli (Bologna, Italy), 3: 435–436

J

J. Collins Warren Laboratory, 1: 87
J. Robert Gladden Orthopaedic Society, 4: *265*
Jackson, Charles T., 1: 57, 60, 306

Index

Jackson, G. H., 3: 35
Jackson, George H., Jr., 2: 140
Jackson, Henry, 2: 20
Jackson, J. B. S., 1: 67
Jackson, James
    founding of MGH, 1: 31, 40–42; 3: 5, *5*, *6b–7b*, 12–13
    on George Hayward, 1: 302
    George Parkman and, 1: 296
    Harvard Medical teaching, 1: 299
    John Collins Warren and, 1: 37, 40, 66
    medical studies in London, 1: 37
    publications of, 1: 38–39
    support for House of the Good Samaritan, 1: 124
Jackson, James, Jr., 1: 73
Jackson, Robert W., 2: 279; 3: 446
Jaffe, Henry, 3: 382, 385, 392
Jaffe, Norman, 2: 422
Jagger, Thomas A., 3: 338
James, J. I. P., 2: 333–335, 399
James H. Herndon Resident Teaching and Mentoring Award, 3: 463
James Lawrence Kernan Hospital, 4: 157
Janeway, Charles A., 2: 215
Jasty, Murali, 3: 398, *460b*, *464b*
JDW (Jigme Dorji Wangchuk) National Referral Hospital, 3: 418
Jeffries, John, 1: 292
Jenkins, Roger, 4: 281
Jennings, Ellen Osgood, 2: 138
Jennings, L. Candace (1949–)
    cancer fatigue and, 3: 405–406
    education and training, 3: 405
    HCORP and, 3: 405
    Hospice and Palliative Medicine fellowship, 3: 407
    as MGH surgeon, 3: 405
    orthopaedic oncology and, 3: 405, *460b*
    publications and research, 3: 405–406
    ulnar nerve compression case, 3: 405–406
Jette, Alan, 3: 391
Jewish Hospital (St. Louis), 2: 231
Jewish Memorial Hospital and Rehabilitation Center, 4: 212
Jewish Memorial Hospital (Boston), 4: 212, 215
Jewish patients
    "Hebraic Debility" and, 4: 202, *203b*, *203*
    hospital formation for, 4: 200–202, 223
    limited medical care for, 4: 199–200
    in-patient care for observant, 4: 199, 204–206
Johansson, S., 3: 189
John Ball and Buckminster Brown Clinical Professor of Orthopaedic Surgery, 1: 111, 177; 2: 63–64, *64*, 133, 147, 157; 3: 202, *464b*; 4: *195b*
John E. Hall Professorship in Orthopaedic Surgery (HMS), 2: 347, 438, *439b*
Johns Hopkins Base Hospital Unit, 2: 221; 3: 288, 291
Johns Hopkins Hospital, 1: 185; 4: 429
Johns Hopkins Medical School
    departmental organization at, 1: 175–176
    Flexner Report and, 1: 146–147
    governance and, 1: 177
    trust for, 4: 1, 3
Johnson, Howard, 2: 272
Johnson, J. A., 2: 77–78
Johnson, Lanny, 3: 446
Johnson, Robert W., Jr., 4: 239
Joint Commission on Accreditation of Healthcare Organizations (JCAHO), 3: 146
Joint Commission on Hospital Accreditation, 3: 131
joint disease. *See* bone and joint disorders
Joint Injuries of the Hand (Eaton), 2: 250, *250*
Joint Kinematics Laboratory, 3: 463, *464b*
Jones, Arlene MacFarlane, 3: 291
Jones, Daniel F., 3: *60b*, 313, 371; 4: 274–276
Jones, Deryk, 4: *190b*
Jones, Ezra A., 2: 78
Jones, Howard, 4: 347
Jones, Neil, 3: 431
Jones, Sir Robert, 4: *394*
    on active motion, 2: 68
    BEF Director of Military Orthopedics, 4: 405
    on femur fracture treatment, 4: 408
    on importance of American surgeons, 4: *412b–413b*
    Lovett and, 2: 63, 80–81
    MGH and, 3: 299
    military orthopaedics and, 2: 124, 127; 4: 392–394, 401, 407
    Notes on Military Orthopaedics, 4: 442, *442*, 443
    orthopaedic surgery and, 4: 463
    Orthopedic Surgery, 2: 69, *69*
    Osgood and, 2: 116, 124–125, *125*, 126
    on prevention of deformity, 4: 409
    request for American orthopaedic surgeons, 4: 393, 398
    SICOT and, 2: 81
Jones, William N. (1916–1991), 3: *291*, *461*
    death of, 3: 293
    early life, 3: 291
    education and training, 3: 291
    evolution of the Vitallium mold, 3: *292b*, 293
    "Fracture of the Month" column, 3: 243, 291
    as MGH surgeon, 3: *398b*
    mold arthroplasty and, 3: 291–292
    orthopedic arthritis service, 3: *388t*
    publications and research, 3: 291; 4: 187
    US Army Medical Corps and, 3: 291
Jones splints, 4: 389, 411
Joplin, Robert J. (1902–1983), 3: *293*
    AOFS and, 3: 295, 298
    Boston Children's Hospital and, 2: 274; 3: 293
    Boston VA Hospital and, 3: 298
    death of, 3: 298
    early life, 3: 293
    education and training, 3: 293
    on epiphyseal injuries, 4: 356
    foot surgery and, 3: 294–295, *296b–297b*, 298
    HMS appointment, 3: 293, 298
    legacy of, 3: 298
    memberships and, 3: 298
    as MGH surgeon, 3: 293–294, 298
    publications and research, 3: 293–294, *294*, 295, 341; 4: 63
    RBBH and, 3: 293; 4: 36, 93, 111
    sling procedure and, 3: 294, *294*, 295, *296b–297b*
    Slipped Capital Femoral Epiphysis, 3: 294, 333
    slipped capital femoral epiphysis research, 4: 237–238
Jorevinroux, P., 2: 340
Joseph O'Donnell Family Chair in Orthopedic Sports Medicine, 2: 438, *439b*
Joseph S. Barr Memorial Fund, 3: 214

Joseph S. Barr Visiting Consultantship, 3: 213
Joseph Warren, about 1765 (Copley), 1: *3, 11*
Josiah B. Thomas Hospital, 2: 252
Joslin, Elliott P., 4: 274
Joslin and Overholt Clinic, 4: 279
Journal of Bone and Joint Surgery (JBJS)
   American issues of, 3: 345, 347
   Annual Bibliography of Orthopaedic Surgery, 3: 261
   as British Orthopaedic Association's official publication, 3: 345
   budget deficits and, 3: 345–346
   Charles Painter as acting editor, 4: 50
   David Grice as associate editor, 2: 214
   Elliott Brackett as editor, 2: 130; 3: 157–159, 160*b*, 161
   expansion of editorial board positions, 3: 345
   Frank Ober as associate editor, 2: 165
   H. Winnett Orr as editor, 2: 125
   James Heckman as editor, 1: 233; 2: 240
   John Bell as associate editor, 2: 221
   Jonathan Cohen as editor, 2: 238–239
   as the journal of record, 3: 261–262
   logo for, 3: *261*
   name changes of, 1: xxiv
   ownership reorganization, 3: 346–347
   standards for, 3: 261
   Thornton Brown as editor, 3: 260–262
   Zabdiel Adams as associate editor, 3: 235
Journal of Pediatrics, 2: 7
Joyce, Michael, 1: 217*b*; 4: 189
Judet hip prosthesis, 3: 293
Junghanns, Herbert, 4: 262
Jupiter, Beryl, 3: 411
Jupiter, Jesse B. (1946–), 3: *407, 461*
   Cave Traveling Fellowship and, 1: 217*b*
   Children's Hospital/MGH combined program and, 3: 408
   education and training, 3: 407–408
   fracture treatment and, 3: 408–409

Fractures of the Distal Radius, 3: 409, *409*
   Hand Forum president, 3: 411
   as Hansjorg Wyss/AO Foundation Professor, 3: 464*b*
   HMS appointment, 3: 408–409
   honors and awards, 3: 409
   intra-articular radial nerve entrapment case, 3: 410–411
   memberships and, 3: 411
   as MGH clinical faculty, 3: 464*b*
   MGH hand service and, 3: 396, 410, 460*b*
   as MGH surgeon, 3: 408
   MGH trauma unit and, 3: 399, 408
   named lectures and, 3: 410–411
   public health service and, 3: 408
   publications and research, 3: 408–411
   WRIST and, 3: 410
juvenile rheumatoid arthritis, 2: 171

K

Kaden, D. A., 4: 171
Kadiyala, Rajendra, 4: 190*b*
Kadzielski, John J., 3: 463*b*
Kagno, Marcia, 4: 89
Kanavel, Allan B., 3: 113*b*
Kaplan, Ronald K., 4: 89
Karlin, Lawrence I. (1945–), 2: *369*
   Boston Children's Hospital and, 2: 369–371
   education and training, 2: 369
   HMS appointment, 2: 370
   ISOLA implants and, 2: 371
   Isola Study Group, 2: 371
   orthopaedics appointments, 2: 369
   pediatric orthopaedics, 2: 370
   professional memberships, 2: 370
   publications of, 2: 371
   Scheuermann kyphosis treatment, 2: 371
   Tufts Medical School and, 2: 369
Karp, Evelyn Gerstein, 4: 241
Karp, Meier G. (1904–1962), 4: *240*
   as Beth Israel chief of orthopaedics, 4: 241, 289*b*
   Beth Israel Hospital and, 4: 240
   Boston Children's Hospital and, 4: 240
   death of, 4: 241
   education and training, 4: 240
   HMS appointment, 4: 240–241
   marriage and family, 4: 241
   PBBH and, 4: 18–20, 110, 240
   private medical practice, 2: 313; 4: 240

   professional memberships, 4: 241
   publications and research, 2: 229; 4: 240–241
   Thayer General Hospital and, 4: 241
   US Army and, 4: 241
   West Roxbury Veterans Administration Hospital and, 4: 240
Kasser, James
   Boston Children's Hospital and, 2: 354, 364, 434, 439*b*
   Catharina Ormandy Professorship, 2: 439*b*
   on Griffin, 2: 354
   HCORP and, 1: 224–225
   John E. Hall Professorship in Orthopaedic Surgery, 2: 439*b*
   Karlin and, 2: 369
   as orthopaedic chair, 2: 15*b*, 436
   publications of, 2: 368, 380
   on Zeke Zimbler, 4: 249
Kast, Thomas, 1: 25
Katz, Eton P., 2: 324
Katz, Jeffrey N., 2: 375; 4: 184–186, 195*b*, 269
Katzeff, Miriam (1899–1989), 2: *273*
   arthrogryposis multiplex congenita case, 2: 274–275
   Boston Children's Hospital and, 2: 222, 252, 273–275
   death of, 2: 275
   education and training, 2: 273
   as first female orthopaedic surgeon in Mass., 1: 239; 2: 275
   New England Hospital for Women and Children and, 2: 274
   orthopaedics appointments, 2: 274
   Osgood tribute, 2: 275
   professional memberships, 2: 275
   publications of, 2: 275
Kawalek, Thaddeus, 3: 282
Keats, John, 1: 36
Keely, John L., 2: 220
Keen, William W., 2: 72, *73*; 3: 103; 4: 411
Keep, Nathan C., 1: 308
Keeting, Mr., 1: 97
Kehinde, Olaniyi, 4: 169
Keith, Arthur, 2: 39
Keller, Joseph Black, 2: 126
Keller, Robert B. (ca. 1937–), 2: *371*
   Boston Children's Hospital and, 2: 286, 371
   Brigham and Women's Hospital and, 4: 193
   carpal tunnel syndrome research, 2: 375; 4: 184–185

Index

Dartmouth Atlas of Health Care in Virginia, The, 2: 375
Dartmouth-Hitchcock Medical Center and, 2: 371
education and training, 2: 371
Harrington rods and, 2: 316, 371
health care policy and, 2: 371–376
Health Security Act and, 2: 374–375
HMS appointment, 2: 371
low-back pain research, 2: 371–372
Maine Carpal Tunnel Study, 2: 375
Maine Lumbar Spine Study Group, 2: 373, *373*
Maine Medical Assessment Foundation, 2: 372
Maine Medical Practice of Neurosurgery and Spine, 2: 376
MGH/Children's Hospital residency, 2: 371
PBBH and, 4: 22, 116, 128
private medical practice, 2: 371, 376
professional memberships, 2: 371, 376
publications of, 2: 372, *372*, 374–375, *375*, 376
scoliosis and spine surgery, 2: 371–374
University of Massachusetts and, 2: 371
Keller, William L., 3: 168; 4: 416
Kellogg, E. H., 1: 307
Kelly, Robert P., 4: 158
Kelsey, Jennifer, 4: 264
Kennedy, Edward, 3: 275
Kennedy, John F., 3: 191
Kennedy, Robert H., 4: 473
Kennedy Institute of Rheumatology, 4: 268, *268*
Kenzora, John E. (1940–)
 avascular necrosis of the femoral head research, 4: 154–156, *156*
 Beth Israel Hospital and, 4: 154
 Boston Children's Hospital and, 4: 154, 157
 Children's Hospital/MGH combined program and, 4: 154
 education and training, 4: 153
 HMS appointment, 4: 157
 hospital appointments, 4: 157
 hydroxylysine-deficient collagen disease case, 4: 155
 as MGH research fellow, 2: 328; 4: 153–154
 osteonecrosis of the femoral head research, 4: 156–157
 PBBH and, 4: 154, 157, 163
 publications and research, 2: 328, *328*; 4: *153*, 154–156, *156*, 157
 RBBH and, 4: 154
 University of Maryland appointment, 4: 157
Keogh, Alfred, 2: 68
Kermond, Evelyn Conway, 3: 299
Kermond, William L. (1928-2012), 3: *298*, *461*
 death of, 3: 299
 early life, 3: 298
 education and training, 3: 298–299
 HMS appointment, 3: 299
 marriage and family, 3: 299
 as MGH surgeon, 3: 299, 398b
 mold arthroplasty and, 3: 292b
 private medical practice, 1: 284; 4: 169
 publications and research, 3: 299
 White 9 Rehabilitation Unit and, 3: 299
 Winchester Hospital and, 3: 299
Kettyle, William M., 2: 277
Kevy, Shervin, 2: 234
Key, Einer, 1: 263
Key, John Albert, 1: 189; 2: 171; 4: 237, 453, 473
Kibler, Alison, 3: 328
Kidner, Frederick C., 2: 78; 4: 473
Kilfoyle, Richard, 1: 202; 2: 314; 4: 341, 378
Kim, S., 4: 251
Kim, Saechin, 4: 286
Kim, Young-Jo, 2: 390, 439b
Kinematic knee prosthesis, 4: 138–139, 147, 149–150
Kiner, Ralph, 4: 342
King, Donald S., 2: 195; 3: 301
King, Graham J.W., 3: 431
King, Martin Luther, Jr., 4: 262
King, Thomas V., 1: 217b
King Faisal Specialist Hospital, 2: 424, 425
King Report (MGH), 3: 301–302
King's College (Nova Scotia), 2: 284, *284*
Kirk, Norman T., 4: 471, 472b, 473
Kirkby, Eleanor, 3: 246
Kirkland House (Harvard University), 2: *358*
Kite, J. Hiram, 4: 158
Klein, Armin (1892-1954), 4: *231*
 as Beth Israel chief of orthopaedics, 4: 236, 239, 289b
 Beth Israel Hospital and, 4: 208b
 Chelsea Survey of posture, 4: 234–235
 death of, 4: 239
 education and training, 4: 231
 histology laboratory and, 2: 322
 HMS appointment, 4: 236
 Klein's Line, 4: 238–239, *239*
 legacy of, 4: 239
 MGH and, 4: 231, 236
 as MGH surgeon, 3: 375, 456b
 Orthopedics and Body Mechanics Committee, 4: 236
 posture research and, 4: 84, 233–235, *235*–236
 private medical practice, 4: 231
 professional memberships, 4: 239, 239b
 publications and research, 2: 136–137; 4: 231–233, *236*, *237*, 239
 scoliosis research and, 4: 231–233
 Slipped Capital Femoral Epiphysis, 3: 294; 4: 238
 slipped capital femoral epiphysis research, 3: 331, 333; 4: 237–239
 Tufts Medical School appointment, 4: 236
 US Army Medical Corps and, 4: 231
 US General Hospital No. 3 and, 4: 452
Kleinert, Harold E., 3: 408
Klein's Line, 4: 238–239, *239*
Kleweno, Conor, 4: 190b
Kloen, Peter, 4: 190b
Klopsteg, Paul E., 3: 376
Klumpke paralysis, 2: 90
Knee Biomechanics and Biomaterials Laboratory, 3: 463, 464b
knee flexion contracture
 before and after treatment, 1: *99*, *125*
 apparatus for, 1: *98*, 107
 Bradford's appliance for, 2: *20*, *21*
 iliotibial band and, 3: 374
 iron extension hinge for, 2: *123*
 leg brace for, 1: *124*
 osteotomies for, 2: 117
 physical therapy and, 3: 375
 plaster shells for, 2: 265
 prevention and, 4: 61
 surgical approach to, 3: 374–375, *375*
 treatment of, 1: 126–127
Knee Society, 4: 150
knees. *See also* total knee replacement

ACL injuries, 1: 277–278, 285–286
amputations and, 1: 61, 65, 84
ankylosis, 4: 64
arthroplasty of, 4: 64, 70b–71b, 103, 129–130, 131t, 179t
arthroscopic simulator, 4: 173
arthroscopy and, 1: 279; 4: 129
arthrotomy and, 3: 165, 165b, 166, 351
bilateral knee valgus deformities, 1: *125*
bone tumors and, 3: 389
cautery and, 1: 73
central-graft operation, 3: 368
discoid medial meniscus tear, 3: 422
dislocated patella treatment, 2: 294–296; 3: 79, 79b, 80, *81*
gait and, 2: 408
hamstring lengthening and, 2: 172
internal derangement of, 1: xxii; 4: 48
joint injuries in Harvard sports, 1: 268t
lateral tibial plateau fracture, 4: *312*
ligament rupture treatment, 1: 278
meniscectomy and, 1: 279
mold arthroplasty and, 3: 291–292
nylon arthroplasty in arthritic, 4: *65*, 66, 66b, 69, 91, 93–94
Osgood-Schlatter disease and, 2: 115
outcomes with duopatellar prostheses, 4: 180t
patella dislocations, 2: 294–296; 3: 79, 79b, 80, *81*
patella fractures, 4: 320
patellar turndown procedure, 4: 373–374
pes anserinus transplant, 1: 279
posterior cruciate ligament (PCL) deficiency, 3: 450
resection and, 1: 81
rheumatoid arthritis and, 4: 188–189
splint for knock, 2: 247
sports medicine and, 1: 267–268, 287; 2: 387
synovectomy in rheumatoid arthritis, 4: 40, 102–103
torn ligaments in, 3: 272
torn meniscus, 1: 278
treatment of sports injuries, 1: 277–279
trigger/jerking, 4: 311–312

tuberculosis and, 1: 73; 4: 225
valgus deformity, 2: *21*
Kneisel, John J., 4: 489
Knirk, Jerry L., 3: 409; 4: 194, 195b, 262–263
Kocher, Mininder S. (1966–), 2: *376*
ACL research, 2: 378–379
Beth Israel Deaconess Medical Center (BIDMC) and, 2: 377
Boston Children's Hospital and, 2: 377, 379, 439b
Brigham and Women's Hospital and, 2: 377
clinical research grants, 2: 377–378
education and training, 2: 377
on ethics of ghost surgery, 2: *380*, 381
on ethics of orthopaedic research, 2: *381*, 381
HCORP and, 2: 377
hip research, 2: 380
HMS appointment, 2: 377
honors and awards, 2: 377, 377b, 381
humeral fracture research, 2: 368, 379
New England Baptist Hospital and, 2: 377
outcomes research, 2: 379–380
professional memberships, 2: 382b
publications and research, 2: 378, *378*, 379–381
sports medicine and, 2: 377–378
team physician positions, 2: 382b
Kocher, Theodor, 2: 146
Kocher approach, 2: 347
Köhler's disease, 4: 240
Kopta, Joseph, 1: 232
Korean War
deferment during, 4: 125, 221
physician volunteers and, 4: 220–221
US Army physicians, 2: 218
Koris, Mark J., 4: 193, 195b
Kornack, Fulton C., 1: 217; 3: 460b, 464b
Krag, Martin, 3: 249
Kramer, D. L., 3: 420
Krane, Stephen, 2: 321; 3: 458b
Krause, Fedor, 4: 215
Krebs, David E., 3: 460b, 464b
Kreb's School, 2: 38
Krida, Arthur, 2: 111
Krisher, James, 4: 40
Kronenberg, Henry, 2: 330
Krukenberg procedure, 2: 425
Kubik, Charles, 3: *203*, 204
Kuhn, George H., 2: 5

Kühne, Willy, 3: 142
Kuhns, Jane Roper, 4: 66
Kuhns, John G. (1898–1969), 4: *59*
amputations research, 3: 373, *373*; 4: 60
arthritis research and, 4: 60–61, *61*, 63
Body Mechanics in Health and Disease, 3: *90*, 91; 4: 62
Boston Children's Hospital and, 2: 222, 274; 4: 59–61
on congenital flatfoot, 4: 63
correction of fixed foot deformities, 4: 62, 62t, 63
death of, 4: 66
education and training, 4: 59
end-results clinic, 1: 194
on Goldthwait, 3: 82, 92
HMS appointment, 2: 223; 4: 59–61
HMS medical student teaching, 4: 35
knee arthroplasty and, 4: 64
lymphatic supply of joints research, 1: 193; 4: 59–60
marriage and family, 4: 66
on medical education, 1: 93
on nylon arthroplasty in arthritis, 4: 65, *65*, 66, 66b, 69
private medical practice, 4: 62
professional memberships, 4: 66
publications and research, 4: 60–66, 93
RBBH and, 3: 91, 293; 4: 31–32, 35, 38, 60–62
as RBBH chief of orthopaedics, 4: 63–66, 79, 89, 196b
on roentgenotherapy for arthritis, 4: 64, *64*
scoliosis treatment, 2: 223; 4: 62, 65
on Swaim, 4: 58
Küntscher, Gerhard, 3: 272
Küntscher femoral rod, 3: 272
Kurth, Harold, 4: 360
kyphoscoliosis, 1: 97, 105; 4: 155
kyphosis, 2: 343–345, 359, 366; 3: 239–240; 4: *317*

L

La Coeur's triple osteotomy, 2: 390
Laboratory for Skeletal Disorders and Rehabilitation (HMS), 2: 413
Ladd, William E., 1: 264; 3: 64
Laënnec, René, 1: 74
Lahey, Frank, 4: 275–276, 277b
Lahey Clinic, 4: 275–277, 281, 378
Lahey Clinic Integrated Orthopaedic Program, 4: 378–379

Index

Lahey Clinic Medical Center, 4: 279
Lahey Hospital and Medical Center, 4: 214
Laing, Matthew, 2: 371
Lakeville State Hospital, 4: 378
Lakeville State Sanatorium, 2: 102; 3: 235, 365, 367
LaMarche, W. J., 3: 269
Lambert, Alexander, 4: 416
Lambert, Alfred, 1: 60
Lambrinudi stabilization, 2: 229
laminectomy, 3: 204, 206–208
Landfried, M., 3: 433
Landsteiner, Karl, 3: 313
Lane, Timothy, 1: 217b
Lange, Thomas, 3: 390
Langenbeck, Bernhard von, 1: 82; 2: 146
Langmaid, S. G., 2: 6, 9
Langnecker, Henry L., 3: 266
laparotomy, 3: 55
LaPrade, Robert F., 1: 287
Larson, Carroll B. (1909–1978), 3: 300, 303
   AAOS subcommittee on undergraduate teaching, 1: 162
   Calderwood's Orthopedic Nursing, 3: 303
   Children's Hospital/MGH combined program and, 3: 301
   death of, 3: 303
   early life, 3: 300
   education and training, 3: 300
   foot deformity treatment, 2: 229
   hip arthroplasty research, 3: 302
   hip surgery and, 3: 238, 240
   Iowa Hip Score, 3: 219
   King Report and, 3: 301–302
   kyphosis treatment, 3: 239
   legacy of, 3: 303
   marriage and family, 3: 300
   as MGH surgeon, 3: 74, 192, 302
   mold arthroplasty and, 3: 238–239, 241, 302
   nursing education and, 3: 302–303
   private medical practice, 3: 301
   professional roles, 3: 303, 303b
   publications and research, 3: 239, 241–242, 244, 302–303
   Santa Clara County Hospital and, 3: 300
   septic wounds in osteomyelitis case, 3: 301
   Smith-Petersen and, 3: 237
   University of Iowa orthopaedics chair, 3: 303
   US Army ROTC and, 3: 300
   World War II service, 3: 301
Larson, Charles Bernard, 3: 300
Larson, Ida Caroline, 3: 300
Larson, Nadine West Townsend, 3: 300
Larson, Robert L., 1: 279
Lateral Curvature of the Spine and Round Shoulders (Lovett), 2: 79, *79*, 227
Lattvin, Maggie, 4: 80
Latvian Medical Foundation, 3: 451
laudanum, 1: 10
Laurencin, Cato T., 4: 266b
Lavine, Leroy S., 3: 386, 388, 462, *463*
Law, W. Alexander, 3: 192, 199
law of osteoblasts, 1: xxiii
Lawrence, Amos, 2: 3–4
Lawrence, John, 2: 425
Lawrence, William P., 2: 3
Le, Hai V., 3: 463b; 4: 190b
Leach, Robert E., 4: 89, *342*, 379
Leadbetter, Guy W., 4: 473
Lee, Henry, 3: 24
Lee, Olivia, 4: 190b
Lee, Roger I., 4: 84, *84*, 233–234, 420
Lee, Sang-Gil P., 3: 460b, 464b
Leffert, Adam, 3: 415
Leffert, Linda Garelik, 3: 415
Leffert, Lisa, 3: 415
Leffert, Robert D. (1923–2008), 3: *412*, 461
   Brachial Plexus Injuries, 3: 414
   brachial plexus injuries and, 3: 412, *412*, 413–414
   death of, 3: 415
   diabetes presenting as peripheral neuropathy case, 3: 413
   education and training, 3: 412
   HMS appointment, 3: 413, 415
   Hospital for Joint Diseases and, 3: 413
   memberships and, 3: 415
   as MGH clinical faculty, 3: 464b
   as MGH surgeon, 3: 320–321, 385, 395, 398b, 413
   Mount Sinai Medical School and, 3: 413
   orthopaedics education and, 3: 415
   pianist hand treatment and, 3: 414
   publications and research, 3: 412–415
   rehabilitation and, 3: 386, 388t, 413, 461
   shoulder treatment and, 3: 386, 412–414, 460b
   thoracic outlet syndrome treatment, 3: 415
   US Navy and, 3: 412
leg length
   discrepancy in, 2: 170, 191, 193, 350
   distal femoral physeal fractures, 2: 400
   effects of irradiation on epiphyseal growth, 3: 331
   epiphyseal arrest, 2: 170–171
   fractures and, 2: 350
   lengthening procedures, 2: 110
   muscle strength and, 3: 332
   prediction techniques for, 2: 193
   research in, 2: 191, 350
   teleroentgenography and, 2: 170, 170t
   use of sympathetic ganglionectomy, 3: 332
Legg, Allen, 2: 101
Legg, Arthur T. (1874–1939), 2: *84*, *105*, 255
   Boston Children's Hospital and, 2: 13, 40, 101–102, 106, 252, 274, 282; 4: 338
   Clinics for Crippled Children and, 2: 230
   as consulting orthopaedic surgeon, 2: 102
   on coxa plana research, 3: 166
   death of, 2: 112
   education and training, 2: 101
   foot research, 2: 107–108
   gait laboratory, 2: 107
   Georgia Warm Springs Foundation board and, 2: 78
   Harvard Infantile Paralysis Clinic director, 2: 107, 188
   on hip disease, 2: 108
   HMS appointment, 2: 102; 4: 59–60
   identification of coxa plana, 2: 102–106; 3: 165
   on joint disease, 2: 110
   leg lengthening and, 2: 110
   marriage and, 2: 111–112
   military surgeon training and, 2: 42, 66; 4: 396
   on muscle atrophy in children, 2: 110
   orthopaedic surgery advances, 2: 79
   pediatric orthopaedics and, 2: 101, 106–107
   Physical Therapy in Infantile Paralysis, 2: 107
   poliomyelitis treatment, 2: 107, 109

professional memberships, 2: 110–111
public health and, 2: 107
publications of, 2: 107
Section for Orthopedic Surgery (AMA), 2: 110–111
on tendon transplantation, 2: 108, *108*, 109
testing of foot strength apparatus, 2: 102
Tufts appointment, 2: 102
Legg, Charles Edmund, 2: 101
Legg, Emily Harding, 2: 101
Legg, Marie L. Robinson, 2: 111–112
Legg-Calvé-Perthes disease
case reports, 2: 103, *103*, 104
epiphyseal extrusion measurement, 2: *354*
etiology of, 2: 104
identification of, 2: 13, 102, *102*, 103–106
long-term study of, 2: 425
research in, 2: 351; 3: 165–166
treatment of, 2: 105
Legg-Perthes Study Group, 2: 425; 4: 250
legs. *See also* leg length
acute thigh compartment syndrome, 3: 417–418
correction of bowleg, 1: *101*; 2: 247
fasciotomies, 3: 417
limb deformities, 2: 23, 334, 354, 413; 3: 58
limb-salvage procedure, 2: 422, 423*b*
radiculitis in, 3: 204
Lehigh Valley Hospital, 3: 407
Leidholt, John, 2: 314
Leinonen, Edwin, 4: 244
Leland, Adams, 3: 313
Leland, George A., 1: 154; 3: 60; 4: 433
Lemuel Shattuck Hospital, 3: 246, 253
Leonard, Ralph D., 4: *359*
L'Episcopo, James B., 2: 90, 96, 417
LeRoy, Abbott, 2: 78
Lest We Forget (Rowe), 3: 61, 70*b*, 187, *347*, *357*, 360
"Letter to the Honorable Isaac Parker" (J.C. Warren), 1: *45*
Letterman Army Hospital, 3: 336
Letterman General Hospital, 4: 451
LeVay, David, 4: 383
Levine, Leroy, 3: 397, 398*b*, 461
Levine, Philip T., 2: 324
Lewinnek, George, 4: 262
Lewis, Frances West, 2: 4

Lewis, William H., 1: 252
Lewis, Winslow, Jr., 1: 308
Lewis H. Millender Community of Excellence Award, 4: 168
Lewis H. Millender Occupational Medicine Conference, 4: 168
Lexington, Mass., 1: 17–18
Lhowe, David W. (1951–), 3: *416*
acute thigh compartment syndrome research, 3: 417, *417*, 418
Cambridge Hospital clinic and, 3: 399, 416
education and training, 3: 416
Harborview Medical Center and, 3: 416
HCORP and, 3: 416
HMS appointment, 3: 416
hospital appointments, 3: 416
humanitarian work and, 3: 416–418
IMSuRT and, 3: 417–418
as MGH clinical faculty, 3: 464*b*
as MGH surgeon, 3: 416
Pristina Hospital (Kosovo) and, 3: 416–417
Project HOPE and, 3: 417
publications and research, 3: 416
trauma care and, 3: 399, 416–418, 460*b*
Winchester Hospital and, 3: 417
Li, Guoan, 3: 462
Liaison Committee on Graduate Medical Education (LCGME), 1: 210–212
Liang, M. H., 4: 26
Liberating Technologies, Inc., 2: 326
Liberty Mutual Insurance Company, 3: 287; 4: 352–353
Liberty Mutual Research Center, 2: 326
Lidge, Ralph, 3: 448
Life of John Collins Warren, The (Edward Warren), 1: 46
Lifeso, Robert, 2: 424
ligatures, 1: 10, 55, 85
limb deformities
internal fixation of fractures to prevent, 3: 58
pediatric orthopaedics and, 2: 334, 354
thalidomide and, 2: 413
traction treatment for, 2: 23
limb salvage surgery, 3: 390–391, 433
Lincoln, Joan Tozzer, 3: 276
Lindbergh, Charles, 2: 232
Linenthal, Arthur J., 4: 210
Lingley, James, 3: 331

Linker, Beth, 4: 233
Linn, Frank C., 3: 324–325
Lippiello, Louis, 3: 383, 385–386
Lippman, Walter, 4: 469
Lipson, Jenifer Burns, 4: 271
Lipson, Stephen J. (1946–2013), 4: 116*b*, 163, *267*
on back surgery, 4: 270
Berg-Sloat Traveling Fellowship and, 4: 268
as Beth Israel chief of orthopaedics, 1: 233; 4: 223, 268, 270, 289*b*
as BIDMC chief of orthopaedics, 4: 268, 270–271, 281, 289*b*
BIDMC teaching program and, 1: 166–167, 220, 224, 226; 4: 286
Cave Traveling Fellowship and, 1: 217*b*
death of, 4: 271
development of multiple sclerosis, 4: 271
education and training, 4: 267
HCORP and, 4: 267
HMS appointment, 4: 271
honors and awards, 4: 268, 272
Kennedy Institute of Rheumatology and, 4: 268
legacy of, 4: 271–272
Mankin on, 4: 267–268
marriage and family, 4: 271
MGH and, 4: 267
PBBH and, 4: 268
publications and research, 4: 268–269, *269*, 270–271
spinal stenosis due to epidural lipomatosis case, 4: 269
spine research, 4: 268–271
Lisfranc, Jacque, 1: 73–74
Lister, Joseph
antisepsis principles, 1: 55, 81, 84–85; 3: 45
carbolic acid treatment, 1: 82–83, *83*, 85
treatment of compound fractures, 1: 84
Liston, Robert, 1: 76, 84
litholapaxy, 3: 41
lithotrite, 3: 41
Litterer-Siewe disease, 2: 171
Little, Moses, 1: 95
Little, Muirhead, 4: 402
Little, William John, 1: xxiii, 98, 106; 2: 26; 3: 54
Little Orthopaedic Club, 4: 74
Littlefield, Ephraim, 1: 303, *303*, 304, 309
Littler, J. William, 2: 248, 250
Lloyd, James, 1: 6, 8, 10

Lloyd Alpern–Dr. Rosenthal Physical Therapy Fund, 2: 439*b*
Locke, Edward, 4: 296
Locke, Joseph, 4: 100, *100*
Loder, Halsey B., 4: 438
Loh, Y. C., 3: 317
Long, Crawford W., 1: 56–57, 60, 63
Long Island Hospital, 2: 284
Longfellow, Frances (Fannie), 1: 297, 306
Longfellow, Henry Wadsworth, 1: 297, 302, 306
Longwood Medical Building Trust, 1: 264
Lord, J. F., 1: 177
Lorenz, Adolf, 2: 34, 242; 3: 234
Lorenz, Hans, 1: 264
Los Angeles Orthopaedic Hospital, 2: 266
Losina, Elena, 4: 195*b*
Loskin, Albert, 4: 280
Louis, Dean, 4: 168, 183
Louis, Pierre Charles Alexander, 1: 73–74
Louise and Edwin F. Cave Traveling Fellowship, 1: 217, 217*b*; 3: 274
Lovell General Hospital, 4: 482*b*
Lovett, Elizabeth Moorfield Storey, 2: 80, 230
Lovett, John Dyson, 2: 45
Lovett, Mary Elizabeth Williamson, 2: 45
Lovett, Robert Williamson (1859–1924), 1: *190*; 2: 45
   address to the American Orthopaedic Association, 2: 51
   Advisory Orthopedic Board and, 3: 157
   AOA and, 2: 48, *48*
   on astragalectomy, 2: 93–94
   Beth Israel Hospital and, 4: 208, 208*b*, 223
   birth palsies research, 2: 415
   Boston Children's Hospital and, 1: 188, 190–192; 2: 1, 10, 12–13, 40, 49, 54, *62*, 64, 68
   Boston City Hospital and, 1: 141, 143; 2: 45–47; 4: 298, 305*b*
   Boston Dispensary and, 2: 49
   Bradford and, 2: 49
   Brigham and Women's Hospital and, 4: 195*b*
   "Case of Glanders," 2: 46
   cerebral palsy cases, 2: 51
   "Certain Aspects of Infantile Paralysis," 2: *70*
   clinical surgery teaching and, 1: 141, 143
   Dane and, 2: 242, 246–247
   death of, 2: 80–81
   Department for Military Orthopedics and, 4: 406
   on departmental organization, 1: 176
   diaries of, 2: 45–46, *46*, 47, *47*, 48
   on disabled soldiers, 2: 67–68
   donations to Boston Medical Library, 2: 271
   early life, 2: 45
   education and training, 2: 45
   endowment in memory of, 2: 81–82
   Fiske Prize, 2: 52
   FitzSimmons and, 2: 144
   foot treatment, 2: 54–55, *55*, 56
   Harvard orthopaedic clinic and, 1: 174
   hip disease treatment and research, 2: 32, 49, *49*, 52, *52*, 53–54
   History of the Orthopedic Department at Children's Hospital, 2: 247
   as HMS chief of orthopaedics, 2: 64, 68
   House of the Good Samaritan and, 2: 49
   on incision and drainage of psoas abscesses, 2: 53–54
   Infantile Paralysis Commission, 2: 68, 99, 107
   John Ball and Buckminster Brown Professorship, 2: 63–64, *64*; 4: 195*b*
   Lateral Curvature of the Spine and Round Shoulders, 2: 79, *79*, 227
   legacy of, 2: 80
   Lovett Board, 2: *59*
   marriage and family, 2: 80, 230
   Mellon Lecture (Univ. of Pittsburgh), 2: 66–67
   military surgeon training by, 2: 42, 65–69
   New England Peabody Home for Crippled Children and, 2: 270
   at New York Orthopaedic Dispensary and Hospital, 2: 47–48
   obituary, 1: 93
   orthopaedic apprenticeship, 1: 186
   as orthopaedic chair, 2: 15*b*
   orthopaedic surgery, 2: 34, 51
   orthopaedics contributions, 2: 69–71
   Orthopedic Surgery, 2: 69, *69*; 4: 318
   PBBH and, 4: 10, 12
   pedagogy and, 2: 68–69
   as physician to Franklin D. Roosevelt, 2: 71–73, *73*, 74, *74*, 75, *75*, 76–77, 271
   poliomyelitis treatment, 2: 61–63, *63*, 70–79, 147–148, 264
   private medical practice and, 1: 176
   professional memberships, 2: 80, 80*b*
   as professor of orthopaedic surgery, 1: 147, 151, 171
   public health and, 2: 61
   publications and research, 2: 223, 246; 4: 259, 310
   scoliosis treatment, 2: 56–61, 79–80, 86, 223–225
   SICOT and, 2: 80
   social events and, 2: 49
   spina bifida treatment, 2: 51–52
   spring muscle test, 2: 70–71
   study of spine mechanics, 2: 57, *57*, 58, *58*, 59
   Surgery of Joints, The, 2: 52
   teaching hospitals and, 1: 187
   tracheostomy results, 2: 49, 51
   Treatise on Orthopaedic Surgery, A, 1: 108, 143; 2: 29–30, 43, 50, *50*, 51
   tuberculosis treatment, 2: 32
   turnbuckle jacket and, 2: 80, 224, *224*, 225
   US Army Medical Reserve Corps and, 2: 66
   use of radiographs, 2: 54
Lovett Board, 2: *59*, 86
Lovett Fund Committee, 2: 81–82
Low, Harry C. (1871–1943)
   acetonuria associated with death after anesthesia case, 3: 305
   Boston Children's Hospital and, 3: 304
   Boston City Hospital and, 3: 304
   Burrage Hospital and, 4: 226
   Children's Sunlight Hospital and, 3: 307
   Committee on Occupational Therapy chair, 3: 304–306
   death of, 3: 307
   early life, 3: 304
   education and training, 3: 304
   European medical studies, 3: 304
   marriage and, 3: 304
   on the MGH orthopaedic outpatient clinic, 3: 304, *304*, 306*b*–307*b*

as MGH surgeon, 3: 269, 304, 306
New England Home for Little Wanderers and, 3: 307
as poliomyelitis surgeon, 3: 306–307
"Progress in Orthopaedic Surgery" series, 2: 297
publications and research, 3: 304
Low, Mabel C. Chapman, 3: 304
Lowell, Abbott Lawrence, 1: 174, 176; 2: 41–42, 64
Lowell, Charles
 hip dislocation case, 1: 42, 44–49, 49b, 50; 3: 13, 13b, 36
 hip dislocation close-up, 1: 49
 letter of support for, 1: 45
 malpractice suit against John Collins, 1: 44, 50–51, 68
 x-ray of pelvis and hips, 1: 49
Lowell, J. Drennan (1922–1987), 4: 158, 161
 bladder fistula case, 4: 162
 Boston Children's Hospital and, 2: 384
 as BWH assistant chief of orthopaedic surgery, 4: 163
 BWH medical staff president, 4: 163
 Children's Hospital/MGH combined program and, 4: 158
 death of, 4: 164
 education and training, 4: 158
 Emory University Hospital and, 4: 158
 Fracture course and, 3: 273
 hip fracture research, 4: 160
 HMS appointment, 4: 162
 marriage and family, 4: 164
 MGH and, 3: 244; 4: 158–159
 on MGH approach to hip fractures, 4: 159b–160b
 PBBH and, 4: 116, 116b, 128–129
 as PBBH chief of clinical orthopaedics, 4: 161–163
 private medical practice, 4: 158
 professional memberships, 4: 162–163, 163b
 publications and research, 4: 159, 161–164
 RBBH and, 4: 114
 reconstructive hip surgery and, 4: 159
 train hobby and, 4: 160
 US Army and, 4: 158
 on use of ultraviolet light, 4: 162–163, 163, 164
Lowell, Olivia, 1: 263
Lowell, Ruth, 4: 164

Lowell General Hospital, 4: 243
Lower Extremity Amputations for Arterial Insufficiency (Warren and Record), 1: 90; 3: 330
Lowry, Robert, 4: 277
LTI Digital™ Arm Systems for Adults, 2: 326
lubrication, 3: 324–325
Lucas-Championniere, Just, 1: xxiii
Ludmerer, Kenneth, 1: 146
lumbago, 3: 203
lumbar spinal stenosis, 2: 373–374
lunate dislocation, 3: 101–102
Lund, F. B., 4: 331
Lund, Fred, 4: 220
Lycée Pasteur Hospital, 4: 388, 389b, 390
Lynch, Peter, 2: 414
Lynn General Hospital, 3: 253
Lyon, Mary, 2: 276
Lysholm Knee Scoring Scale, 2: 380

M

MacArthur, Douglas, 2: 232
MacAusland, Andrew R., 3: 308
MacAusland, Dorothy Brayton, 3: 308
MacAusland, Frances Prescott Baker, 3: 308
MacAusland, William R., Jr. (1922–2004), 3: 308
 as AAOS president, 3: 311, 311, 312
 ABC traveling fellowship and, 3: 309
 Carlos Otis Stratton Mountain Clinic and, 3: 311
 Carney Hospital and, 3: 308; 4: 45
 death of, 3: 312
 early life, 3: 308
 education and training, 3: 308
 Emergency Care and Transportation of the Sick and Injured, 3: 310, 311
 emergency responder training and, 3: 310–311
 HMS appointment, 3: 308
 knee arthroplasty and, 4: 64
 love of skiing and, 3: 311
 marriage and family, 3: 308, 312
 memberships and, 3: 309
 as MGH surgeon, 3: 266, 398b
 Orthopaedics, 3: 310
 Orthopaedics Overseas and, 3: 310
 private medical practice, 3: 308, 310

publications and research, 2: 248; 3: 308–310, 376, 377–378
 Rocky Mountain Trauma Society and, 3: 311
 on sepsis after intramedullary fixation of femoral fractures, 3: 309–310
 trauma research and, 3: 309
 as Tufts University professor, 3: 308
 US Air Force and, 3: 308
 West Roxbury Veterans Administration Hospital and, 3: 312
MacAusland, William R., Sr., 3: 308
Macdonald, Ian, 4: 102
MacEwen, Dean, 2: 304
Macewen, William, 1: xxiii
MacFarlane, Arlene, 3: 291
MacFarlane, J. A., 4: 468–469, 471
MacIntosh prothesis, 4: 69, 71b, 129, 188
Mackin, Evelyn J., 4: 168
Macknight, Jane, 1: 289
Maddox, Robert, 2: 121
Magee, James, 4: 471
Magill, H. Kelvin, 4: 376
magnetic resonance imaging (MRI), 3: 255
Magnuson, Paul B., 4: 473
Maine Carpal Tunnel Study (Keller, et al.), 2: 375, 375
Maine Carpal Tunnel Syndrome Study, 4: 184
Maine Lumbar Spine Study Group, 2: 373, 373, 374
Maine Medical Assessment Foundation, 2: 372, 374; 4: 184–185
Maine Medical Association, 2: 372
Maine Medical Practice of Neurosurgery and Spine, 2: 376
Maine Medical Society, 1: 49
Maisonneuve, Jacques, 1: 82
malaria treatment, 4: 491
Malchau, Henrik, 3: 219
Malenfant, J., 3: 45
Mallon, William J., 3: 143, 145
Mallory, Tracy B., 2: 254
malpractice suits
 Charles Lowell and, 1: 44, 50
 early concerns about, 1: 24
 fractures and, 1: 50–51; 3: 63
 increase in, 1: 50–51
 insurance and, 1: 51
 Joseph Warren on, 1: 12
 orthopaedics and, 1: 50; 3: 378–379
Malt, Ronald, 3: 217
Management of Fractures and Dislocations (Wilson), 3: 62, 273

Index

Mankin, Allison, 3: 393
Mankin, Carole J. Pinkney, 1: 218;
  3: 382, 385, 393
Mankin, David, 3: 393
Mankin, Henry J. (1928–2018),
  1: *210, 212*; 3: *381, 386, 393, 461*
  AAOS and, 3: 388
  articular cartilage research,
    3: 383, *383*, 384, *385*, 388,
    442
  BIH Board of Consultants,
    4: 262–263
  breakfast meetings with residents,
    1: 213, *214*
  on Chandler, 3: 279
  chordoma of the spinal column
    and, 3: 390
  core curriculum and, 1: 215
  death of, 3: 393
  early life, 3: 381
  Edith M. Ashley Professor,
    3: 464*b*
  education and training,
    3: 381–382
  establishment of the Institute of Health Professions,
    3: 391–392
  femoral allograft transplantation,
    3: 389, *389*, 390
  HCORP and, 1: 210–221, 239;
    3: 387, 397
  histologic-histochemical grading
    system, 3: 384, 384*t*, 385
  HMS appointment, 3: 385
  honors and awards, 3: 392, 393*b*
  Hospital for Joint Diseases and,
    3: 382–383, 385, 389
  Korean War and, 3: 382
  limb salvage surgery and,
    3: 390–391
  on Lipson, 4: 267–268
  marriage and family, 3: 382, 385
  memberships and, 3: 392
  MGH Bone Bank and, 3: 386,
    388, 396, 439
  as MGH clinical faculty, 3: 464*b*
  MGH operations improvement
    and, 3: 387, 395–399
  as MGH orthopaedics chief,
    1: 180; 3: 11*b*, 219, 228, 320,
    378, 385–388, 395–399, 459,
    461
  MGH residents and, 3: *387, 460*
  Mount Sinai Medical School and,
    3: 383, 385
  NIH and, 3: 383, 387–388, 392
  Orthopaedic Biology and Oncology Laboratories, 3: 464*b*

orthopaedic oncology and,
    3: 386, 388, 388*t*, 390,
    392–393, 460*b*
  orthopaedic research support,
    1: 218
  orthopaedics education and,
    3: 386
  pathology course and, 3: 396
  *Pathophysiology of Orthopaedic
    Diseases*, 4: 226
  publications and research,
    3: 383–385, 387–392, 433,
    440
  as residency program director,
    1: 181, 210–211, 213–221
  on rickets and osteomalacia,
    3: 388
  on Rowe, 3: 360
  specialty services at MGH under,
    3: 388*t*, 459, 460*t*, 461–462
  on sports medicine clinic, 2: 384
  Such a Joy for a Yiddish Boy,
    3: 392, *392*
  University of Chicago clinics and,
    3: 382
  University of Pittsburgh appointment, 3: 382–383
  US Navy and, 3: 382
Mankin, Hymie, 3: 381
Mankin, Keith, 3: 392, *392*, 393,
  398*b*, 401, 460*b*, 464*b*
Mankin, Mary, 3: 381
Mankin System, 3: 384, 384*t*, 385
Mann, Robert W., 2: 326; 3: 397,
  398*b*
Mansfield, Frederick L. (1947–),
  3: *419*
  education and training, 3: 419
  HCORP and, 3: 419
  HMS appointment, 3: 419
  memberships and, 3: 421
  as MGH clinical faculty, 3: 464*b*
  as MGH surgeon, 3: 419
  open anterior lumbosacral fracture dislocation case, 3: 420
  orthopaedics education and,
    3: 421
  publications and research,
    3: 419–421
  sciatica treatment and, 3: 254
  spine surgery and, 3: 397,
    419–421, 460*b*
  use of chymopapain, 3: 254,
    419, *421*
Manson, Anne, 2: 277
Manson, James G. (1931–2009)
  Boston Children's Hospital and,
    2: 276–277
  death of, 2: 277
  early life, 2: 275

education and training, 2: 276
  hemophilia clinic, 2: 276
  HMS appointment, 2: 276
  marriage and family, 2: 276–277
  MGH residency, 2: *276*
  MIT Medical and, 2: 276–277,
    290
  Mount Auburn Hospital and,
    2: 276
  PBBH and, 4: 22
Manson, Mary Lyon, 2: 276
*Manual of Bandaging, Strapping and
  Splinting, A* (Thorndike), 1: 268
Manual of Chemistry (Webster),
  1: 299, 301
Manual of Orthopedic Surgery, A
  (Thorndike), 2: 311, *312*
Manual of Orthopedic Surgery (Bigelow), 3: 25–26, *26*
Manuel II, King, 4: 399–401, *401*,
  402–403, 442
marathon runners, 1: 250
Marble, Alice Ingram, 3: 316
Marble, Henry C. (1885–1965),
  3: *312*
  AAST and, 3: 315, *315*
  American Mutual Liability Insurance Company and, 3: 314,
    316
  American Society for Surgery of
    the Hand and, 3: 316
  anatomy education and, 3: 314
  Base Hospital No. 6 and,
    4: 433–434, 436
  Bedford Veterans Administration
    Hospital and, 3: 314
  blood transfusion work, 3: 313
  Chelsea Memorial Hospital and,
    3: 314
  death of, 3: 316
  early life, 3: 312
  education and training,
    3: 312–313
  Faulkner Hospital and, 3: 314
  as Fracture Clinic chief, 3: 60*b*
  fracture research and, 3: 340
  Fractures, 3: 315
  Hand, The, 3: 316
  HMS appointment, 3: 313
  legacy of, 3: 316
  marriage and family, 3: 316
  Massachusetts Regional Fracture
    Committee, 3: 64
  memberships and, 3: 316
  MGH Fracture Clinic and, 3: 60,
    313–315
  MGH Hand Clinic and, 3: 314
  as MGH surgeon, 3: 313–315
  orthopaedics education and,
    3: 315

publications and research, 3: 314–316
Scudder Oration on Trauma, 3: 63
Surgical Treatment of the Motor-Skeletal System, 3: 316
US Army Medical Corps and, 3: 313
US General Hospital No. 3 and, 4: 452
Marcella Street Home, 2: 242, 247
March of Dimes, 2: 315
Marcove, Ralph, 3: 382
Margliot, Z., 3: 409
Marian Ropes Award, 4: 100
Marie-Strumpell disease, 3: 239
Marion B. Gebbie Research Fellowship, 4: 127
Marjoua, Youssra, 4: 190*b*
Marlborough Medical Associates, 2: 146, 269, 299
Marmor modular design prosthesis, 4: 130
Marnoy, Samuel L., 4: 208*b*
Marshall, H. W., 3: 155
Martin, Edward, 3: 112, 113*b*
Martin, Ernest, 2: 70, *70*, 71
Martin, Franklin H., 3: 113*b*; 4: 324
Martin, Geraldine, 4: 389*b*
Martin, Joseph, 1: 181, 232–234; 4: 284–285
Martin, Scott D., 1: 230; 4: 193, 195*b*
Martin, Tamara, 4: 193
Marvin, Frank W., 4: 407
Mary Alley Hospital, 2: 269
Mary Hitchcock Memorial Hospital, 3: 363–364
Mary Horrigan Conner's Center for Women's Health, 4: *194*
Mary MacArthur Memorial Respiratory Unit (Wellesley Hospital), 2: 189, 315
Maslin, Robert, 2: 354
Mason, Jonathan, 1: 38
Mason, Susan Powell, 1: 37–38, 72
Masons, 1: 10–12, 29
Mass General Brigham (MGB), 3: 462
Massachusetts Agricultural Society, 1: 29
Massachusetts Arthritis Foundation, 4: 100
Massachusetts Board of Registration in Medicine, 3: 423
Massachusetts Eye and Ear Infirmary, 2: 252; 3: 331, 339; 4: 113–114

Massachusetts General Hospital, 1955–1980, The (Brown), 3: 299
Massachusetts General Hospital, Its Development, 1900–1935, The (Washburn), 3: 1
Massachusetts General Hospital (MGH)
apothecary position, 1: 184
arthritis research program at, 2: 82
Base Hospital No. 6 and, 4: 420*t*, 429–432
blood transfusions at, 3: 313
clinical surgery curricula at, 1: 151
End-Result Idea, 3: 112, 114
expansion of staff, 3: 14–15
faculty model at, 1: 174, 176
fee structures, 3: 16, 21–22
first orthopaedic case at, 1: 42, 44
first patients at, 1: 42; 3: 11
General Hospital No. 6 and, 3: 239, 362; 4: 474, 485*b*
HMS clinical teaching at, 3: 13
house physicians/surgeons, 1: 184
house pupils (pups) at, 1: 80, 184, *185*; 2: 20
impact of World War II on, 4: 467
innovation at, 3: 216–217
institutional racism and, 3: 15–16
internes/externs, 1: 184–185
James Jackson and, 1: 31, 41–42; 3: 5, *5*, 6*b*–7*b*, 12–13
John Ball Brown and, 3: 12
John Collins Warren and, 1: 31, 41–42, 52–55, 57–58; 3: 5, *5*, 6*b*–7*b*, 12–13
King Report, 3: 301–302
military surgeon training at, 4: 396
modernization of, 3: 453
nursing school at, 4: 467
occupational rehabilitation and, 4: 444
105th General Hospital and, 4: 493
ophthalmology service at, 3: 13
performance-based promotions at, 3: 123–124
postgraduate education and, 2: 157–159
rehabilitation clinic and, 1: 273
reserve units for army service, 4: 429–430
roentgenology department, 3: 21
surgical residencies, 1: 184, *185*

surgical volume due to ether use, 1: 63, 64*t*
treatment categories, 1: 54, 54*t*
treatment of children in, 2: 4, 8
treatment of soldiers, 3: 21
treatment outcomes reporting, 1: 54; 3: 112
treatments and techniques at, 3: 20–22
use of ether anesthesia, 1: 57–63, 85; 3: 15, 22, 27–28, 28*b*, 29, 29*b*, 30–34
use of ligatures, 1: 85
use of radiographs, 2: 54
visiting surgeons at, 3: *31*
Warren family and, 1: 71
women surgeons at, 1: 239
World War II and, 4: 493
x-rays and, 3: 20, *20*
Massachusetts General Hospital. Facilities
Allen Street House, 3: 17–18
Ambulatory Care, 3: 396, 399
Baker Memorial, 3: *73*, 75
Bigelow Building, 3: 15–17
Bulfinch Building, 1: *41*; 3: *9*, 13, 15, *16*, 22, *60*, 70*b*
Children's Ward, 3: *71*
East Wing, 3: *14*, 15, *60*
Ellison Tower, 3: 75
Ether Dome, 1: *59*, *63*, *84*; 3: *14*, 16
expansion of, 3: 14, *14*, 15, *15*, 16–18, 18*b*, 20–21, 74–75
Gay Ward (outpatient building), 3: *19*, 265
Henry J. Bigelow Operating Theater, 1: *84*
medical school, 3: *15*
Moseley Memorial Building, 3: 70*b*, 75
Nerve Room, 3: 20
Out-Patient Department, 3: 75
pathological laboratory, 3: 21
Patient Ward, 3: *74*
Pavilion Wards, 3: *17*
Phillips House, 1: 86, 204; 3: *72*, *73*, 75
Physical Therapy Department, 3: 269
plot plans for, 3: *10*, *17*, *22*, *71*, *72*, *461*
Treadwell Library, 3: 70*b*
view in 1840, 1: *54*
Wang ACC building, 3: 75
Ward 5, 1: 203
Ward A (Warren), 3: 17, *17*, 18
Ward B (Jackson), 3: 17, *17*
Ward C (Bigelow), 3: 17–18
Ward D (Townsend), 3: 18, *18*

Index

Ward E (Bradlee), 3: 18–19, *19*
Ward F (George A. Gardner building), 3: 19
wards in, 3: *12*
Warren Building, 3: 17
West Wing, 3: 15, *60*
White Building (George Robert White), 3: *74*, 75
Massachusetts General Hospital. Founding of
 advocacy for, 1: 41; 3: 3–5, *5*, *6*, 6*b*–7*b*
 Almshouse site, 1: 41
 Bulfinch design for, 1: 41; 3: 10–11
 construction of, 3: 9–10
 funding for, 1: 41–42; 3: 6–7, 9, 14, 18–19, 21
 grand opening of, 3: 11–12
 Province House and, 3: 6–7, 9
 seal of, 3: *10*, 11, *11*
 state charter authorizing, 3: 6–7, *8*
Massachusetts General Hospital. Orthopaedics Department
 adults and, 2: 157
 approach to hip fractures, 4: 159*b*–160*b*
 Biomaterials and Innovative Technologies Laboratory, 3: 463
 Biomotion Laboratory, 3: 463, 464*b*
 bone bank for allografts and, 3: 388, 396, 440–441, 443
 Cambridge Hospital clinic, 3: 396, 399
 Clinical and Research Programs, 3: 464*b*
 clinical faculty, 3: 464*b*
 clinical service rotations, 1: 198
 continuing medical education and, 3: 396
 creation of, 3: 67–69
 expansion of, 3: 286
 facilities for, 3: 68–69, 70*b*, 71, *72*, 73, *73*, 75, 80
 femoral replacement prosthesis, 4: 129
 Fracture Clinic at, 2: 130; 3: 60, 60*b*, 62, 241–242, 245, 273, *273*, 313–315, 371, 373, 378, 456*b*; 4: 464
 Fracture Course at, 3: 62
 Frederick and Joan Brengle Learning Center, 3: 463
 gait laboratory and, 3: 397
 growth in, 3: 227–228
 Hand Clinic at, 3: 314

Harris Orthopaedic and Biomaterials laboratory, 3: 463
HCORP and, 1: 213–215
house officers at, 1: 189
internships at, 1: 196
Joint Kinematics Laboratory, 3: 463, 464*b*
Joseph S. Barr and, 3: 453, 453*b*–456*b*
Knee Biomechanics and Biomaterials Laboratory, 3: 463, 464*b*
Melvin J. Glimcher and, 3: 453, 455*b*–458*b*
opening of, 3: 68
Orthopaedic Biochemistry and Osteoarthritis Therapy Laboratory, 3: 464*b*
Orthopaedic Biology and Oncology Laboratories, 3: 463, 464*b*
Orthopaedic Biomechanics and Biomaterials Laboratory, 3: 464*b*
orthopaedic chairpersons at, 3: 11*b*
Orthopaedic Oncology Unit, 3: 440
orthopaedic rehabilitation and, 3: 459
Orthopaedic Research Laboratories, 2: 321–324; 3: 211–212
orthopaedic specialties, 3: 459, 460*b*, 461–462
orthopaedic staff in 1984, 3: 398*b*
orthopaedic surgery department, 1: 171, 180
orthopaedics curriculum and, 1: 136–137, 157–158, 167
orthopaedics fellowships, 1: 241
orthopaedics instruction at, 1: 190
orthopaedics residencies, 1: 186, 199, 204, 207, 217–218, 221–225, 241–242; 2: *249*, *278*, *290*, *320*, *327*; 3: 74
Orthopedic Biomechanics Laboratory, 3: 463
outpatient services and, 3: 80, 227, 304, 306*b*–307*b*
pediatric orthopaedics and, 3: 388*t*, 400
physical therapy and, 3: 454*b*
podiatry service and, 3: 396–398
Problem Back Clinic, 3: 254
professorships, 3: 464*b*
research activities, 3: 455*b*, 458*b*
Research Building, 3: *454*
Research Laboratory Centers, 3: 464*b*

Sarcoma Molecular Biology Laboratory, 3: 464*b*
specialty services under Mankin, 3: 388*t*, 396–398
sports medicine and, 3: 397
Sports Medicine Service, 3: 356, 448
surgeon-scholars at, 3: 228, 395–398, 398*b*, 399, *461*
surgical appliance shop, 3: 73
surgical residencies, 1: 198; 3: 455*b*, 457*b*–458*b*
Thornton Brown on changes at, 3: 453*b*–458*b*
transition in, 3: 461–463
Ward 1, 1: 273; 2: 116; 3: *67*, 68, *68*, 70*b*, 74–75, *80*
White 9 Rehabilitation Unit, 3: 286, 299, 455*b*, 459, 461
Zander Room (Medico-Mechanical Department), 3: 71, 227, 264–268
Massachusetts General Hospital Physicians Organization (MGPO), 3: 256
Massachusetts General Orthopaedic Group, 3: 246
Massachusetts General/Boston Children's Hospital residency program, 1: 210; 2: 144
Massachusetts Homeopathic Hospital, 3: 120
Massachusetts Hospital Life Insurance Company, 3: 9
Massachusetts Hospital School for Crippled Children, 2: 38–39, *39*, 384; 3: 319–320
Massachusetts Humane Society, 1: 29
Massachusetts Industrial Accident Board, 2: 92; 4: 325, 327
Massachusetts Infantile Paralysis Clinic, 2: 188–189, 191, 208, 212, 314
Massachusetts Institute of Technology (MIT), 2: 321; 4: 152
Massachusetts Medical Association, 1: 184
Massachusetts Medical College of Harvard University, 1: 6, 40, *40*, 41, *135*; 3: 35, 38
Massachusetts Medical Society, 1: 25–26, 29, 38, 99, 272–273, 277; 2: 164, 208, 230; 3: 35; 4: 162, 366*b*, 367, 367*b*
Massachusetts Memorial Hospital, 4: 347
Massachusetts Orthopaedic Association (MOA), 3: 421; 4: 253

513

Massachusetts Regional Fracture Committee, 3: 64
Massachusetts Rehabilitation Hospital, 3: 387, 396
Massachusetts Services for Crippled Children, 2: 208
Massachusetts Society of Examining Physicians, 4: 324
Massachusetts State Board of Health, 2: 61
Massachusetts State Hospital, 2: 102
Massachusetts Volunteer Aid Association, 2: 43
Massachusetts Women's Hospital, 4: 447–448
Massachusetts Workingmen's Compensation Law, 4: 325
massage
    avoidance of tender muscles, 1: 267; 2: 73
    congenital dislocated hips (CDH) and, 2: 178
    foot problems and, 2: 56, 245
    injured soldiers and, 2: 56, 67, 118, 120
    obstetrical paralysis and, 2: 90, 94
    physical therapy and, 1: 100; 3: 266, 297
    poliomyelitis and, 2: 62, 73, 109
    therapeutic, 3: 264–266
Massage (Böhm), 3: 266
Matson, Donald, 2: 301
Matza, R. A., 2: 279, 280*b*
Mayer, Leo, 1: 1, 107, 114; 2: 24, 33, 51, 70, 99, 165; 3: 156*b*, 196; 4: 291, 463
Mayfield, F. H., 3: 210
Mayo, Charles W., 4: 411
Mayo, Richard, 3: 310
Mayo, William J., 2: 69; 3: 40–41, 44–45, 50, 113*b*
Mayo Clinic, 3: 50, 289
McBride, Earl D., 3: 295
McCabe, Charles, 1: 167
McCall, M. G., 2: 212
McCall, Samuel W., 3: 134
McCarroll, H. Relton, 1: 162; 4: 237
McCarthy, Clare, 2: 178–180, 182, 204, 230, 287–288
McCarthy, E. A., 2: 230
McCarthy, Eddie, 3: 97
McCarthy, Joseph, 2: 368
McCarthy, Ralph, 4: 342
McCharen, Littleton L., 4: 489
McClellan, George, 3: 43
McCombs, Betsy, 3: 280
McCord, David, 4: 3, 9, 20

McDermott, Leo J., 2: 171–172, 229, 299, 438; 3: 74
McDermott, William, Jr., 4: 277–279, 303
McDonagh, Eileen, 1: 285
McDonald, John L., 2: 183
McDougall, Jean, 3: 288
McGibbon, Chris, 3: 460*b*
McGill University School of Medicine, 3: 253
McGinty, Beth A. Dignan, 2: 277–278
McGinty, John B. (1930–2019), 2: *278*, *281*
    AAOS chairman, 2: 281
    Arthroscopic Surgery Update, 2: 279
    arthroscopy and, 2: 279, 280*b*, 281; 3: 448
    Boston Children's Hospital and, 2: 278–279; 4: 22
    Brigham and Women's Hospital and, 4: 163, 193
    death of, 2: 281
    education and training, 2: 277
    Green and, 2: 178, 205, 279
    marriage and family, 2: 277–278
    Medical University of South Carolina and, 2: 281
    MGH and, 2: 278
    MGH/Children's Hospital residency, 2: 278
    military service, 2: 278–279
    Newton-Wellesley Hospital and, 2: 279
    Operative Arthroscopy, 2: 279
    Orthopaedics Today editor, 2: 281
    PBBH and, 2: 278–279; 4: 22, 116, 128, 163
    professional memberships, 2: 281
    publications and research, 2: 279
    Tufts University and, 2: 279
    Valley Forge Army Hospital and, 2: 279
    Veterans Administration Hospital and, 2: 279; 4: 22
McIndoe Memorial Research Unit, 2: 422, *422*
McKay, Douglas, 2: 304, 351
McKeever, Duncan, 4: 40
McKeever prothesis, 4: 40, 69, 70*b*–71*b*, 129–130, 177, 188–189
McKittrick, Leland S., 3: 301; 4: 276, 277*b*
McLaughlin, F. L., 3: 210
McLean, Franklin C., 3: 211
McLean Hospital, 1: 294
McMahon, Mark S., 3: 449
McMahon, Vince, 4: 252
McRae, Ronald, 1: 167

Meals, Roy, 3: 431
measles, 1: 7; 2: 4
Mechanic, Gerald L., 2: 324
Mechanism of Dislocation and Fracture of the Hip, The (Bigelow), 3: 35, *35*, 38
Medearis, Donald N., 3: 397
Medical and Orthopaedic Management of Chronic Arthritis, The (Osgood and Pemperton), 4: 32
Medical College of Virginia, 4: 153
medical degrees, 1: 6–7
medical education. *See also* Harvard Medical School (HMS); orthopaedics residencies
    admission requirements, 1: 146
    American, 1: 138, 142, 146–147
    apprenticeships and, 1: 6, 8, 15
    approved teaching hospitals, 1: 196, 198
    clinical facilities for, 1: 40
    curricular reform, 1: 169
    development of medical schools, 1: 25–28
    dressers, 1: 6, 33, 36–37
    early orthopaedic surgery training, 1: 186–189
    early surgical training, 1: 183–186
    in Edinburgh, 1: 7, 37, 76
    in England, 1: 6, 33, 37, 73, 142
    examinations for physicians, 1: 15, 21, 29
    Flexner Report and, 1: 146–147
    governance and, 1: 177
    graduate education, 1: 196, 196*b*, 197–199, 213
    graduate orthopaedic surgery, 2: 160–162, 162*b*
    hospitals and, 1: 41, 52
    human dissections and, 1: 21, 24, 26–27, 32, 34, 38, 52
    impact of World War II on, 4: 467
    inclusiveness in, 2: 146
    internships and, 1: 189–190
    leaders of, 1: 147
    military hospitals and, 1: 24
    musculoskeletal medicine in, 1: 168–170
    orthopaedics curriculum in, 1: 153–155, 159–162; 2: 183–184, 184*b*, 185, 185*b*, 186
    in Paris, 1: 34, 37, 73–76
    postgraduate, 2: 157–160
    reform of, 1: 139–140
    regulation of, 1: 196–200, 211–213
    regulations and milestones of, 1: 196*b*

Index 515

specialization in, 1: 189;
  4: 300–301
supervised training in,
  1: 198–199
surgery in, 1: 29, 33–36
teaching program in, 1: 40; 4: 3
treating and teaching of fractures
  in, 1: 161
use of audio-visual aids in, 1: 161
Veterans Administration hospitals
  and, 1: 91
walkers, 1: 33
Medical Institution of Harvard
  College (1782–1816), 1: 25–26.
  See also Harvard Medical School
  (HMS)
Medical Institution of Liverpool,
  2: 135
*Medical Malpractice in Nineteenth-
  Century America* (De Ville), 1: 47
Medical Research Council of Great
  Britain, 2: 71
Medical University of South Carolina, 2: 281
*Medical War Manual No. 4 Military
  Orthopaedic Surgery*, 4: 473, *474*
Meeks, Berneda, 4: 255
Meeks, Laura, 4: 256
Meeks, Louis W. (1937–2015),
  4: *254*
  as Beth Israel acting chief of orthopaedics, 4: 223, 255, 289*b*
  as Beth Israel chief of sports medicine, 4: 255
  Beth Israel Hospital and, 4: 263
  BIDMC teaching program and,
    4: 286–287
  community organizations and,
    4: 255, 256*b*
  death of, 4: 256
  education and training, 4: 254
  HCORP and, 4: 255
  HMS appointment, 4: 263
  marriage and family, 4: 255
  orthopaedics education and,
    4: 254–255
  outpatient arthroscopic ACL
    reconstructions, 4: 255
  private medical practice, 4: 254
  publications and research, 4: 255
  US Army and, 4: 254
Meigs, Joe V., 2: 254
Meigs, Sarah Tyler, 3: 257
Meisenbach, Roland O., 4: 188
Mellon, William, 3: 135
Mellon Lecture (Univ. of Pittsburgh),
  2: 66–67
Melrose Hospital, 4: 343
Meltzer, S. J., 3: 212
Merrick, Phiny, 1: 307

Merrill, Ed, 3: 224
Merrill, Janet, 2: 107; 4: 60, 396
Messner, Marie Blais, 2: 170, 191,
  193–194
metal implants, 2: 237–238
metatarsalgia, 4: 188
Metcalf, Carleton R., 4: 440–441,
  441*b*
methylmethacrylate (bone cement),
  3: 220, 222; 4: 133, 171
Meyer, George von L., 2: 432
Meyerding, Henry W., 3: 340
MGH. *See* Massachusetts General
  Hospital (MGH)
MGH Institute of Health Professions, 3: 391, *391*, 392, 397
MGH School of Nursing, 3: 302,
  391
MGH Staff Associates, 3: 241
MGH Surgical Society Newsletter, 3: 1
Michael G. Ehrlich, MD, Fund for
  Orthopedic Research, 3: 401
Micheli, Lyle J. (1940–), 2: *383*
  on ACL reconstruction in young
    athletes, 2: 385, *385*, 386, *386*
  athletic spine problems and,
    2: 385
  as Boston Ballet attending physician, 2: 384
  Boston Children's Hospital and,
    2: 354, 383–385, 436, 439*b*
  Brigham and Women's Hospital
    and, 4: 163, 193
  education and training, 2: 383
  HMS appointment, 2: 383–384
  honors and awards, 2: 387*b*
  Joseph O'Donnell Family Chair
    in Orthopedic Sports Medicine,
    2: 439*b*
  Massachusetts Hospital School
    and, 2: 384
  MGH/Children's Hospital residency, 2: 383
  military service, 2: 383
  New England Deaconess Hospital
    and, 4: 280
  orthopaedics appointments,
    2: 384
  orthopaedics leadership, 2: 387
  PBBH and, 4: 163
  private medical practice, 2: 338
  publications and research,
    2: 359, 378–379, 385
  rugby and, 2: 383–385
  sports medicine and, 2: 287,
    384–385, 387
  *Sports Medicine Bible for Young
    Adults, The*, 2: 385
  Sports Medicine Bible, The,
    2: 385, *385*

Middlesex Central District Medical
  Society, 3: 319
Miegel, Robert, 4: 194, 195*b*
Mignon, M. Alfred, 4: 102
Milch, R. A., 4: 21
Milgram, Joseph, 3: 382
Military Orthopaedic Surgery (Orthopaedic Council), 2: 68, 69
military orthopaedics. *See also* base
  hospitals
  amputations and, 1: 23;
    4: 418–419
  bone and joint injuries, 4: 419
  camp work, 2: 258; 4: 452–453
  casualty clearing stations (CCS),
    4: 414, *415*, 421, 424–425
  compound fractures and, 4: 391,
    392
  curative workshops and, 4: 399–
    403, *403*, 404, 442, 448, *448*,
    449
  documentation and, 4: 407–408
  evacuation hospital care,
    4: 417–418
  expanded role of orthopaedists
    and, 4: 453–454
  facilities for, 4: 414–416
  Goldthwait and, 2: 127–128;
    4: 443
  Goldthwait units, 4: 440
  Harvard Medical School surgery
    course, 4: 455–462
  manual of splints and appliances
    for, 2: 126
  massage and, 2: 56, 67, 120, 188
  medical categories for,
    4: 412–414
  Medical Officer instructions for,
    4: 410*b*
  necessary equipment for, 4: 393*b*
  nerve lesions and, 4: 392
  open-bone fractures, 4: *400*
  Orthopaedic Centers and, 2: 127
  Osgood and, 2: 120–128;
    4: 423*b*
  patient flow process and,
    4: 435–436
  reconstruction and occupational
    aides, 4: 436*b*
  reconstruction hospitals and,
    4: 439–443, 447–449
  rehabilitation and, 1: 270–272;
    2: 121, 127; 3: 232; 4: 411,
    454
  standardization of equipment for,
    2: 124
  Thomas splint and, 2: 20
  Thorndike and, 1: 270–272
  trauma surgery and, 3: 274, 301;
    4: 393

use of splints in, 2: 120; 4: 389, *391*, 408–409, 411, 416–417
war injuries and, 2: 124, 126, 128; 4: 391
World War I volunteer orthopaedic surgeons, 2: 117–119, 124–127, 145; 4: 386–396, 398–399, *399*, 402, 404, 406–409, 412*b*–413*b*, 425, 452
World War II and, 4: 463–464, 473, 485, 493
wound treatment and, 4: 392–393, 435–436
Military Orthopedics for the Expeditionary Forces, 3: 156
military reconstruction hospitals. *See also* Reconstruction Base Hospital No. 1 (Parker Hill, Boston)
    amputation services, 4: 451
    Canadian, 4: 443
    Cotton on, 4: 449–451
    gyms in, 4: 444
    Harvard orthopaedic surgeons and, 4: 452
    as models for civilian hospitals, 4: 450–451
    occupational rehabilitation and, 4: 444
    organization of British, 4: 441*b*
    orthopaedics services in, 4: 439, 451
    rehabilitation of wounded soldiers and, 4: 439–444, 447–450
    in the United Kingdom, 4: 440–441
Millender, Bonnie Cobert, 4: 168
Millender, Lewis H. (1937–1996), 4: *165*
    Beth Israel Hospital and, 4: 262
    Brigham and Women's Hospital, 4: 163, 167
    death of, 4: 168
    education and training, 4: 165
    Entrapment Neuropathies, 4: 168
    hand therapy and, 4: 97–98, 132, 165, 168
    HMS appointment, 4: 165
    honors and awards, 4: 168
    hospital appointments, 4: 167
    marriage and family, 4: 168
    Nalebuff on, 4: 167
    New England Baptist Hospital and, 4: 165, 167
    Occupational Disorders of the Upper Extremity, 4: 168, 183
    occupational medicine and, 4: 167–168
    PBBH and, 4: 116, 129, 161, 163
    posterior interosseous syndrome case, 4: 165–166
    publications and research, 4: 165, *165*, 166–167, *167*
    RBBH and, 4: 132, 165, 167
    Tufts appointment, 4: 167
    US Public Health Service and, 4: 165
    West Roxbury Veterans Administration Hospital and, 4: 167
Miller, Bill, 2: 339, 358, *359*
Miller, Richard H., 3: 60; 4: 475
Millet, Peter, 4: 194
Milligan, E. T. C., 4: 385
Millis, Michael B. (1944–), 2: *388*
    acetabular dysplasia case, 2: 389, *389*, 390
    Boston Children's Hospital and, 2: 338, 354, 388–389
    Boston Concept and, 2: 391, *391*
    Brigham and Women's Hospital and, 4: 163, 193
    computer-simulated planning and, 2: 389
    education and training, 2: 358, 388
    Hall and, 2: 347, 388
    HCORP and, 2: 388
    hip and pelvis research, 2: 389–394
    HMS appointment, 2: 388–389
    honors and awards, 2: 388, 390
    metacarpal phalangeal joint replacement, 4: 132
    military service, 2: 388
    orthopaedics appointments, 2: 389
    orthopaedics education and, 2: 394
    on Pappas, 2: 289
    pediatric orthopaedics, 2: 394
    periacetabular osteotomy research, 2: 390–394
    professional memberships, 2: 392–393
    publications and research, 2: 389–394
Milton Hospital, 1: 264; 3: 257, 287
Milwaukee Brace, 2: 265–266, 336
Minas, Thomas, 4: 193, 195*b*
Minot, Charles S., 3: 94; 4: 2–3, *6*
Miriam Hospital, 3: 401
MIT Medical, 2: 276–277, 290
Mital, Mohinder A., 2: 234; 3: 320
Mitchell, William, Jr., 4: 286
Mixter, Charles G., 4: 283*t*, 468
Mixter, Samuel J., 2: 117; 3: *19*, 184
Mixter, William J.
    back pain research and, 3: 203, *203*, 204–207
    Beth Israel Hospital and, 1: 158
    publications and research, 3: 302
    ruptured intervertebral disc research, 3: 204; 4: 352–353
Mizuno, Schuichi, 4: 194
mobile army surgical hospitals (MASHs), 2: 231, *232*; 4: 468–469, *470*
Mock, Harry, 1: 271
Moe, John, 2: 335
Moellering, Robert, 4: 279
Mohan, Alice, 1: 62
Molasses Act, 1: 11
mold arthroplasty
    evolution of the Vitallium, 3: 292, 292*b*, 293
    hip surgery and, 3: 218, 242, *242*, 243–244
    historical evolution of, 3: *194*
    knee and, 3: 291–292
    original design of, 3: 193*b*
    postoperative roentgenogram, 3: *195*, *196*
    preoperative roentgenogram, 3: *196*
    problems with cup, 3: 241
    results of, 3: 242*t*, 243*b*
    Smith-Petersen and, 3: 181, 182*b*, 183, 192, *192*, 193–196, 198
    Vitallium, 3: 193*b*, *195*, *196*, 238–239, 243*b*
Molloy, Maureen K., 1: 239; 3: 208
mononucleosis, 3: 324–325
Monson State Hospital, 4: 350
Montgomery, James B., 4: 407
Moody, Dwight, 4: 257
Moody, Ellsworth, 3: 165–166
Moore, Belveridge H., 2: 78, 172
Moore, Francis D.
    on Banks, 4: 72
    burn care and, 3: 336
    as BWH chief of surgery, 3: 135
    family of, 1: 90
    as Moseley Professor of Surgery, 2: 421
    PBBH 50th anniversary report, 4: 21*b*
    PBBH and, 4: 79
    as PBBH chief of surgery, 4: 8, 18, 22, 74*b*, 75
    on Sledge, 4: 114
    on surgery residents, 4: 19
Moore, Howard, 4: 372
Moral Re-Armament program (Oxford Group), 4: 57
Morales, Teresa, 3: 462, 464*b*
Moratoglu, Orhun, 3: 460*b*

Morgan, John, 1: 23
Morris, Katherine, 2: 284
Morris, Miriam Morss, 2: 282
Morris, Richard B., 1: 317
Morris, Robert H. (1892–1971), 2: *283*
  on arthrodesis procedures, 2: 282–283
  BCH Bone and Joint Service, 4: 380*b*
  Boston Children's Hospital and, 1: 194; 2: 222, 231, 252, 274, 284
  death of, 2: 284
  education and training, 2: 282
  Fitchet and, 2: 282
  on foot stabilization, 2: 282–284
  HMS appointment, 2: 223, 282; 4: 60–61
  King's College and, 2: 284
  Long Island Hospital and, 2: 284
  marriage and family, 2: 282, 284
  professional memberships, 2: 284
  publications of, 2: 282
  RBBH and, 4: 36, 93, 111
  World War I service, 2: 282
Morrison, Gordon M. (1896–1955), 4: *346*
  AAST president, 4: 349
  Boston City Hospital and, 4: 347
  boxing and, 4: 347
  Cotton and, 4: 330
  death of, 4: 349
  education and training, 4: 346–347
  football coaching and, 4: 347
  hip fracture treatment, 4: 319
  hospital appointments, 4: 347
  ischaemic paralysis case, 4: 348
  Joseph H. Shortell Fracture Unit, 4: 307
  Massachusetts Regional Fracture Committee, 3: 64
  New England Society of Bone and Joint Surgery, 4: 347
  professional memberships, 4: 347–349
  publications and research, 4: 316, 347
  Royal Flying Corps and, 4: 346–347
  on trauma treatment, 4: 349
Morrison, H., 4: 202, 203*b*, *203*
Morrison, Sidney L., 4: 64, *64*
Morrissey, Raymond, 2: 438
Morrow, Edward R., 2: 272
Morss, Miriam, 2: 282
Morton, William T. G., 1: *57*
  ether composition, 1: 61
  ether inhaler, 1: *58*, 63
  ether patent and, 1: 60
  ether use, 1: 55, 57–60, 62; 3: 27–29, 32–33
  as witness for Webster, 1: 310
Morton's neuroma, 2: 287
Moseley, William, 3: 74
Moseley's growth charts, 2: 194, *194*
Moss, H. L., 4: 261–262
Moss, William L., 3: 313
Mott, Valentine, 1: xxiv
Mount Auburn Cemetery, 3: 23; 4: 2
Mount Auburn Hospital, 2: 276; 3: 327
Mount Sinai Monthly magazine, 4: *201*, 202
Moyer, Carl, 4: 125
Mt. Sinai Hospital (Boston)
  Chambers Street location, 4: 201*b*, 202, *202*
  closing of, 4: 205, 223
  Compton Street location, 4: 201*b*, 202, *202*
  financial difficulties, 4: 203–205
  fundraising for, 4: 202
  Jewish patients at, 4: 199–200, 202
  Jewish physicians and, 4: 202, 204
  non-discrimination and, 4: 199, 201
  orthopaedic treatment at, 4: 202, 204, 204*t*
  outpatient services at, 4: 203–204
  planning for, 4: 200–201
  Staniford Street location, 4: 202
Mt. Sinai Hospital (New York)
  Jewish patients at, 4: 200
  orthopaedics residencies and, 4: 88
  World War II and, 4: 88
Mt. Sinai Hospital Society of Boston, 4: 200–201
Mt. Sinai Medical School, 3: 383, 385, 413, 435
Mueller, Maurice, 4: 263
Mueller Professorship, 4: 263
Muir, Helen, 4: 116*b*, 268
Multicenter Arthroscopy of the Hip Outcomes Research Network (MAHORN), 2: 380
multiple cartilaginous exostoses, 4: 218–219, *219*, 220
Mumford, E. B., 4: 452
Mumford, James, 4: 52
Muratoglu, Orhun, 3: 224
Muro, Felipe, 2: 309
Murphy, Eugene, 3: 317
Murphy, Steven, 2: 389–392; 4: 286
Murray, Martha, 2: 439
Murray S. Danforth Oration of Rhode Island Hospital, 3: 275
Muscle Function (Wright), 2: 70
muscle training
  heavy-resistance exercise, 3: 282–285
  poliomyelitis and, 2: 62–63, 78, 109; 3: 284–285
  progressive resistance exercises, 3: 285
Muscular Dystrophy Association of America, 2: 266
Musculoskeletal Imaging Fund, 2: 439*b*
musculoskeletal medicine
  apparatus for, 2: 27
  biomechanics and, 2: 410
  disease and, 2: 439
  early treatment, 1: xxiii
  in medical education, 1: 168–170
  orthopaedics curriculum and, 1: 168–170; 2: 184–186
  orthopaedics research and, 2: 439
  pathology and, 3: 432
  sarcomas and, 2: 424
  spinal disorders and, 2: 337
  sports injuries and, 1: 288
  surgery advances for, 2: 36
  tissue banks for, 3: 442–443
  tumors and, 3: 432–433, 436
Musculoskeletal Outcome Data Evaluation and Management System (MODEMS), 4: 186
Musculoskeletal Tissue Banking (Tomford), 3: 443
Musculoskeletal Tumor Society, 3: 390, 436, *436*
Musnick, Henry, 4: 91
Myelodysplasia Clinic (Children's Hospital), 2: 359, 402
Myers, Grace Whiting, 3: 10
myositis ossificans, 1: 266–267

N

Nachemson, Alf, 2: 373; 4: 262
Nadas, Alex, 2: 234
Nalebuff, Edward A. (1928–2018), 4: *94*
  art glass collection, 4: 100, *100*
  Boston Children's Hospital and, 4: 95
  Brigham and Women's Hospital, 4: 163
  death of, 4: 100

education and training, 4: 94–95
hand surgery and, 4: 96, 98–100
hand surgery fellowship, 4: 95–96
HMS appointment, 4: 97–98
hospital appointments, 4: 99
implant arthroplasty research, 4: 99–100
Marian Ropes Award, 4: 100
marriage of, 4: 100
metacarpal phalangeal joint replacement, 4: 132
MGH and, 4: 95
New England Baptist Hospital and, 4: 99
PBBH and, 4: 95, 116, 129, 161, 163
professional memberships, 4: 100
publications and research, 4: 40, 95–99, 99, 166, 167
RBBH and, 4: 38, 41b, 42, 68–69, 95–97, 100, 102, 116b, 131
RBBH hand clinic and, 4: 42
as RBBH hand service chief, 4: 97–98
rheumatoid arthritis of the hand research and surgery, 4: 96, 96, 97–98, 98, 131
rheumatoid thumb deformity classification, 4: 97
surgical procedures performed, 4: 131t
Tufts appointment, 4: 98
Tufts hand fellowship, 2: 250; 4: 98–99
US Air Force and, 4: 95
Veterans Administration Hospital and, 4: 95
Nalebuff, Marcia, 4: 100
Nathan, David, 2: 234
"Nation and the Hospital, The" (Osgood), 2: 137–138, 138b–139b
National Academy of Medicine, 3: 405
National Academy of Sciences, 3: 405
National Birth Defects Center, 2: 370
National Collegiate Athletic Association (NCAA), 1: 248, 253
National Foundation for Infantile Paralysis, 2: 188–189, 191, 260
National Foundation for Poliomyelitis, 2: 188, 191
National Institute of Arthritis and Metabolic Diseases, 3: 323
National Institutes of Health (NIH), 3: 383, 387–388, 392; 4: 38–39

National Intercollegiate Football, 1: 253
National Rehabilitation Association, 2: 266
National Research Council, 2: 215–216
Natural History of Cerebral Palsy, The (Crothers and Paine), 2: 172
Naval Fleet Hospital No. 109, 4: 490
Naval Medical Research Institute, 3: 439, 440
Navy Regional Medical Center (Guam), 3: 446
necks, 2: 256
Nélaton, Auguste, 1: 82
nerve injuries, 2: 67, 120, 140, 393; 3: 157, 353
Nerve Injuries Committee (Medical Research Council of Great Britain), 2: 71
Nesson, H. Richard, 2: 272
Nestler, Steven P., 1: 215, 218, 220, 232–233; 3: 435–436, 436
neuritis, 3: 324–325
neurofibromatosis, 2: 172, 174–175
Neusner, Jacob, 4: 220
New England Baptist Hospital (NEBH)
  affiliation with BIDMC, 4: 214
  affiliation with New England Deaconess Hospital, 4: 280
  Aufranc and, 3: 246–247
  Ben Bierbaum and, 1: 233–234, 236
  Bone and Joint Institute Basic Science Laboratory, 4: 271, 286
  Brackett and, 3: 153
  Edward Kennedy and, 3: 275
  Emans and, 2: 358
  Fitchet and, 2: 252
  Hall and, 2: 338
  Hresko and, 2: 364
  Kocher and, 2: 377
  Morris and, 2: 284
  Nalebuff and, 4: 98–100
  New England Bone and Joint Institute, 4: 280
  orthopaedics residencies, 3: 247
  Painter and, 4: 47
  Pathway Health Network and, 4: 280
  Pedlow and, 3: 426
  Potter and, 4: 69, 116
  purchase of RBBH buildings and land, 4: 26, 114, 121
  reconstructive hip surgery and, 3: 246
  Runyon and, 2: 290
  Schiller and, 2: 369

  Smith-Petersen and, 3: 362
  Swaim and, 4: 58
New England Bone and Joint Institute, 4: 280
New England Deaconess Association, 2: 219–220
New England Deaconess Home and Training School, 4: 273
New England Deaconess Hospital (NEDH), 4: *273, 274, 275*
  admissions and occupancy at, 4: 279
  bed allocation at, 4: 277t
  early history of, 4: 275, 276t
  foot and ankle service, 4: 279
  founding of, 4: 273
  Harvard Fifth Surgical Service and, 4: 279
  Lahey Clinic and, 4: 275–277
  long-range planning at, 4: 278b
  maps of, 4: 276
  medical and surgical (sub) specialties in, 4: 274
  merger with Beth Israel Hospital, 4: 214, 223, 270, 281, 283
  orthopaedics department at, 4: 279–280
  Palmer Memorial Hospital and, 4: 275–276
  Pathway Health Network and, 4: 280
  physician affiliations at, 4: 277, 277t, 278
  relationship with HMS, 4: 277–279
  as a specialized tertiary-care facility, 4: 279
New England Dressings Committee (Red Cross Auxiliary), 4: *10*
New England Female Medical College, 2: 273; 4: 296
New England Home for Little Wanderers, 3: 307
New England Hospital for Women and Children, 2: 274
New England Journal of Medicine, 1: 39
New England Medical Center, 4: 249, *311*
New England Medical Council, 2: 157–158
New England Muscular Dystrophy Association Clinic Directors, 2: 403
New England Organ Bank, 3: 443
New England Orthopedic Society, 3: 319
New England Patriots, 3: 348, 397, 399, 448

New England Peabody Home for Crippled Children, 2: 37, 165, 183, 191, 230–231, 269–270; 3: 174, 202, 209, 329, 362
New England Pediatric Society, 2: 13
New England Regional Committee on Fractures, 4: 341, 347
New England Rehabilitation Center, 1: 272
New England Revolution, 3: 348, 450
New England Society of Bone and Joint Surgery, 4: 347
New England Surgical Society, 1: 90; 2: 136; 3: 63
New York Bellevue Hospital, 2: 111
New York Hospital for the Ruptured and Crippled, 1: 89
New York Orthopaedic Dispensary and Hospital, 2: 20, 47–48
New York Orthopaedic Hospital, 2: 47
Newcomb, Sarah Alvord, 1: 107
Newhall, Harvey F., 3: 266
Newhauser, E. B. D., 2: 215
Newman, Erik T., 3: 463*b*; 4: 190*b*
Newton-Wellesley Hospital (NWH), 1: 225; 2: 279; 3: 240, 331, 334, 426
Nichol, Vern, 3: 248
Nichols, Edward H. (1864–1922), 1: *252*; 4: *302*
   Base Hospital No. 7 and, 1: 256; 4: 301–302, 438–439
   Boston Children's Hospital and, 2: 247, 307
   Boston City Hospital and, 1: 174, 252; 4: 301–302
   death of, 1: 256–257
   as football team surgeon, 1: 252–256
   Harvard baseball team and, 1: 251–252
   HMS appointment, 4: 302
   HMS Laboratory of Surgical Pathology and, 2: 90
   legacy of, 1: 257
   offices of, 4: *302*
   orthopaedic research and, 1: 252
   osteomyelitis research and, 4: 301
   PBBH teaching and, 4: 10, 12
   as professor of surgery, 1: 174
   study of football injuries, 1: 254–256
   Surgery of Joints, The, 2: 52
   tuberculosis treatment, 2: 32
   vascular anastomosis and, 4: 216
   World War I medical unit, 1: 256; 4: 391
Nichols, Emma, 4: 438
Nickel, Vernon, 2: 315; 3: 249, 319, 321
Nightingale, Florence, 2: 5; 4: 274*b*
nitrous oxide, 1: 56–59, 63; 3: 15
Noall, Lawrence, 3: 208
Noble, Nick, 3: 94
non-hinged metal–polyethylene prosthesis, 4: 145–146
Nordby, Eugene J., 3: 255
North Charles General Hospital, 4: 157
North Shore Children's Hospital, 2: 269
Northwestern University, 2: 302
Norton, Margaret, 3: 320
Norton, Paul L. (1903–1986)
   adjustable reamer and, 3: 317
   Children's Hospital/MGH combined program and, 3: 317
   Clinics for Crippled Children and, 2: 230; 3: 317
   death of, 3: 320
   early life, 3: 317
   education and training, 3: 317
   Emerson Hospital and, 3: 317, 319
   HMS appointment, 3: 317
   as honorary orthopaedic surgeon, 3: 398*b*
   legacy of, 3: 320
   marriage and family, 3: 320
   Massachusetts Hospital School and, 3: 319–320; 4: 378
   memberships and, 3: 319
   as MGH surgeon, 3: 70*b*, 192, 317
   New England Orthopedic Society president, 3: 319
   Norton-Brown spinal brace, 3: 317–319
   paraplegia research and, 3: 319
   publications and research, 3: 258–259, 317–320, 455*b*; 4: 95
Norton-Brown spinal brace, 3: 317–319
Norwalk train wreck, 1: 77, *78*
nose reconstructions, 1: 71, 75–76
Notes on Military Orthopaedics (Jones), 4: 442, *442*, 443
Nuffield Orthopaedic Centre (Oxford), 3: 412
Nursery and Child's Hospital (New York), 2: 3, 5
Nursery for Children (New York), 2: 3
nursing
   Cadet Nursing Corps, 4: 467
   Children's Island Sanitorium and, 4: 87
   Deaconess training and, 4: 274*b*
   early training in, 1: 41; 2: 6–8, 13–14
   foot problems, 2: 54–56
   impact of World War II on, 4: 467
   for Jewish women, 4: 208
   Larson and, 3: 302–303
   MGH School of Nursing and, 3: 302, 391
   New England Deaconess Hospital and, 4: 273
   reforms in, 3: 142
nutrition, 2: 361–362
Nydegger, Rogert C., 4: 489

O

Ober, Ernest, 2: 144, 166
Ober, Frank R. (1881–1960), 1: *188*, *195*; 2: *143*, 147, 255
   AAOS and, 4: 337
   as AOA president, 2: 161
   "Back Strains and Sciatica," 2: 151–152
   Barr and, 3: 201
   Base Hospital No. 5 and, 4: 420, *422*
   Bell and, 2: 220
   on biceps-triceps transplant, 2: 154
   Boston Children's Hospital and, 1: 153, 155, 158, 178, 188, 195–196, 198–199; 2: *143*, 144–147, 149, 163, 217, 252, 274, 282; 4: 338, 468
   brachioradialis transfer for triceps weakness, 2: 153–154, *154*
   Brigham and Women's Hospital and, 4: 195*b*
   Children's Hospital/MGH combined program and, 1: 210
   club foot treatment, 2: 145
   death of, 2: 166
   on diagnosis, 2: 155–156
   education and training, 2: 143–144
   expert testimony and, 2: 164–165
   on FitzSimmons, 2: 256, 258
   Georgia Warm Springs Foundation board and, 2: 78, 165
   graduate education in orthopaedic surgery and, 2: 160–162, 162*b*
   graduate education review, 1: 196–197

Green and, 2: 168
Harvard Unit and, 4: 419
HCORP and, 1: 192, 195–199
Hibbs spinal fusion procedure, 2: 164
hip abductor paralysis treatment, 2: 149–150
hip and knee contractures, 2: 153, *153*
HMS appointment, 2: 144, 146–147, 156; 4: 59
honorary degrees, 2: 165
Hugenberger and, 2: 269, 271
iliotibial band tightness and, 2: 151–152
John Ball and Buckminster Brown Professorship, 2: 147, 157; 4: 195*b*
Journal of Bone and Joint Surgery editor, 2: 165
lectures at Tuskegee Institute, 2: 146
Lovett and, 2: 144
Lovett Fund Committee and, 2: 82
Marlborough Medical Associates and, 2: 299
marriage and, 2: 144
Massachusetts Medical Society and, 2: 164
Massachusetts Regional Fracture Committee, 3: 64
medical education, 2: 155
military orthopaedics and, 4: 473
military surgeon training and, 2: 42
modification of use of sacrospinalis, 2: 146–147
Mount Desert Island practice, 2: 143–145
New England Peabody Home for Crippled Children and, 2: 270
as orthopaedic chair, 2: 15*b*
on orthopaedic problems in children, 2: 164
orthopaedics education and, 2: 155–157, 163
on orthopaedics training at Harvard, 1: 195–196
Orthopedic Surgery revisions, 2: 166
on Osgood, 2: 148
on paralysis of the serratus anterior, 2: 154–155
PBBH and, 4: 18
poliomyelitis treatment, 2: 147–148, 154–155
posterior approach to the hip joint approach, 2: 146
postgraduate education and, 2: 157–159, 164
private medical practice and, 1: 176; 2: 146, 313; 3: 454*b*
professional memberships, 2: 165
publications of, 2: 227
RBBH and, 4: 15
rehabilitation planning and, 1: 273
Roosevelt and, 2: 77
surgery techniques, 2: 177
teaching department plan, 1: 157
on tendon transplantation, 2: 108, 147–148, *148*, 149
triple arthrodesis and, 2: 149
use of shelf procedure for CDH, 2: 151
Vermont poliomyelitis rehabilitation program, 2: 149
on wartime medical education, 4: 397
weakness/paralysis of the foot and ankle treatment, 2: 150–151
World War I and, 2: 125–126
"Your Brain is Your Invested Capital" speech, 2: 156, 158*b*–159*b*
Ober, Ina Spurling, 2: 144, 166
Ober, Melita J. Roberts, 2: 143
Ober, Otis Meriam, 2: 143
Ober abduction sign, 2: 151
Ober Research Fund, 2: 436
Ober Test, 2: 151–152
Ober-Yount fasciotomy, 2: 153, 172
Objective Structure Clinical Examination (OSCE), 1: 168
O'Brien, Michael, 4: 287
O'Brien, Paul, 4: 333, 378
obstetrical paralysis
  brachial plexus injuries, 2: 91, *91*
  Lange's theory, 2: 91
  massage and exercise for, 2: 90
  Sever-L'Episcopo procedure, 2: 90, 100
  Sever's study of, 2: 90, *90*, 94–96
  subscapularis tendon, 2: 95, *95*
  tendon transfers and, 2: 96
  treatment of, 2: 89–90, 94–95, *95*, 96
Occupational Disorders of the Upper Extremity (Millender et al.), 4: 168, 183
occupational therapy, 4: 28, *29*, 358–359
O'Connor, Frank, 4: 116*b*
O'Connor, Mary I., 4: 266*b*
O'Connor, Richard, 3: 446
O'Donoghue, Don, 3: 272
O'Donovan, T., 4: 167
Ogden, John, 2: 302
O'Hara, Dwight, 1: 273
Ohio State Medical Association, 3: 58
Ohio State University School of Medicine, 2: 407–408
O'Holleran, James, 4: 190*b*
Okike, Kanu, 2: *381*
Olcott, Christopher W., 4: 180
Oliver, Henry K., 1: 47, 49–50
Oliver Wendell Holmes Society, 4: 264
Ollier, Louis Xavier Edouard Leopold, 1: xxiii
O'Malley, Peter, 4: 264
O'Meara, John W., 2: 230
Omni Med, 3: 379
Oneida Football Club, 1: 247
O'Neil, Edward, Jr., 3: 379
O'Neil, Eugene, 4: 371
O'Neill, Eugene, 2: 272
Ontario Crippled Children's Center, 2: 334–335
opera-glass hand deformity, 4: 99
Operative Arthroscopy (McGinty et al.), 2: 279
Operative Hand Surgery (Green), 4: 98
Operative Nerve Repair and Reconstruction (Gelberman), 3: 404
ophthalmology, 1: 138; 3: 13
optical coherence tomography (OCT), 4: 194
Order of St. John of Jerusalem in England, 4: 401
Orr, Bobby, 3: 357, 357*b*
Orr, H. Winnett, 2: 125; 3: 159, 235, 340; 4: 383, 393, 400, 409
Orthopaedia (Andry), 1: xxi
Orthopaedic Biochemistry and Osteoarthritis Therapy Laboratory, 3: 464*b*
Orthopaedic Biology and Oncology Laboratories, 3: 463, 464*b*
Orthopaedic Biomechanics and Biomaterials Laboratory, 3: 464*b*
Orthopaedic Centers (Great Britain), 2: 127, 127*b*
Orthopaedic Fellow Education Fund, 2: 439*b*
Orthopaedic In-Service Training Exam (OITE), 1: 231
Orthopaedic Journal at Harvard Medical School, The, 1: 231–232
Orthopaedic Journal Club, 3: 369
orthopaedic oncology
  allografts and, 3: 389
  bone sarcomas and, 3: 136–137, 137*t*, 138–140, 140*b*, 141–142

Index

chondrosarcoma of bone, 3: 406
data digitization and, 3: 392–393
flow cytometry and, 3: 388
giant-cell tumors and, 3: 390
limb salvage surgery and, 3: 390–391
Mankin and, 3: 386, 388
osteosarcoma and, 2: 422; 3: 391
sacrococcygeal chordoma, 3: 390
Orthopaedic Research and Education Foundation, 2: 241; 3: 213, 215, 360
Orthopaedic Research Laboratories (MGH), 2: 321–324; 3: 211–212
Orthopaedic Research Society, 2: 240, 316, 327; 3: 262
orthopaedic surgeons
    advancement of the field, 2: 26, 50, 81, 99
    assistive technology and, 2: 408
    blue blazers and, 3: 30
    board certification of, 4: 324, 377
    diagnostic skills, 2: 155–156
    education and training, 2: 133–135
    evaluation and treatment, 2: 48
    extremity injuries and, 2: 122
    fracture care and, 4: 463–464
    general surgery foundations and, 2: 24
    graduate education and, 1: 197–199
    on hip disease, 2: 52
    interest in visceroptosis, 3: 83–84, 84*b*, 86–88
    logical thinking and, 2: 155
    military and, 2: 42, 65–68, 118–120
    minimum requirements for, 2: 134
    observational skills, 2: 155
    orthopaedic physician versus, 4: 47*b*
    recruitment of, 2: 39–40
    scientific study and, 2: 32
    as surgeon-scholars, 2: 217, 357; 3: 228, 395; 4: 43, 79, 143, 163, 193–194, 195*b*
    transformation of profession, 2: 130*b*–131*b*
    volunteer wartime, 2: 124–127
    war injuries and, 2: 124
    x-rays and, 2: 56
orthopaedic surgery
    advances in, 2: 14–15, 20, 25–28
    approved teaching hospitals, 1: 198
    Boylston Medical School and, 1: 138
    certification in, 1: 189, 196–198, 200, 231
    characteristics of, 2: 132
    computer-simulated planning, 2: 389
    conditions for, 4: 451
    development of, 2: 78
    early 20th century, 2: 36
    early training in, 1: 186–189
    founding of, 1: xxiii; 2: 26–27
    growth-sparing, 2: 360–361
    Harvard athletics and, 1: 284
    knee joint resections, 1: 81
    in London, 1: 106
    minimal requirements for specialization, 1: 191–192
    naming of, 1: xxiv
    orthopaedics curriculum and, 1: 141, 143, 147, 158, 162
    outcomes of, 2: 372
    personalities in early, 2: 99
    public reporting of, 1: 102
    rehabilitation and, 2: 172
    residencies, 1: 186–187, 198–199; 2: 160–161
    seminal text on, 2: 29–30, 50
    tracing of deformities, 2: *53*
    traction treatment for, 2: 21–23, 25, 27
    training in, 1: 101
    transformation of, 2: 130*b*–131*b*
    trauma and, 3: 275; 4: 393
    in the United States, 1: 100–101, 107; 2: 23; 4: 393
    use of traction, 2: 27
    women in, 1: 200, 239
    World War I and, 2: 119–126
    World War II and, 4: 463–464, 473, 485, 493
Orthopaedic Surgery at Tufts University (Banks), 4: 77
Orthopaedic Surgery in Infancy and Childhood (Ferguson), 2: 188, 303
"Orthopaedic Surgery in the United States of America" (Mayer), 1: 114
Orthopaedic Surgical Advancement Fund, 2: 439*b*
Orthopaedic Trauma Association Visiting Scholars Program, 3: 418
orthopaedic wards
    Boston Children's Hospital and, 1: 205
    Boston City Hospital and, 2: 24
    House of the Good Samaritan, 1: 123, 125–130; 2: 25
    Massachusetts General Hospital and, 1: 193, 203, 273; 2: 116, 322; 3: 62, 68, 272, 304, 343
"Orthopaedic Work in a War Hospital" (Osgood), 2: 120
orthopaedics
    18th century history of, 1: xxi, xxii
    19th century history of, 1: xxii, xxiii, xxiv
    20th century specialty of, 1: 189–192
    advances in, 4: 466–467
    diversity initiatives in, 4: 264–265
    established as separate specialty, 1: 83, 95–96, 98–99, 119
    first case at MGH, 1: 42, 44
    impact of World War I on, 4: 453–454, 463–464
    impact of World War II on, 4: 473, 493
    malpractice suits and, 1: 50
    mechanical devices and, 1: 107–108, *108*
    opening of first specialty hospital, 1: 99
    radiology and, 2: 16–17
    rehabilitation and, 4: 454
    respect for field, 4: 453, 463–464
    scientific study of, 2: 51
    specialization in, 1: 187, 193; 4: 300–301
    as specialty course at HMS, 1: 141–143
    spelling of, 1: xxiv, xxv, *177*
    standards of practice and, 4: 463–464
Orthopaedics (MacAusland and Mayo), 3: 310
orthopaedics apparatus
    Abbott Frame, 4: 232, *232*
    Adam's machine, 2: 86
    adjustable reamer, 3: 317
    Austin Moore prosthesis, 3: 213
    Balkan Frame, 3: 317, 357*b*
    basket plasters, 2: *122*
    Boston Arm, 2: 326, *326*; 3: 287
    Boston brace, 2: 339–340, 358–359, *360*, *361*, 423
    brace shop, 2: *22*
    braces, 3: 318–319
    Bradford Frame, 2: 27, *27*, 30–31, *31*, 32
    Bradford's method of reducing the gibbus, 3: *149*
    Buckminster Brown and, 1: 105–107

celastic body jackets, 2: 178
celluloid jackets, 2: *85*
charitable surgical appliances, 2: *14*
clover leaf rod, 3: 272
club foot device, 1: 98, 100, 106; 2: 23, *23*, 24
De Machinamentis of Oribasius, 3: *149*
Denis Browne splint, 2: 208
fluoroscope, 2: 307
foot strength tester, 2: 101–102
fracture table, 2: *121*
Goldthwait irons, 3: 89, *89*, *149*
Harrington rods, 2: 316, *317*, 325, 335
hyperextension cast, 3: *69*
inclinometers, 2: 366, *367*
interpedicular segmental fixation (ISF) pedicle screw plate, 3: 420
iron extension hinge, 2: *123*
iron lung, 2: 78, *79*, *190*, 191, 260, 264, 314
ISOLA implants, 2: *370*
Jewett nail-plate, 3: 320
knee flexion contracture appliance, 2: *20*
Küntscher femoral rod, 3: 272
Lovett Board, 2: *59*, 86
MacIntosh prothesis, 4: 69, *71b*
McKeever prothesis, 4: 40, 69, *70b*–*71b*
McLaughlin side plate, 3: 320
metal implants, 2: 237–238
Milwaukee Brace, 2: 265–266, 336
Norton-Brown spinal brace, 3: 317–319
pedicle screws, 2: 343; 3: 420
pelvic machine design, 2: 86
Pierce Collar, 3: 321
Pierce Fusion, 3: 321
Pierce Graft, 3: 321
plaster casts, 2: *122*–*123*
portable traction device, 2: 297
pressure correction apparatus (Hoffa-Schede), 3: *151*, *152*
Relton-Hall frame, 2: 334–335, *335*
Risser cast, 2: 178
rocking beds, 2: 314, *315*
Sayre jacket, 1: 107
for scoliosis, 2: 35, *35*, 36, *36*, 296
scoliosis jackets, 2: 59–61, 85–87
scoliosometer, 2: 36
Smith-Petersen Vitallium mold, 3: *195*, *196*
for spinal deformities, 1: 107; 2: *31*
splints, 3: 167, *167*, 168
spring muscle test, 2: *70*
Steinmann pin, 2: 237–238
surgical scissors, 3: *138*
Taylor back brace, 2: 247
Thomas splint, 2: *123*, *247*; 3: *168*
triflanged nail, 3: 62, 185–186, *186*, 187, 189, 189b, 190, 320
turnbuckle jacket, 2: 80, 223–224, *224*, 225, *225*, 226–227, 316, *336*; 3: 209
VEPTR (Vertical Expandable Prosthetic Titanium Rib), 2: 360, 362
wire arm splints, 2: *122*
wire drop foot splints, 2: *123*
World War I and, 2: 124
Zander chair, 3: *153*
Zander tilt table, 3: *152*
Zander's medico-mechanical equipment, 3: *69*, *71*, 264, *264*, 265, *265*, 266–267, *267*, 268b
"Orthopaedics at Harvard" (Brown), 1: 195
orthopaedics curriculum
  Allison on, 2: 134; 3: 171–173
  anatomy lectures in, 1: 134, 136
  cadaver dissection, 1: *142*
  case method and, 4: 299
  case-based discussions, 1: 167
  competency examinations, 1: 168
  development of, 1: 140–141
  early medical instruction, 1: 134, 136–138
  electives in, 1: 143, 144t, 148–151, 164–166
  evolution of, 1: 143, 147, 148b–151b, 152–170
  examination questions, 1: 140–141, 144b
  fractures in, 1: 154
  graduate training, 2: 187b
  Jack Warren and, 1: 40, 134
  John Collins Warren and, 1: 40, 136–137
  Massachusetts General Hospital (MGH) and, 1: 136–137
  medical education and, 2: 183–184, 184b, 185, 185b, 186
  military orthopaedic surgery course, 4: 455–462
  musculoskeletal medicine in, 1: 168–170; 2: 184–186
  ophthalmology and, 1: 138
  orthopaedic clerkship in, 1: 167–169
  orthopaedic surgery in, 1: 141, 143, 147, 158, 162
  recommendations for, 1: 162–163
  reform of, 1: 140
  required courses, 1: 143
  sample curriculum for, 1: 159–161
  sports medicine elective, 1: 165–166
  surgical pedagogy, 1: 137–138
  teaching clinics, 1: 155–157, 163, 170, 194
  teaching modalities, 3: 172
  for third- and fourth-year students, 1: 144t–146t
  undergraduate, 2: 183–186, 202
Orthopaedics Overseas, 3: 310
orthopaedics residencies. *See also* Harvard Combined Orthopaedic Residency Program (HCORP)
  ABOS board and, 4: 377–379
  AOA survey on, 2: 160–161
  approved hospitals for, 1: 196–200
  BCH and, 2: *413*; 4: 377–379
  BCH Bone and Joint Service, 4: 377
  Carney Hospital and, 4: 378
  certification examinations and, 1: 198, 231
  core competencies in, 1: 238–239
  examinations for, 1: 210, 231
  grand rounds, 1: 189, 203, *203*, 204, *204*, 205, 218, 232
  history of, 1: 183–186
  hospital internships and, 1: 186–188
  internal review of, 1: 239
  Lahey Clinic and, 4: 378
  Lakeville State Hospital and, 4: 378
  Massachusetts General/Boston Children's Hospital residency program, 1: 210; 2: 144
  MGH and, 2: *249*, *276*, *278*, *290*, *320*, *327*
  minimum surgical case requirements for, 3: 435–436, *436*
  pediatric, 1: 210–211
  program length and, 1: 215–216, 218–220, 222–223
  restructuring at MGH, 1: 198–199
  RRC for, 1: 211–213, 215, 217–220, 224, 232–233, 241–242

Index

West Roxbury Veterans Administration Hospital and, 4: 378–379
Orthopaedics Today, 2: 281
Orthopedic Nursing (Funsten and Calderwood), 3: 303
Orthopedic Surgery (Bradford and Lovett), 4: 318
Orthopedic Surgery (Jones and Lovett), 2: 69, *69*, 166
Orthopedic Treatment of Gunshot Injuries, The (Mayer), 3: 156*b*
L'Orthopédie (Andry), 3: 90
orthoroentgenograms, 2: 171
os calcis fractures, 4: 313, 314*b*, 335–336
Osgood, John Christopher, 2: 113
Osgood, Margaret Louisa, 2: 138
Osgood, Martha E. Whipple, 2: 113
Osgood, Robert B. (1873–1956), 1: *193*, *194*; 2: 113, *118*, 125, 140, 222, 255; 4: *404*, *417*
    adult orthopaedics and, 2: 157
    on AEF medical care organization, 4: 417
    AEF splint board, 4: 416
    American Ambulance Hospital and, 2: 117–123; 4: 386, 389*b*, 390, 392–393
    on Andry's *Orthopaedia*, 1: xxii
    AOA preparedness committee, 4: 394
    on arthritis and rheumatic disease, 4: 58
    back pain research and, 3: 203
    Base Hospital No. 5 and, 4: 420, 421*b*, 422, 422*b*, *422*
    Beth Israel Hospital and, 4: 208*b*, 247
    Boston Children's Hospital and, 1: 192; 2: 16, 40–41, 114, 132–133, 140, 247, 274, 282; 3: 99
    Brigham and Women's Hospital and, 4: 195*b*
    British Expeditionary Forces and, 4: 420
    Burrage Hospital and, 4: 226
    Carney Hospital and, 2: 116
    as chief at MGH, 1: 151, 192
    chronic disease treatment and, 4: 52
    as clinical professor, 1: 158
    curative workshops and, 4: 403–404
    death of, 2: 140
    Department for Military Orthopedics and, 4: 405
    Diseases of the Bones and Joints, 2: 117; 3: 81–82
    education and training, 2: 113–114
    on Edward H. Bradford, 2: 44
    elegance and, 2: 138–140
    end-results clinics and, 1: 194
    European medical studies, 2: 116
    faculty salary, 1: 177, 179
    on FitzSimmons, 2: 258–259
    on foot problems, 2: 56, 123–124
    foot strength apparatus and, 2: 101–102
    Fundamentals of Orthopaedic Surgery in General Medicine and Surgery, 2: 135–136
    George W. Gay Lecture, 4: 324
    Georgia Warm Springs Foundation and, 2: 78
    hand-washing policy, 1: 193
    Harvard Unit and, 2: 119–121, 123–124; 3: *180*, 369, *370*; 4: 386–387, 421*b*
    HCORP and, 1: 192–195
    as head of HMS orthopaedic surgery department, 1: 174–175, 177, 192
    HMS appointment, 2: 116, 133–135
    honorary degrees, 2: 137
    House of the Good Samaritan and, 2: 113–114
    identification of Osgood-Schlatter disease, 2: 115, *116*, 117
    John Ball and Buckminster Brown Professorship, 2: 133; 4: 195*b*
    Journal of Bone and Joint Surgery editor, 2: 130
    Katzeff and, 2: 275
    King Manuel II and, 4: 401
    on Legg-Calve-Perthes disease, 2: 105
    Lovett Fund and, 2: 82
    marriage and family, 2: 138
    MGH and, 2: 116–117, 129–134; 3: 67
    MGH crystal laboratory, 2: 322
    MGH Fracture Clinic and, 3: 313; 4: 464
    as MGH orthopaedics chief, 3: 11*b*, 227, 266, 268; 4: 472*b*
    MGH surgical intern, 1: 189
    military orthopaedics and, 2: 124–128; 4: 403, 406–407, 412, 417–419, 423*b*, 453
    on mobilization of stiffened joints, 4: 27*b*
    "Nation and the Hospital, The," 2: 137–138, 138*b*–139*b*
    New England Surgical Society president, 2: 136
    Ober on, 2: 148
    as orthopaedic chair, 2: 15*b*
    orthopaedic research support, 1: 193, 195
    orthopaedic surgery and, 1: xxiii; 2: 79, 106, 116–117, 132, 140
    "Orthopaedic Work in a War Hospital," 2: 120
    orthopaedics education and, 1: 152; 2: 133–136
    Orthopedics and Body Mechanics Committee, 4: 235
    poetry of, 2: 128–129, 129*b*, 140
    poliomyelitis treatment, 2: 77, 264
    on preventative measures, 2: 122–123
    private medical practice and, 1: 176; 3: 338
    professional memberships, 2: 136–137
    as professor of orthopaedic surgery, 1: 172
    "Progress in Orthopaedic Surgery" series, 2: 43, 297
    publications and research, 2: 135–137; 4: 32, 65, 421*b*
    as radiologist, 2: 114–115
    RBBH and, 4: 25–26, 28, 31, 56
    on rehabilitation of wounded soldiers, 4: 451
    roentgenograms and, 2: 54, 116
    on sacroiliac joint fusion, 3: 184–185
    scoliosis treatment, 2: 87
    on synovial fluid diagnosis, 3: 175
    on transformation of orthopaedic surgeons, 2: 130*b*–131*b*, *132*
    treatment of fractures, 3: 61
    US Army Medical Corps and, 3: 61
    on visceroptosis, 3: 87–88
    war injury studies and, 2: 128–129
    World War I and, 2: 65, 117–128; 3: 157, 166; 4: 403, 406–407, 412, 417, 421*b*
    World War II volunteers and, 4: 363
Osgood Visiting Professors, 2: 141*b*
Osgood-Schlatter disease, 2: 89, 115, *116*, 117
Osler, Sir William, 1: 1, 185, 275; 3: 2; 4: vii, 6
osteoarthritis

articular cartilage structure research, 3: 383–384, *385*
bilateral, 3: 244, 279
biomechanical factors in, 3: 322, 326–328, 383
etiology of, 3: 327
femoral neck fractures and, 3: 383–384
hip surgery and, 3: 155
histologic-histochemical grading systems, 3: 384, 384*t*, 385
knee arthroplasty and, 4: 70*b*–71*b*
Mankin System and, 3: 384, 384*t*
mold arthroplasty and, 3: 195–196
nylon arthroplasty in, 4: 65
periacetabular osteotomy and, 2: 389
total hip replacement and, 3: 221, *222*
total knee replacement and, 4: 177
Osteoarthritis Cartilage Histopathology Assessment System (OARSI), 3: 384–385
osteoarthrosis, 3: 328
osteochondritis, 3: 363
osteochondritis deformans juvenilis, 2: 103–104. *See also* Legg-Calvé-Perthes disease
osteochondritis dissecans, 2: 194–195
osteogenic sarcoma, 4: 102
osteolysis
after total hip replacement, 3: 220, *220*, 221–222, *222*, 223, 225
associated with acetabular replacement, 3: 279
rapid postoperative in Paget Disease, 3: 441
osteomalacia, 3: 388
osteomyelitis
in children, 2: 169
following intramedullary nailing of femoral shaft fractures, 2: 249
Green and, 2: 169–170
in infants, 2: 169–170
of the metatarsals and phalanges, 1: 120
orthopaedic research and, 1: 193, 252, 256
pyogenic spinal, 3: 254
radical removal of diseased bone and, 1: 252
septic wounds in, 3: 301
Staphylococcus and, 2: 169

Streptococcus and, 2: 169
treatment of, 2: 169–170
osteonecrosis
acetabular, 2: 392–394
of the femoral head, 2: 328–329; 3: 434; 4: 156–157
osteoarticular allografts and, 3: 433
pinning of the contralateral hip and, 2: 380
osteosarcoma
adjuvant therapy and, 3: 432
allografts and, 3: 433
amputations and, 3: 136, 391, 432
chemotherapy and, 2: 422
hip disarticulation for, 1: 78
limb salvage surgery and, 3: 391, 432–433
of the proximal humerus, 2: 398
wide surgical margin and, 3: 433
osteotomies
Bernese periacetabular, 2: 391–392
Boston Concept, 2: 391–392
Chiari, 2: 345
club foot and, 2: 28–29, 36
Cotton, 4: 329
derotation, 2: 34
derotational humeral, 2: 419
femoral derotation for anteversion, 2: 33–34
hips and, 4: 171
innominate, 2: 345
for knee flexion contractures, 2: 117
knee stabilization and, 1: 279
kyphosis and, 3: 239–240
La Coeur's triple, 2: 390
lateral epicondyle, 3: 441
leg lengthening and, 2: 110
Meisenbach's procedure, 4: 188
metatarsal, 4: 188
paralytic flat foot deformities, 2: 210
periacetabular, 2: 389–394
Salter innominate, 2: 390–391
scoliosis treatment, 2: 342
subtrochanteric femur, 1: 68
subtrochanteric hip, 2: 293
total hip replacement and, 3: 221
trochanteric, 4: 133, 145
Van Nes rotational, 2: 345
VCR procedure, 2: 362
Wagner spherical, 2: 390–392
Osterman, A. Lee, 3: 431
Otis, James, 1: 13, 15
Ottemo, Anita, 4: 266
Otto Aufranc Award, 3: 224

Outline of Practical Anatomy, An (John Warren), 1: 88
Oxland, Thomas R., 4: 266*b*
Ozuna, Richard, 1: 230; 4: 193, 195*b*

P

Pace, James, 2: 379
Paget, James, 1: 81; 2: 172, 194; 3: 25
Paget Disease, 3: 441
Paine, R. S., 2: 172
Painter, Charles F. (1869–1947), 4: *44*
as AOA president, 2: 64; 4: 46–47
back pain research and, 3: 203
Beth Israel Hospital and, 4: 208*b*
bone and joint disorders, 3: 82
on Brackett, 3: 150, 161
Burrage Hospital and, 4: 226
Carney Hospital and, 2: 102; 4: 44–45
clinical congress meeting, 3: 116
death of, 4: 51
Diseases of the Bones and Joints, 2: 117; 3: 81; 4: 45
education and training, 4: 44
HMS appointment, 4: 44
hospital appointments, 4: 48
internal derangement of knee-joints case, 4: 48
Journal of Bone and Joint Surgery editor, 3: 161, 344; 4: 50
Massage, 3: 266
on medical education, 4: 49, 49*b*, *49*, 50
MGH and, 4: 45
on orthopaedic surgeon versus physician, 4: 47*b*
on physical therapy, 3: 266*b*
private medical practice, 2: 116
professional memberships, 4: 50*b*, 51
publications and research, 4: 44–46, 48, 50
RBBH and, 4: 25–26, 28, 31, 39*b*, 45, 56, 79, 406
as RBBH chief of orthopaedics, 4: 45–48, 79, 196*b*
rehabilitation of soldiers and, 4: 444
sacroiliac joint treatment, 3: 183
Tufts Medical School appointment, 4: 44–45, 48
World War I and, 4: 47
Paley multiplier method, 2: 194
Palmer Memorial Hospital, 2: 219, *219*, 220; 4: 275, *275*, 276

Index

Panagakos, Panos G., 4: 22, 116, 128, 193
Pancoast, Joseph, 1: 79
Panjabi, Manohar M., 4: 260–262
Papin, Edouard, 3: 233–234
Pappano, Laura, 1: 285
Pappas, Alex, 2: 285
Pappas, Arthur M. (1931–2016), 2: *286*, *288*
   athletic injury clinic and, 2: 287
   "Biomechanics of Baseball Pitching," 2: *288*
   Boston Children's Hospital and, 2: 277, 285–287
   Boston Red Sox and, 2: 288
   Brigham and Women's Hospital and, 4: 193
   on combined residency program, 1: 192, 210
   community organizations and, 2: 289
   Crippled Children's Clinic and, 2: 287
   death of, 2: 289
   education and training, 2: 285
   famous patients of, 2: 288
   as interim orthopaedic surgeon-in-chief, 2: 285–286
   MGH/Children's Hospital residency, 2: 285
   military service, 2: 285
   as orthopaedic chair, 2: 15*b*, 371
   Pappas Rehabilitation Hospital, 2: 39
   PBBH and, 2: 285; 4: 22, 116, 128
   private medical practice and, 2: 313
   professional leadership positions, 2: 289, 289*b*
   publications of, 2: 285, *287*, 288, 368
   on residency program, 1: 208
   sports medicine and, 2: 287–288
   on sports medicine clinic, 2: 384
   University of Massachusetts and, 2: 286–288, 371
   Upper Extremity Injuries in the Athlete, 2: 288
Pappas, Athena, 2: 285
Pappas, Martha, 2: 289
Pappas Rehabilitation Hospital, 2: 39
paralysis. *See also* obstetrical paralysis; poliomyelitis
   brachial plexus, 2: 96
   Bradford frame and, 2: 30
   of the deltoid muscle, 2: 148, 230
   exercise treatment for, 3: 265
   foot and ankle treatment, 2: 150–151
   of the gluteus maximus, 2: 146
   hip abductor treatment, 2: 149–150
   nerve lesions and, 2: 120
   Pott's Disease and, 3: 148–149
   radial nerve, 3: 64
   Roosevelt and, 2: 71–78
   spinal cord injury, 3: 347
   spinal tuberculosis and, 2: 309
   treatment of spastic, 2: 36, 172, 196
Paraplegia Hospital (Ahmadabad, India), 3: 423
Paré, Ambrose, 1: 55; 3: 48
Parfouru-Porel, Germaine, 3: 369–370
Park Prewett Hospital, 4: 363
Parker, Isaac, 1: 45–46
Parker Hill, 4: 23*b*, *24*, 35
Parker Hill Hospital, 2: 358; 4: 327, *328*
Parkman, Francis, 1: 298, 307
Parkman, George (1790–1849), 1: *292*
   care of the mentally ill, 1: 293–295
   dental cast, 1: *308*
   disappearance of, 1: 298, 303–304
   education and training, 1: 292–293
   Harvard Medical School and, 1: 296
   home of, 1: *313*
   on John Collins Warren, 1: 296
   John Webster and, 1: 302–303
   money-lending and, 1: 297, 302–303
   murder of, 1: 291, 304–312, 315, *315*, 318; 3: 40
   philanthropy and, 1: 295–297
   remains found, 1: 304, *305*, 306, *306*, 307–308
Parkman, George F., 1: *313*, 314
Parkman, Samuel (businessman), 1: 292
Parkman, Samuel (surgeon), 1: 60, 62; 3: 15
Parkman Bandstand, 1: *313*, 314
Parks, Helen, 4: 389*b*
Parran, Thomas, Jr., 4: 467
Parsons, Langdon, 3: 301
Partners Department of Orthopaedic Surgery, 1: 181
Partners Healthcare, 3: 462; 4: 192–194
Partners Orthopaedics, 4: 284
Partridge, Oliver, 1: 13

Pasteur, Louis, 1: 82
Patel, Dinesh G. (1936–), 3: *421*, *424*, *461*
   arthroscopic surgery and, 3: 422–423, 448
   Center of Healing Arts and, 3: 423
   Children's Hospital/MGH combined program and, 3: 422
   discoid medial meniscus tear case, 3: 422
   early life, 3: 421
   education and training, 3: 422
   HCORP and, 1: 230; 3: 423
   HMS appointment, 3: 422, 424
   honors and awards, 3: 424
   hospital appointments, 3: 422
   Massachusetts Board of Registration in Medicine and, 3: 423
   as MGH clinical faculty, 3: 464*b*
   as MGH surgeon, 3: 398*b*, 423
   Patient Care Assessment (PCA) Committee, 3: 423
   professional memberships and, 3: 422–423
   publications and research, 3: 424
   sports medicine and, 3: 388*t*, 396, 422, 448, 460*b*
Patel, Shaun, 4: 190*b*
patella. *See* knees
Pathophysiology of Orthopaedic Diseases (Mankin), 4: 226
Pathway Health Network, 4: 280
Patient Care Assessment (PCA) Committee, 3: 423
patient-reported outcomes (PRO), 4: 186
Patton, George S., 4: 478
pauciarticular arthritis, 2: 171, 350
Paul, Igor, 2: 407; 3: 326–328
Pauli, C., 3: 384
Payson, George, 3: 237
PBBH. *See* Peter Bent Brigham Hospital (PBBH)
Peabody, Francis, 2: 72; 3: 244; 4: 297
Peale, Rembrandt, 1: *23*
Pearson, Ruth Elizabeth, 1: 276
Pediatric Orthopaedic International Seminars program, 2: 304
Pediatric Orthopaedic Society (POS), 2: 304, 351
Pediatric Orthopaedic Study Group (POSG), 2: 351, 425
pediatric orthopaedics. *See also* Boston Children's Hospital (BCH)
   ACL reconstruction and, 2: 385–386
   Bradford Frame and, 2: 30

children's convalescence and, 2: 9
children's hospitals and, 2: 3–9
congenital dislocated hips (CDH) and, 2: 34
congenital kyphosis and, 2: 366
"Dark Ages" of, 2: 15
early medical literature on, 2: 7
flat feet treatment, 2: 107–108
Goldthwait and, 2: 101
Green and, 2: 168
hip disease and, 2: 108
Hresko and, 2: 365
infant and neonatal mortality, 2: 15
Karlin and, 2: 370
leg lengthening and, 2: 110
Legg and, 2: 101, 106–107
managing fractures, 2: 379
polio treatment, 2: 109–110
societies for, 2: 351
sports injuries and, 2: 287, 385–387
Tachdjian and, 2: 300–304
trauma and, 2: 365, 368, 385
tuberculosis of the spine and, 2: 11
valgus deformity treatment, 2: 209
Pediatric Orthopedic Deformities (Shapiro), 2: 403, *404*
Pediatric Orthopedic Society of North America (POSNA), 2: *346, 347,* 351, *351,* 363, *363,* 364, 403, 425
Pediatric Orthopedics (Tachdjian), 2: 188, 303, *303*
pedicle screws, 2: 343; 3: 420
Pedlow, Francis X, Jr. (1959–), 3: *424*
  anterior vertebral reconstruction with allograft research, 3: 426, *426*
  early life, 3: 424–425
  education and training, 3: 425
  HCORP and, 3: 426
  HMS appointment, 3: 426
  as MGH clinical faculty, 3: 464*b*
  as MGH surgeon, 3: 426
  open anterior lumbosacral fracture dislocation case, 3: 425
  professional memberships and, 3: 426
  publications and research, 3: 426
  spinal surgeries and, 3: 425–426, 460*b*
Pedlow, Francis X, Sr., 3: 424
Pedlow, Marie T. Baranello, 3: 424
Pedrick, Katherine F., 3: 154

Peking Union Medical College, 3: 365
Pellicci, Paul, 4: 134–135
Peltier, L. F., 1: 106
Pemperton, Ralph, 4: 32
Peninsular Base Station (PBS), 4: 481–482
Pennsylvania Hospital, 1: 183
periacetabular osteotomy, 2: 389–391
Perkins, Leroy, 2: 159–160
Perkins Institution and the Massachusetts School for the Blind, 1: 273
Perlmutter, Gary S., 1: 166–167; 3: 415, 460*b*, 464*b*
Perry, Jacqueline, 3: 248
Pershing, John J., 3: 168
Person, Eleanor, 3: 281
Perthes, George, 2: 103, 105; 3: 165
Perthes disease. *See* Legg-Calvé-Perthes disease
Peter Bent Brigham Hospital Corporation, 4: 2–3
Peter Bent Brigham Hospital (PBBH), 4: *2, 7, 8, 9, 11, 15, 117*
  Administrative Building, 4: *115, 191*
  advancement of medicine and, 4: 5
  affiliation with RBBH, 4: 34, 36, 39
  annual reports, 4: 6, 16, 18
  Banks on, 4: 73*b*–74*b*
  Base Hospital No. 5 and, 4: 420*t*
  blood bank, 4: 107
  board of overseers, 4: 132
  bone and joint cases, 4: *16*
  Boston Children's Hospital and, 4: 10, 14
  Brigham Anesthesia Associates, 4: 22
  cerebral palsy cases, 2: 172
  Clinical Research Center floor plan, 4: *21*
  construction of, 4: 4, *4,* 5
  faculty group practice, 4: 13, 21–22
  faculty model at, 1: 176
  50th anniversary, 4: 20–21, 21*b*
  founding of, 2: 42; 4: 2–3
  fracture treatment and, 4: 18–19, 22, 108
  Francis Street Lobby, 4: *119*
  general surgery service at, 4: 8–10, 14, 16
  grand rounds and, 4: 118
  growth of, 4: 20, 22
  history of, 4: 1

  HMS and, 4: 1–4, 12, *12,* 13–14
  Industrial Accident Clinic, 4: 21–22
  industrial accidents and, 4: 19, 21
  internships at, 1: 189, 196
  leadership of, 4: 4–5, 9–11, 14–19, 22, 99, 127
  opening of, 4: *6*
  orthopaedic service chiefs at, 4: 43
  orthopaedic surgeons at, 4: 116–117
  orthopaedic surgery at, 1: 171; 4: 8, 11, 16–18, 22, 115–116
  orthopaedics as specialty at, 4: 1, 18
  orthopaedics diagnoses at, 4: 6–8
  orthopaedics residencies, 1: 199, 204, 207; 4: 19
  outpatient services at, 1: 173; 4: 5–6, 14, 20, 22
  patient volume at, 4: 124*t,* 129
  Pavilion C (Ward I), 4: *8*
  Pavilion F, 4: *7*
  Pavilion Wards, 4: *115*
  plans for, 4: *7*
  professors of surgery at, 1: 174
  report of bone diseases, 4: 13, 13*t*
  research program at, 4: 75*b*
  Spanish Flu at, 4: *11*
  staffing of, 4: 5, 9, 18–19, 21–22, 128–129, 161–163
  surgeon-scholars at, 4: 43, 79
  surgery specialization at, 4: 10–12, 15–16, 18–20
  surgical research laboratory, 4: 12, *12*
  surgical residencies, 1: 90
  teaching clinics at, 1: 155, 157–158, 194; 4: 14
  transition to Brigham and Women's Hospital, 4: 42, 69, 113–114, 116, 116*b,* 117–119, 121, 127, 132
  trust for, 4: 1, 3
  World War I and, 4: 9–10, 79
  World War II and, 4: 17–18
  Zander Room at, 4: 14
Peter Bent Brigham Hospital Surgical Associates, 4: 21–22
Peters, Jessica, 3: 328
Petersdorf, Robert G., 4: 121
Peterson, L., 3: 210
Petit Lycée de Talence, 4: *429, 430, 432*
Pfahler, George E., 3: 142
Pharmacopoeia of the United States, 1: 300
Phelps, A. M., 2: 99
Phelps, Abel, 4: 463
Phelps, Winthrop M., 1: 193; 2: 294

Index

Phemister, D. B., 2: 170–171, *192*
Phillips, William, 1: 41; 3: 5, 75
Phillips House (MGH), 1: 86, 204; 3: 72, *73*, 75
phocomelia, 2: 334
Phoenix Mutual Insurance Company, 2: 267
phrenicectomy, 4: 215
physical therapy
    athletic training and, 1: 258, 266; 3: 348
    DeLorme table and, 3: 284
    early 20th century status of, 3: 266, 266*b*
    Elgin table, 3: 284, *287*
    knee flexion contracture and, 3: 375
    Legg and, 2: 107
    massage and, 1: 100; 3: 266, 297
    medical schools and, 4: 396–397
    for paralyzed children, 2: 61, 107
    RBBH patient in, 4: *28*, *29*
    rehabilitation equipment for, 2: 107
    Roosevelt and, 2: 74
    sports medicine and, 2: 287
    tenotomy and, 1: 100
    Zander's medico-mechanical equipment, 3: 71, *71*
Physical Therapy in Infantile Paralysis (Legg and Merrill), 2: 107
physicians
    bleeding and, 1: 9
    board certification of, 4: 324, 377
    18th century demand for, 1: 7–8
    examinations for, 1: 15, 21, 29
    Jewish, 1: 158; 4: 199–200, 202
    licensing of, 1: 184, 190
    medical degrees and, 1: 6–7, 26–28
    standards for, 1: 26
    surgical training and, 1: 184
Physicians' Art Society of Boston, 4: 329–330
Pierce, Donald S. (1930–), 3: *461*
    Amputees and Their Prostheses, 3: 320
    Cervical Spine Research Society president, 3: 321
    early life, 3: 320
    education and training, 3: 320
    electromyogram use, 3: 320
    familial bilateral carpal tunnel syndrome case, 3: 321
    Halo Vest, 3: 321
    HMS appointment, 3: 320
    marriage and, 3: 321
    as MGH clinical faculty, 3: 464*b*
    as MGH surgeon, 3: 248, 320, 398*b*
    orthopaedics treatment tools and, 3: 321
    on pressure sores management, 3: 321
    publications and research, 3: 320–321, 355
    rehabilitation and, 3: 388*t*, 459, 461
    spine surgery and, 3: 460*b*
    Total Care of Spinal Cord Injuries, The, 3: 321
Pierce, F. Richard, 1: 264
Pierce, Janet, 3: 321
Pierce, R. Wendell, 1: 284; 3: 299
Pierce, Wallace L., 4: 39*b*
Pierce Collar, 3: 321
Pierce Fusion, 3: 321
Pierce Graft, 3: 321
Pierson, Abel Lawrence, 1: 60, 62
Pilcher, Lewis S., 4: 318
Pinel, Philippe, 1: 293–294
Pinkney, Carole, 3: 382
Pio Istituto Rachitici, 2: 36
Pittsburgh Orthopaedic Journal, 1: 232
plantar fasciitis, 3: 437–438
plantar fasciotomy, 2: 24
Plaster-of-Paris Technique in the Treatment of Fractures (Quigley), 1: 277
plastic surgery
    development of, 1: 76
    introduction to the U.S., 1: 71–72, 77
    orthopaedics curriculum and, 1: 150, 218
Plath, Sylvia, 2: 272
Platt, Sir Harry, 1: 114; 3: 369; 4: 464
Ploetz, J. E., 3: 440
pneumonia, 1: 74; 2: 4, 306
Poehling, Gary G., 2: 279
Polavarapu, H. V., 1: 186
poliomyelitis
    Berlin epidemic of, 2: 260, 264
    Boston epidemic of, 2: 213, 314–315
    calcaneus deformity, 2: 189–190
    children's hospitals and, 3: 307
    circulatory changes in, 2: 316
    electricity and, 2: 62
    epidemics of, 1: 191; 2: 61
    ganglionectomy in, 3: 332
    Green and, 2: 188–191
    Grice and, 2: 208
    Harrington rods, 2: 316, *317*
    heavy-resistance exercise and, 3: 284–285
    hip contracture treatment, 2: 294, 295*b*
    hot pack treatment, 2: 264
    importance of rest in, 2: 63, *63*
    intraspinal serum, 2: 72
    iron lung and, 2: 78, *190*, 191, 260, 264, 314
    Legg and, 2: 107, 109
    Lovett and, 2: 61–63, *63*, 70–72, 74–75, 77, 147–148
    massage treatment for, 2: 62, 73
    moist heat treatment for, 2: 264
    muscle training for, 2: 62–63, 78
    muscle transfers, 2: 154
    nonstandard treatments and, 2: 77
    Ober and, 2: 147–148
    orthopaedic treatment for, 2: 78
    paralysis of the serratus anterior, 2: 154–155
    paralytic flat foot deformities, 2: 210–212
    patient evaluation, 2: 315
    patient reaction to, 2: 261*b*–263*b*
    prevention of contractures, 2: 78
    research in, 3: 209
    rocking beds, 2: 314, *315*
    Roosevelt and, 2: 71–78
    second attacks of, 1: 276
    shoulder arthrodesis, 2: 154
    spinal taps and, 2: 72, 78
    spring muscle test, 2: 70, *70*, 71
    study of, 2: 61–62
    tendon transfers and, 2: 96, 108, *108*, 109, 147–149; 3: 332–333
    treatment of, 2: 61–63, 71–79, 109–110, 188–191
    Trott and, 2: 314, *314*, 315
    unequal limb length and, 3: 331–332
    vaccine development, 2: 189, 191, 264, 315
    Vermont epidemic of, 2: 61–62, 71
Polivy, Kenneth, 3: 254
Pongor, Paul, 4: 279
Pool, Eugene H., 3: 338
Pope, Malcolm, 2: 371
Porter, C. A., 3: 313
Porter, Charles A., 3: 116
Porter, G. A., 1: 174
Porter, John L., 2: 78; 3: 157; 4: 406, 464
Porter, W. T., 4: 216
Poss, Anita, 4: 174
Poss, Robert (1936–), 4: *169*
    ABOS board and, 4: 173

Ames Test and, 4: 171
Brigham and Women's Hospital and, 4: 163, 172, 193, 195*b*
Brigham Orthopaedic Foundation (BOF) and, 4: 172
Brigham Orthopedic Associates (BOA) and, 4: 123, 172
as BWH orthopaedics chief, 4: 143, 193, 196*b*
Children's Hospital/MGH combined program and, 4: 169
Deputy Editor for Electronic Media at *JBJS*, 4: 173–174
education and training, 4: 169
hip arthritis research, 4: 170
hip osteotomy research, 2: 390; 4: 171
HMS appointment, 4: 171–172
on Hylamer acetabular liner complications, 4: *171*, 172
marriage and family, 4: 174
MIT postdoctoral biology fellowship, 4: 169–170
PBBH and, 4: 163
private medical practice, 4: 169
professional memberships, 4: 174
publications and research, 4: 169–170, *170*, 171–172, 174
RBBH and, 4: 132, 134, 169–171
on total hip arthroplasty, 3: 223; 4: 134, 170–172, 174
US Navy and, 4: 169
Post, Abner, 4: 307
posterior cruciate ligament (PCL)
avulsion of, 2: 386
biomechanical effects of injury and repair, 3: 448
pediatric orthopaedics and, 2: 381
retention in total knee replacement, 4: 130, 138–139, 147, 180–181
robotics-assisted research, 3: 450
posterior interosseous syndrome, 4: 165–166
posterior segment fixator (PSF), 3: 420
posture. *See also* body mechanics
body types and, 4: 235, *236*
Bradford on, 2: 36
chart of normal and abnormal, 4: *84, 234*
Chelsea Survey of, 4: 234–235
children and, 2: 36; 3: 83
contracted iliotibial band and, 2: 152
Goldthwait and, 3: 80–81, 83, 85–91; 4: 53

Harvard study in, 4: 84, *84,* 85–86, 234, *234*
high-heeled shoes and, 2: 317
impact on military draft, 4: 233
medical conflict and, 3: 83
Ober operation and, 2: 153
research in, 4: 233–235, *235*
school children and, 4: 233–234, *234, 235, 236*
scoliosis and, 1: 109
standards for, 4: *236*
Swaim on, 4: 52–54
types of, 4: 85–86
Potter, Constance, 4: 69
Potter, Theodore A. (1912–1995), 4: *67*
arthritis treatment, 4: 67
Boston University appointment, 4: 67
Children's Hospital/MGH combined program and, 4: 68
death of, 4: 69
education and training, 4: 67
HMS appointment, 4: 69
knee arthroplasty and, 4: 64, *65,* 68–69, 70*b*–71*b*
marriage and family, 4: 69
on McKeever and MacIntosh prostheses, 4: 189
nylon arthroplasty in arthritic knees, 4: 65–66, 69
orthopaedic research and, 4: 38
private medical practice, 4: 67
professional memberships, 4: 69
publications and research, 4: 67, *68,* 69, 96
RBBH and, 4: 35, 37–38, 67–68, 89, 93, 116*b*, 187
as RBBH chief of orthopaedics, 4: 40, 41*b*, 63, 66–69, 79, 102, 196*b*
Tufts appointment, 4: 69
Pott's Disease, 1: xxiii, 97, *97,* 105, 108–109; 2: 25, *31,* 247; 3: 148, *149, 154, 155*
Pott's fracture, 4: *317,* 318
Prabhakar, M. M., 3: 423
Practical Biomechanics for the Orthopedic Surgeon (Radin et al.), 3: 328
PRE (Progressive Resistance Exercise) (DeLorme and Watkins), 3: *286*
Presbyterian Hospital, 2: 74–75
Prescott, William, 1: 18
press-fit condylar knee (PFC), 4: 180, 180*t*
pressure correction apparatus (Hoffa-Schede), 3: *151, 152*
pressure sores, 3: 321
Preston, Thomas, 1: 14

Price, Mark, 4: 190*b*
Price, Mark D., 3: 463*b*
Priestley, Joseph, 1: 56
Principles of Orthopedic Surgery for Nurses, The (Sever), 2: 92, *93*
Principles of Orthopedic Surgery (Sever), 2: 92, *93*
Pristina Hospital (Kosovo), 3: 416–417
Pritchett, Henry S., 1: 147
Problem Back Clinic (MGH), 3: 254
"Progress in Orthopaedic Surgery" series, 2: 43, 297
progressive resistance exercises, 3: 285–286
Project HOPE, 3: 417, *417*
prospective payment system (PPS), 3: 397
Prosperi, Lucia, 1: *59*
Prosperi, Warren, 1: *59*
Prosser, W.C.H., 4: 482*b*
prostheses
all-plastic tibial, 4: 148
Austin Moore, 3: 213, 241, 354*b*
biomechanical aspects of hip, 2: 407
bone ingrowth, 3: 220–223
Brigham and Women's Hospital and, 4: 122
Buchholz shoulder, 2: 423
capitellocondylar total elbow, 4: 145, *145,* 146–147
Cohen and patents for, 2: 237
distal humerus, 2: 250
Duocondylar, 4: 178
duopatellar, 4: 130, 180*t*
electromyographic (EMG) signals and, 2: 326
femoral replacement, 4: 69
femoral stem, 3: *293*
hinged elbow, 4: 147
hip replacement, 2: 407
internal, 2: 423
Judet hip, 3: 293
Kinematic knee, 4: 138–139, 147, 149–150
knee arthroplasty and, 3: 292
LTI Digital™ Arm Systems for Adults, 2: 326
MacIntosh, 4: 69, 71*b*, 129, 188
Marmor modular design, 4: 130
McKeever, 4: 40, 69, 70*b*–71*b*, 129–130, 177, 188–189
metal and polyethylene, 4: 148
metallic, 3: 433
myoelectric, 2: 326
nonconstrained total elbow, 4: 145
non-hinged metal–polyethylene, 4: 145–146

Index

PFC unicompartmental knee, 4: 177
press-fit condylar knee (PFC), 4: 180, 180*t*
suction socket, 1: 273
temporary, 3: 374
total condylar, 4: 130
total knee, 4: 137
unicompartmental, 4: 176, 178
used in knee arthroplasty, 4: 179*t*
Prosthetic Research and Development Unit (Ontario Crippled Children's Center), 2: 335
Province House, 3: 6–7, 9, *9*
psoas abscesses, 2: 53–54; 4: 225
psoriatic arthritis, 4: 99
Ptasznik, Ronnie, 3: 437
public health, 2: 61, 107, 425
Pugh, J., 3: 327
pulmonary embolism (PE), 3: 196, 218, 362
pulmonary function
    anterior and posterior procedures, 2: 360
    corrective casts and, 2: 265
    Milwaukee Brace and, 2: 265–266
    scoliosis and, 2: 343
    spine fusion and, 2: 265
    thromboembolism pathophysiology, 1: 82
pulmonary tuberculosis, 1: 56; 2: 9, 16; 3: 25, 128
Pulvertaft, Guy, 3: 427; 4: 95
Putnam, George, 1: 312–313, 317
Putnam, Israel, 1: 18
Putnam, James Jackson, 2: 20
Putti, Vittorio, 2: 80; 3: 203; 4: 14, 65
pyloric stenosis, 3: 49–50

Q

Quain, Jones, 2: 242
Quain's Anatomy (Quain et al.), 2: 242
Queen Victoria Hospital, 2: *421*, 422
quiet necrosis, 2: 194
Quigley, Daniel Thomas, 1: 275
Quigley, Ruth Elizabeth Pearson, 1: 276, 282
Quigley, Thomas B. (1908–1982), 1: *275*, *281*; 4: *342*
    on acromioclavicular joint dislocation in football, 1: 268
    AMA Committee on the Medical Aspects of Sports, 1: 280
    Athlete's Bill of Rights and, 1: 280–281
    athletic injury clinic and, 2: 287
    Boston City Hospital and, 4: 297
    on Dr. Nichols, 1: 257
    education and training, 1: 276
    5th General Hospital and, 4: 484
    Harvard athletics surgeon, 1: 276–279
    Harvard University Health Service and, 1: 277
    as HMS professor, 1: 277
    legacy of, 1: 282–283
    PBBH and, 1: 204, 276–277; 2: 279; 4: 18–21, 116
    pes anserinus transplant, 1: 279
    Plaster-of-Paris Technique in the Treatment of Fractures, 1: 277
    publications of, 1: 268, 276–282; 2: 220
    sports medicine and, 1: 277–283
    US General Hospital No. 5 and, 4: 485
    WWII active duty and, 1: 270, 277; 4: 17
Quinby, William, 4: 11
Quincy, Josiah, 1: 14
Quincy City Hospital, 2: 256

R

Rabkin, Mitchell, 4: 255, 281
radiation synovectomy, 4: 64, 136
Radin, Crete Boord, 3: 328
Radin, Eric L. (1934–2020), 3: *322*, *323*, *328*
    Beth Israel Hospital and, 3: 325
    biomechanics research, 3: 326–328
    Boston Children's Hospital and, 3: 325
    Children's Hospital/MGH combined program and, 3: 322
    death of, 3: 328
    early life, 3: 322
    education and training, 3: 322
    fracture research and, 3: 322–324
    on Glimcher, 2: 326
    on Green, 2: 177
    Henry Ford Hospital and, 3: 328
    HMS appointment, 3: 325, 327
    joint lubrication research, 3: 324–325, *325*, 326, *326*, 327
    marriages and family, 3: 328
    MIT appointment, 3: 325
    Mount Auburn Hospital and, 3: 327
    neuritis with infectious mononucleosis case, 3: 324–325
    Practical Biomechanics for the Orthopedic Surgeon, 3: 328
    publications and research, 2: 396, *396*, *397*, 406; 3: 322–326, *326*, 327–328
    subchondral bone research, 3: 326–327, *327*
    Tufts Medical School and, 3: 328
    University of Michigan appointment, 3: 328
    US Air Force Hospital and, 3: 323
    West Virginia University School of Medicine and, 3: 328
Radin, Tova, 3: 328
radiography
    diagnostic value of, 2: 56
    growth calculation and, 2: 194
    Harvard Athletic Association and, 1: 258
    in hip disease, 2: 54
    leg-length discrepancy and, 3: 299
    scoliosis treatment, 2: 366
radiology. *See also* roentgenograms
    Boston Children's Hospital and, 2: 16, *16*, 17, 17*t*
    HMS and, 2: 16
    Osgood and, 2: 114–116
Radius Management Services, 4: 212
Radius Specialty Hospital, 4: 212
Ragaswamy, Leela, 2: 439*b*
Ralph K. Ghormley Traveling Scholarship, 3: 290
Ramappa, Arun, 4: 287
Ranawat, Chit, 4: 130, 134
Rancho Los Amigos, 4: 129, 151, *151*
Rand, Frank, 4: 279–280
Rand, Isaacs, 1: 25
Rand, Jessie Sophia, 3: 79
Ranvier, Louis Antoine, 1: 82; 3: 142
Rappleye, W. C., 1: 189
Ratshesky, Abraham, 3: 134–135
Ray, Robert D., 1: 162
RBBH. *See* Robert Breck Brigham Hospital (RBBH)
Ready, John, 1: 167
Ready, John E., 4: 193, 195*b*
Rechtine, G. R., 3: 420
Reconstruction Base Hospital No. 1 (Parker Hill, Boston), 4: *328*, *445*, *446*. *See also* US General Hospital No. 10
    Benevolent Order of Elks funding for, 4: 447
    development of, 4: 444–445
    physiotherapy at, 4: *447*
    RBBH and, 4: 447–448

rehabilitation goals and,
4: 446–447
Record, Emily, 3: 330
Record, Eugene E. (ca.1910–2004),
3: *329*
as AAOS fellow, 2: 215
amputation research, 3: 330
ankle arthrodesis case, 3: 330
Boston Children's Hospital and,
2: 299; 3: 329
Children's Hospital/MGH combined program and, 3: 329
death of, 3: 330
early life, 3: 329
education and training, 3: 329
Lower Extremity Amputations for Arterial Insufficiency, 1: 90;
3: 330
Marlborough Medical Associates and, 2: 269
marriage and family, 3: 330
as MGH surgeon, 1: 203;
3: 329
New England Peabody Home for Crippled Children and, 3: 329
private medical practice, 2: 146;
3: 329
publications and research, 3: 330
US Army Reserve and, 3: 329
Record, Eugene E., Jr., 3: 329
Redfern, Peter, 1: xxii
Reed, John, 1: 307; 3: 347
reflex sympathetic dystrophy, 2: 68.
See also chronic regional pain syndrome (CRPS)
Registry of Bone Sarcoma,
3: 136–142
Rehabilitation Engineering and Assistive Technology Society of North America (RESNA), 2: 408, *408*
Rehabilitation Engineering Research Center, 2: 406
Reid, Bill, 1: 252–253, 255
Reidy, Alice Sherburne, 3: 334
Reidy, John A. (1910–1987)
early life, 3: 331
education and training, 3: 331
effects of irradiation on epiphyseal growth, 3: 331
Faulkner Hospital and, 3: 331
fracture research and, 3: 334
ganglionectomy in polio patient case, 3: 332
as honorary orthopaedic surgeon,
3: 398*b*
marriage and family, 3: 334
as MGH surgeon, 3: 74, 331
Newton-Wellesley Hospital and,
3: 331
polio research, 3: 331–333

professional memberships and,
3: 334
publications and research,
3: 209, 331–334
RBBH and, 4: 35, 38, 89, 93
Slipped Capital Femoral Epiphysis,
3: 294, 333
slipped capital femoral epiphysis research, 3: 331, 333–334;
4: 237–238
on tendon transfers in lower extremities, 3: 332–333, *333*
Reilly, Donald, 4: 286
Reinertsen, James L., 4: 283
Reitman, Charles A., 4: 272*b*
Relton, J. E. S., 2: 334–335, *335*
Relton-Hall frame, 2: 334, *335*
Remarks on the Operation for the Cure of Club Feet with Cases (Brown), 1: 100
Remembrances (Coll Warren), 1: 83
Report of Cases in the Orthopedic Infirmary of the City of Boston (J.B. Brown), 1: *120*
Reports of Cases Treated at the Boston Orthopedic Institution (Brown and Brown), 1: *120*
Residency Review Committee (RRC), 1: 211
RESNA. *See* Rehabilitation Engineering and Assistive Technology Society of North America (RESNA)
Resurrectionists (Browne), 1: *21*
Reverdin, Jaques-Louis, 4: 216
Revere, Anne, 2: 272
Revere, John, 1: 293
Revere, Paul, 1: 8, 13–17, 19–20,
22, 28, *28*; 2: 272
Reynolds, Edward, 3: 42
Reynolds, Fred, 4: 125
Reynolds, Fred C., 1: 162
rheumatic fever, 2: 171
Rheumatism Foundation Hospital,
4: 96
rheumatoid arthritis
body mechanics and, 4: 82–83
boutonniere deformities of the hand, 4: 98
children and, 2: 164, 171, 350
foot surgery and, 4: 188, *188*
gene therapy and, 2: 82
genetics in, 4: 169
of the hand, 4: 96–98, *98*
hindfoot pain, 4: 188, *189*
knee arthroplasty and,
4: 70*b*–71*b*
MacIntosh prosthesis and, 4: 188
McKeever prothesis and,
4: 188–189

metacarpophalangeal arthroplasty,
4: 97
mold arthroplasty and, 3: 239
nylon arthroplasty in, 4: *65*
opera-glass hand deformity, 4: 99
radiation synovectomy and,
4: 136
release of contractures in arthroplasty, 4: 166
swan neck deformity, 4: 98
synovectomy of the knee in,
4: 102
thumb deformities, 4: 97
total hip replacement and, 4: 134
total knee replacement and,
4: 181
treatment for, 4: 97, 138
upper extremities and, 2: 137
wrist joint damage in, 4: 166–167, *168*
rheumatoid synovitis, 4: 166
rheumatology, 2: 321
Rhinelander, Frederic W., Jr. (1906–1990), 3: *335*
Boston Children's Hospital and,
3: 335
burn care and, 3: 336
Case Western Reserve University School of Medicine and,
3: 337
death of, 3: 337
early life, 3: 335
education and training, 3: 335
HMS appointment, 3: 335
honors and awards, 3: 337, 337*b*
Letterman Army Hospital and,
3: 336
marriage and family, 3: 337
as MGH surgeon, 3: 74, 335
private medical practice, 3: 336
publications and research,
3: 335–336, *336*, 337
Shriners Hospital for Children and, 3: 335
University of Arkansas College of Medicine and, 3: 337
University of California Hospital and, 3: 336–337
US Army and, 3: 336
US Army Legion of Merit,
3: *337*
Rhinelander, Julie, 3: 337
Rhinelander, Philip Mercer, 3: 335
Rhode Island Hospital, 3: 401
Rhodes, Jonathan, 1: 90
Richard J. Smith Lecture, 3: 431
Richards, Thomas K. (1892–1965)
Boston City Hospital and, 1: 258
as football team physician,
1: 258–262

as Harvard athletics surgeon, 1: 258, 262; 4: 303
Harvard Fifth Surgical Service and, 4: 303
on physician's role, 1: 259–262
scientific studies, 1: 262
as team physician for the Boston Red Sox, 1: 258
Richardson, Frank, 1: 255
Richardson, Lars C., 4: 287
Richardson, Mary R., 3: 75
Richardson, Maurice H., 3: 18, 94; 4: 274–275
Richardson, William, 4: 3
rickets, 1: 129; 2: 36, 114; 3: 83, 388
Riley, Donald, 1: 225; 4: 193
Riley, Maureen, 2: 414
Ring, David, 1: 167; 3: 410, 463
Riseborough, Bruce, 2: 400
Riseborough, Edward J. (1925–1985), 2: *395*
  Boston Children's Hospital and, 2: 286, 399; 4: 127
  Brigham and Women's Hospital and, 4: 163, 193
  congenital kyphosis case, 2: 399–400
  death of, 2: 400
  distal femoral physeal fractures research, 2: 400
  education and training, 2: 395
  fat embolism syndrome research, 2: 397, *397*, 398
  HMS appointment, 2: 395, 399
  intercondylar fractures of the humerus research, 2: 397, *397*
  marriage and family, 2: 400
  MGH and, 2: 395; 4: 127
  orthopaedics appointments, 2: 399
  orthopaedics education and, 2: 398–399
  PBBH and, 4: 163
  professional memberships, 2: 400
  publications and research, 2: 385, 396, *396*, 397, 399–400, *400*; 3: 322–323
  rugby and, 2: 385, 400
  Scoliosis and Other Deformities of the Axial Skeleton, 2: 398, *398*
  scoliosis research, 2: 395–396, 399–400, *400*; 4: 127
  trauma research, 2: 396, *396*, 397, 399
Riseborough, Jennifer, 2: 400
Risser, Joseph, 2: 335
Risser cast, 2: 178
RMS *Aurania*, 4: 431

Robbins, Anne Smith, 1: 123–125; 2: 114
Robbins, Chandler, 2: 5
Robert Breck Brigham Hospital Corporation, 4: 23–24, 25*b*
Robert Breck Brigham Hospital for Incurables, 4: 22, 23*b*, 30, 36
Robert Breck Brigham Hospital (RBBH), 4: *26, 28, 31, 35, 37, 40, 42*
  affiliation with PBBH, 4: 34, 36, 39
  annual reports, 4: *37*
  arthritis clinic and, 3: 371; 4: 36
  arthroplasties at, 4: 64
  board of overseers, 4: 132
  Chief of Orthopedic Service report, 4: 41*b*
  chronic disease treatment at, 4: 23*b*, 25*b*, 27–28, 30, 30*b*, 32, 32*b*, 33, 36, 39*b*, 46
  as Clinical Research Center, 4: 38, 40
  clinical teaching at, 4: 32–33
  Emergency Campaign speech, 4: 32, 32*b*
  financial difficulties, 4: 25–26, 28–29, 31–32, 34, 35*b*, 37, 42
  founding of, 4: 22–24
  Goldthwait and, 3: 81, 84, 91–92; 4: 24–25, 25*b*, 26–28, 31, 36–38, 39*b*
  Goldthwait Research Fund, 4: 27
  grand rounds and, 4: 118
  growth in patient volume, 4: 124*t*
  history of, 4: 1
  HMS students and, 4: 30, 69
  laboratory at, 4: 35
  lawsuit on hospital mission, 4: 29–30, 30*b*
  leadership of, 4: 31–33, 35–36, 38, 39*b*, 40, 41*b*, 42, 99, 127
  Lloyd T. Brown and, 3: 257; 4: 25, 30–34, 36
  military reconstruction hospital and, 4: 443–444
  occupational therapy department, 4: 28, *29*
  orthopaedic advancements at, 4: 40
  orthopaedic research and, 4: 38, 41*b*
  orthopaedic service chiefs at, 4: 43
  orthopaedic surgery at, 1: 171; 4: 28, 31, 40, 41*b*, 115
  orthopaedics and arthritis at, 4: 26–28, 43
  orthopaedics as specialty at, 4: 1

orthopaedics instruction at, 1: 157; 4: 41*b*, 68
orthopaedics residencies, 1: 207–208; 4: 30, 40, 131
patient conditions and outcomes, 4: 29*t*
patient outcomes, 4: 31*t*
physical therapy and, 4: *28, 29*
professorship in orthopedic surgery, 4: 114
Reconstruction Base Hospital No. 1 and, 4: 445, 447–448
rehabilitation service at, 4: 37, *38*
research at, 4: 33, 42, 117, 132
residencies at, 4: 34–35, 39–40, 42
rheumatic disease treatment, 4: 47, 136, 188
as specialty arthritis hospital, 4: 122–123
staffing of, 4: 25, 28, 32, *34*, 35–38, 45, 68, 131–132
statistics, 1945, 4: 34*t*
surgeon-scholars at, 4: 43, 79
surgery at, 4: *132*
surgical caseloads at, 4: 131, 131*t*, 132
total knee arthroplasty and, 4: 129–130, 131*t*
transition to Brigham and Women's Hospital, 4: 42, 69, 113–114, 116, 116*b*, 117–119, 121, 127, 132
World War I and, 4: 25–26, 79
World War II and, 4: 33
Robert Brigham Multipurpose Arthritis and Musculoskeletal Disease Center, 4: 184
Robert C. Hinckley and the Recreation of The First Operation Under Ether (Wolfe), 1: 59
Robert Jones and Agnes Hunt Orthopaedic Hospital, 3: 426
Robert Jones Orthopaedic Society, 2: 132
Robert Leffert Memorial Fund, 3: 415
Robert Salter Award, 2: 415
Robert W. Lovett Memorial Unit for the Study of Crippling Diseases, 2: 82
Robert W. Lovett Professorship, 2: 166; 4: 195*b*
Roberts, Ada Mead, 3: 338
Roberts, Elizabeth Converse, 3: 339
Roberts, Melita Josephine, 2: 143
Roberts, Odin, 3: 338
Roberts, Sumner N. (1898–1939), 3: *338*

cervical spine fracture research, 3: 340–341, *341*
Children's Hospital/MGH combined program and, 3: 338
congenital absence of the odontoid process case, 3: 340
death of, 3: 342
early life, 3: 338
education and training, 3: 338
fracture research and, 3: 339–341, *342*
HMS appointment, 2: 223; 3: 338–339; 4: 61
marriage and family, 3: 339
Massachusetts Eye and Ear Infirmary and, 3: 339
as MGH surgeon, 3: 187, 270, 339
private medical practice, 3: 338
professional memberships and, 3: 341–342
publications and research, 3: 339–341; 4: 63
RBBH and, 3: 339; 4: 31, 60
World War I and, 3: 338
Robinson, James, 1: 248
Robinson, Marie L., 2: 111–112
Robson, A. W. Mayo, 2: 91
Rockefeller Foundation, 1: 147
Rockefeller Institute, 2: 72
rocking beds, 2: *315*
Rocky Mountain Trauma Society, 3: 311
Rodriguez, Edward, 3: 410
Rodriquez, Ken, 4: 287
Roentgen Diagnosis of the Extremities and Spine (Ferguson), 4: 110
Roentgen Method in Pediatrics, The (Rotch), 2: 170
roentgenograms. *See also* x-rays
arthritis and, 4: 64, *64*
in curriculum, 1: 161
diagnosis and, 2: 155; 3: 99
discovery of, 2: 24, 54; 3: 57, 96
MGH and, 3: 20–21
Osgood and Dodd on, 2: 116
slipped capital femoral epiphysis and, 4: 238
total knee arthroplasty-scoring system, 4: 150
ROFEH International, 2: 363, *363*
Rogers, Carolyn, 1: 239
Rogers, Elizabeth Grace, 2: 258
Rogers, Emily, 3: 350
Rogers, Emily Ross, 4: 230
Rogers, Fred A., 1: 180
Rogers, Horatio, 4: 475
Rogers, Margaret, 4: 371

Rogers, Mark H. (1877–1941), 4: *224*
American Journal of Orthopedic Surgery editor, 4: 226
AOA resolution on orthopaedics, 4: 227
as Beth Israel chief of orthopaedics, 4: 220, 223, 228–230, 289*b*
Beth Israel Hospital and, 4: 208*b*
as Boston and Maine Railroad orthopaedic surgeon, 4: 225
Boston City Hospital and, 4: 229–230, 328
Burrage Hospital and, 4: 226
Clinics for Crippled Children and, 2: 230
education and training, 4: 224
Fort Riley base hospital and, 4: 452–453
HMS appointment, 4: 226, 226*b*
legacy of, 4: 230
marriage and family, 4: 230
Massachusetts Regional Fracture Committee, 3: 64
MGH orthopaedics and, 1: 189; 3: 266, 268; 4: 224, 226, 226*b*
as MGH orthopaedics chief, 3: 11*b*, 173, 227
New England Deaconess Hospital and, 4: 225
New England Regional Committee on Fractures, 4: 341
orthopaedics education and, 4: 228–230
professional memberships and roles, 4: 229*b*
psoas abscess in the lumbar retroperitoneal lymph glands case, 4: 225
publications and research, 4: 224–225, *225*, 226, 228–229, 242
RBBH and, 4: 406
rehabilitation of soldiers and, 4: 444
Trumbull Hospital and, 4: 225
tuberculosis research and, 4: 224–226
Tufts appointment, 4: 226, 226*b*
US Army Medical Corps and, 4: 226–227
Rogers, Orville F., Jr., 2: 119; 4: 389*b*
Rogers, Oscar H., 3: 343
Rogers, W. B., 3: 420
Rogers, William A. (1892–1975), 3: *343*

closed reduction of lumbar spine facture-dislocation case, 3: 347
death of, 3: 350
early life, 3: 343
education and training, 3: 343
fracture research and, 3: 343, 347–348
HMS appointment, 2: 223; 4: 60–61
honors and awards, 3: 350
Journal of Bone and Joint Surgery editor, 2: 165; 3: 161, 260, 344–347
legacy of, 3: 349
marriage and family, 3: 349–350
on mental attitude and spine fractures, 3: 349*b*
as MGH surgeon, 1: 158; 3: 187, 192, 270, 343–344, 348, 375
publications and research, 2: 297; 3: 184–185, 294, 347–349
RBBH and, 4: 31, 36, 93, 111
sacroiliac joint arthrodesis and, 3: 184–185
sling procedure for the foot and, 3: 294
spinal fusion and, 3: 321, 344
spinal research and, 3: 343–344, 347–349, *349*
Rogers, William Allen, 4: *200*
Roi Albert I Anglo-Belgian Hospital, 4: 401
Rokitanasky, Karl, 1: 82
Romney, Mitt, 3: 424
Roosevelt, Eleanor, 2: 72
Roosevelt, Franklin D.
chair lift design, 2: 76, *76*
Lovett and, 2: 72, *73*, *74*, 75–76, 271
Lovett's diagram of muscle exam, 2: *75*
nonstandard treatments and, 2: 77
onset of poliomyelitis, 2: 71–72
poliomyelitis treatment, 2: 72–78
suggestions on treatment, 2: 76–77
and Warm Springs Foundation, 2: 77–78
World War II and, 4: 465–466, *466*
Roosevelt, James, 2: 72
Roosevelt, Theodore, 1: 248, 253; 4: 361
Roosevelt Hospital, 2: 248, 250–251
Root, Howard F., 4: 229
Roper, Jane, 4: 66
Ropes, Marian W., 3: 336

Rose, P., 3: 327
Rose, Robert M., 2: 407;
   3: 327–328
Rosenau, Milton J., 4: 6, 210
Rosenberg, Benjamin, 2: 368
Rosenthal, Robert K. (1936–2021),
   2: *401*
   Boston Children's Hospital and,
      2: 401–402
   Brigham and Women's Hospital
      and, 4: 163, 193
   Cerebral Palsy Clinic and, 2: 402
   cerebral palsy research, 2: 401,
      401, 402
   education and training, 2: 401
   HMS appointment, 2: 401
   PBBH and, 4: 163
   professional memberships, 2: 402
   publications and research,
      2: 401–402
Rossier, Alain B., 4: 152
Rotch, Thomas Morgan, 2: 13–14,
   170
Roussimoff, André (Andre the
   Giant), 4: *251*, 252–253
Rowe, Carter R. (1906–2001),
   3: *350*, *359*, *360*, *361*, *447*, *461*;
   4: *491*
   as AOA president, 3: 355, 355b,
      360
   Bankart procedure and, 3: 351,
      351, 352–354, 357–359, *359*,
      360
   Children's Hospital/MGH com-
      bined program and, 3: 237
   dead arm syndrome and,
      3: 359–360
   death of, 3: 361
   early life, 3: 350
   education and training,
      3: 350–351
   on Ernest Codman, 3: 143
   on Eugene Record, 3: 330
   Fracture course and, 3: *273*
   fracture research and, 3: 354
   on fractures in elderly patients,
      3: *353*, 354, 354b
   Harvard Unit and, 1: 270, *270*
   HMS appointment, 3: 354, 360
   on Klein, 4: 236
   knee arthrotomy research, 3: 351
   legacy of, 3: 360–361
   Lest We Forget, 3: 61, 187, 257,
      347, *357*, 360
   on Mankin, 3: 387
   marriage and family, 3: 361
   MGH Fracture Clinic and,
      4: 464
   as MGH surgeon, 3: 354, 360,
      398b

   MGH Ward 1 and, 3: 70b, 74
   105th General Hospital and,
      3: 351; 4: 489, 490b–491b
   as orthopaedic surgeon for the
      Boston Bruins, 3: 356–357,
      357b
   private medical practice, 3: 271,
      448
   professional memberships and,
      3: 354–355, 360
   publications and research,
      3: 350–359, 448–449
   Shoulder, The, 3: 360
   shoulder dislocations and,
      3: 352, *352*, 353, 355–356,
      356
   shoulder surgery and, 3: 352–
      354, 356
   on Smith-Petersen, 3: 187
   sports medicine and, 3: 356,
      388t
   34th Infantry Division and,
      4: 484
   on Thornton Brown, 3: 257
   US Army Medical Corps and,
      3: 351
   voluntary shoulder dislocation
      case, 3: 355–356
   on William Kermond, 3: 299
   on William Rogers, 3: 347, 349
   World War II service, 4: 17
Rowe, George, 4: 3
Rowe, Mary, 3: 361, *361*
Roxbury Clinical Record Club
   (R.C.R.C.), 3: 161
Roxbury Ladies' Bikur Cholim Asso-
   ciation, 4: 212
Roxbury Latin School, 1: 6, 20
Royal National Orthopaedic Hospital
   (London), 1: 106; 2: 333–334,
   334; 3: 412, 426
Royal Orthopaedic Hospital (Bir-
   mingham, England), 2: 181
Rozental, Tamara D., 3: 410;
   4: 288
RRC. *See* Residency Review Commit-
   tee (RRC)
Rubash, Harry E.
   Edith M. Ashley Professor,
      3: 464b
   HCORP and, 1: 224–225
   Knee Biomechanics and Biomate-
      rials Laboratory, 3: 464b
   as MGH clinical faculty, 3: 464b
   as MGH orthopaedics chief,
      3: 11b, 228, 399, 462–463
Rubidge, J. W., 1: *34*
Rubin, S. H., 4: 199
Ruby, Leonard, 2: 250; 4: 99
Rudman, Warren, 2: 414

Rudo, Nathan, 2: 173, 175–176,
   438
Ruggles, Timothy, 1: 13
Ruggles-Fayerweather House, 1: 22,
   22
Rugh, J. T., 3: 158
Rumford, Count Benjamin,
   1: 292–293
Runyon, Lucia, 2: 291
Runyon, Robert C. (1928–2012),
   2: *290–291*
   Boston Children's Hospital and,
      2: 289–290
   death of, 2: 291
   education and training, 2: 289
   marriage and family, 2: 291
   MGH/Children's Hospital resi-
      dency, 2: 289
   MIT Medical and, 2: 277,
      290–291
   private medical practice, 2: 289
   publications of, 2: 291
   sports medicine and, 2: 290
Runyon, Scott, 2: 291
Rush, Benjamin, 1: 25, 293; 3: 23
Russell, Stuart, 3: 364
Ruth Jackson Orthopaedic Society,
   2: 413, *414*
Ryerson, Edwin W., 1: 197; 2: 160;
   4: 394
Ryerson, W. E., 2: 105

S

Sabatini, Coleen, 4: 190b
Sabin, Albert, 2: 191, 264, 315
sacrococcygeal chordoma, 3: 390
sacroiliac joint
   arthrodesis of, 3: 183–185
   fusion for arthritis, 3: 184–185
   fusion for tuberculosis, 3: 185
   ligamentous strain of, 3: 191
   low-back and leg pain, 3: 184
   orthopaedic surgeon opinions on
      fusion of, 3: 184–185
sacrospinalis, 2: 146–147
Saint Joseph Hospital, 4: 157
Salem Hospital, 1: 220, 224–225;
   2: 270–272
Salib, Philip, 3: 238, 239, 460b
Salk, Jonas, 2: 189
Salter, Robert B., 1: 167; 2: 209,
   302, 334–335; 4: 351, 355–356
Salter innominate osteotomy,
   2: 390–391
Salter–Harris classification system,
   4: 351, 355–356
Saltonstall, Francis A. F. Sherwood,
   3: 89
Salvati, Eduardo, 4: 134

Salve Regina College, 1: 216
Salzler, Matthew, 3: 463*b*
Salzman, Edwin W., 4: 251
Samilson, Robert, 3: *293*
San Diego Naval Center, 4: 246
Sancta Maria Hospital, 4: 342, 346
Sandell, L. J., 3: 445
Sanders, Charles, 3: 391
Sanders, James, 2: 378
Sanderson, Eric R., 4: 489
Sanderson, Marguerite, 4: 444
Sanhedrin, Mishnah, 4: 197
Santa Clara County Hospital, 3: 300
Santore, R. F., 4: 176, *176*, 177
Santurjian, D. N., 1: 179
sarcoidosis, 4: 98
Sarcoma Molecular Biology Laboratory, 3: 464*b*
Sargent, John Singer, 4: *424*
Sarmiento, Augusto, 3: 249
Sarni, James, 3: 463, 464*b*
Sarokhan, Alan, 2: 249
Sayre, Lewis A., 1: 119; 2: 26, 30, 48, 50–51, 63, *227*
Sayre, Reginald H., 2: 52
Scannell, David D., 4: 207, 439
scaphoid fracture, 3: 101–102; 4: 359–361, 368–369
Scardina, Robert J., 3: 396, 398*b*, 460*b*, 464*b*
scarlet fever, 1: 7; 2: 4, 52
Scarlet Key Society (McGill), 3: 253, *253*
Schaffer, Jonathan L., 4: 193, 195*b*
Schaffer, Newton M., 2: 47–48
Schaller, Bill, 4: 284
Scheuermann kyphosis, 2: 343, 359
Schiller, Arnold, 2: 369
Schlatter, Carl B., 2: 115
Schlens, Robert D., 2: 266
Schmitt, Francis O., 2: 321, 323; 3: 248, 455*b*
Schmorl, Georg, 3: 204; 4: 262
Schneider, Bryan, 2: 439*b*
School for Health Officers (HMS), 2: 42, 65–66
Schurko, Brian, 4: 190*b*
Schussele, Christian, 1: *57*
Schwab, Robert, 3: 286
Schwab, Sidney I., 3: 164
Schwamm, Lee, 3: 412–413
Schwartz, Felix, 4: 489
Schwartz, Forrest, 3: 463*b*
sciatica
   herniated disc as cause of, 3: 184
   laminectomy and, 3: 204, 206
   low-back pain research, 2: 396; 3: 184, 203–206
   nonoperative treatment of, 2: 373–374

   ruptured intervertebral disc and, 3: 205–207, *207*
   surgery for, 2: 373–374, 396
   treatment of, 2: 152–153; 3: 203
   use of chymopapain, 3: 254–255, 419, *421*
scoliosis
   Abbott Frame, 4: 232, *232*
   Adam's machine, 2: 86
   Boston brace, 2: 339–340, 358–359
   brace management of, 2: 339–340, 367
   Bradford and, 2: 35, *35*, *36*, 58
   Brewster and, 2: 223–228
   cadaver studies, 2: 56, 58, *58*
   celluloid jackets, 2: *85*
   collagen and, 2: 328
   congenital, 4: 62, 65
   devices for, 2: 35, *35*, *36*, 296–297, *297*
   diastematomyelia in, 2: 399–400
   Dwyer instrumentation, 2: 336
   Dwyer procedure, 2: 328
   early onset (EOS), 2: 360–361
   exercises for, 2: 59
   Forbes method of correction, 2: 87, *87*; 3: 229; 4: 232, *232*
   forward flexion test, 2: *367*
   Galeazzi method, 2: 227
   genetic background and, 2: 399, *400*
   growth-sparing surgery, 2: 360–361
   Hall and, 2: 334–335
   Harrington rods, 2: 316, 325, 335, 340
   Hibbs spinal fusion procedure, 2: 164
   idiopathic, 1: xxiii; 2: 334, 339, 341, 343, 358–359, 366–367, 399
   jackets for, 2: 59, *59*, 60, *60*, 61, 85–87
   kyphoscoliosis, 1: 97, 105
   latent psoas abscess case, 2: 365
   Lovett and, 2: 56–61, 79, 86, 223–225
   Lovett Board, 2: *59*, 86
   Lovett-Sever method, 2: 87
   measurement methods, 2: 366, *367*
   Milwaukee Brace, 2: 336
   pedicle screws, 2: 343
   pelvic machine design, 2: 86
   photography and, 2: 247
   posterior spinal fusion, 2: 341
   pressure correction apparatus (Hoffa-Schede), 3: *151*, 152

   Relton-Hall frame, 2: 334
   right dorsal, 3: *229*
   self-correction of, 2: *297*
   Sever and, 2: 84–86
   Soutter and, 2: 296
   spinal surgery and, 2: 334–335, 337–338, 340–343
   surgical procedures for, 2: *369*
   suspension and, 2: *336*
   tibial osteoperiosteal grafts, 2: 316
   treatment of, 1: xxi, xxii, 100, 106, 109, *116*; 2: 35, 84–88, 296, 316, 334, 366–367, 396; 3: 208–209, 229; 4: 232–233
   turnbuckle jacket, 2: 80, 223–226, 226*b*, 227, 227*b*, 316, *336*; 3: 209
   use of photographs, 2: 84
   vertebral transverse process case, 3: 229–230
   x-rays and, 2: 79
   Zander apparatus for, 3: *152*, 153
Scoliosis and Other Deformities of the Axial Skeleton (Riseborough and Herndon), 2: 398, *398*
Scoliosis Research Society (SRS), 2: 338, 342, 347, 370, 400, 411, *411*
scoliosometer, 2: 36
Scollay, Mercy, 1: 19
Scott, Catherine, 4: 175
Scott, Dick, 1: 167
Scott, Richard D. (1943–), 4: 175
   Brigham and Women's Hospital and, 4: 163, 181, 193
   CHMC and, 4: 176
   education and training, 4: 175
   HCORP and, 4: 175
   hip and knee reconstructions, 4: 175–178
   HMS appointment, 4: 176, 178
   honors and awards, 4: 180
   on importance of PCL preservation, 4: 181
   on metal tibial wedges, 4: 180, *180*
   metallic tibial tray fracture case, 4: 177
   MGH and, 4: 175
   New England Baptist Hospital and, 4: 181
   New England Deaconess Hospital and, 4: 280
   PBBH and, 4: 163
   PFC unicompartmental knee prothesis, 4: 177
   publications and research, 4: 176, *176*, 177–178, *178*, 180, *180*, 181, *181*, 189
   RBBH and, 4: 132, 175–176

Index

Total Knee Arthroplasty, 4: 176
  on total knee replacement outcomes, 4: 178, 180–181
  unicompartmental prothesis and, 4: 176
Scott, S. M., 2: 212
Scudder, Abigail Taylor Seelye, 3: 55
Scudder, Charles L. (1860–1949), 3: *53, 57, 63,* 65
  ACS Committee on Fractures, 3: 64
  American College of Surgeons Board of Regents and, 3: 62–63
  Boston Children's Hospital and, 2: 438; 3: 54
  Boston Dispensary and, 2: 306
  clinical congress meeting, 3: 118
  club foot research and, 3: 54
  "Coll" Warren and, 3: 54–55
  death of, 3: 65
  early life, 3: 53
  education and training, 3: 53–54
  fracture treatment and, 3: 55–56, 56*b*, 58–65; 4: 340*b*
  HMS appointment, 3: 58, 61
  legacy of, 3: 64–65
  marriage and family, 3: 55, 64
  at MGH case presentation, 3: *54*
  MGH Fracture Clinic and, 2: 130; 3: 60, 60*b*, 371; 4: 464
  as MGH house officer, 1: 189; 3: 54
  as MGH surgeon, 3: 54, 58, 64, 266; 4: 472*b*
  New England Deaconess Hospital and, 4: 274
  professional memberships and, 3: 65
  publications and research, 1: 264; 3: 55–58, 64–65; 4: 335
  Treatment of Fractures, 1: 147; 3: 55–56, *57, 58,* 64, 99; 4: 312, 350
  Tumors of the Jaws, 3: 64
Scudder, Evarts, 3: 53
Scudder, Sarah Patch Lamson, 3: 53
Scudder Oration on Trauma, 3: 63
Scutter, Charles L., 2: 66
Seal of Chevalier du Tastevin, 2: 348, *348*
Sears, George, 4: 303
Seattle Children's Hospital, 4: 250
Section for Orthopedic Surgery (AMA), 2: 110–111, 176
Seddon, Herbert, 2: 135, 140; 3: 412
Sedgwick, Cornelius, 4: 276–277, 279

Seeing Patients (White and Chanoff), 4: *265*
Seelye, Abigail Taylor, 3: 55
Segond, Paul, 2: 91
Seider, Christopher, 1: 14
Sell, Kenneth, 3: 439
Selva, Julius, 2: 31
Semmelweis, Ignaz, 1: 81, 84, 193
sepsis. *See also* antisepsis
  amputations and, 3: 373
  ankle arthrodesis case, 3: 330
  following intramedullary fixation of femoral fractures, 2: 248; 3: 309–310
  hip fractures and, 3: 218
  infectious research and, 1: 91
  recurrence of, 3: 196, 301
septic arthritis, 2: 79
Sevenson, Orvar, 2: 302
Sever, Charles W., 2: 83
Sever, Elizabeth Bygrave, 2: 92, 97
Sever, James T., 2: 252
Sever, James W. (1878–1964), 2: *84, 98, 255*
  on astragalectomy, 2: 92–93
  on back disabilities, 2: 92
  birth palsies research, 2: 415, 417
  Boston Children's Hospital and, 1: 187; 2: 13, 40, 84, 90, 92, 274, 282, 296; 4: 338
  Boston City Hospital and, 4: 305*b*, 307–308, 308*b*, 328
  brachial plexus injury study, 2: 90, 96
  on Bradford, 2: 44, 92
  as Browne & Nichols School trustee, 2: 97
  calcaneal apophysitis study, 2: 88–90, 100
  clinical congress meeting, 3: 116
  death of, 2: 100
  early life, 2: 83
  foot research, 2: 107
  fracture research, 3: 340
  HMS appointment, 2: 92, 97; 4: 59
  HMS Laboratory of Surgical Pathology and, 2: 90
  on improvement of medicine, 2: 98
  marriage and family, 2: 92, 97
  Massachusetts Industrial Accident Board examiner, 2: 92
  Massachusetts Regional Fracture Committee, 3: 64
  medical appointments, 2: 84
  as medical director of the Industrial School, 2: 97
  medical education, 2: 83

  military surgeon training and, 4: 396
  New England Regional Committee on Fractures, 4: 341
  obstetrical paralysis study, 2: 89–90, *90,* 91, 94–96, 100
  on occupational therapy, 4: 359
  on orthopaedic surgery advances, 2: 99–100
  pelvic machine design, 2: 86
  Principles of Orthopedic Surgery, 2: 92, *93*
  Principles of Orthopedic Surgery for Nurses, The, 2: 92, *93*
  professional memberships, 2: 97–98
  publications of, 2: 84, 92, 223
  schools for disabled children, 2: 97
  scoliosis treatment, 2: 59, 61, 84–86
  Textbook of Orthopedic Surgery for Students of Medicine, 2: 92, *93*
  tibial tuberosity fracture treatment, 2: 91, 96–97
Sever, Josephine Abbott, 2: 97
Sever, Mary Caroline Webber, 2: 83
Sever procedure, 2: 90
Sever-L'Episcopo procedure, 2: 90, 100, 417
Sever's disease. *See* calcaneal apophysitis (Sever's Disease)
Seymour, N., 2: 211
Shaffer, Newton M., 2: 43, 48, *49,* 57, 99
Shanbhag, Arun, 3: 462, 464*b*
Shands, Alfred, 1: 99, 114, 180
Shands, Alfred R., Jr., 2: 165, 183; 3: 208, 290
Shands Hospital, 3: 432
Shapiro, Frederic (1942–), 2: *402*
  Boston Children's Hospital and, 2: 354, 403, 403*b*, 439*b*; 4: 280
  education and training, 2: 402–403
  HMS appointment, 2: 403, 403*b*
  honors and awards, 2: 403–404
  Pediatric Orthopedic Deformities, 2: 403, *404*
  professional memberships, 2: 403–405
  publications and research, 2: 400, 403–404, *404*
Sharpey, William, 1: 84
Sharpey-Schafer, Edward A., 2: 242
Shattuck, Frederick C., 2: 20, 39, 43; 3: 94
Shattuck, George Cheever, 4: 414–415

Shaw, A., 2: 115
Shaw, Amy, 1: 85
Shaw, Benjamin S., 2: 8
Shaw, Lemuel, 1: 302, 307, 310–311
Shaw, Robert Gould, 1: 303, 308
Shaw, Robert S., 3: 287
Shea, William D., 4: 163
Sheehan, Diane, 1: 239
Sheltering Arms (New York), 2: 5
Shephard, Margaret, 3: 219
Shepherd's Bush Military Hospital, 4: 398, *398*, 399, 402, 411, 444
Shepherd's Bush Orthopaedic Hospital, 3: 365
Sherman, Henry M., 3: 234
Sherman, William O'Neill, 3: 60–61; 4: 338, 339*b*, 340, 340*b*, 342
Sherrill, Henry Knox, 3: 1
Shields, Lawrence R., 4: 116, 116*b*, 117, 128, 163
Shippen, William, 1: 25
shock, 4: 373
Shortell, Joseph H. (1891–1951), 4: *338*
    AAOS and, 4: 337
    American Expeditionary Forces and, 4: 338
    athletic injury treatment, 4: 342
    BCH Bone and Joint Service, 4: 307, 328, 333–334, 341, 380*b*
    BCH residencies and, 4: 377
    Boston Bruins and, 4: 342
    Boston Children's Hospital and, 2: 252, 274; 4: 338
    Boston City Hospital and, 1: 199; 3: 64; 4: 242, 338, 341
    death of, 4: 342
    education and training, 4: 338
    fracture treatment and, 4: 339*b*, 342
    hip fractures in elderly case, 4: 341
    HMS appointment, 4: 338, 341
    on industrial accidents, 4: 338, 341
    New England Regional Committee on Fractures, 4: 341
    professional memberships, 4: 341
    publications and research, 4: 338, 341
    Ted Williams and, 4: 342
Shortkroff, Sonya, 4: 136, 194
Shoulder, The (Codman), 2: 239; 3: 105, *105*, 115, 122, 140*b*
Shoulder, The (Rowe), 3: 360
shoulders
    acromioclavicular dislocation, 3: 449
    amputations, 1: 23
    anterior subluxation of, 3: 360
    arthrodesis outcomes, 2: 154
    Bankart procedure, 3: 351–354, 357–358, *359*, 450
    Bankart procedure rating sheet, 3: 358*t*
    brachial plexus injuries, 2: 90–91, 96; 3: 412, *412*, 413–414
    cleidocranial dysostosis, 2: 254
    Codman's Paradox, 3: 105
    dislocations and, 3: 352, *352*, 353, 355–356, *356*
    fracture treatment and, 3: 339
    frozen shoulder, 1: 277–278
    glenoid labrum composition, 3: 449
    instability and, 3: 352, 448–450, *450*
    posterior dislocations, 2: 417–418
    ruptures of the serratus anterior, 2: 253
    sports injuries and, 2: 288
    subacromial bursitis, 3: 104–105, 107–109
    subdeltoid bursa, 3: 95, 98, 103–105, 108
    supraspinatus tendon, 3: 108–109
    surgery, 1: 29
    transfers for, 2: 154
    transient subluxation of, 3: 359
    treatment of, 3: 107–110
Shriners Hospital for Crippled Children, 4: 378
Shriners Hospitals for Children, 2: 110, 212, 424; 3: 335
Sibley, John, 1: 307
sickle cell disease, 3: 403
SICOT. *See* International Society of Orthopaedic Surgery and Traumatology (SICOT)
Siffert, R. S., 1: 126
Silen, William, 1: 167; 4: 262, 283, 283*t*
silicone flexible implants, 4: 132, 166–167, *167*
Siliski, John M., 1: 217*b*; 3: 399, 460*b*, 464*b*
Silver, David, 2: 31, 64, 67, 87; 3: 87, 156, 158, 375; 4: 405, 412, 451
Simcock, Xavier C., 3: 463*b*; 4: 190*b*
Simmons, Barry P. (1939–), 4: *182*
    AO trauma fellowship, 4: 182
    Beth Israel Hospital and, 4: 182, 262
    Brigham and Women's Hospital and, 2: 375; 4: 163, 183, 193, 195*b*
    carpal tunnel syndrome research, 2: 375; 4: 183–184, *184*, 185, *185*, 186
    Children's Hospital/MGH combined program and, 4: 182
    CHMC and, 4: 182
    education and training, 4: 182
    focal scleroderma of the hand case, 4: 183
    hand surgery fellowship, 4: 116*b*, 182
    Hands, 4: 183
    Harvard University Athletics Department and, 4: 183
    HMS appointment, 4: 183
    honors and awards, 4: 186
    New England Baptist Hospital and, 4: 183
    Occupational Disorders of the Upper Extremity, 4: 168, 183
    orthopaedics education and, 4: 186
    outcomes movement and, 4: 186
    PBBH and, 4: 163, 182
    professional memberships, 4: 186
    publications and research, 4: 182–185, *185*, 186
    RBBH and, 4: 182, 184
    residency rotations, 4: 182, 182*b*
    Richard J. Smith Lecture, 3: 431
    US Navy and, 4: 182
    West Roxbury Veterans Administration Hospital and, 4: 182–183
Simmons, C. C., 4: 102
Simmons College, 2: 213, 413
Simon, Michael A., 3: 435–436, *436*
Simon, Sheldon R. (1941–), 2: *405*
    Albert Einstein College of Medicine and, 2: 408
    Boston Children's Hospital and, 2: 406–407
    Brigham and Women's Hospital, 4: 163
    Cave Traveling Fellowship and, 1: 217*b*
    cerebral palsy research, 2: 406–407
    computer-simulated planning and, 2: 389
    education and training, 2: 405–406
    foot and ankle treatment, 2: 407
    gait research, 2: 406–408, 439
    Glimcher and, 2: 406
    HMS appointment, 2: 406–407
    honors and awards, 2: 406–407, 407*b*
    MGH and, 2: 406

Ohio State University School of Medicine and, 2: 407–408
orthopaedics appointments, 2: 408
PBBH and, 4: 163
Practical Biomechanics for the Orthopedic Surgeon, 3: 328
professional memberships, 2: 407, 407b
publications and research, 2: 406, 406, 407–408; 3: 326
RESNA and, 2: 408
study of Swiss method of treating fractures, 2: 406
West Roxbury Veterans Administration Hospital and, 2: 406
Simon, William H., 3: 377
Simpson, Sir James, 1: 84
69th Field Ambulance, 4: 405b
Skaggs, David, 2: 379
skeletogenesis, 2: 439
skiagraphy, 2: 16
Skillman, John J., 4: 251
skin grafts, 1: 75, 77; 3: 310; 4: 204, 216–217
Skoff, Hillel, 4: 263, 286
Sledge, Clement (1930–), 4: *126, 128, 133*
　AAOS and, 4: 139–141
　Affiliated Hospitals Center board and, 4: 119
　articular cartilage research, 4: 133, 136
　on avascular necrosis, 4: 238
　on Barr, 3: 213
　BIH Board of Consultants, 4: 262–263
　Boston Children's Hospital and, 2: 354–355
　Brigham Orthopaedic Foundation (BOF) and, 4: 123, 191
　Brigham Orthopedic Associates (BOA) and, 4: 123, 191
　BWH chair of orthopaedic surgery, 1: 180, 284; 4: 132–133, 143, 191–193, 195b–196b
　Children's Hospital/MGH combined program and, 1: 210; 4: 126
　chondrocyte metabolism in cell culture research, 4: 133
　on Codman, 4: 141
　on diastematomyelia, 2: 236
　education and training, 4: 125–127
　embryonic cartilage research, 4: 127, *127*
　Hip Society president, 4: 141
　HMS appointment, 4: 127
　honors and awards, 4: 142
　John Ball and Buckminster Brown Professorship, 3: 202; 4: 132, 195b
　joint replacement research and treatment, 4: 40, 133, *133*, 134–135, *135*
　knee arthroplasty and, 4: 129–130, 147, 149
　mandate to unify orthopaedics at Brigham Hospitals, 4: 116, 116b, 117–118
　Marion B. Gebbie Research Fellowship, 4: 127
　on merger of RBBH and PBBH, 4: 128
　as MGH honorary orthopaedic surgeon, 3: 398b
　MGH orthopaedics department and, 1: 210–211; 4: 127
　on orthopaedic basic and clinical research, 4: 141, *141*, 142
　as PBBH chief of orthopaedic surgery, 2: 269, 279; 4: 43, 115–117, 128–129, 132, 143, 191, 196b
　as PBBH orthopaedic surgery professor, 4: 43, 114–115
　publications and research, 4: 127, 129–130, *130*, 131, 133–139, *139*
　radiation synovectomy research, 4: 64, 136, *136*, 137
　RBBH board of overseers, 4: 132
　as RBBH chief of surgery, 2: 279; 4: 43, 115, 128–129, 131–132, 143, 191, 196b
　as RBBH orthopaedic surgery professor, 4: 43, 114–115
　as research fellow in orthopaedic surgery, 4: 126
　rheumatoid arthritis treatment, 4: 138–139
　Strangeways Research Laboratory fellowship, 4: 126
　US Navy and, 4: 125
Slipped Capital Femoral Epiphysis (Joplin et al.), 3: 294, 333
Slipped Capital Femoral Epiphysis (Klein et al.), 4: 238
slipped capital femoral epiphysis (SCFE)
　acetabular morphology in, 2: 392
　Howorth procedure and, 4: 243
　impingement treatment, 3: 189
　internal fixation of, 2: 176
　Klein's Line and, 4: 238–239, *239*
　open reduction of, 2: 168; 4: 237
　recommendations for, 2: 176
　research in, 3: 294, 331, 333; 4: 237–238, 243
　treatment of, 2: 137
　treatment outcomes, 2: 380
　use of roentgenology in, 3: 334
Slocum, Donald B., 1: 279
Slowick, Francis A., 2: 230
smallpox, 1: 8–9, 295; 2: 4
Smellie, William, 1: 6
Smith, Dale C., 4: 464
Smith, Ethan H., 3: 160b
Smith, Gleniss, 3: 427
Smith, H., 3: 210
Smith, H. W., 1: *31*
Smith, Homer B., 1: 253–254
Smith, Ida, 2: 431–432
Smith, J. V. C., 1: 97
Smith, Jacob, 3: 427
Smith, Job L., 2: 7
Smith, Lyman, 3: 254
Smith, Nellie, 3: 247
Smith, Richard J. (1930–1987), 3: *427, 428, 430*
　ASSH and, 3: 428–429, *430*
　death of, 3: 399, 429–430
　early life, 3: 427
　education and training, 3: 427
　factitious lymphedema case, 3: 429
　hand surgery and, 3: 385–386, 388t, 427–429, 460b
　HMS appointment, 3: 428
　Hospital for Joint Diseases and, 3: 413, 427
　legacy of, 3: 430–431
　Mankin on, 3: 427, 429–430
　as MGH surgeon, 3: 395, 398b, 413, 428
　professional memberships and, 3: 428, 430
　publications and research, 3: 427–429
　Smith Day lectures, 3: 431
　Tendon Transfers of the Hand and Forearm, 3: 428
Smith, Robert M., 2: 177, 234, 432
Smith, Rose, 3: 427
Smith, Theobold, 4: 6
Smith-Petersen, Evelyn Leeming, 3: 362
Smith-Petersen, Hilda Dickenson, 3: 198
Smith-Petersen, Kaia Ursin, 3: 179
Smith-Petersen, Marius N. (1886–1953), 3: *174, 179, 197, 198*
　AAOS and, 4: 337
　AAOS Fracture Committee and, 3: 191
　adjustable reamer and, 3: 317
　American Ambulance Hospital and, 4: *388, 389b, 390*

approach to wrist during arthrodesis, 3: 191
Brackett and, 3: 180–181
death of, 3: 198
early life, 3: 179
education and training, 3: 179–181
femoral neck fracture treatment, 3: 185–186, *186*, 189, *189b*, 190
femoral stem prothesis, 3: *293*
femoroacetabular impingement treatment, 3: 188–189
Harvard Surgical Unit and, 2: 119, 123–124; 3: 180, *180*, *370*
hip nailing and, 3: 237
hip surgery and, 3: 244
HMS appointment, 3: 183, 187, 192; 4: 59
innovation and, 3: 216–217
Knight's Cross, Royal Norwegian Order of St. Olav, 3: *198*
kyphosis treatment, 3: 239
legacy of, 3: 198–199
on Legg-Calve-Perthes disease, 2: 103
marriage and family, 3: 198
MGH Fracture Clinic and, 3: 60*b*, 315
MGH orthopaedics and, 1: 179, 189, 203–204; 2: 297; 3: 183, 269, 456*b*
as MGH orthopaedics chief, 3: 11*b*, 187–188, 191, 227, 375
MGH physical chemistry laboratory, 2: 322
military orthopaedics and, 4: 473
mold arthroplasty and, 3: 181, 183, 192, *192*, 193, 193*b*, 194, *194*, 195, *195*, 196, *196*, 198, 216, 238–239, 241, 292, 292*b*, 293
New England Rehabilitation Center and, 1: 272
orthopaedic surgery and, 1: 158
personality of, 3: 187–188
pillars of surgical care, 3: 187
private medical practice, 3: 183, 192
professional memberships and, 3: 197, 197*b*
publications and research, 2: 136; 3: 188, 192–193, 241–242, 302, 366
RBBH and, 4: 31, 36, 93, 111
sacroiliac joint treatment, 3: 183–185, 191
supra-articular subperiosteal approach to the hip, 3: 181, *181*, 182*b*
treatment of fractures, 3: 62
triflanged nail development, 3: 62, 185–186, *186*, 187, 189–190; 4: 237
World War II and, 3: 191
Smith-Petersen, Morten (1920–1999), 3: *361*
Children's Hospital/MGH combined program and, 3: 361
death of, 3: 362
early life, 3: 361
education and training, 3: 361
hip surgery and, 3: 362
HMS appointment, 3: 362
marriage and family, 3: 362
New England Baptist Hospital and, 3: 362
publications and research, 3: 362
Tufts appointment, 3: 362
US Naval Reserves and, 3: 361
Smith-Petersen, Morten, Sr., 3: 179
Smith-Petersen Foundation, 3: 198
Snedeker, Lendon, 2: 191
Snyder, Brian D. (1957–), 2: *409*
biomechanics research, 2: 410–411
Boston Children's Hospital and, 2: 409–411
Cerebral Palsy Clinic and, 2: 409
contrast-enhanced computed tomography and, 2: 411
education and training, 2: 409
fracture-risk research, 2: 411, *411*
HCORP and, 2: 409
HMS appointment, 2: 409
honors and awards, 2: 411
hospital appointments, 2: 409
modular spinal instrumentation device patents, 2: 412
orthopaedics appointments, 2: 409
professional memberships, 2: 412
publications and research, 2: 410, *410*, 411
Society for Medical Improvement, 3: 35
Society of Clinical Surgery, 3: 113*b*
Söderman, P., 3: 219
Sohier, Edward H., 1: 307, 310
Solomon, Dr., 4: 210
Soma Weiss Prize, 2: 319
somatosensory evoked potentials (SSEPs), 2: 342
Sons of Liberty, 1: 11, 13, 15–16
Soule, D., 2: 372
Southern Medical and Surgical Journal, 1: 63
Southmayd, William W., 1: 279; 4: 163, 193
Southwick, Wayne, 4: 258, 261
Soutter, Anne, 2: 292
Soutter, Charlotte Lamar, 2: 292
Soutter, D. R., 2: 34
Soutter, Helen E. Whiteside, 2: 292
Soutter, James, 2: 292
Soutter, Lamar, 2: 292, 293*b*
Soutter, Robert (1870–1933), 2: *292*, *293*
Boston Children's Hospital and, 2: 34, 292; 4: 338
Boston City Hospital and, 4: 305*b*
Bradford and, 2: 292, 297
cartilage transplantation, 2: 294
critique of shoes, 2: 293
death from blood poisoning, 2: 299, *299*
dislocated patella treatment, 2: 294–296
education and training, 2: 292
hip contracture treatment, 2: 294, 295*b*
hip disease treatment, 2: 293–294
HMS appointment, 2: 223, 298; 4: 59–60
hot pack treatment, 2: 264
letter to Catherine A. Codman, 1: *129*, 130
marriage and family, 2: 292, 293*b*
military surgeon training by, 2: 42, 66
New England Peabody Home for Crippled Children and, 2: 270, 292
orthopaedic device innovations, 2: 296–297
orthopaedic surgery and, 1: 171
orthopaedics appointments, 2: 292
professional memberships, 2: 292, 292*b*
"Progress in Orthopaedic Surgery" series, 2: 297
publications of, 2: 61, 293, 297
scoliosis treatment, 2: 296
surgical procedure innovations, 2: 294–296
Technique of Operations on the Bones, Joints, Muscles and Tendons, 2: 294, 297–298, *298*
Soutter, Robert, Jr., 2: 292
Soutter, Robert, Sr., 2: 292
Spalding, James Alfred, 1: 47, 49, 49*b*, 50
Spanier, Suzanne, 3: 390

Index

Spanish American War, 4: 310–311, *311*
Spanish Flu, 4: *11*
Sparks, Jared, 1: 310
Spaulding Rehabilitation Hospital, 1: 217, 225; 3: 387–388, 396, 426, 461
Spear, Louis M., 4: 23, 26–28, 31–32, 45, 79
"Special Orthopedic Hospital–Past and Present, The" (Platt), 1: 114
Spector, Myron, 4: 194, 195*b*
Speed, Kellogg, 4: *319*
Spencer, Herbert, 4: 466–467
Spencer, Hillard, 2: 367
Spencer, Upshur, 4: 190*b*
spina bifida
    Lovett on, 2: 51–52
    research in, 2: 370
    ruptures of sac, 2: 309–310
    treatment of, 2: 51–52
    University of Massachusetts clinic, 2: 364
Spinal Deformity Study Group, 2: 365
spinal dysgenesis, 2: 366
spinal fusion wake-up test, 2: 340–342
Spinal Surgery Service (Children's Hospital), 2: 359
spinal taps, 2: 72, 78
spinal tuberculosis, 1: *109*
    operative treatment for, 4: 343
    pediatric patients, 2: 11, 308–309; 3: 289
    research in, 3: 289
    treatment of, 1: 100, 106, 108–109; 2: 308–309; 4: 225
spine. *See also* scoliosis
    advances in, 2: 338
    anterior and posterior procedures, 2: 343–345, 360, 366; 3: 426
    apparatus for, 1: 107; 2: *35, 36*
    athletes and, 2: 385
    benefits of, 2: 373
    Boston Children's Hospital and, 2: 337–338, 338*t*
    Bradford Frame and, 2: 30
    cerebral palsy and, 2: 370
    children and, 1: 123; 2: 385
    closed reduction of lumbar facture-dislocation, 3: 347
    community-based physicians and, 2: 373
    computed tomography and, 3: 254
    congenital absence of the odontoid process, 3: 340
    degenerative stenosis, 4: 269–270
    Down syndrome and, 2: 370
    Dwyer instrumentation and, 2: 336
    for early-onset, 2: 360
    fractures and dislocations, 3: 349*b*, *349*
    fusion in tubercular, 3: 148–149, 157–158, 158*b*; 4: 343
    halo-vest apparatus, 4: *152*, 153
    Harrington rods and, 2: 316, 325, 335–336, 338
    Hibbs spinal fusion procedure, 2: 164; 3: 155
    instability of lower cervical, 4: 261
    interpedicular segmental fixation (ISF) pedicle screw plate, 3: 420–421
    lumbar spinal stenosis, 2: 373–374
    measurement of, 2: *31*
    mental attitude and, 3: 349*b*
    MRI and, 3: 255
    myelodysplasia, 2: 359
    neurologic effects after surgery, 4: 269
    nutritional status and, 2: 361–362
    open anterior lumbosacral fracture dislocation, 3: 420, 425
    paraplegia and, 3: 319
    pedicle screws in, 2: 343; 3: 420
    posterior segment fixator (PSF), 3: 420
    Pott's Disease, 1: 97, 108–109; 3: 148–150
    pressure and pain, 2: 271
    prosthetic titanium rib and, 2: 360, *362*
    research in, 2: 343
    sacrococcygeal chordoma, 3: 390
    Scheuermann kyphosis, 2: 343, 359
    somatosensory evoked potentials (SSEPs), 2: 342
    spinal dysgenesis, 2: 366
    spinal fusion, 2: 271, 334–335, *335*, 343, 369; 3: 207–208
    spinal fusion wake-up test, 2: 340–342
    spinal height increases, 2: 367
    spondylolisthesis, 3: 421
    strengthening exercises for, 1: 100
    study of, 2: 57, *57*, 58, *58*, 59
    thoracic insufficiency syndrome, 2: 360
    tibial fracture, 4: 365
    treatment of, 1: 97–98, 100, 106; 2: 359; 4: 152
    vertebral column resections (VCRs), 2: 362–363
Spine Care Medical Group, 4: 263
Spine Patient Outcomes Research Trial (SPORT), 2: 371, 373
Spitzer, Hans, 2: 80
splints
    for drop-foot deformity, 4: *418*
    Eames molded plywood leg, 4: *470*
    first aid, 4: *418*
    Jones splints, 4: 389, 411
    manufacture of, 3: *167*, 168
    military orthopaedics and, 2: 120; 4: 389, 408–409, 416–417, *418*
    standardization of, 3: 167–168
    Thomas, 2: 20, *123*, 257; 3: *168*; 4: 389, *391*, *408*, 409, 411, 417, *418*
    use during transportation, 3: 169, 169*b*; 4: 389
sports medicine. *See also* Harvard athletics
    acromioclavicular joint dislocation in, 1: 268, 277
    acute ligament injuries, 1: 277–278
    ankle injuries and, 1: 281
    assessment and treatment in, 1: 274
    athlete heart size, 1: 262, 267, 288
    athletic training and, 1: 248, 250–251, 258, 265–266
    BCH clinic for, 2: 287, 384
    caring for athletic injuries, 1: 268
    concussions in, 1: 247, 254, 275, 286–287; 2: 385
    dieticians and, 1: 258
    fatigue and, 1: 264–265
    foot and ankle treatment, 3: 348
    football injuries and, 1: 247–248, 252–255, 255*t*, 256, 258–262, 288
    frozen shoulder, 1: 277–278
    guidelines for team physicians, 1: 287
    Harvard athletics and, 2: 287
    ice hockey and, 1: 275, 286
    injury prevention and, 1: 265, 285–286
    knee joint injuries, 1: 267–268, 268*t*, 278–279, 285–287
    knee problems and, 2: 387
    MGH and, 3: 397
    Morton's neuroma, 2: 287
    musculoskeletal injuries, 1: 288
    myositis ossificans and, 1: 266–267
    neuromusculoskeletal genius and, 1: 279

orthopaedics curriculum and, 1: 165–166
pediatric, 2: 287, 385–387
physical therapy and, 3: 348
preventative strappings, 1: *269*, 274
professional teams and, 3: 348, 356–357, 397, 399, 448, 450
progress in, 1: 267
reconditioning and, 1: 271
rehabilitation and, 1: 275
scientific study of, 1: 250–251, 254–256, 262, 267–269, 277–278
spinal problems, 2: 385
sports teams and, 1: 248, 250–251
tenosynovitis of the flexor hallucis longus, 3: 348
torn meniscus, 1: 278
women basketball players and, 1: 285–286
Sports Medicine Bible for Young Adults, The (Micheli), 2: 385
Sports Medicine Bible, The (Micheli), 2: 385, *385*
Sports Medicine Fund, 2: 439*b*
Sports Medicine Service (MGH), 3: 356
Sprengel deformity, 2: 195, *196*
spring muscle test, 2: 70, *70*, 71
Springfield, Dempsey S. (1945–), 1: *242*; 3: *431*
  allograft research and, 3: 433, 435
  Association of Bone and Joint Surgeons and, 3: 436
  education and training, 3: 431–432
  Gaucher hemorrhagic bone cyst case, 3: 434
  HCORP and, 1: 242–243; 3: 435
  HMS appointment, 3: 432
  honors and awards, 3: 431, 436
  limb salvage surgery and, 3: 433
  as MGH surgeon, 3: 432
  Mount Sinai Medical School and, 3: 435
  Musculoskeletal Tumor Society and, 3: 436
  orthopaedic oncology and, 3: 399, 432, 435, 460*b*
  orthopaedics education and, 3: 435–436
  publications and research, 3: 432–433, 435–436
  on resident surgical case requirements, 3: 435–436, *436*
  Shands Hospital and, 3: 432
  surgical treatment of osteosarcoma, 3: 432–433
  University of Florida and, 3: 432
  US Army and, 3: 432
Spunkers, 1: 21, 32, 133
Spurling, Ina, 2: 144, 166
St. Anthony Hospital, 2: 111
St. Botolph Club (Boston), 2: *284*
St. George's Hospital, 1: 81, 83, 106
St. Louis Children's Hospital, 3: 165
St. Louis Shriners Hospital for Crippled Children, 3: 173
St. Luke's Home for Convalescents, 2: *307*
St. Luke's Hospital (New York), 2: 5, 20
St. Margaret's and Mary's Infant Asylum, 2: 256
St. Mary's Hospital (Nairobi, Kenya), 3: 379
St. Thomas's Hospital, 1: 37
Stack, Herbert, 2: 249
Stagnara, P., 2: 340
Staheli, Lynn, 2: 302; 4: 250
Stamp Act, 1: 11–13
Stamp Act Congress, 1: 13
Stanish, William, 2: 423
Stanton, Edwin, 3: 43
Staples, Mable Hughes, 3: 362
Staples, Nellie E. Barnes, 3: 362
Staples, O. Sherwin (1908–2002)
  Boston Children's Hospital and, 2: 438
  Children's Hospital/MGH combined program and, 3: 362
  Dartmouth Medical School appointment, 3: 363–364
  death of, 3: 364
  early life, 3: 362
  education and training, 3: 362
  on Edwin Cave, 3: 276
  as first orthopaedic surgeon in NH, 3: 363–364
  marriage and family, 3: 362
  Mary Hitchcock Memorial Hospital and, 3: 363–364
  as MGH surgeon, 3: 74, 362
  New England Peabody Home for Crippled Children and, 3: 362
  on osteochondritis in a finger, 3: 363
  private medical practice, 3: 271, 362
  publications and research, 3: 362
  6th General Hospital and, 4: 482
  White River Junction VA Hospital, 3: 364
  World War II service, 3: 362
Staples, Oscar S., Sr., 3: 362

Star and Garter Hospital, 4: 402
State Hospital School for Children (Canton), 2: 308
Statement by Four Physicians, 2: 6, *6*, *7*
Steadman, Richard, 3: 446
Steadman Hawkins Clinic, 2: 378
Stearns, Peter N., 3: 83
Steele, Glenn, 4: 279
Steele, Mrs., 4: *128*
Steindler, Arthur, 2: 94; 3: 303; 4: 362
Steiner, Mark, 1: 217*b*, 289; 4: 194, 195*b*
Steinmann pin, 2: 237–238; 4: 166
Stelling, Frank H., 2: 351; 4: 19
Stephen J. Lipson, MD Orthopaedic and Spine lectureship, 4: 272, 272*b*
Stern, Peter, 3: 431
Stern, Walter, 1: xxiv
stethoscope, 1: 74
Stevens, James H., 2: 96, 415; 3: 109
Stevens, Samuel, 1: 6
Stevens, W. L., 3: 133
Stillman, Charles F., 2: 50–51
Stillman, J. Sidney, 4: 37, 40, 79
Stillman, James, 2: 253
Stillman Infirmary, 2: 253, *254*
Still's disease, 2: 171
Stimson, Lewis A., 1: 147
Stinchfield, Allan, 3: 332
Stinchfield, Frank, 3: 275
Stirrat, Craig, 4: 194, 195*b*
Stone, James S., 2: 146, 230, 307, 438; 4: 310
Stone, James W., 1: 308
Storer, D. Humphries, 3: 42
Storey, Elizabeth Moorfield, 2: 80
Strammer, Myron A., 4: 208*b*
Strangeways Research Laboratory, 4: 126
Stromeyer, Georg Friedrich Louis, 1: xxiii, 101, 105–106
Strong, Richard P., 4: 389*b*, 422*b*
Stryker, William, 3: 249; 4: 246
Stubbs, George, 1: *136*
Study in Hospital Efficiency, A (Codman), 3: 125, *125*, 127*b*, 128–131
Sturdevant, Charles L. (b. ca. 1913)
  Boston Children's Hospital and, 2: 299
  Crippled Children's Clinic and, 2: 299
  education and training, 2: 299
  HMS appointment, 2: 299
  Marlborough Medical Associates and, 2: 146, 269, 299

MGH orthopaedics residency, 3: 74
PBBH and, 4: 18–20, 110
publication contributions, 2: 300
Sturgis, Susan, 3: 30
Sturgis, William, 3: 30
subacromial bursitis, 3: 104–105, 108–109
subdeltoid bursa, 3: 95, 98, 103–105, 108
Subjective Knee Form (IKDC), 2: 381
Subjective Shoulder Scale, 2: 380
subscapularis tendon, 2: 95, *95*
subtrochanteric osteotomy, 2: 293
Such a Joy for a Yiddish Boy (Mankin), 3: 392, *392*
suction socket prosthesis, 1: 273
Suffolk District Medical Society, 3: 120–122
Sugar Act, 1: 11
Suk, Se Il, 2: 343
Sullivan, James T., 4: 233
Sullivan, Louis, 4: 266*b*
Sullivan, Patricia, 3: 460*b*
Sullivan, Robert, 1: 317
Sullivan, Russell F. (1893–1966), 4: *343*
BCH Bone and Joint Service, 4: 343–344, 346, 380*b*
Boston City Hospital and, 4: 307
Boston Red Sox and, 4: 345
Carney Hospital and, 4: 343
death of, 4: 346
education and training, 4: 343
elbow joint fracture-dislocation case, 4: 345
Lahey Clinic and, 4: 345
marriage and family, 4: 346
Melrose Hospital and, 4: 343
private medical practice, 4: 344
professional memberships, 4: 346
publications and research, 4: 343, 344*b*
spinal tuberculosis research, 4: 343, 344*b*
Ted Williams and, 4: 345–346
Tufts Medical School appointment, 4: 343
Sullivan, Thelma Cook, 4: 346
Sullivan, W. E., 3: 86
Sumner Koch Award, 2: 415
Sunnybrook Hospital, 2: 334
SUNY Downstate Medical Center, 3: 388
supraspinatus tendon, 3: 108–109
Surgeon's Journal, A (Cushing), 3: 369
surgery. *See also* orthopaedic surgery
abdominal, 1: 81
antisepsis principles and, 1: 85, 141
Astley Cooper and, 1: 34, 36, 42, 44
Clavien-Dindo classification in, 2: 393
Coll Warren and, 1: 81–84
early training in, 1: 183–186
fracture care and, 4: 463–464
general anesthesia and, 1: 141
HMS curriculum for, 1: 140–141
infection from dirty, 3: 60
Jack Warren and, 1: 22–23, 25, 29, 40
John Collins Warren and, 1: 36–37, 53, 68
Joseph Warren and, 1: 6, 9, 15
long-bone fractures, 3: 60–61
pedagogy and, 1: 34, 137–138
plastic, 1: 71, 76–77
Richard Warren and, 1: 90
shoulder and, 1: 29
use of ether, 1: 55–65
Surgery (Keen), 3: 103
Surgery (Richard Warren), 1: 90
Surgery of Joints, The (Lovett and Nichols), 2: 52
Surgical After-Treatment (Crandon and Ehrenfried), 4: 217, *217*
surgical instruments, 3: 40–41
Surgical Observations with Cases and Operations (J. M. Warren), 1: 47, 75, 78
Surgical Treatment of the Motor-Skeletal System (Bancroft), 3: 316
Sutterlin, C. E., 3: 420
Sutton, Silvia Barry, 3: 259
Suzedell, Eugene, 2: 233
Swaim, Caroline Tiffany Dyer, 4: 51
Swaim, Joseph Skinner, 4: 51
Swaim, Loring T. (1882–1964), 4: *51*
American Rheumatism Association and, 4: 57–58
Arthritis, Medicine and the Spiritual Law, 4: 58, *58*
back pain research and, 3: 203
Body Mechanics in Health and Disease, 4: 53
Buchmanism and, 4: 57
chronic arthritis growth disturbances case, 4: 56
chronic arthritis treatment and, 4: 54–58
chronic disease treatment and, 4: 52–53
Clifton Springs Sanatorium and, 3: 88; 4: 52–53
death of, 4: 40, 59
early life, 4: 51
education and training, 4: 52
HMS appointment, 2: 223; 4: 57, 59–60
on importance of posture, 4: 52–54
marriage and family, 4: 59
MGH and, 3: 269; 4: 52, 54
Moral Re-Armament program and, 4: 57
on patient care, 4: 54, 55*b*, 58
private medical practice, 4: 53
professional memberships, 4: 58–59
publications and research, 2: 136, 297; 3: 91; 4: 52–55, 57–58, 60–61
RBBH and, 4: 93, 406
as RBBH chief of orthopaedics, 4: 48, 55–57, 79, 196*b*
RBBH orthopaedic surgeon, 4: 28, 31, 33, 35, 63
rehabilitation of soldiers and, 4: 444
World War I and, 4: 54
Swaim, Madeline K. Gill, 4: 59
Swartz, R. Plato, 2: 438
Sweet, Elliot, 3: 242, 243*b*
Sweetland, Ralph, 3: 396
Swinton, Neil, 2: 232
Swiontkowski, Marc, 2: 424–425
Syme, James, 1: 56, 84
synovectomy, 4: 64, 102, 371–372
synovial fluid, 3: 174, *174*, 175
syringes, 1: 80, *80*
System of Surgery (Holmes), 1: 81
systemic lupus erythematosus (SLE), 4: 98
systemic sclerosis, 4: 98

T

Tachdjian, Jason, 2: 305
Tachdjian, Mihran O. (1927–1996), 2: *300*
birth palsies research, 2: 417
Boston Children's Hospital and, 2: 301–302
cerebral palsy treatment, 2: 300–301, *301*
Children's Memorial Hospital (Chicago) and, 2: 302
course on congenital hip dysplasia, 2: 302
death of, 2: 305
education and training, 2: 300
Green and, 2: 301–304
honors and awards, 2: 305*b*
intraspinal tumors in children case, 2: 301–302
marriage and family, 2: 305

Northwestern University and, 2: 302
PBBH and, 4: 20
Pediatric Orthopaedic International Seminars program, 2: 304
Pediatric Orthopaedic Society and, 2: 351
pediatric orthopaedics and, 2: 300–304
Pediatric Orthopedics, 2: 188, 303, *303*
professional memberships, 2: 304, 305*b*
publications and research, 2: 300–303, 303*b*, 304
Tachdjian, Vivian, 2: 305
Taft, Katherine, 4: 286
Taitsman, Lisa, 4: 190*b*
tarsectomy, 2: 23
Taylor, Charles Fayette, 1: 107; 2: 20, 22, 26, 47
Taylor back brace, 2: 247
Tea Act, 1: 15
Technique of Operations on the Bones, Joints, Muscles and Tendons (Soutter), 2: 294, 297–298, *298*
Tegner Activity Scale, 2: 380
teleroentgenography, 2: 170, 170*t*
Temperance Society, 1: 40
tendon transfers
    ankles and, 2: 148
    flexor carpi ulnaris transfer procedure, 2: 172, 188, *199*
    hands and forearms, 3: 428
    iliotibial band and, 2: 109
    Ober on, 2: 147–149
    obstetrical paralysis and, 2: 96
    patella, 2: 294
    polio and, 2: 108–109
    polio patient lower extremities, 2: 265; 3: 332–333
    quadriplegic patient hands and, 2: 265
    Trendelenburg limp and, 2: 108, *108*
    for wrist flexion and pronation deformity, 2: 172
Tendon Transfers of the Hand and Forearm (Smith), 3: 428
tenosynovitis, 2: 89; 3: 315, 414, 438
tenotomy
    Achilles, 1: 100–101, 106; 2: 25
    club foot and, 1: 106, 118; 2: 25–26
    early study of, 1: xxiii, 100
    Guérin's, 1: 118
    physical therapy and, 1: 100
    Stromeyer's subcutaneous, 1: 118, *118*
    technique for, 1: 100–101
Terrono, A., 4: 167
Textbook of Disorders and Injuries of the Musculoskeletal System (Salter), 1: 167
Textbook of Orthopedic Surgery for Students of Medicine (Sever), 2: 92, *93*
thalidomide, 2: 334, *334*
Thane, George D., 2: 242
Thayer General Hospital, 4: 241, *241*
Theodore, George H. (1965–), 3: *437*
    education and training, 3: 437
    extracorporeal shockwave therapy (ESWT) research, 3: 437–438, *438*
    foot and ankle treatment, 3: 460*b*
    HCORP and, 3: 437
    HMS appointment, 3: 437
    as MGH clinical faculty, 3: 464*b*
    as MGH surgeon, 3: 348, 437
    plantar fasciitis treatment, 3: 437–438
    professional sports teams and, 3: 348
    publications and research, 3: 437–438
Theodore, Harry, 3: 437
Theodore, Marie, 3: 437
Therapeutic Exercise and Massage (Bucholz), 3: 269
Thibodeau, Arthur, 4: 91, 95, 333, 378
Thilly, William G., 4: 171
Thomas, Charles, 4: 187
Thomas, Claudia L., 4: 266*b*
Thomas, Hugh Owen, 1: xxiii; 2: 20, 22, 116
Thomas, John Jenks, 2: 90
Thomas, Leah C., 4: *235*, 236
Thomas, Margaret, 4: 189
Thomas, William H. (1930–2011), 4: *187*
    Brigham and Women's Hospital, 4: 163, 187
    Brigham Orthopedic Associates (BOA) and, 4: 123
    Children's Hospital/MGH combined program and, 4: 187
    death of, 4: 189
    education and training, 4: 187
    Florida Civil Air Patrol and, 4: 189
    on foot surgery and rheumatoid arthritis, 4: 188, *188*, 189
    HMS appointment, 4: 187–188
    honors and awards, 4: 189
    marriage and family, 4: 189
    on McKeever and MacIntosh prostheses, 4: 188–189
    MGH and, 4: 187
    PBBH and, 4: 116, 128–129, 161, 163, 187
    publications and research, 4: 69, 70*b*–71*b*, 134, 187–188, *189*
    RBBH and, 4: 40, 68, 116*b*, 129, 131, 187–188
    rheumatoid clinic and, 4: 188
    West Roxbury Veterans Administration Hospital and, 4: 187
Thomas B. Quigley Society, 1: *282*, 283
Thomas splint, 2: 20, *123*, 247; 3: *168*; 4: 389, *391*, *408*, 409, 411, 417, *418*
Thompson, Milton, 3: 192
Thompson, Sandra J. (1937–2003), 2: *412*, 413
    arthritis clinic and, 2: 413
    Boston Children's Hospital and, 2: 413
    death of, 2: 414
    education and training, 2: 412–413
    HMS appointment, 2: 413
    humanitarianism and, 2: 413
    Laboratory for Skeletal Disorders and Rehabilitation and, 2: 413
    pediatric orthopaedics and, 2: 414
    professional memberships, 2: 413–414
    prosthetic clinic and, 2: 413
    publications of, 2: 414
    Ruth Jackson Orthopaedic Society and, 2: 413
    Simmons College and, 2: 413
Thomson, Elihu, 2: 114; 3: 97–98
Thomson, Helen, 1: 317
thoracic insufficiency syndrome, 2: 360
thoracic outlet syndrome, 3: 415
thoracic spine, 4: 259–260
thoracostomy, 2: 360
Thorn, George W., 4: 79
Thorndike, Alice, 2: 312
Thorndike, Augustus (1863–1940), 2: *305*
    address to the American Orthopaedic Association, 2: 311
    Bar Harbor Medical and Surgical Hospital and, 2: 312
    Boston Children's Hospital and, 2: 34, 40, 307
    Boston Dispensary and, 2: 306

Index

Boston Lying-in-Hospital and, 2: 306
death of, 2: 312
disabled children and, 2: 307–308
education and training, 2: 305–306
hip infection treatment, 2: 108
HMS appointment, 2: 307
House of the Good Samaritan and, 2: 114, 115*b*, 306
Manual of Orthopedic Surgery, A, 2: 311, *312*
marriage and family, 2: 312
MGH and, 2: 306
on orthopaedic supervision in schools and sports, 2: 310
orthopaedic surgery and, 1: 171; 2: 311
poliomyelitis treatment, 2: 264
professional memberships, 2: 306–307, 312
publications and research, 2: 61, 308–309
rupture of the spina bifida sac case, 2: 309–310
schools for disabled children, 2: 36, 38, 308, 310–311; 3: 151
St. Luke's Home for Convalescents, 2: 307
tuberculosis treatment, 2: 308
Thorndike, Augustus, Jr. (1896–1986), 1: *263, 270*; 3: *450*; 4: *491*
on acromioclavicular joint dislocation in football, 1: 268
AMA Committee on the Medical Aspects of Sports, 1: 274, 280
Athlete's Bill of Rights and, 1: 279–281
Athletic Injuries. Prevention, Diagnosis and Treatment, 1: 265, *266*
Boston Children's Hospital and, 1: 264
clinical congress meeting, 3: 118
education and training, 1: 263–264
5th General Hospital and, 4: 484
first aid kit, 1: *270*
Harvard Department of Hygiene and, 2: 253
Harvard football team and, 1: 259, 263
Harvard University Health Service and, 1: 274, 277
legacy of, 1: 274–275
Manual of Bandaging, Strapping and Splinting, A, 1: 268
Massachusetts Regional Fracture Committee, 3: 64
military orthopaedics and, 1: 270–272
New England Regional Committee on Fractures, 4: 341
105th General Hospital and, 4: 489–491
preventative strappings, 1: *269*, 274
publications of, 1: 263–268, 271–274, 280–281
rehabilitation and, 1: 271–274
sports medicine and, 1: 264–269, 274–275
study of fracture treatment, 1: 264
suction socket prosthesis and, 1: 273
34th Infantry Division and, 4: 484
World War II active duty and, 1: 270–272; 2: 232; 4: 17
World War II civilian defense and, 1: 269–270
Thorndike, Charles, 3: 338
Thorndike, George, 4: 297
Thorndike, Olivia Lowell, 1: 263
Thorndike, William, 4: 297
Thornhill, Thomas S.
Brigham and Women's Hospital and, 4: 143, 163, 193–194, 195*b*
as BWH orthopaedics chief, 4: 172, 196*b*
John Ball and Buckminster Brown Professorship, 4: 195*b*
New England Deaconess Hospital and, 4: 280
PFC unicompartmental knee prothesis and, 4: 176–177
publications and research, 4: 180, *180*
Thrasher, Elliott, 2: 277, 290
Three Star Medal of Honour, 3: 451, *451*
thrombocytopenia, 3: 434
tibia
anterolateral bowing of, 2: 173
congenital pseudarthrosis of, 2: 173–176
pseudofracture of, 3: 341, *342*
tibial tubercle
lesions during adolescence, 2: 115, *116*, 117
nonunion of the humerus, 2: 96, *96*, 97, *97*
Osgood-Schlatter disease and, 2: 115, *116*, 117
Sever's study of, 2: 91, 96–97
treatment of, 2: 91, 96
Ticker, Jonathan B., 3: *145*
Tobin, William J., 3: 74
Toby, William, 4: 266*b*
Toldt, C., 2: 170
Tomaselli, Rosario, 4: 41*b*
Tomford, William W. (1945–), 3: *439, 461*
adult reconstruction and, 3: 460*b*
articular cartilage preservation research, 3: 442, *442*
on bone bank procedures, 3: 440–441, *442*
Children's Hospital/MGH combined program and, 3: 439
early life, 3: 439
education and training, 3: 439
HMS appointments, 3: 440, 440*b*
leadership of, 3: 443
MGH Bone Bank and, 3: 396, 439–441, 443
as MGH clinical faculty, 3: 464*b*
as MGH orthopaedics chief, 3: 11*b*, 228, 399, 443
as MGH surgeon, 3: 398*b*, 440, 440*b*
Musculoskeletal Tissue Banking, 3: 443
Naval Medical Research Institute and, 3: 439
orthopaedic oncology and, 3: 440
orthopaedic tumor fellowship program and, 3: 388
publications and research, 3: 440–443
rapid postoperative osteolysis in Paget Disease case, 3: 441
tissue banks and, 3: 386
transmission of disease through allografts research, 3: 442–443, *443*
US Navy and, 3: 439
Toom, Robert E., 2: 408
Toronto General Hospital, 2: 334
torticollis brace, 1: *99*, 100, *124*
Tosteson, Daniel, 4: 119
Total Care of Spinal Cord Injuries, The (Pierce and Nickel), 3: 321
total condylar prosthesis, 4: 130
total hip replacement
bladder fistula after, 4: 162
bone stock deficiency in, 3: 279
cemented/uncemented, 3: 223–224
Charnley and, 3: 218–219
Gibson posterior approach, 4: 170
Harris and hybrid, 3: 220
Hylamer acetabular liner complications, 4: *171*, 172
infections and, 4: 170
introduction to the U.S., 3: 218

osteoarthritis and, 3: 221, *222*
osteolysis after, 3: 220, *220*, 221–222, *222*, 223, 225
patient outcomes, 4: 134–135
pelvic osteolysis with acetabular replacement, 3: 279
radiographs of uncemented, 3: *223*
RBBH and, 4: 129
renal transplant infarction case, 4: 252–253
rheumatoid arthritis complications, 4: 134
sensitivity to heparin and, 3: 362
surgeon preferences in, 4: 170*b*
trochanteric osteotomy in, 4: 133–134
ultraviolet light and, 4: 162
use of bone ingrowth type prostheses, 3: 222–223
use of methylmethacrylate (bone cement), 3: 220, 222; 4: 129, 133, 171
total joint replacement
  BWH registry for, 4: 141, *172*, 173
  continuing medical education and, 3: 225
  implant design, 4: 137–138
  infection rates, 4: 164
  metals for use in, 2: 234
  patellofemoral joint, 4: 137
  patient outcomes and, 3: 277; 4: 134
  proximal femoral grafts and, 3: 435
  research in, 3: 326; 4: 133–134, 136
  tibial component fixation, 4: 137, 148
  ultraviolet light and, 4: 164
Total Knee Arthroplasty (Scott), 4: 176
total knee replacement
  Duocondylar prostheses and, 4: 178
  duopatellar prosthesis, 4: 180*t*
  gait and, 2: 408
  giant cell synovitis case, 4: 148
  inflammatory reactions, 3: 223
  kinematic, 4: 138–139
  Kinematic prosthesis, 4: 138–139, *139*, 147, 149–150
  Maine Medical Assessment Foundation, 2: 372
  McKeever prosthesis, 4: 40, 130
  metal and polyethylene prosthesis, 4: 147–148, *148*
  metallic tibial tray fracture, 4: 177

osteoarthritis and, 4: 177
preservation of PCL, 4: 130, 138–139, 147, 180–181
press-fit condylar knee (PFC), 4: 180, 180*t*
prosthesis development, 4: 137, 179*t*
at RBBH, 1950–1978, 4: 131*t*
research in, 4: 133, 135
roentgenographic arthroplasty-scoring system, 4: 150
soft tissue balancing and, 4: 139
tibial component fixation, 4: 148
tourniquet, 1: 55
Towle, Chris, 3: 386
Townsend, Nadine West, 3: 300
Townsend, Solomon Davis, 1: 59; 3: 14, 18, *31*
Townshend, Charles, 1: 13
Townshend Acts, 1: 13–15
tracheostomy, 2: 49, 51
traction
  Buck's, 1: 80
  continuous, 1: 108; 2: 32
  femoral neck fractures and, 3: 186, 189–190
  flexion injuries and, 3: 348–349
  for fractures and limb deformities, 2: 23, 25
  halo-femoral, 2: 342, 344, 399
  hip disease and, 2: 21–22, 32–33, 52–54; 3: 148
  lumbar fracture-dislocation and, 3: 347
  modification of, 2: 27
  reductions of dislocations and, 1: 10, *43*, 44, 52, 68
  scoliosis and, 2: 35, 296–297
  slipped capital femoral epiphysis (SCFE) and, 2: 176
  Sprengel deformity and, 2: 195–196
  Thomas splint, 3: *168*, 169
Tracy, Edward A., 4: 204
Trahan, Carol, 3: 386, 392
Training Administrators of Graduate Medical Education (TAGME), 1: 238
transmetatarsal amputation, 4: 276
trauma
  acute compartment syndrome of the thigh and, 3: 417
  amputations and, 3: 373
  bone cysts and, 2: 236
  cartilaginous labrum and, 3: 352
  in children, 2: 359, 365, 368, 378, 385
  coxa plana, 2: 104
  to the epiphysis, 2: 176, 193

fracture treatment and, 4: 339*b*–340*b*
fractures of the radial head and, 2: 396–397
hip dislocations, 2: 352–353
ischemia-edema cycle and, 2: 200
laparotomy and, 3: 55
lesions of the atlas and axis, 2: 117
military orthopaedics and, 3: 274, 301; 4: 393
olecranon fractures and, 3: 309
orthopaedic surgery and, 3: 220, 275, 376, 416; 4: 393
paralysis and, 2: 71
Sever's disease and, 2: 88–89
sports injuries and, 2: 279, 385
thoracic spine and, 4: 259
tibial tubercle and, 2: 115
treatment deficiencies, 4: 349
Trauma Management (Cave, et al.), 3: 62, 253, 273
Travis, Dorothy F., 2: 324
Travis Air Force Base, 3: 337
Treadwell, Ben, 3: 386
Treatise on Dislocations and Fractures of Joints, A (Cooper), 1: 35, 36, *42*, *43*
Treatise on Orthopaedic Surgery, A (Bradford and Lovett), 1: 108; 2: 29–30, *30*, 43, 50, *50*, 51
Treatise on the Disease of Infancy and Childhood (Smith), 2: 7
Treatment of Fractures, The (Scudder), 1: 147; 3: 55–56, *57*, *58*, 64, 99; 4: 312, 350
"Treatment of Infantile Paralysis, The" (Lovett), 2: 71
Tremont Street Medical School, 3: 26, 42
Trendelenburg limp, 2: 33, 108, *108*, 151
triceps
  brachioradialis transfer for weakness, 2: 148, 153–154, *154*
  tendon repair, 3: 309
  transfers for deltoid muscle paralysis, 2: 230
triflanged nail, 3: 62, 185–186, *186*, 187, 189, 189*b*, 190; 4: 237
triple arthrodesis
  foot deformities and, 2: 197, 228–229
  heel-cord lengthening and, 2: 172
  modification of, 2: 180–181
  Ober and, 2: 149
  stabilization of polio patients by, 2: 265

Index

tendon transplantations and, 3: 333
weakness/paralysis of the foot and ankle, 2: 150–151
Trippel, Stephen B. (1948–), 3: *444*
  adult reconstruction and, 3: 460*b*
  articular cartilage research, 3: 445
  Cave Traveling Fellowship and, 1: 217*b*
  education and training, 3: 444
  Gordon Research Conference and, 3: 445
  growth-plate chondrocytes research, 3: *444*, 445
  HCORP and, 3: *444*
  HMS appointment, 3: 444–445
  as MGH clinical faculty, 3: 464*b*
  as MGH surgeon, 3: 444–445
  professional memberships and, 3: 445
  publications and research, 3: 444–445
  University of Indiana School of Medicine and, 3: 445
trochanteric osteotomy, 4: 133, 145
Trott, Arthur W. (1920–2002), 2: *179*, 313–314
  AAOS and, 2: 314
  Boston Children's Hospital and, 2: 233, 301, 313–316
  Boston polio epidemic and, 2: 314–315
  Brigham and Women's Hospital and, 4: 163, 193
  on circulatory changes in poliomyelitis, 2: 264
  Crippled Children's Clinic and, 2: 314
  death of, 2: 318
  education and training, 2: 313
  Foot and Ankle, The, 2: 317
  foot and ankle treatment, 2: 316–317
  Green and, 2: 177, 286, 317–318
  on Grice, 2: 214
  Korean War and, 2: 313
  March of Dimes and, 2: 315
  marriage and family, 2: 313
  military service, 2: 313
  as naval hospital surgical consultant, 2: 313–314
  PBBH and, 2: 313; 4: 19–20, 22, 116, 128, 163
  poliomyelitis research and treatment, 2: 190, 314, *314*, 315–316
  private medical practice and, 2: 313
  publications and research, 4: 243
  publications of, 2: 316–317
Trott, Dorothy Crawford, 2: 313, 318
Trout, S., 2: 417
Trowbridge, William, 2: 114
Truax, R., 1: 15
Trumble, Hugh C., 3: 367
Trumble, Thomas E., 3: 431
Trumbull, John, 1: *19*
Trumbull Hospital, 4: 225
Truslow, Walter, 2: 84; 3: 229
Tseng, Victor, 1: 217*b*
tuberculosis. *See also* spinal tuberculosis
  amputations and, 3: 374
  bone and joint, 2: 11, 16, 25, 308–309; 3: 148, 166
  decline due to milk pasteurization, 2: 16
  hip disease and, 2: 21–22
  of hips, 2: 52–53, *54*
  infected joints and, 1: 61, 73, 75, 81; 4: 225
  of the knee, 1: 73; 4: 225
  mortality due to, 2: 4
  open-air treatment of, 4: 363, 367
  pulmonary, 1: 56; 2: 16
  sacroiliac joint fusion for, 3: 185
  spinal, 1: 100, 106, 108–109, *109*; 2: 11; 3: 289; 4: 225
  synovial joints and, 4: 226
  treatment advances in, 2: 32
Tubiana, Raoul, 4: 182
Tucker, Sarah, 1: 4
Tufts Medical Center Hospital, 2: 306; 4: *311*
Tufts University School of Medicine
  affiliation with Beth Israel Hospital, 4: 213–214, 214*b*, 228
  affiliation with Boston City Hospital, 4: 228, 296–297
  Aufranc and, 3: 247
  Boston Pathology Course at, 1: 230
  Fitchet and, 2: 252
  hand fellowships and, 2: 250
  Karlin and, 2: 369–370
  Legg and, 2: 102
  Lovett and, 2: 64
  MacAusland and, 3: 308
  Ober and, 2: 165
  orthopaedics residencies, 4: 377–379
  Painter and, 3: 266
  Radin and, 3: 328
  Smith-Petersen and, 3: 362
  Webber and, 2: 9
Tukey, Marshall, 1: 304, 309
tumors
  Barr and Mixter on, 3: 204
  bone irradiation and, 2: 237
  Codman on, 3: 110
  femoral allograft transplantation, 3: 389–390
  giant-cell, 3: 390
  intraspinal in children, 2: 301–302
  knee fusion with allografts, 3: 435
  musculoskeletal, 3: 433, 435
  research in, 2: 236–237
  sacrococcygeal chordoma, 3: 390
Tumors of the Jaws (Scudder), 3: 64
turnbuckle jacket, 2: 80, 223–224, *224*, 225, *225*, 226, 226*b*, 227, 227*b*, 316, *336*; 3: 209
Turner, Henry G., 4: 434
Turner, Roderick H., 2: 397; 3: 246; 4: 187
Tyler, Charles H., 4: 303
typhoid fever, 2: 4

U

Ulin, Dorothy Lewenberg, 4: 244
Ulin, Kenneth, 4: 244
Ulin, Robert (1903–1978), 4: *242*
  BCH surgeon-in-chief, 4: 333
  as Beth Israel chief of orthopaedics, 4: 243–244, 289*b*
  Beth Israel Hospital and, 4: 242, 247
  Boston City Hospital and, 4: 242
  Boston VA Hospital and, 4: 242
  death of, 4: 244
  education and training, 4: 242
  Faulkner Hospital and, 4: 242
  fender fracture case, 4: 242
  HMS appointment, 4: 244
  Lowell General Hospital and, 4: 243
  marriage and family, 4: 244
  private medical practice, 4: 242–243
  professional memberships, 4: 244
  publications and research, 4: 229, 242–243
  silverwork by, 4: *242*, *243*, 244, *244*
  slipped capital femoral epiphysis research, 4: 243
  subdeltoid bursitis research, 4: 243
  Tufts Medical School appointment, 4: 242, 244
  US Army and, 4: 242–243
ultraviolet light, 4: 162–164, 164*t*
unicompartmental prothesis, 4: 176, 178

Unit for Epidemic Aid in Infantile Paralysis (NFP), 2: 188–189
United Cerebral Palsy Association, 2: 401
United States General Hospital (Readville, Mass.), 2: 5
University of Arkansas College of Medicine, 3: 337
University of California Hospital, 3: 336–337
University of California in San Diego (UCSD), 3: 402
University of Chicago, 3: 382
University of Edinburgh, 1: 7
University of Florida, 3: 432
University of Indiana School of Medicine, 3: 445
University of Iowa, 3: 303
University of Maryland Health Center, 4: 263–264
University of Maryland Medical Center, 4: 157
University of Massachusetts, 2: 286–288, 364
University of Massachusetts Medical School, 2: 293, 371
University of Miami Tissue Bank, 3: 442
University of Michigan Medical Center, 4: 254–255
University of Missouri, 4: 372
University of Pennsylvania Medical School, 1: 7; 2: 424
University of Pittsburgh School of Medicine, 3: 382–383, 385; 4: 111
University of Southern California, 2: 266
Upper Extremity Injuries in the Athlete (Pappas and Walzer), 2: 288
Upton, Joseph, III, 3: 431
Urist, Marshall R., 3: 433
US Air Force Hospital, 3: 323
US Army
  Boston-derived base hospitals, 4: 420t
  curative workshops and, 4: 403
  Division of Orthopedic Surgery, 2: 65; 4: 411–412
  Harvard Unit and, 1: 270
  hospital reconditioning program, 1: 271–272
  Hospital Train, 4: *414*
  levels of medical care by distance, 4: 475t
  Medical Officer instructions for, 4: 410b
  recruiting poster, 4: *397*
  staffing of ambulances with medics, 4: 387
US Army 3rd General Hospital (Mt. Sinai), 4: 88
US Army 3rd Southern General Hospital (Oxford), 3: 365
US Army 7th General Hospital (St. Alban's, England), 4: 90
US Army 11th General Hospital, 4: 420, 422b, *424–425*
US Army 13th General Hospital (Boulogne, France), 4: 422b
US Army 22nd General Hospital, 4: 415
US Army 42nd General Hospital, 4: 488, 490
US Army 105th General Hospital, 4: *490*
  Biak Island deployment, 4: 491, 491b, 492, *492*
  camaraderie at, 4: 492
  Cave and, 3: 271; 4: 489
  closing of, 4: 493
  construction of, 4: 489
  in Gatton, Australia, 1: 270; 4: 488–489, *489*
  Harvard Unit and, 1: 270–271; 2: 231–232; 4: 484, 487–489
  hospital beds at, 4: 490
  malaria treatment and, 4: 491
  MGH and, 4: 493
  orthopaedic staff at, 4: 489–490
  patient rehabilitation and, 1: 271; 4: 490–491
  plaque commemorating, 4: *492*
  Rowe and, 3: 351; 4: 489, 490b–491b
  Sheldon Hall Surgical Building, 4: *490*
  tent ward, 4: *491*
  Thorndike and, 4: 489–491
US Army 118th General Hospital, 4: 488
US Army 153rd Station Hospital (Queensland), 4: 488
US Army Base Hospital No. 5 (Boulogne, France), 4: *424*, *426*
  commemoration of Harvard Unit, 4: *428*
  Cushing and, 4: 420, 420t, 422–423
  demobilization of, 4: 426
  first two years at, 4: 422b
  Harvard Unit and, 1: 270; 4: 420, 423–424, *428*
  hazards and mortality rate at, 4: 424–425
  map of, 4: *427*
  Ober and, 2: 145
  officers of, 4: 422
  operating room at, 4: *427*
  Osgood and, 2: 125; 4: 405, 421b, 422
  patient ward in, 4: *428*
  PBBH and, 4: 420t
  training in, 4: 420–421
  US and British medical staff in, 4: 422–423, 425
US Army Base Hospital No. 6 (Talence, France)
  Adams and, 3: 232; 4: 433–434
  buildings at, 4: *432*
  demobilization of, 4: 437
  expansion of, 4: 433–434
  map of, 4: *429*
  MGH orthopaedists and, 3: 313; 4: 420t, 429–432
  operating room at, 4: *431*
  patient census at, 4: 436, 436t, 437
  patient flow process at, 4: 435–436
  patients treated at, 4: *434*
  reconstruction and occupational aides, 4: 436b
  release of equipment to Base Hospital No. 208, 4: 437
  surgical & orthopaedic wards, 4: *431*
  surgical ward at, 4: *433*
  use of the Petit Lycée de Talence, 4: *429*, 432
  Ward in Lycée building, 4: *430*
  WWII reactivation of, 4: 474
US Army Base Hospital No. 7 (Tours, France), 4: *438*
  Boston City Hospital and, 1: 256; 4: 420t, 438–439
  Harvard Unit and, 4: 437–439
  Nichols and, 4: 438–439
  Ward 6, 4: *437*
US Army Base Hospital No. 8 (Savenay, France), 3: 365
US Army Base Hospital No. 9 (Chateauroux, France), 4: 409
US Army Base Hospital No. 10 (Roxbury, Mass.), 2: 258
US Army Base Hospital No. 18 (Bazoilles-sur-Meuse, France), 2: 221–222
US Army Base Hospital No. 114 (Beau-Desert, France), 3: 232
US Army Base Hospital No. 208, 4: 437
US Army Evacuation Hospital No. 110 (Argonne), 4: 439
US Army Hospital (Landstuhl, Germany), 3: 418
US Army 34th Infantry Division, 4: 484

Index

US Army Medical Board, 2: 124; 3: 168
US Army Medical Corps, 2: 124, 130, 220, 222; 3: 282, 288, 291, 313, 351, 365, 370; 4: 387, 420
US Army Medical Reserve Corps, 2: 66, 268; 3: 61, 89, 232
US Army Mobile Unit No. 6 (Argonne), 4: 426
US Army Nurse Corps, 4: 492
US Army ROTC, 3: 300
US Food and Drug Administration (FDA), 3: 249
US General Hospital No. 2 (Fort McHenry, Maryland), 4: 452
US General Hospital No. 3 (Camp Shanks, Orangeburg, New York), 4: 88
US General Hospital No. 3 (Colonia, N.J.), 4: 452
US General Hospital No. 5, 4: *487*
 in Belfast, Ireland, 4: 484–485
 closing of, 4: 487
 construction of, 4: *486*
 facilities at, 4: 485–486
 Fort Bragg and, 4: 484
 Harvard Unit and, 1: 270, 277; 3: 271; 4: 484
 in Normandy, France, 4: 486, *486*, 487
 nursing at, 4: *487*
 in Odstock, England, 4: 486
 operating room at, 4: *487*
 personnel and training, 4: 484
 ward tent, 4: *486*
US General Hospital No. 6
 Aufranc and, 3: 239, 240*b*
 bivouac and staging area in Maddaloni, Italy, 4: *479*
 in Bologna, Italy, 4: *481*, 482
 Camp Blanding and, 4: 474–475
 Camp Kilmer and, 4: 475
 in Casablanca, 4: 476–477, *477*, 480*b*
 closing of, 4: 482, 484
 commendation for, 4: 485*b*
 experiences at, 4: 483*b*
 hospital ward in Naples, 4: *479*
 Instituto Buon Pastore and, 4: *480*, 481
 leadership of, 4: 482*b*
 main entrance, 4: *481*
 medical staff, 4: *476*
 MGH and, 3: 239, 362; 4: 474, 485*b*
 mobilization of, 4: 475–476
 operating room at, 4: *481*
 organization of, 4: 477
 orthopaedics section of, 4: 482, 483*b*
 Peninsular Base Station and, 4: 481–482
 personnel and training, 4: 474–475
 prisoners of war and, 4: 484
 relocation of, 4: 479, 481
 in Rome, Italy, 4: 481–482
 surgical services at, 4: 478, *478*
 temporary camp in Italy, 4: *480*
 wards at, 4: *478*
US General Hospital No. 10, 4: *328*, *445*, *446*
 Cotton and, 4: 452
 Elks' Reconstruction Hospital and, 4: 447–448
 Massachusetts Women's Hospital and, 4: 447–448
 as a model for civilian hospitals, 4: 450–451
 RBBH and, 4: 447–448
 West Roxbury plant (Boston City Hospital), 4: 447–448
US Medical Department, 4: 439
US Naval Hospital, 3: 201, 207
US Naval Medical Corps, 3: 248
US Navy Tissue Bank, 3: 439–440, 442
US Public Health Service, 4: 165
US War Department, 4: 474
USS *Arizona*, 4: *465*
USS *Okinawa*, 3: 446, *447*
USS *West Point*, 4: 488

V

Vail Valley Medical Center, 3: 446
Vainio, Kauko, 4: 96
Valley Forge Army Hospital, 2: 279
Van Dessel, Arthur, 1: 193
Van Gorder, George W. (1888–1969), 3: *364*
 arthrodesis procedures, 3: 368, *368*
 Brackett and, 3: 365
 Cave on, 3: 368
 chronic posterior elbow dislocation case, 3: 366
 Clinics for Crippled Children and, 2: 230; 3: 365
 death of, 3: 368
 early life, 3: 364
 education and training, 3: 364–365
 femoral neck fracture research and treatment, 3: 185–186, *186*, 367, *367*
 fracture research and, 3: 334, 366–367
 hip nailing and, 3: 237
 HMS appointment, 3: 365
 hospital appointments, 3: 365
 marriage and family, 3: 365
 MGH Fracture Clinic and, 3: 60*b*, 314, 366
 as MGH house officer, 1: 189
 as MGH orthopaedics chief, 1: 199; 3: 11*b*
 as MGH surgeon, 3: 187, 192, 365, 367–368
 Peking Union Medical College and, 3: 365
 private medical practice, 3: 365
 professional memberships and, 3: 368
 publications and research, 3: 365–368
 Trumble technique for hip fusion and, 3: 367, *367*
 US Army Medical Corps and, 3: 365
 World War I volunteer orthopaedics, 4: 407
Van Gorder, Helen R. Gorforth, 3: 365
Vanguard, The, 4: *421*
Vanishing Bone (Harris), 3: 225, *225*
vascular anastomosis, 4: 216
vastus slide, 3: 278
Vauzelle, C., 2: 340
Venel, Jean-Andrew, 1: xxii
VEPTR (Vertical Expandable Prosthetic Titanium Rib), 2: 360, *362*
Verdan, Claude, 4: 96
Vermont Department of Health, 2: 221
Vermont Medical Association, 2: 221
Vermont State Medical Society, 2: 147
vertebral column resections (VCRs), 2: 362–363
Veterans Administration Hospital (La Jolla, Calif.), 3: 402
Veterans Administration Medical Center (Richmond, Virginia), 4: 153
Veterans Administration Prosthetic and Sensory Aids Service, 1: 273
Veterans Administration Rehabilitation Research and Development Programs, 4: 152
Vincent, Beth, 2: 119; 4: 389*b*
Virchow, Rudolf, 1: 82
visceroptosis, 3: 83–84, 84*b*, 86–88
Vogt, E. C., 3: 341, *342*
Vogt, Paul, 2: 115
volar plate arthroplasty, 2: 248
Volkmann ischemic contracture, 2: 200–201, *201*, 249–250

Volunteer Aid Association, 3: 152–153
Von Kessler, Kirby, 2: 325
Vose, Robert H., 4: 389*b*
Vrahas, Mark, 1: 167, 235; 3: 462, 464*b*; 4: 194
Vresilovic, Edward J., Jr., 4: 288

W

Wacker, Warren E .C., 4: 132
Wagner, Katiri, 3: 410
Wagner spherical osteotomy, 2: 390–392
Waite, Frederick C., 4: 50
Waldenström, Johann H., 2: 104
Waldo County General Hospital, 2: 371
Walford, Edward, 1: *34*
Walker, C. B., 4: 10
Walker, Irving, 4: 305
Walker, Peter, 4: 130, 137–138, 147, 152, 176, 178
Walker, Thomas, 3: 132–133
Wallis, Oscar, 3: 25
Walsh, Francis Norma, 2: 333
Walter, Alice, 4: 109
Walter, Carl, 4: 109
Walter, Carl Frederick, 4: 104
Walter, Carl W. (1905–1992), 4: *104, 106, 108*
    aseptic technique interest, 4: 105–106
    Aseptic Treatment of Wounds, 4: 106, *106,* 107*b*
    blood storage bag, 4: 107, *107,* 108
    canine surgical scenarios and, 4: 105
    death of, 4: 109
    education and training, 4: 104
    fracture treatment and, 1: 204; 4: 16, 18
    HMS appointment, 4: 105, 107*b*
    HMS Surgical Research Laboratory, 4: 105, *106,* 107–108
    marriage and family, 4: 109
    medical device development, 4: 107–108
    PBBH and, 4: 16, 18–20, 79, 104–105
    PBBH blood bank and, 4: 107–108
    PBBH fracture service, 4: 108–109
    professional memberships, 4: 109
    publications and research, 4: 106
    renal dialysis machine modification, 4: 108
    on ultraviolet light use, 4: 164
Walter, David, 4: 109
Walter, Leda Agatha, 4: 104
Walter, Linda, 4: 109
Walter, Margaret, 4: 109
Walter, Margaret Davis, 4: 109
Walter, Martha, 4: 109
Walter Reed General Hospital, 3: 168; 4: 327, *450,* 451, 488, *488*
Walzer, Janet, 2: 288
War of 1812, 1: 40–41
Ware, John, 1: 296, 299, 302
Warman, Matthew, 2: 439, 439*b*
Warner, Jon J. P., 3: *145,* 462, 464*b*; 4: 194, 195*b*
Warren, Abigail Collins, 1: 24, 28, 31
Warren, Amy Shaw, 1: 85, 87
Warren, Anne Winthrop, 1: 55
Warren, Annie Crowninshield, 1: 76–78
Warren, Edward (author), 1: 46, 68
Warren, Edward (son of Jack), 1: 24, 28, 31
Warren, Elizabeth, 1: 4
Warren, Elizabeth Hooton, 1: 9, 15, 21
Warren, Gideon, 1: 4
Warren, Howland (1910–2003), 1: 90–91
Warren, Howland Shaw, Jr. (1951–), 1: 71, 91
Warren, John (1874–1928), 1: *88*
    anatomical atlas and, 1: 88–89
    anatomy instruction at Harvard Medical School, 1: 71, 88; 2: 296; 4: 82
    enlistment in WWI, 1: 88
    injury and death of, 1: 89
    medical education, 1: 87–88
    Outline of Practical Anatomy, An, 1: 88
Warren, John (ca. 1630), 1: 4
Warren, John Collins (1778–1856), 1: *31, 33, 67, 68*
    American mastodon skeleton and, 1: 51, *51,* 52
    amputations and, 1: 52–53, 61
    apprenticeship with father, 1: 33
    birth of, 1: 24, 31
    on chloroform, 3: 31
    community organizations and, 1: 69
    daily routine of, 1: 39
    death of, 1: 66–67, 77
    diagnostic skills, 1: 52–53
    dislocated hip treatment, 3: 13, 13*b*
    donation of anatomical museum, 1: 66
    early life, 1: 31
    educational organizations and, 1: 38–39
    Etherization, 1: 62, *62;* 3: 33
    European medical studies, 1: 33–37, 54
    on father's death, 1: 29–30
    first use of ether at MGH, 1: 56–59, *59,* 60–62, *63,* 64–65, 77; 3: 27–28, 28*b,* 29, 29*b,* 30, 32–34
    founding of Boston Medical Association, 1: 38
    founding of MGH, 1: 31, 41–42, 71; 3: 5, *5,* 6*b*–7*b,* 12–13
    fundraising for hospital in Boston, 1: 41
    Genealogy of Warren, 1: 4
    at Harvard College, 1: 31–32
    Harvard Medical School and, 1: 38–40, 66, 68–69, 299; 3: 30, 94
    as Hersey Professor of Anatomy and Surgery, 1: 29, 66, 68
    hip dislocation case, 1: 42, 44–46, *46,* 47–50, 68; 3: 36
    home of, 1: *38, 51*
    influence of Astley Cooper on, 1: 36–37
    influence on Mason, 1: 72, 75
    interest in exercise, 1: 54
    John Ball Brown and, 1: 97–99
    legacy of, 1: 68–69
    "Letter to the Honorable Isaac Parker," 1: 45, *45*
    marriage to Anne Winthrop, 1: 55
    marriage to Susan Powell Mason, 1: 37–38
    medical and surgical practice, 1: 37–39, 51–55, 66
    medical studies at Harvard, 1: 32–33
    orthopaedics curriculum and, 1: 136–137
    orthopaedics specialty and, 1: 99–100, 119
    Parkman on, 1: 296
    postsurgical treatment and, 1: 52–53
    publications of, 1: 46, 52, *52, 53,* 62, *62,* 69*b*
    reputation of, 1: 51–53
    retirement and, 1: 65–66
    Spunkers and bodysnatching, 1: 32–33
    surgical apprenticeship, 1: 33–37
    surgical practice at MGH, 1: 52–55, 57–58, 65
    Temperance Society and, 1: 40
    thumping skills, 1: 37

Index

Warren, John Collins "Coll" (1842–1927), 1: *79, 80, 82*; 3: *19*
   antisepsis principles and, 1: 85–86; 3: 45
   Charles L. Scudder and, 3: 54–55
   as Civil War hospital surgeon, 1: 79–80
   death of, 1: 87
   European medical studies, 1: 81–84
   fundraising for cancer research, 1: 87
   fundraising for Harvard Medical School, 1: 85, 87; 4: 3
   Harvard Medical School campus and, 1: 87
   Henry Bowditch and, 1: 82
   honorary degrees, 1: 87
   as house pupil at MGH, 1: 80–81
   influence of father on, 1: 80
   influence of Lister on, 1: 84
   Lowell hip dislocation and, 1: 49
   medical and surgical practice, 1: 84–85, *85*, 86; 2: 3
   medical education, 1: 79–81
   professorship at Harvard Medical School, 1: 87; 2: 32
   publications of, 1: 87
   Remembrances, 1: 83
   research laboratory at MGH, 1: 71
   study of tumors, 1: 85
   as supervisor at MGH, 2: 20
   surgical training, 1: 81–84
   treatment of tumors and, 1: 82
Warren, John "Jack" (1753–1815), 1: *23*
   admission tickets to lectures, 1: *27*
   anatomical studies, 1: 22–25
   anatomy lectures, 1: 24, 26–29
   anti-slavery sentiment, 1: 24
   apprenticeships by, 1: 15, 21, 25, 33
   attendance certificates, 1: *28*
   community affairs and, 1: 29
   death of, 1: 29–30, 41
   early life, 1: 21
   establishment of medical board, 1: 29
   father's death and, 1: 3–4
   founding of Boston Medical Association, 1: 25
   founding of Harvard Medical School, 1: 21, 25–29, 40, 71
   at Harvard College, 1: 21
   institutionalization of Boston medicine and, 1: 30
   marriage and family, 1: 24, 28, 31
   Masons and, 1: 29
   medical studies at Harvard, 1: 6
   military service, 1: 22
   orthopaedics curriculum and, 1: 134
   as pioneer of shoulder surgery, 1: 29
   private medical practice, 1: 22, 24, 28
   publications of, 1: 29
   as senior surgeon for Continental Army, 1: 22–24
   smallpox inoculations and, 1: 9, 29
   Spunkers and bodysnatching, 1: 21
Warren, Jonathan Mason (1811–1867), 1: *71, 76*
   birth of, 1: 38
   chronic illness, 1: 72, 76–78
   European medical studies, 1: 53, 73–76
   fracture care and, 1: 76
   influence of father on, 1: 72, 75
   influence on Coll, 1: 80
   instrument case, 1: *77*
   introduction of plastic surgery to the U.S., 1: 71–72, 77
   legacy of, 1: 78–79
   on Lowell's autopsy, 1: 47–50
   medical practice with father, 1: 76–77
   medical studies at Harvard, 1: 72
   MGH and, 1: 53; 3: 15, *31*
   Norwalk train accident and, 1: 77
   orthopaedic surgery and, 1: 81
   plastic surgery techniques, 1: 76–77
   publications of, 1: 78
   scientific method and, 1: 71, 74
   support for House of the Good Samaritan, 1: 124
   Surgical Observations with Cases and Operations, 1: 47, 75, 78
   use of ether, 1: 57, 63
   as visiting surgeon at MGH, 1: 77
   Warren Triennial Prize and, 1: 78
Warren, Joseph (1663–1729), 1: 4
Warren, Joseph (1696–1755), 1: 3–4
Warren, Joseph (1741–1775), 1: *3, 11*, 18
   apprenticeships by, 1: 15
   Boston Massacre oration, 1: 15–16
   Boston Massacre report, 1: 14
   Bunker Hill battle, 1: 18–19
   command of militia, 1: 18
   death at Bunker Hill, 1: 3, 19, *19*, 20, 22
   early career, 1: 6
   father's death and, 1: 3–4
   as founder of medical education in Boston, 1: 15
   marriage to Elizabeth Hooten, 1: 9
   Masons and, 1: 10–12
   medical studies at Harvard, 1: 6
   Mercy Scollay and, 1: 19
   obstetrics and, 1: 9
   orthopaedic practice and, 1: 10
   physician apprenticeship, 1: 6, 8
   as physician to the Almshouse, 1: 15
   as president of the Third Provincial Congress, 1: 18
   private medical practice, 1: 8–10, 15
   publications and, 1: 12
   as Revolutionary War leader, 1: 10–20
   smallpox inoculations and, 1: 8–9
   Suffolk Resolves and, 1: 16
   tea party protest and, 1: 16
Warren, Joseph (1876–1942), 1: 87, 90
Warren, Margaret, 1: 4
Warren, Martha Constance Williams, 1: 90
Warren, Mary, 1: 19
Warren, Mary Stevens (1713–1803), 1: 3–4, 10
Warren, Peter, 1: 4
Warren, Rebecca, 1: 96
Warren, Richard (1907–1999), 1: 71, 90–91, 270; 3: 330; 4: 20
Warren, Richard (d. 1628), 1: 4
Warren, Shields, 4: 277*b*
Warren, Susan Powell Mason, 1: 37–38, 72
Warren Anatomical Museum, 1: 28, 49–50, 52, 66; 3: 38
Warren family
   early years in Boston, 1: 4
   Harvard Medical School (HMS) and, 1: 71
   history of, 1: 4*b*
   lineage of physicians in, 1: 3, 5, 6, 71
   Massachusetts General Hospital (MGH) and, 1: 71
Warren Russet (Roxbury) apples, 1: 3, *4*
Warren Triennial Prize, 1: 78
Warren's Atlas, 1: 89
Warshaw, Andrew, 3: 146

Washburn, Frederick A., 1: 188; 3: 1, 70*b*, 174; 4: 420*t*, 429–430, *432*, 433
Washington, George, 1: 19, 22–23
Washington University, 3: 163–165
Washington University Base Hospital No. 21, 3: 166
Washington University School of Medicine, 3: 165, 170, 404–405
Watanabi, Masaki, 2: 279
Waterhouse, Benjamin, 1: 25, 40
Waters, Peter (1955–), 2: *414*
    birth palsies research, 2: 415, 417, *417*, 418–419, *419*, 420
    Boston Children's Hospital and, 2: 415, 415*b*, 420, 439*b*
    education and training, 2: 414
    hand surgery and, 2: 414–415
    hand trauma research, 2: 415
    HMS appointment, 2: 415, 415*b*
    honors and awards, 2: 415
    John E. Hall Professorship in Orthopaedic Surgery, 2: 439*b*
    as orthopaedic chair, 2: 15*b*
    orthopaedics curriculum and, 1: 216, 225
    orthopaedics education and, 2: 416*b*
    posterior shoulder dislocation case, 2: 417–418
    professional memberships, 2: 416*b*
    publications and research, 2: 415, 417, *417*, 418–420
    radiographic classification of glenohumeral deformity, 2: 419*t*
    on Simmons, 4: 186
    visiting professorships and lectures, 2: 415, 416*b*
Watkins, Arthur L., 1: 273; 3: 269, 285–286, *286*, 454*b*
Watts, Hugh G. (1934–), 2: *420*
    Boston brace and, 2: 423–424, *424*
    Boston Children's Hospital and, 2: 422–423
    Brigham and Women's Hospital and, 4: 193
    Children's Hospital of Philadelphia and, 2: 424
    education and training, 2: 420
    on gait laboratories, 2: 424
    global public health and, 2: 421, 424–425
    HMS appointment, 2: 422
    humanitarianism and, 2: 421
    on the Krukenberg procedure, 2: 425
    limb-salvage procedure by, 2: 422, 423*b*
    McIndoe Memorial Research Unit and, 2: 422
    PBBH and, 4: 163
    on pediatric orthopaedics, 2: 303–304
    professional memberships, 2: 425
    publications and research, 2: 421–422, *422*, 423–424, *424*, 425
    scoliosis research, 2: 423
    University of California and, 2: 425
    University of Pennsylvania and, 2: 424
Wayne County Medical Society, 2: 135
Weaver, Michael J., 3: 463*b*
Webber, S. G., 2: 5, 9
Webster, Daniel, 1: 54, 307
Webster, Hannah White, 1: 298
Webster, Harriet Fredrica Hickling, 1: 299
Webster, John W., 1: *299*
    confession of, 1: 312–313
    debt and, 1: 302–303
    detection of arsenic poisoning, 1: 301–302
    education and training, 1: 299
    Ephraim Littlefield and, 1: 303–304
    execution of, 1: *313*, 314
    on guilt of, 1: 314–318
    HMS chemistry professorship, 1: 296, 298–301
    home of, 1: *302*
    letters on behalf of, 1: 309, *309*, 310–311
    Manual of Chemistry, 1: 299, 301
    murder of George Parkman, 1: 305–312, 315, *315*, 318
    publications of, 1: 299–301
    trial of, 1: *307*, *307*, 308–311, 314–316; 3: 40
Webster, Redford, 1: 298
Weed, Frank E., 4: 409
Weigel, Louis A., 2: 56
weight training, 3: 281–282
Weiland, Andrew J., 3: 431
Weiner, David, 2: 436
Weiner, Norbert, 2: 326
Weinfeld, Beverly D. Bunnin, 4: 101, 103
Weinfeld, Marvin S. (1930–1986), 4: *101*
    Beth Israel Hospital and, 4: 247
    Brigham and Women's Hospital, 4: 163
    death of, 4: 103
    education and training, 4: 101
    HMS appointment, 4: 102–103
    hospital appointments, 4: 102
    knee arthroplasty evaluation, 4: 103
    marriage and family, 4: 101, 103
    on McKeever and MacIntosh prostheses, 4: 189
    MGH and, 4: 101
    osteogenic sarcoma research, 4: 102
    PBBH and, 4: 163
    private medical practice, 4: 102
    professional memberships, 4: 103
    publications and research, 4: 102–103
    RBBH and, 4: 41*b*, 68, 80, 102–103, 116*b*, 131
    synovectomy of the knee research, 4: 40, 102–103
    total elbow replacement and, 4: 129
    US Army Medical Corps and, 4: 101
Weinstein, James N., 2: 371; 4: 266*b*
Weiss, Charles, 3: 385–386, 395, 413, 460*b*
Weiss, Soma, 3: 350; 4: 79
Weissbach, Lawrence, 3: 460*b*
Weld, William, 3: 424
Weller, Thomas, 2: 234
Wellesley Convalescent Home, 2: 9, 189, 191
Wellington, William Williamson, 1: 59
Wells, Horace, 1: 56–57, 60
Welsh, William H., 1: 185
Wenger, Dennis, 2: 403
Wennberg, Jack, 2: 372, 374, *374*
Wennberg, John, 4: 185
Wesselhoeft, Walter, 3: 120
West Roxbury Veterans Administration Hospital
    DeLorme and, 3: 285
    Ewald and, 4: 144
    HCORP residencies and, 1: 199–200, 206–208, 218, 220, 224–225
    MacAusland and, 3: 312
    McGinty and, 2: 279; 4: 22
    orthopaedic biomechanics laboratory, 4: 137
    orthopaedics residencies, 4: 378
    RBBH and, 4: 36
    Simon and, 2: 406
    spinal cord injury research and treatment, 4: 152
    Spinal Cord Injury Service, 4: 152–153
    training program at, 4: 117

Index

West Virginia University School of Medicine, 3: 328
Weston, Craig, 1: 217*b*
Weston, G. Wilbur, 2: 438
Weston, Nathan, 1: 44–45, 50
Weston Forest and Trail Association, 4: 91, *91*
Whipple, John Adams, 1: *31*
Whipple, Martha Ellen, 2: 113
White, Anita Ottemo, 4: 266
White, Arthur H., 4: 263
White, Augustus A., III (1936–), 4: *257, 263*
    "Analysis of the Mechanics of the Thoracic Spine in Man," 4: 259, *259*
    AOA Alfred R. Shands Jr. lecture, 4: 264
    back pain research and, 4: 258
    as Beth Israel chief of orthopaedics, 4: 262–264, 289*b*
    as Beth Israel chief of surgery, 4: 223, 255
    BIDMC teaching program and, 4: 286
    BIH annual reports, 4: 262–263
    biomechanics research, 4: 260–261
    Brigham and Women's Hospital and, 4: 163, 193
    Cervical Spine Research Society president, 4: 265
    Clinical Biomechanics of the Spine, 4: 262
    clinical research protocols at BIH and, 4: 262
    Delta Upsilon fraternity and, 4: 258
    diversity initiatives in orthopaedics, 4: 264–265
    education and training, 4: 257–258
    Ellen and Melvin Gordon Professor of Medical Education, 4: 264, 266
    Federation of Spine Associations president, 4: 265
    Fort Ord US Army Hospital and, 4: 259
    HMS appointment, 4: 262, 264, 266
    honors and awards, 4: 264–265
    legacy of, 4: 265–266
    marriage and family, 4: 266
    MGH and, 3: 398*b*
    nonunion of a hangman's fracture case, 4: 261
    Oliver Wendell Holmes Society and, 4: 264
    orthopaedic biomechanics doctorate, 4: 259
    professional memberships and activities, 4: 265
    publications and research, 4: 259–262, 264
    Seeing Patients, 4: 265
    spine fellowship program and, 4: 263
    spine research, 4: 259–261, *261*, 262, 264
    University of Maryland Health Center presidency offer, 4: 263–264
    US Army Medical Corps and, 4: 258–259
    Yale University School of Medicine and, 4: 259–260, 262
White, D., 1: 258
White, George Robert, 3: 75
White, Hannah, 1: 298
White, J. Warren, 2: 197
White, John, 3: 191
White, Kevin, 4: 379
White, Paul Dudley, 4: 431
Whitehill, W. M., 2: 11
White's Apothecary Shop, 1: 39–40
Whiteside, Helen E., 2: 292
Whitman, Armitage, 4: 233
Whitman, Royal, 2: 31, 93
Whitman's foot plate, 2: 244–245
Whitman's operation (astragalectomy), 2: 92–94
Whittemore, Wyman, 4: 211, 283*t*
whooping cough, 2: 4
Wickham, Thomas W., 4: 371
Wiggin, Sidney C., 4: 330
Wigglesworth, George, 3: 124
Wigglesworth, Marian Epes, 4: 83
Wilcox, C. A., 3: 34
Wilcox, Oliver D., 3: 34
Wild, Charles, 1: 96
Wilensky, Charles F., 1: 158
Wilkins, Early, 3: 448
Willard, DeForest P., 1: 197; 2: 78, 160
Willard, Joseph, 1: 25
Willard Parker Hospital, 1: 276
Willert, H. G., 3: 220
William H. and Johanna A. Harris Professorship, 3: 464*b*
William H. Thomas Award, 4: 189, 190*b*
William T. Green Fund, 2: 436
William Wood and Company, 2: 50–51
Williams, Harold, 1: 250
Williams, Henry W., 1: 138
Williams, Ted, 1: 258; 4: 342, 345–346
Wilson, Edward, 3: 369
Wilson, George, 1: 56
Wilson, Germaine Parfouru-Porel, 3: 370
Wilson, H. Augustus, 3: 234
Wilson, James L., 2: 78, 191
Wilson, John C., Sr., 1: 189
Wilson, Louis T., 4: 313
Wilson, Marion, 4: 389*b*
Wilson, Michael G., 3: 248; 4: 193–194, 195*b*
Wilson, Philip D., Sr. (1886–1969), 3: 369, 375
    American Ambulance Hospital and, 4: 389*b*, 390
    American Appreciation, An, 3: 369
    amputation expertise, 3: 371, 373–374; 4: 472*b*
    arthroplasty of the elbow, 4: 63
    back pain research and, 3: 204
    on Cobb, 2: 225–226
    death of, 3: 376
    displacement of proximal femoral epiphysis case, 3: 372
    early life, 3: 369
    education and training, 3: 369
    Experience in the Management of Fractures and Dislocations, 3: 376
    fracture research and, 3: 371–373
    Fractures, 3: 315
    Fractures and Dislocations, 3: 371, *371*
    Harvard Unit and, 2: 119, 123; 3: *180*, 369
    HMS appointment, 3: 371
    Hospital for the Ruptured and Crippled, 3: 376
    Human Limbs and Their Substitutes, 3: 376
    knee flexion contracture approach, 3: 374–375, *375*
    Management of Fractures and Dislocations, 3: 62, 273
    marriage and family, 3: 370
    MGH Fracture Clinic and, 3: 60*b*, 61, 314, 371, 373, 376
    as MGH house officer, 1: 189
    as MGH surgeon, 3: 187, 269, 370
    military orthopaedics and, 4: 473
    New York Hospital for the Ruptured and Crippled and, 1: 89
    on Osgood, 2: 138
    private medical practice, 3: 338
    professional memberships and, 3: 376

publications and research, 2: 136, 297; 3: 371–373, *373*, 374–376; 4: 60, 363
RBBH and, 4: 28, 31, 55
Robert Breck Brigham Hospital and, 3: 370
Scudder Oration on Trauma, 3: 63
slipped capital femoral epiphysis treatment, 4: 237
US Army Medical Corps, 3: 370
World War II volunteers and, 4: 363
Wilson, Philip, Jr., 4: 134
Wiltse, Leon, 3: 249
Wimberly, David, 1: 233
Winchester Hospital, 2: 218–219; 3: 299, 417; 4: 169, 214
Winter, R. B., 2: 343
Winthrop, Anne, 1: 55
Winthrop Group, 2: 317
Wirth, Michael, 2: 288
Wislocki, George B., 1: 179
Wistar, Casper, 1: 39
Wittenborg, Dick, 2: 234
Wojtys, Edward, 1: 286
Wolbach, S. Burt, 2: 234; 4: *6*
Wolcott, J. Huntington, 2: 5
Wolfe, Richard J., 1: 59
Wolff, Julius, 1: xxiii
women
   ACL injuries, 1: 285–286
   admission to HMS, 1: 138, 138*b*, 239
   chronic illness treatment, 1: 123–124, 129
   as MGH house officers, 1: 239
   nursing training, 1: 41; 2: 7–8; 4: 208
   opposition to medical studies by, 3: 44
women orthopaedic surgeons
   first HCORP resident, 1: 239
   limited teaching residencies for, 1: 200
   Ruth Jackson Orthopaedic Society and, 2: 413
Wong, David A., 4: 272*b*
Wood, Bruce T., 4: 117, 129, 163, 193
Wood, Edward Stickney, 3: 94
Wood, G. W., 3: 420
Wood, Leonard, 4: 337
Woodhouse, Charles, 4: 378
Woods, Archie S., 2: 82
Worcester, Alfred, 1: 259, 262–263
workers' compensation
   Aitken and, 4: 353–354
   carpal tunnel syndrome and, 2: 375; 4: 186

   Cotton and, 4: 325, 444
   major medical problems and, 3: *379*
   rehabilitation goals and, 4: 354
   surgical interventions and, 2: 373; 4: 352
   treatment protocols and, 4: 353–354
   Yett and, 4: 253
World Health Organization, 1: 168
World War I. *See also* American Expeditionary Forces (AEF); British Expeditionary Forces (BEF)
   American Ambulance Hospital (Neuilly, France), 2: 117–119, *119*, 120; 3: 166, 180, *180*; 4: 9, 386, *386*, 387, *387*
   American base hospitals, 4: 419–420
   American Expeditionary Forces, 2: 126, 128, 221
   American experience in, 4: 405*b*
   American Field Service Ambulance, 4: 386, *386*, 387, *387*, 388
   American medical volunteers, 1: 256; 2: 117–119; 4: 387–396, 398–399, *399*, 402, 404, 406–409, 412*b*–413*b*, 425
   AOA and orthopaedic hospitals, 2: 64
   British Expeditionary Forces, 4: 10
   curative workshops, 4: 399–403, *403*
   end of, 4: *453*
   facilities for wounded soldiers, 4: 414–416
   femur fracture treatment, 4: 408
   field ambulances, 4: 414–415, *415*
   field hospital equipment, 4: 393*b*
   field hospitals, 4: *414*
   First Goldthwait Unit, 4: *399*
   Harvard Medical School and, 2: 41, 64, 117–120, 125, 145
   hospital trains, 4: *414*, 416
   impact of posture-related conditions, 4: 233
   impact on medical education, 4: 397
   impact on orthopaedics, 4: 453–454, 463–464
   impact on US economy, 4: 465
   military hospitals and, 1: 270
   military reconstruction hospitals and, 4: 439–441
   military surgeon training and, 1: 148; 2: 65–69

   New England Dressings Committee (Red Cross Auxiliary), 4: *10*
   orthopaedic contributions before, 2: 50–63
   orthopaedic surgery, 2: 119–126
   postural treatments and, 3: 83
   recruiting poster, 4: 397
   rehabilitation of soldiers and, 2: 67–68; 4: 396
   scheme of British hospitals, 4: *414*
   splints and, 3: 167–169, 169*b*; 4: 389, *391*, 408, 409, 411, 416–417
   standardization of equipment, 2: 124; 3: 167–168
   transport of injured, 3: 169, 169*b*, 170
   trench warfare in, 4: 385, 389, *390*
   US Army Hospital Train, 4: *414*
   US declaration of war on Germany, 4: *396*
   US entry into, 4: 409
   wound treatment during, 4: 385, 389, *390*, 391, 395–396, 407, 471
World War II
   American medical volunteers, 4: 363
   bombing of Pearl Harbor, 4: *465*, 466
   civilian defense and, 1: 269–270
   civilian surgery specialists, 4: 471–472
   field hospitals and, 4: 468
   Fifth Portable Surgical Hospital, 4: 489
   Fourth Portable Surgical Hospital (4PSH), 2: 232–233; 4: 489
   Harvard Unit (5th General Hospital), 1: 270, 277; 3: 271; 4: 17, 484
   Harvard Unit (105th General Hospital), 1: 270–271; 2: 231–232; 4: 488–489
   HMS surgeons and, 1: 270; 2: 232
   Hospital Trains, 4: *478*
   impact on training programs, 4: 467
   impact on US economy, 4: 465
   impact on US hospitals, 4: 467–468
   military hospitals in Australia, 4: 488–489
   military surgery and, 4: 469–470
   mobile army surgical hospitals (MASHs), 2: 231–232, *232*, 233; 4: 468–469, *470*
   mobile warfare in, 4: 468–469

Index 553

orthopaedic surgery and, 4: 463, 473, 493
physician preparation for war injury treatment, 3: 367
US Army 5th General Hospital, 4: 484–487
US Army 6th General Hospital, 4: 474–478, *478*, *479*, 480*b*, 481–482, 483*b*, 484, 484*b*
US Army 105th General Hospital, 1: 270; 2: 232; 3: 351; 4: 487–493
US Army levels of medical care, 4: 475*t*
US entry into, 4: *466*, *467*
wound management and, 3: 274; 4: 469, 469*b*, 470–473
wound management
amputations, 4: *469*
aseptic treatment of, 4: 107*b*, 469
changes from WWI to WWII, 4: 471, 473
evidence-based practices and, 2: 379
gunshot injuries, 2: 66, 119, 161, 233; 3: 43; 4: 437, 441
impact of World War II on, 3: 274; 4: 469, 469*b*, 470–472
military orthopaedics and, 2: 121, 128, 233; 3: 43
in osteomyelitis, 3: 301
standardization of, 4: 470
wounded soldiers and, 4: 385, 391, 398–399, 432, 434–435, 437, 451
WWI Medical Officer instructions for, 4: 410*b*
Wright, John, 1: 216, 224–225; 2: 378
Wright, R. John, 4: 193, 195*b*
Wright, Wilhelmine, 2: 70
Wrist and Radius Injury Surgical Trial (WRIST), 3: 409–410
wrists. *See also* hands
arthrodesis procedures, 3: 191, 239; 4: 166–167
avascular necrosis case, 3: 403
carpal injuries, 3: 101–102
distal radius fractures, 3: 408–409
flexor carpi ulnaris transfer procedure, 2: 172, 188, 198–199, *199*, 200
fusion and, 2: 198, 200; 4: 167
lunate dislocation, 3: 101–102
reconstruction of, 2: 248
rheumatoid arthritis and, 4: 166–167, *167–168*
scaphoid fracture, 4: 361

tendon transfers and, 2: 172
ulnar nerve compression and, 3: 405–406
vascularity and, 3: 403
Wry neck, 2: 256
Wulfsberg, Karen M., 1: 231
Wyman, Edwin T., Jr. (1930–2005), 3: *377*, *378*, *380*, *461*
Children's Hospital/MGH combined program and, 3: 376
death of, 3: 380
education and training, 3: 376
fracture research and, 3: 376–378
fracture service and, 3: 388*t*
HMS appointment, 3: 380
medical cost research, 3: 379, 379*t*
metastatic pathological fracture case, 3: *376*, 377–378
as MGH clinical faculty, 3: 464*b*
MGH Fracture Clinic and, 3: 378
MGH operations improvement and, 3: 378–379
as MGH surgeon, 3: 376, 398*b*
MGH trauma unit and, 3: 396, 399, 460*b*
Omni Med and, 3: 379
orthopaedics education and, 3: 378
private medical practice, 3: 310
publications and research, 3: *376*, 377–379, *379*
Wyman, James, 1: 308
Wyman, Jeffries, 1: 306, *306*; 3: 25
Wyman, Stanley, 3: 241
Wynne-Davies, Ruth, 2: 399, *400*

X

x-rays. *See also* roentgenograms
accidental burns, 3: 100
American Surgical Association on, 3: 58
bone disease diagnosis and, 3: 101–103
bone lesions and, 4: 110
of bullet fragments, 3: *98*
calcaneal apophysitis (Sever's Disease) and, 2: *88*
clinical use of, 3: 97, 99–100
discovery of, 3: 58
Dodd and, 3: 20, *20*, 21, 96, 99
experiments with, 3: 96
fluoroscope and, 3: 96–97
MGH and, 3: 20
orthopaedic surgeons and, 2: 56
publication of, 3: 97, *97*, 98, *99*
safety of, 3: 99–100
scoliosis and, 2: 79

skin injury and, 3: 97–98

Y

Yale University School of Medicine, 4: 259–260
Yanch, Jacquelyn C., 4: 136
Yee, Lester B. K., 3: 351; 4: 489
Yett, Harris S. (ca. 1934–), 4: *250*
Andre the Giant and, 4: 252–253
as Beth Israel chief of orthopaedics, 4: 251, 289*b*
Beth Israel Hospital and, 4: 248, 251, 253, 262–263
BIDMC and, 4: 253
BIDMC teaching program and, 4: 286–287
Boston Orthopaedic Group, 4: 251
Children's Hospital/MGH combined program and, 4: 250–251
deep vein thrombosis research, 4: 251–252
education and training, 4: 250
HMS appointment, 4: 251
honors and awards, 4: 251
hospital appointments, 4: 251
MGH and, 4: 251
professional memberships, 4: 253
publications and research, 4: 251–253
renal transplant infarction case, 4: 252–253
Y-ligament, 3: 35–36, 38
Yoo, Won Joon, 2: 379
Yorra, Alvin, 3: 258
Yosifon, David, 3: 83
Young, E. B., 2: 115
Young, Thomas, 1: 14
Yount, Carl, 2: 153, 294
youth sports, 2: 384–385, *385*, 386
Yovicsin, John, 1: 275
Yun, Andrew, 1: 217*b*

Z

Zaleske, David J., 3: 401, 460*b*, 464*b*
Zander, Gustav, 3: *69*, *71*, 152, 264–265
Zarins, Antra, 3: 383, 386
Zarins, Bertram (1942–), 3: *359*, 388*t*, *446–447*, *461*
anterior interosseous nerve palsy case, 3: 449
arthroscopic surgery and, 3: 422, 446, 448
as Augustus Thorndike Professor, 3: 464*b*

Cave Traveling Fellowship and, 1: 217*b*
Children's Hospital/MGH combined program and, 3: 446
early life, 3: 446
education and training, 3: 446
glenoid labrum composition research, 3: 449
Harvard University Health Services and, 3: 450
HMS appointment, 3: 448, 450
honors and awards, 3: 450–451
Latvian Medical Foundation and, 3: 451
leadership roles, 3: 451*b*
as MGH clinical faculty, 3: 464*b*
as MGH surgeon, 3: 398*b*, 450
posterior cruciate ligament (PCL) research, 3: 450
private medical practice, 3: 448
professional sports teams and, 3: 448, 450
publications and research, 3: 359, 448–450, *450*
shoulder surgery and research, 3: 448–450

sports medicine and, 3: 396, 399, 422, 446, 448, 450, 460*b*
sports medicine fellowship program director, 3: 448
Three Star Medal of Honour and, 3: 451
US Navy and, 3: 446
Vail Valley Medical Center and, 3: 446
as Winter Olympics head physician, 3: 448
Zausmer, Elizabeth, 2: 260, *260*
Zechino, Vincent, 2: 299
Zeiss, Fred Ralph, 2: 438
Zeleski, David, 1: 225
Zevas, Nicholas T., 3: 420
Zilberfarb, Jeffrey, 4: 286–287
Zimbler, Seymour "Zeke" (ca. 1932–2021), 4: *245*, 247
as Beth Israel chief of orthopaedics, 4: 247–249, 251, 289*b*
Beth Israel Hospital and, 4: 246–247
Boston Children's Hospital and, 2: 279, 439*b*; 4: 245–250
breast carcinoma and chondrosarcoma case, 4: 247–249

Charleston Naval Hospital and, 4: 246
Children's Hospital/MGH combined program and, 4: 245
education and training, 4: 245
on Green, 2: 182
HCORP and, 4: 247–248
HMS appointment, 4: 247
Legg-Perthes Study Group and, 2: 425; 4: 250
MGH and, 3: 401; 4: 250
New England Medical Center and, 4: 249
pediatric orthopaedics and, 4: 248–250
private medical practice, 4: 247, 249
publications and research, 4: 246–247, 250
on shoes with correctives, 4: 250
Simmons College physical therapy lectures, 4: 246
Tufts Medical School appointment, 4: 248–249
US Navy and, 4: 246
Zimmerman, C., 4: 253
Zurakowski, D., 2: 380

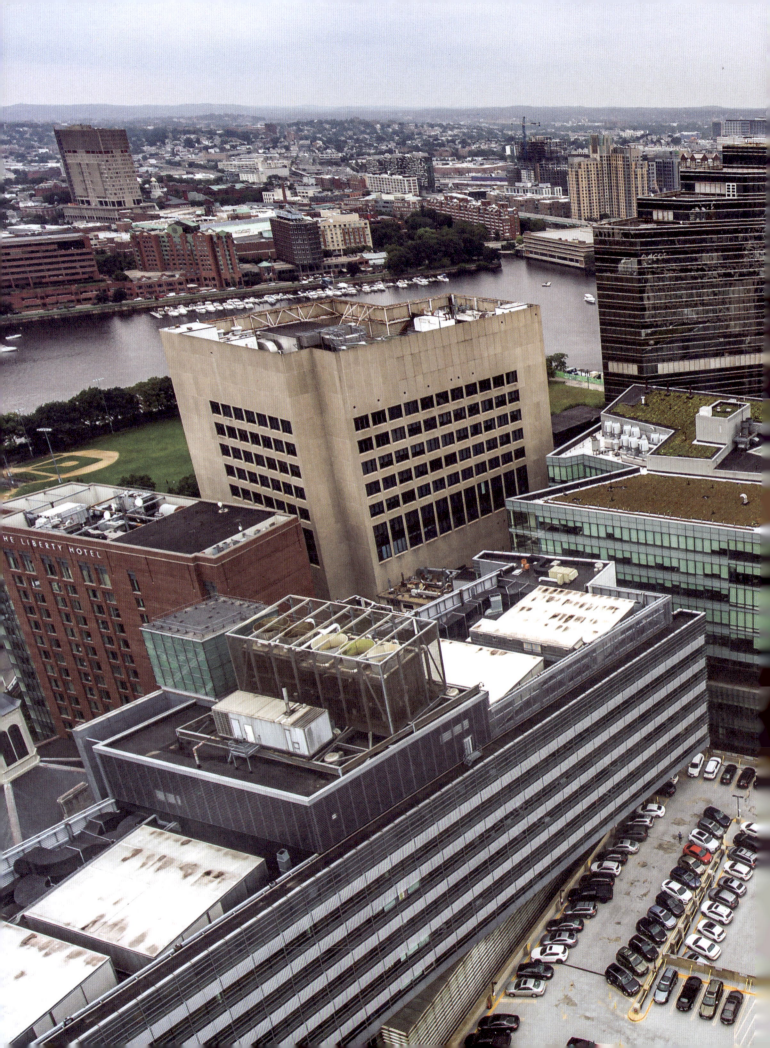